WHAT WORKS IN TACKLING HEALTH INEQUALITIES?

Pathways, policies and practice through the lifecourse

Sheena Asthana and Joyce Halliday

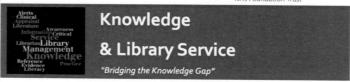

First published in Great Britain in March 2006 by

The Policy Press
University of Bristol
Fourth Floor
Beacon House
Queen's Road
Bristol BS8 1QU
UK

Tel +44 (0)117 331 4054
Fax +44 (0)117 331 4093
e-mail tpp-info@bristol.ac.uk
www.policypress.org.uk

© Sheena Asthana and Joyce Halliday 2006

British Library Cataloguing in Publication Data
A catalogue record for this book is available from the British Library.

Library of Congress Cataloging-in-Publication Data
A catalog record for this book has been requested.

ISBN 10-1 86134 674 3 paperback
ISBN 13-978 1 86134 674 2 paperback
ISBN 10-1 86134 675 1 hardcover
ISBN 13-978 1 86134 675 9 hardcover

Sheena Asthana is Professor of Health Policy and **Joyce Halliday** is RCUK Academic Fellow, both in the School of Sociology, Politics and Law, University of Plymouth, UK.

Cover design by Qube Design Associates, Bristol.
Front cover: photograph supplied by kind permission of www.JohnBirdsall.co.uk
Printed and bound in Great Britain by MPG Books, Bodmin.

For our children
Rosalind, Ellen, John, Angus and Leela Gibson
and
Edward and Eleanor Lewis

in the hope that your lifecourses
are blessed
with health and happiness

Contents

List of tables, boxes and figure

Tables

Boxes

Figure

Acknowledgements

Joyce Halliday has been funded by an Economic and Social Research Council (ESRC) Research Fellowship (Res-000-27-0042). We would also like to thank the anonymous referees for their valuable comments and the team at The Policy Press for their patience and support.

List of abbreviations

ABI   area-based initiative
ADHD   Attention Deficit/Hyperactivity Disorder
AHC   after housing costs
ALSPAC   Avon Longitudinal Study of Parents and Children
ASBO   Anti-Social Behaviour Order
ASH   Action on Smoking and Health
BFI   Baby Friendly Initiative
BFHI   Baby Friendly Hospital Initiative
BGOP   Better Government for Older People
BHC   before housing costs
BHPS   British Household Panel Survey
BIBS   Breastfeeding is Best Supporters Project
BMI   body mass index
CAB   Citizens' Advice Bureau
CAMHS   Child and Adolescent Mental Health Service
CAP   Common Agricultural Policy
CBT   cognitive behavioural therapy
CDRP   Crime and Disorder Reduction Partnership
CEBPP   Centre for Evidence-based Policy and Practice
CHD   coronary heart disease
CHQ   Child Health Questionnaire
COPD   chronic obstructive pulmonary disease
CPAG   Child Poverty Action Group
CRH   corticotropin-releasing hormone
CSA   childhood sexual abuse
CTC   Child Tax Credit
CYPU   Children and Young People's Unit
DAT   Drug Action Team
DCMS   Department for Culture, Media and Sport
DfEE   Department for Education and Employment
DfES   Department for Education and Skills
DH   Department of Health
DoE   Department of the Environment
DSH   deliberate self-harm
DSS   Department of Social Security
DWP   Department for Work and Pensions
EAZ   Education Action Zone
EFNEP   Expanded Food and Nutrition Education Program
EMA   Education Maintenance Allowance

EPIC	European Prospective Investigation into Cancer
EPNDS	Edinburgh Postnatal Depression Scale
EPPE	Effective Provision of Pre-School Education Project
EPPI-Centre	Evidence for Policy and Practice Information and Coordination Centre
ESRC	Economic and Social Research Council
ETS	environmental tobacco smoke
EU	European Union
EZ	Employment Zone
FAC	Families and Children Study
FAS	Foetal Alcohol Syndrome
FE	further education
FFT	functional family therapy
FNS	Fourth National Survey
FSA	Food Standards Authority
FSM	free school meals
FTE	full-time equivalent
GDP	Gross Domestic Product
GEM	geriatric evaluation and management
GHQ	General Health Questionnaire
GHS	General Household Survey
GP	general practitioner
GUM	genitourinary medicine
HAS	home assessment services
HAZ	Health Action Zone
HCHS	Hospital and Community Health Services
HDA	Health Development Agency
HE	higher education
HIA	Home Improvement Agency
HPA	Health Protection Agency
HSE	Health Survey for England
ICD	International Classification of Diseases
IFI	Infant Feeding Initiative
IHD	ischaemic heart disease
ILM	intermediate labour market
IMD 2000	Index of Multiple Deprivation 2000
LEA	local education authority
LETS	Local Exchange Trading Scheme
LRNI	Lower Reference Nutrient Intake
LSP	Local Strategic Partnership
LTP	Local Transport Plan
MEWS	Midwifery Education for Women who Smoke
MIG	Minimum Income Guarantee

MRC	Medical Research Council
MST	multi-systemic treatment
NAO	National Audit Office
ND25plus	New Deal for 25 plus
ND50plus	New Deal for 50 plus
NDC	New Deal for Communities
NDDP	New Deal for Disabled People
NDLP	New Deal for Lone Parents
NDNS	National Diet and Nutrition Survey
NDYP	New Deal for Young People
NESS	National Evaluation of Sure Start
NFPI	National Family and Parenting Institute
NICHD	National Institute for Child Health and Human Development
NHS	National Health Service
NHSS	National Healthy School Standard
NICE	National Institute for Clinical Excellence
NRF	Neighbourhood Renewal Fund
NRT	nicotine replacement therapy
NRU	Neighbourhood Renewal Unit
NSF	National Service Framework
NSNR	National Strategy for Neighbourhood Renewal
NSPCC	National Society for the Prevention of Cruelty to Children
NS-SEC	National Statistics Socio-economic Classification
NVQ	National Vocational Qualification
OECD	Organisation for Economic Co-operation and Development
ONS	Office for National Statistics
PCT	primary care trust
PDU	Programme Development Unit
PE	Physical Education
PHSE	personal health and social education
PID	pelvic inflammatory disease
PIPPIN	Parents in Partnership–Parent Infant Network
PISA	Programme for International Student Assessment
PMHW	Primary Mental Health Worker
PSA	Public Service Agreement
RCT	randomised controlled trial
RSI	Rough Sleepers' Initiative
SCIE	Social Care Institute for Excellence
SEN	special educational needs
SIR	Standardised Illness Ratio
SMR	Standardised Mortality Ratio
SRB	Single Regeneration Budget
SSLP	Sure Start Local Programme

STEP	Systematic Training for Effective Parenting Programme
STI	sexually transmitted infection
STP	School Travel Plan
UNICEF	United Nations Children's Fund
WFTC	Working Families' Tax Credit
WHO	World Health Organization
WIC	Women, Infants and Children Program of special supplemental nutrition
WTC	Working Tax Credit
YOT	Youth Offending Team

ONE

Introduction

Tackling health inequalities has become a key policy objective in the UK in recent years. While the 1980 Black Report received international attention but had a limited impact on national policy, the 1998 Acheson Independent Inquiry into Inequalities in Health has stimulated a wide-ranging policy response. For the first time ever, health inequalities have been made a priority for the National Health Service (NHS). Indeed, the principle that the "NHS will help keep people healthy and work to reduce health inequalities" was established as one of the service's 10 core principles in the Labour government's *NHS Plan* (DH, 2000).

The extent to which the British government will succeed in these goals rests on a number of factors including a *sufficient understanding* of the causes of health inequalities, a well-founded *knowledge* of the policies and interventions that can effectively address those causes and a *political will* to invest in those policies. Amid continued uncertainty about how the broad policy recommendations that arise from health inequalities research should be translated into practice and about the specific health outcomes of many NHS and socio-economic interventions, these three issues are the focus of this book.

One key area of uncertainty concerns the *role of local-level initiatives*. Many propose that health inequalities can only be addressed through a significant redistribution of income or wealth. This does appear in the government's agenda through tax and benefit reform. However, as evidenced by the emphasis on area-based initiatives and the expected role of primary care trusts, local authority bodies and community groups in taking forward the public health agenda, health inequality policies are primarily targeted at local areas. One aim of this book is to examine what this means in practice. Given what we know about the causes of health inequalities, what can local policy makers, practitioners and agencies do to narrow the health gap between the most and least deprived groups? What evidence exists about the potential impact of local initiatives on health outcomes and what factors shape the effectiveness of such interventions? Can local agencies be given clearer advice about the best ways to respond to the government's health inequalities agenda? Indeed, is it possible to overcome uncertainty about the effectiveness of the government's strategy? Through a detailed examination of theoretical evidence, national policies and local practice, the book aims to address some of the most intractable issues in the health inequalities field.

There were a number of ways of potentially structuring a book of this type – around, for example, major health outcomes (such as coronary heart disease [CHD], cancer and diabetes), health risk factors (such as smoking, diet and sexual health) or policy sectors (such as education, employment and transport). All three of these dimensions have appeared in key public health initiatives, from *The health of the nation* (DH, 1992), launched by the Conservative government in 1991 to HM Treasury's 2002 Cross-cutting Review, *Tackling health inequalities* (HM Treasury and DH, 2002). In practice, however, strategies framed around disease and/or disease risk factors have tended to have a medical rather than a social focus and to target individuals rather than communities or populations. By contrast, a sectoral approach explicitly acknowledges the underlying determinants of health but is not always clear about the mediating factors that link broad areas of welfare to individual health outcomes.

In view of these problems, we rejected more conventional approaches to categorising public health policy areas in favour of a *lifecourse perspective*. This not only reflects the theoretical orientation of health inequalities research in recent years; it has also allowed us to explore the links between social determinants of health, mediating biological factors and a range of health outcomes; to assess research evidence of the role of both social and medical interventions; and to tease out key areas of debate (pertaining, for example, to critical periods of vulnerability and intervention). Within the lifecourse framework we have been able to make explicit links between theory, policy and practice as they relate to health inequalities. Thus, for each period of the lifecourse, we have explored the pathways and processes giving rise to health inequalities before examining key government strategies and examples of interventions that are designed to address such pathways. Finally, the lifecourse framework is broad enough to encompass more standard public health categories, which means that the role of different policy sectors, of strategies targeting particular risk factors and the potential impact on particular health outcomes has been continually explored.

Structure and content of the book

The book is organised into three parts, the first of which (Chapters Two and Three) examines the *research and policy context* of health inequalities. In Chapter Two we discuss the growth of interest in health inequalities since the publication of the original Black Report. Examining the legacy of the Report to both research and policy, we find that it provided a springboard for a remarkable body of research that is both theoretically innovative and empirically robust. In the second part of the chapter, we look at key theoretical 'landmarks' since the 1990s and explore the way in which different explanations for health inequalities give rise to different policy responses. This is examined practically in Chapter Three, which traces the evolution of policy responses to health inequalities research under New Labour.

The second and largest section of the book (Chapters Four to Thirteen) examines *health inequalities pathways, policies and practice* throughout the lifecourse. Four critical periods are examined (early life, childhood and youth, adulthood and older age). For each period, companion chapters are devoted respectively to research evidence and to evidence on policies and interventions. Thus, the research chapters explore the pathways that give rise to health inequalities. By linking epidemiological evidence of key risk factors to evidence of the social context of risk, these highlight the areas where, theoretically, policy interventions need to be developed to address health inequalities. Picking up on these areas, each companion policy chapter assesses research evidence of 'what works', examines the limitations of the existing evidence base and describes the recent development of key policy initiatives. In what is to become an important theme of the book, the tensions that emerge in translating policy recommendations into actual policy mechanisms are explored and the point made that outcomes vary according to a wide range of factors such as content, process, context and the characteristics of the intervention group.

As well as highlighting what we have included in Part 2, it is important to acknowledge what has been excluded. In each of the chapters concerning research evidence of health inequalities and the pathways that give rise to health inequalities, the focus of interest has been explicitly on *socio-economic status* whether measured, as in the past, by social class, by individual variables such as housing tenure or educational qualifications, or by the new National Statistics Socio-economic Classification (NS-SEC). Throughout the course of the book, rather less attention has been paid to health differences between *socio-demographic* groups (although where the strength of evidence demands it, we have made reference to health exclusion issues facing teenage mothers, black and minority ethnic groups and women). Our choice of emphasis reflects the focus on socio-economic differentials within health inequalities research and policy. It was also guided by pragmatism. As it stands, the book provides a fairly comprehensive account of the factors that link poverty and deprivation to health exclusion during the course of a lifetime. Within this account, very little space was left for detailed examination of other sources of vulnerability.

It is also important to note the geographical limitations to the book. One of our aims was to examine the UK government's response to health inequalities with respect both to policy and practice. However, the establishment of the Scottish Executive, the National Assembly for Wales and the Northern Ireland Assembly has meant that legislative, executive and financial responsibilities are differentially devolved across the UK and there are now important and growing differences with respect to policy and practice between the four countries. The scope of this book has meant that it has not always been possible to address these permutations. When this has been the case, our focus has been primarily on policy in England.

In Part 3 (Chapter Fourteen), we take up and develop a theme that has become familiar throughout the book's discussion of policy and practice, namely the *many limitations that exist to the current evidence base of health inequalities policies*. Indeed, many commentators question the current approach to evidence-based policy on the basis that this all too often leads to a narrow focus on so-called 'downstream' interventions with an individualised/medical rather than a community/social focus; underestimates the role of context in shaping health, health-related behaviour and responses to health interventions; and establishes impossibly stringent criteria by which to measure programme success. The question arises, however, of how 'upstream' initiatives that target the wider determinants of health can be designed that fulfil basic effectiveness criteria. Chapter Fourteen attempts to address this question by setting out a new research agenda for evidence-based public health, one that, drawing on a number of traditions including comparative social policy, involves the analysis of *public health regimes*. Examining significant dimensions of the public health regime in Britain, we question whether the government's strategy for reducing health inequalities is as far-reaching as policy rhetoric would have us believe. Paying explicit attention to indicators of structural reform, we conclude that the UK still has some way to go before developing the social, political, cultural and economic structures that, on the basis of international evidence, are key to promoting health equity.

This conclusion should not lead readers to presume that this is a polemic text or one that has little to say for those who are struggling with the daily realities of implementing the government's health inequalities policies. We have worked hard to produce a comprehensive, rigorous, relevant and up-to-date text (and gratefully acknowledge the efforts of our publishers to minimise the time between typescript delivery and publication) that, in addition to appealing to academic colleagues and their students, can be practically used by service planners, managers and professionals. Our professional colleagues suggest that there is a strong perceived need for clearer guidance about how local agencies can take forward the government's health inequalities agenda. As academics involved in policy relevant research, we hope that this book will help service planners who want to know what, within the enabling or constraining environment of national policy initiatives, they might be able to achieve locally.

Health inequalities: the nature and scale of the problem

While the book mainly focuses on pathways giving rise to health inequalities and on policy interventions to address those pathways, it also outlines the nature and scale of the 'problem' of health inequalities itself. Since the publication of the Black Report (see Chapter Two), an extensive body of research has documented the extent and magnitude of socio-economic differentials in health. This growth in evidence in part reflects improvements in our ability to measure health inequalities. Because early studies relied heavily on vital registration data, most evidence of health inequalities related to differences in mortality according to social class (as defined by the Registrar General). Relatively few studies examined variations in morbidity and certain groups were largely overlooked by researchers. These included children and young people (where lower rates of mortality made it difficult to establish statistically significant social variations), minority ethnic groups and older people.

Since 1980, data sources for the analysis of health inequalities have increased significantly. The Census now includes questions on self-reported health and, from 1991 onwards, the Health Survey for England (HSE) has collected detailed health data. The General Household Survey (GHS) provides information on both self-reported health and use of health services and a number of more detailed local surveys have been implemented which focus on more specific groups (for example, the Avon Longitudinal Study of Parents and Children [ALSPAC]) or conditions (for example, the British Regional Heart Surveys). Such datasets allow information on health to be directly linked with information on socio-demographic and socio-economic status. Their design has also responded to concerns about the way in which socio-economic status was captured. The replacement in 2001 of the Registrar General's classification by the NS-SEC and the use of alternative indicators of socio-economic status (for example, income, housing tenure and educational qualifications) have been important developments in this respect, although there remains debate about the extent to which the social status of groups other than paid workers is effectively captured (see, for example, Chapter Six for a discussion about measuring the social status of children and young people).

Improvements in data sources and indicators of health and social status have therefore given rise to a large volume of research describing the nature and scale of health inequalities in Britain. This suggests that health inequalities are pervasive throughout society, pertain to a wide range of diseases and conditions and, if anything, are widening with time.

Demography and health inequalities

Differences in health status according to socio-economic status are found across all age groups, from birth to old age, although the scale of inequality varies – in both absolute and relative terms – between different stages of the lifecourse. In England and Wales in 2002, the percentage of low birth weight births was 6.0% in children whose fathers were in higher managerial and professional occupations, compared with 12.1% whose fathers were in routine and semi-routine occupations (ONS, 2004), suggesting that even before birth, children from more deprived households are at higher risk of being disadvantaged with regard to their physical development (see Chapter Four). The smallest babies are more likely to die in the first few weeks and months of life. Thus, social inequalities in infant mortality reflect inequalities in low birth weight. In 2002, the estimated infant mortality rate among children whose fathers were in higher managerial and professional occupations was 3.1 per 1,000 live births compared with 9.2 whose fathers were in routine and semi-routine occupations (ONS, 2004).

After infancy and early childhood, mortality rates fall, making 5-14 the ages at which death is least likely to occur. Nevertheless, social differences in risk of death during childhood were highlighted in the 1997 *Decennial Supplement* on health inequalities (Botting, 1997). This found that, between 1991 and 1993, death rates among boys and girls aged 5-9 in Social Class V were twice as high as in Social Class I. Among boys aged 10-14 this ratio increased to 2.7 although it closed among girls of this age. Throughout childhood and youth, class gradients in mortality are predominantly attributable to accidents and injuries. By contrast, mortality due to other causes shows much less variation. Evidence of socio-economic variations in physical health is also equivocal, although mental health status during childhood and youth varies significantly according to socio-economic status, gender and ethnicity (see Chapter Six). For example, children who live in low-income households, in social sector housing and whose parents have no educational qualifications are at increased risk of suffering from conduct, emotional and attention deficit disorders. Mental health problems in childhood often mark the early stages of difficulties that continue into adult life and addressing the pathways that give rise to poor mental health in young people should be a key issue for health inequalities policies.

In relative terms, social class differences in premature death are widest during early adulthood, becoming narrower as retirement age approaches (Blane, 1999, p 23). During 1991-93, mortality rates in Social Class V were 4.7 times greater than those in Social Class I in 30- to 34-year-old men; 4.1 times greater at ages 35-39, falling to 2.5 times at ages 60-64 (Drever and Bunting, 1997, p 98). This reflects the profound social class differences that exist in mortality rates from suicide and undetermined injury at younger ages (also see Chapter Six). By contrast, deaths from other causes are comparatively rare.

In absolute terms (reflected in numbers of premature deaths) health inequalities are greatest among 45- to 64-year-olds. This is largely accounted for by social differences in risk for premature chronic/degenerative disease (Hertzman, 1999, p 25). Chronic conditions such as heart disease, stroke, arthritis and cancers are prevalent in later years. Indeed, many would describe the development of chronic and/or degenerative conditions as a natural outcome of the ageing process. As such diseases are the major causes of illness and death in the industrialised West, the highest rates of morbidity and mortality occur in the very oldest age cohorts. In 2002, for example, rates of death from all causes were significantly higher among men aged 85+ (18,806 per 100,000) than among 65- to 84-year-olds (4,427 per 100,000) and 45- to 64-year-olds (654 per 100,000) (data derived from the Office for National Statistics [ONS]). Because risk for developing chronic disease rises steeply with age, deaths occurring before the age of 65 are generally classed as 'premature' and associated with risk factors over and above the process of ageing. Such factors are strongly associated with socio-economic status.

The impact of excess premature mortality among lower socio-economic groups and the growing importance of demography relative to socio-economic status as a determinant of health with increasing age results in a narrowing of health differentials in older age. This does not mean that socially mediated risk factors do not play a role in morbidity and mortality in later life. Health inequalities persist after retirement. As in childhood and youth, these appear to be more marked for mental than physical health. However, mortality rates remain subject to significant variation. In the 1971 Longitudinal Study cohort, Standardised Mortality Ratios (SMRs) (1971-92) of those aged 60-74 years ranged from 77 among owner-occupiers to 115 among local authority tenants (the respective range for those aged 74+ was 91-104). The SMR of those owning two or more cars was 77 compared to 115 for those without a car (91 to 104 for 74+ years) (Smith and Harding, 1997).

In addition to age, social inequalities vary according to sex. Across the age range, gradients in mortality are less steep for women than for men. This partly reflects the fact that female mortality rates are lower than male mortality rates at all ages, a difference that has been variously attributed to biological, material, behavioural and psychosocial factors (Carpenter, 2000; Graham, 2000). However, evidence of health inequalities does vary according to the measure of health status used and strong social gradients have been observed with respect to morbidity among women, lower socio-economic status increasing risk of self-reported ill health and disability. Gender-related social changes may also have important consequences for differences in the magnitude of health inequalities between the sexes. As more women benefit from higher qualifications and as the labour market role of women increasingly becomes more important, educational and occupational class gradients among women are likely to become stronger. Changes in the relative importance of women's family and labour market roles may also have important consequences for gender differences in key risk factors (such as heavy drinking, smoking and exposure to job stresses) that have been implicated in health inequalities.

Ethnicity also shapes the relationship between socio-economic status and health. In contrast to social class variations, ethnic variations in health become more pronounced with age. Drawing on the 1999 HSE and the Fourth National Survey (FNS) of Ethnic Minorities, profiles of self-reported health among African-Caribbean and Indian people were found to be similar to each other and to show a worsening in health in comparison with the white English group from the mid-thirties to the mid-forties onwards, while the Pakistani and Bangladeshi groups had the worse profiles of all (Nazroo et al, 2004). This may suggest that adversity experienced by people from certain minority ethnic groups during the course of their lifetimes is greater than would be predicted on the basis of social status at birth alone. The accumulation of disadvantage reflects the extent to which certain minority ethnic groups experience social and economic exclusion. While 28% of people in England and Wales lived in households that had incomes less than half the national average in 1994, this was the case for over 40% of African-Caribbean and Indian people and over 80% of Pakistani and

Bangladeshi people, trends which, according to the government's Social Exclusion Unit, reflect differences in employment rates, although not differences in skills and qualifications. Thus, social exclusion and discrimination are likely to make a contribution to variations in health through their impact on inequalities in material advantage and through psychosocial mechanisms.

Unfortunately, our understanding of the ways in which relationships between socio-economic status, ethnicity and health are mediated remains poor. This partly reflects limitations in available data. In the *Decennial Supplement* on health inequalities, for example, data on ethnicity were based on country of birth, thereby excluding minority ethnic people born in England and Wales. Given the relatively young age distribution of minority ethnic groups compared to the white population in the early 1990s, it is also unlikely that health variations will have been adequately captured through the use of mortality statistics. The *Decennial Supplement* did nevertheless note relatively high rates of death from ischaemic heart disease (IHD) among men born in the Indian subcontinent and higher risks of cerebrovascular disease among West/South African and African-Caribbean people (Harding and Maxwell, 1997). Mental health has been another area in which ethnic variations has been a subject of interest. Claims of a higher prevalence of schizophrenia among African-Caribbean men have been particularly controversial, some questioning whether higher observed prevalence rates are real or reflect bias in the diagnosis and management of the disease (Fernando, 1995). Similarly, significantly higher rates of conduct disorders have been observed among young Black teenagers in mental health surveys, while teenage Pakistani and Bangladeshi boys exhibit higher than average rates of emotional disorders (see Chapter Six). However, the extent to which these reflect material disadvantage, exposure to discrimination and racism or ethnic differences in the way in which psychological response to stressors is expressed, has been debated.

Social gradients in cause-specific mortality and morbidity

While the magnitude of health inequalities varies according to age, sex and ethnicity, social gradients in health are remarkably pervasive with respect to the range of diseases and conditions. The 1997 *Decennial Supplement* noted strong social gradients in male mortality aged 20-64 (1991-93) in each of the International Classification of Diseases (ICD) chapters (Drever et al, 1997). Social class differences were greatest for deaths from mental disorders. Within ICD Chapter V, where deaths were largely related to drug or alcohol dependency, the SMR was 12 times greater in Social Class V than Social Class I. It is important to note, however, that mental disorders are a relatively minor cause of death, accounting for less than 1% of overall mortality.

External causes of death (including accidents and injuries), respiratory diseases and diseases of the digestive system are also subject to very large social class differences. They contribute to larger numbers of deaths (12%, 5.5% and 3.6%

respectively of all deaths to men aged 20-64 between 1991-93) than mental disorders. Profound inequalities were noted in the *Decennial Supplement* in a range of respiratory illnesses, including chronic airway obstruction, bronchitis and emphysema, pneumonia and asthma. Overall, Social Class V had 5.9 times the SMR of Social Class I for respiratory diseases, 5.0 times the rate for external causes of death and 3.6 times the rate for deaths of the digestive system, half of which were due to chronic liver disease and cirrhosis.

Social class differences in premature death from the largest causes of mortality – circulatory disease and cancers – were found to be less pronounced than for the causes described earlier. However, they were not insignificant. In 1991-93, circulatory diseases were responsible for nearly 40% of all deaths to men aged 20-64. Within ICD Chapter VII, the Social Class V SMR was 2.9 times higher than that of Social Class I. For both major contributors to deaths within Chapter VII (IHD and cerebrovascular disease), the differential between Social Classes V and I was around 3. By contrast, social class differences in deaths from cancers (32% of overall mortality) varied widely according to the specific cause of death.

The differential between Social Classes I and V SMRs for all malignant neoplasms was 2.1. Lung cancer, which was responsible for nearly 10% of all deaths to men aged 20-64 in 1991-93, played a very large part in this social gradient. The Social Class V SMR for malignant neoplasms of the trachea, bronchus and lung was 4.6 times higher than that of Social Class I. Stomach and oesophageal cancers also showed increasing SMRs with lower social class, the differential between Social Classes I and V standing at 3.0 and 2.2 respectively. Rectal and pancreatic cancers showed a tendency towards increasing mortality with lower social class (with Social Class I/V differentials of around 1.5-1.6). By contrast, cancers of the colon, prostate and non-Hodgkins lymphoma showed no clear pattern and brain cancer showed an opposite tendency to most conditions, having significantly raised mortality in Social Classes I and IIIN (Drever et al, 1997).

Social differences in cancer incidence are slightly less consistent than differences in cancer mortality (Rosengren and Wilhelmsen, 2004), raising questions about the role that access to effective health services might play in determining disease outcome. Several cancer registration studies indicate excess risks in men in higher social strata for cancers of the colon and prostate and find a weak association between socio-economic status and pancreatic cancer (Rimpela and Pukkala, 1987; Sharp et al, 1993; van Loon et al, 1995; Smith et al, 1996; Brown et al, 1998). Evidence of social gradients in the incidence of rectal and liver cancers is also mixed (van Loon et al, 1995; Faggiano et al, 1997). For the most part, however, international studies of cancer incidence and mortality find more or less consistent excess risks in men in lower social strata for all respiratory cancers (nose, larynx and lung) and cancers of the oral cavity and pharynx, oesophagus and stomach. For women, low-class excesses are consistently encountered for cancers of the oesophagus, stomach and cervix uteri. By contrast, men in higher social strata display excesses of brain cancers and skin melanoma and women in higher socio-economic strata excess rates of cancers of the colon and ovary and skin melanoma (Faggiano et al, 1997). Earlier studies also suggest that breast cancer incidence was higher in women in a higher socio-economic status. This is still evident among older women. At younger ages, however, the pattern of breast cancer incidence may be changing (Harding et al, 1999).

Socio-economic inequalities in morbidity are not confined to cancers but occur across the disease categories covered by different ICD chapters (Eachus et al, 1996; Saul and Payne, 1999). Thus, a positive association has been observed between socio-economic disadvantage and risk of developing Type II diabetes mellitus (Meadows, 1995; Ismail et al, 1999); depression and other mental disorders (Payne et al, 1993; McCormick et al, 1995; Kind et al, 1998; Stansfeld et al, 1998); IHD and cerebrovascular disease (Marmot et al, 1991; Woodward et al, 1992; Lampe et al, 1994; Morrison et al, 1997; Gibson et al, 2002); severe asthma, bronchitis and emphysema (Littlejohns and Macdonald, 1993); and musculoskeletal disease (McCormick et al, 1995). Inequalities in morbidity are not consistent or universal. Diseases where the relationship between morbidity and deprivation appears to be weak, or where contradictory evidence exists, include hypertension (Dong et al, 1994), Type I diabetes mellitus (Meadows, 1995; Ismail et al, 1999), and rheumatoid arthritis (Bankhead et al, 1996). Finally, like some cancers, certain diseases such as inflammatory bowel disease appear to be more prevalent among the more affluent (Montgomery et al, 1998).

The stepwise gradient

The identification of variations in the magnitude of health inequalities according to different causes of morbidity and mortality provides important information for the generation of hypotheses about the causes of health inequalities. The fact that the gradient in health outcomes is continuous across the whole social hierarchy has also informed the development of a number of key theories regarding causal pathways. Applying the new NS-SEC classification to the 1991-93 male mortality dataset, SMRs increase in a stepwise fashion from 55 in socio-economic group 1.1 to 155 in socio-economic group 7 (Donkin et al, 2002). Until relatively recently, more attention focused on the profound difference between mortality rates in the highest and lowest socio-economic groups, highlighting the needs of a disadvantaged minority. From a research point of view, however, the stepwise nature of the social gradient is of particular significance. Why should the mortality rates of large employers and men working in higher managerial occupations be lower than those of higher professionals? Why should intermediate employees, who have a combined labour contract and service relationship (that is, some assurance of security and career opportunities) have higher death rates than those found in lower managerial and professional occupations but lower death rates than small employers and own account workers? As we discuss in Chapter Two, investigating the processes by which social status exerts such a finely tuned effect has been an important focus of work seeking to explain inequalities in adult health.

Geographical patterns of disease distribution

The analysis of geographical variations in health in Britain has a long tradition (Joshi et al, 2000), and evidence suggests considerable historical continuity in the geography of mortality. For example, Britton (1990, cited by Macintyre, 1999) suggests that for the past 150 years, death rates have been consistently higher in the North and West, compared to the South and East, and in highly urbanised areas, compared to rural areas. Evidence of a North–South divide in mortality is particularly strong, higher death rates occurring in Scotland, Northern Ireland, Wales and Northern England, while lower death rates occur in the South of England (Fitzpatrick et al, 2001).

Using parliamentary constituencies to analyse health differences, Shaw et al (1999) found that eight of the 15 'worst health' areas in Britain (constituencies where people are most at risk of premature death) were located in Glasgow, where the chances of dying before the age of 65 ranged from 1.6 to 2.3 times the national average. A total of 52% of the worst-off million people in Britain (that is, those living in the least healthy areas) were in Scotland and a further 40% in the North of England. Thus, only one of the 15 areas with the highest under-65 mortality rates was located in the South of England and this was the Inner London constituency of Southwark and Bermondsey.

As this work and that of others (for example, Drever and Whitehead, 1995; Charlton, 1996; Dorling, 1997) demonstrate, areas with the highest mortality rates tend to be located in urban and declining industrial areas. This reflects the fact that social deprivation tends to be more extreme and geographically concentrated in inner cities than in rural areas where disadvantaged households live among the more affluent. Observed urban/rural differences in health status have given rise to a tendency to depict health inequalities as a specifically 'urban' problem. However, some care should be taken in assuming that people living in rural areas are not subject to health exclusion (Asthana et al, 2002). First, the rural poor may be equally at risk of suffering from health inequalities as the urban poor, but their poorer health outcomes are hidden by favourable averages. Second, a distinction should be drawn between different types of rural area. While it is generally accepted that the populations of suburban and semi-rural areas (particularly those in the South East of the country) are among the most affluent and healthy in the country, the populations of *remote* rural areas suffer distinct disadvantages. For example, limiting long-term illness appears to be subject to a U-shaped pattern of prevalence, the highest rates being observed in the most urban and the most peripheral rural areas (Barnett et al, 2001). Higher rates of mortality for accidents, suicides and undetermined injuries are also observed in remote rural areas (Fitzpatrick et al, 2001).

Analysis of cause-specific mortality (1991-97) reveals that geographical inequalities in health are not entirely the same for different causes of death. Given that IHD and stroke account for such a high proportion of deaths in the UK, it is hardly surprising that the geographical distribution of mortality from these causes was similar to that of all-cause mortality. Patterns of lung cancer mortality and death from respiratory disease were also subject to a North–South divide and concentrated in urban and early industrial areas. However, high mortality rates from other cancers (for example, prostrate and breast and, to a lesser extent, colorectal cancer) and, as already observed, accidents, were less concentrated in urban areas, while deaths from other causes were subject to a distinct regional pattern. London had a particularly high mortality rate from infectious diseases and areas with high mortality rates from alcohol- or drug-related deaths were largely confined to Scotland, London and Manchester (Fitzpatrick et al, 2001).

Historical patterns of disease distribution

There has been considerable historical continuity in the geography of mortality in the UK, reflecting long-standing inequalities in the distribution of poverty and wealth. The plight of the urban poor was highlighted in the early 1840s when the Royal Commission on the Health of Towns described the appalling sanitary conditions in which the poorest lived. In 1843 an editorial in the *Lancet* showed wide differences between different sections of the community in towns and rural districts in average age of death. While gentry and professionals in the city of Bath might expect to live for an average of 52 years, the figure for labourers living in Liverpool, Bethnal Green and Manchester ranged between 15 and 17 years (Whitehead, 1997).

Over the course of the late 19th and early 20th century, there was a marked decline in adult mortality rates and, from the early 20th century a decline in infant mortality rates, leading to a shift from a health profile dominated by infectious diseases to one in which chronic and degenerative diseases have become prominent. During the first three decades of the 20th century, this shift was accompanied by a decline in class inequalities in infant and adult mortality in both absolute and relative terms. However, although mortality rates continued to fall, social class differentials increased from the 1940s (Pamuk, 1985, cited by Whitehead, 1997).

The last few decades have seen a particular widening of the mortality gap. Examining trends in SMRs for deaths under 65 from the early 1950s to the late 1990s, Dorling et al (2000) found that the relative mortality rates of the 10% of people living in the highest mortality areas of the country had progressively risen over the period from an SMR of 131 in 1950-53 to 150 in 1996-98. By contrast, the SMRs of the population decile living in the lowest mortality areas had decreased from 82 to 75. Thus, over the period, the ratio in SMRs between the worst and best areas had increased from 1.6 to 2.0. Updating analysis of social class differences in cause-specific mortality, White et al (2003) also note that health inequalities have continued to widen since the mid-1980s, with some qualifications. First, there is a gender difference in trends, inequalities in mortality increasing for men but decreasing for women between 1986 and 1999. A major contribution to the increasing social class gap in male mortality was made by IHD, cerebrovascular disease and respiratory diseases, where large falls in deaths in Social Classes I and II were not matched by the lower social classes. Second, social class differences in mortality trends have changed over time, at least for IHD. Here, most of the reduction in mortality among non-manual males occurred between 1986-92 and 1993-96, the rate of reduction slowing down significantly between 1993-96 and 1997-99. Among manual males, by contrast, improvements in mortality from IHD have been slower but consistent over time. Consequently, the social class gradient in IHD rose in 1993-96 but fell again in 1997-99 (White et al, 2003). Similar trends were not observed for cerebrovascular and respiratory diseases, where falls in mortality were greater in Social Classes I and II for both periods.

Trends in IHD mortality could suggest that men in Social Class V are beginning to catch up, and that a narrowing of the mortality gap will occur. However, there is no sign of this happening as yet. Recent analysis by Shaw et al (2005) suggests that inequalities in health widened during the 1990s, particularly among men. Using life expectancy data for local authority districts, they find that between 1992-94 and 2001-03, the absolute difference in life expectancy between the top and bottom poverty groups increased from 3.91 to 4.06 years, while the difference between the individual local authority areas with the highest (Kensington and Chelsea) and lowest (Glasgow City) life expectancies increased from 8.9 to 9.4 years. For men, the gap increased even further, the difference in the life expectancy between the top and bottom poverty groups rising from 4.73 to 4.97. The difference in male life expectancy between the highest local authority area (East Dorset) and the lowest (Glasgow City) rose to 11 years, causing the authors to comment that inequalities have not been as high since Victorian times.

The analysis of temporal trends in mortality differentials is important because it can throw light on the processes by which health inequalities are produced. During the period of Conservative rule, the widening mortality gap between the most and least socially advantaged in society was often attributed at the time to government policies that promoted increasing social and economic polarisation. Income inequalities have been sustained during the 1990s and into the 2000s (until very recently when changes to taxation and benefits have been slightly more redistributive) and inequalities in wealth have further deepened (see Chapter Three). At first sight, the fact that these trends have been accompanied by a growing polarisation of health suggests that socio-economic differentials in mortality are sensitive to short-term changes in the distribution of key resources.

In fact, care should be taken before reaching such a conclusion. Linking relatively short-term socio-economic trends to health variations rests on certain assumptions about the relative contribution of early and later life determinants of health outcomes.

In Chapters Two and Four we introduce the theory of biological programming. This suggests that inequalities that occur in adult life are set in place in very early life. If the implications of this theory are followed through, then the increase in health inequalities in the 1980s and 1990s may have been less of a direct consequence of growing social and spatial polarisation during this time than a reflection of the long-term effects of differential exposures by children from different social groups to health risk factors during the inter-war period. Thus, observed associations between income and health polarisation in recent years would not be causal but coincidental. If, by contrast, factors in later life play a more significant role in the production of health inequalities, then the growth in mortality differentials would be a reflection of short-term government policies that have encouraged inequalities in income and wealth. A third explanation is that, because risk of chronic disease reflects the accumulation of disadvantage over time, early and later life determinants have both played a role in the patterns of health that we observe today. If this is the case, then the fact that inequalities in income and wealth have been allowed to flourish has not only resulted in growing inequalities in the current generation; it may well have consequences for health inequalities in the mid-21st century.

If we are to properly understand the implications of social and economic policies for health inequalities now and in the future, we need to develop a more complex understanding of the relative contribution of early and later life determinants of health. This has been a central focus of lifecourse epidemiology and shapes our decision to use this perspective to examine the links between health inequalities pathways and policies. The major theories that have emerged within lifecourse epidemiology are discussed in more detail in Chapter Two and evidence in support of each of these theories described during the course of the book.

References

Asthana, S., Halliday, J., Brigham, P. and Gibson, A. (2002) *Rural deprivation and service need: A review of the literature and an assessment of indicators for rural service planning*, Bristol: South West Public Health Observatory.

Bankhead, C., Silman, A., Barrett, B., Scott, D. and Symmons, D. (1996) 'Incidence of rheumatoid arthritis is not related to indicators of socio-economic deprivation', *Journal of Rheumatology*, vol 23, no 12, pp 2039-42.

Barnett, S., Roderick, P., Martin, D. and Diamond, I. (2001) 'A multilevel analysis of the effects of rurality and social deprivation on premature limiting long term illness', *Journal of Epidemiology and Community Health*, vol 55, pp 44-51.

Blane, D. (1999) 'Adults of working age (16/18 to 65 years)', in D. Gordon, M. Shaw, D. Dorling and G. Davey Smith (eds) *Inequalities in health: The evidence presented to the Independent Inquiry into Inequalities in Health, chaired by Sir Donald Acheson*, Bristol: The Policy Press, pp 23-32.

Botting, B. (1997) 'Mortality in childhood', in F. Drever and M. Whitehead (eds) *Health inequalities: Decennial Supplement*, London: ONS, pp 83-94.

Britton, M. (ed) (1990) *Mortality and geography*, Series DS 9, London: OPCS/ HMSO.

Brown, J., Harding, S., Bethune, A. and Rosato, M. (1998) 'Longitudinal study of socio-economic differences in the incidence of stomach, colorectal and pancreatic cancers', *Population Trends*, vol 94, pp 35-41.

Carpenter, M. (2000) 'Reinforcing the pillars: rethinking gender, social divisions and health', in E. Annandale and K. Hunt (eds) *Gender inequalities in health*, Buckingham: Open University Press, pp 36-63.

Charlton, J. (1996) 'Which areas are healthiest?', *Population Trends*, vol 83, pp 17- 24.

DH (Department of Health) (1992) *The health of the nation: A strategy for health in England and Wales*, London: DH.

DH (2000) *The NHS Plan: A plan for investment, a plan for reform*, Cm 4818-1, London: The Stationery Office.

Dong, W., Colhoun, H. and Lampe, F. (1994) *Blood pressure: Health Survey for England 1994*, London: Joint Health Surveys Unit, UCL.

Donkin, A., Lee, Y.H. and Toson, B. (2002) 'Implications of changes in the UK social and occupational classifications in 2001 for vital statistics', *Population Trends*, vol 107, pp 23-9.

Dorling, D. (1997) *Death in Britain: How local mortality rates have changed: 1950s- 1990s*, York: Joseph Rowntree Foundation.

Dorling, D., Shaw, M. and Brimblecombe, N. (2000) 'Housing wealth and community health: exploring the role of migration', in H. Graham (ed) *Understanding health inequalities*, Buckingham: Open University Press, pp 186-99.

Drever, F. and Bunting, J. (1997) 'Patterns and trends in male mortality', in F. Drever and M. Whitehead (eds) *Health inequalities: Decennial Supplement*, London: ONS, pp 95-107.

Drever, F. and Whitehead, M. (1995) 'Mortality in regions and local authority districts in the 1990s: exploring the relationship with deprivation', *Population Trends*, Winter, no 82, pp 19-26.

Drever, F., Bunting, J. and Harding, D. (1997) 'Male mortality from major causes of death', in F. Drever and M. Whitehead (eds) *Health inequalities: Decennial Supplement*, London: ONS, pp 122-42.

Eachus, J., Williams, M., Chan, P., Davey Smith, G., Grainge, M., Donovan, J. and Frankel, S. (1996) 'Deprivation and cause-specific morbidity: evidence from the Somerset and Avon Survey of Health', *British Medical Journal*, vol 312, pp 287- 92.

Faggiano, F., Partanen, T., Kogevinas, M. and Boffetta, P. (1997) 'Socioeconomic differences in cancer incidence and mortality', *IARC Scientific Publications*, vol 138, pp 65-176.

Fernando, S. (1995) 'Social realities and mental health', in S. Fernando (ed) *Mental health in a multiethnic society: A multidisciplinary handbook*, London: Routledge, pp 12-35.

Fitzpatrick, J., Griffiths, C., Kelleher, M. and McEvoy, S. (2001) 'Descriptive analysis of geographic patterns and trends in adult mortality by cause of death', in C. Griffiths and J. Fitzpatrick (eds) *Geographic variations in health*, London: The Stationery Office, pp 248-325.

Gibson, A., Asthana, S., Brigham, P., Moon, G. and Dicker, J. (2002) 'Geographies of need and the new NHS: methodological issues in the definition and measurement of the health needs of local populations', *Health and Place*, vol 8, pp 47-60.

Graham, H. (2000) 'Socio-economic change and inequalities in men and women's health in the UK', in E. Annandale and K. Hunt (eds) *Gender inequalities in health*, Buckingham: Open University Press, pp 90-122.

Harding, S. and Maxwell, R. (1997) 'Differences in mortality of migrants', in F. Drever and M. Whitehead (eds) *Health inequalities: Decennial Supplement*, London: ONS, pp 108-21.

Harding, S., Brown, J., Rosato, M. and Hattersley, L. (1999) 'Socio-economic differentials in health: illustrations from the Office for National Statistics Longitudinal Study', *Health Statistics Quarterly*, vol 1, pp 5-15.

Hertzman, C. (1999) 'Population health and human development', in D.P. Keating and C. Hertzman (eds) *Developmental health and the wealth of nations*, New York, NY and London: The Guilford Press, pp 21-40.

HM Treasury and DH (Department of Health) (2002) *Tackling health inequalities: Summary of the 2002 Cross Cutting Review*, London: HM Treasury and DH.

Ismail, A.A., Beeching, N.J., Gill, G.V. and Bellis, M.A. (1999) 'Capture-recapture-adjusted prevalence rates of type 2 diabetes are related to social deprivation', *QJM: Monthly Journal of the Association of Physicians*, vol 92, no 12, pp 707-10.

Joshi, H., Wiggins, R., Bartley, D., Mitchell, R., Gleave, S. and Lynch, K. (2000) 'Putting health inequalities on the map: does where you live matter, and why?', in H. Graham (ed) *Understanding health inequalities*, Buckingham: Open University Press, pp 143-55.

Kind, P., Dolan, P., Gudex, C. and Williams, A. (1998) 'Variations in population health status: results from a United Kingdom national questionnaire survey', *British Medical Journal*, vol 316, pp 736-41.

Lampe, F., Colhoun, H. and Dong, W. (1994) *Cardiovascular disease and respiratory conditions: Health Survey For England 1994*, London: Joint Health Surveys Unit, UCL.

Littlejohns, P. and Macdonald, L.D. (1993) 'The relationship between severe asthma and social class', *Respiratory Medicine*, vol 87, pp 139-43.

McCormick, A., Fleming, D. and Charlton, J. (1995) *Morbidity statistics from general practice: Fourth national study, 1991-1992*, London: HMSO.

Macintyre, S. (1999) 'Geographical inequalities in mortality, morbidity and health-related behaviour', in D. Gordon, M. Shaw, D. Dorling and G. Davey Smith (eds) *Inequalities in health: The evidence presented to the Independent Inquiry into Inequalities in Health, chaired by Sir Donald Acheson*, Bristol: The Policy Press, pp 148-54.

Marmot, M.G., Davey Smith, G., Stansfeld, S.A., Patel, C., North, F., Head, J., Brunner, E.J. and Feeney, A. (1991) 'Health inequalities amongst British civil servants: the Whitehall II Study', *The Lancet*, vol 337, pp 1387-93.

Meadows, P. (1995) 'Variation of diabetes mellitus: prevalence in general practice and its relation to deprivation', *Diabetic Medicine*, vol 12, pp 696-700.

Montgomery, S.M., Morris, D.L., Thompson, N.P., Subhani, J., Pounder, R.E. and Wakefield, A.J. (1998) 'Prevalence of inflamatory bowel disease in British 26 year olds: national longitudinal birth cohort', *British Medical Journal*, vol 316, pp 1058-9.

Morrison, C., Woodward, M., Leslie, W. and Tunstall-Pedoe, H. (1997) 'Effect of socioeconomic group on incidence of, management of, and survival after myocardial infarction and coronary death: analysis of community coronary event register', *British Medical Journal*, vol 314, p 541.

Nazroo, J., Bajekal, M., Blane, D. and Grewal, I. (2004) 'Ethnic inequalities', in A. Walker and C. Hennessy (eds) *Growing older: Quality of life in old age*, Buckingham: Open University Press, pp 35-59.

ONS (Office for National Statistics) (2004) *Mortality statistics: Childhood, infant and perinatal. Review of the Registrar General on deaths in England and Wales 2002*, Series DH3 No 35, London: ONS.

Pamuk, E. (1985) 'Social class inequality in mortality from 1921 to 1972 in England and Wales', *Population Studies*, vol 39, pp 17-31.

Payne, J.N., Coy, J., Milner, P.C. and Patterson, S. (1993) 'Are deprivation indicators a proxy for morbidity? A comparison of the prevalence of arthritis, depression, dyspepsia, obesity and respiratory symptoms with unemployment rates and Jarman scores', *Journal of Public Health Medicine*, vol 16, no 1, pp 113-14.

Rimpela, A.H. and Pukkala, E.I. (1987) 'Cancers of affluence: positive social class gradient and rising incidence trend in some cancer forms', *Social Science and Medicine*, vol 24, no 7, pp 601-6.

Rosengren, A. and Wilhelmsen, L. (2004) 'Cancer incidence, mortality from cancer and survival in men of different occupational classes', *European Journal of Epidemiology*, vol 19, pp 533-40.

Saul, C. and Payne, N. (1999) 'How does the prevalence of specific morbidities compare with measures of socio-economic status at small area level?', *Journal of Public Health Medicine*, vol 21, pp 340-7.

Sharp, L., Black, R.J., Harkness, E.F., Finlayson, A.R. and Muir, C.S. (1993) *Cancer registration statistics, Scotland, 1981-1990*, Edinburgh: Common Services Agency.

Shaw, M., Davey Smith, G. and Dorling, D. (2005) 'Health inequalities and New Labour: how the promises compare with real progress', *British Medical Journal*, vol 330, pp 1016-21.

Shaw, M., Dorling, D., Gordon, D. and Davey Smith, G. (1999) *The widening gap: Health inequalities and policy in Britain*, Bristol: The Policy Press.

Smith, D., Taylor, R. and Coates, M. (1996) 'Socioeconomic differentials in cancer incidence and mortality in urban New South Wales, 1987-1991', *Australian and New Zealand Journal of Public Health*, vol 20, pp 129-37.

Smith, J. and Harding, S. (1997) 'Mortality of women and men using alternative social classifications', in F. Drever and M. Whitehead (eds) *Health inequalities: Decennial Supplement*, London: ONS, pp 168-83.

Stansfeld, S., Head, J. and Marmot, M. (1998) 'Explaining social class differences in depression and well-being', *Social Psychiatry and Psychiatric Epidemiology*, vol 33, pp 1-9.

van Loon, A.J., Brug, J., Goldbohm, R.A., van den Brandt, P.A. and Brug, J. (1995) 'Differences in cancer incidence and mortality among socio-economic groups', *Scandinavian Journal of Social Medicine*, vol 23, no 2, pp 110-20.

White, C., van Galen, F. and Huang Chow, Y. (2003) 'Trends in social class differences in mortality by cause, 1986-2000', *Health Statistics Quarterly*, vol 20, pp 25-37.

Whitehead, M. (1997) 'Life and death over the millennium', in F. Drever and M. Whitehead (eds) *Health inequalities: Decennial Supplement*, London: ONS, pp 7-28.

Woodward, M., Shewry, M., Smith, W. and Tunstall-Pedoe, H. (1992) 'Social status and coronary heart disease: results from the Scottish Heart Health Study', *Preventive Medicine*, 21, pp 136-48.

Part I:
The research and policy context of health inequalities

It is doubtful whether the original architects of the welfare state would have predicted that, at the start of the 21st century, health in the UK would be been even more unequal than it was in 1948, the year in which the National Health Service (NHS) was launched. It is, of course, generally accepted today that the health service has a relatively small role to play in the determination of health and well-being in the population. At the time, however, the formation of the NHS reflected a strong sense of social justice and a belief that health was a basic right, the enjoyment of which should not depend on an individual's wealth.

By the late 1970s there was growing awareness that the NHS had not made a marked impact on differences in the health of those at different ends of the social spectrum. The publication of the Black Report in 1980 demonstrated that, with respect to a range of indicators, health differentials between the most affluent and the most impoverished in British society had grown wider. As we discuss in Chapter Two, the Black Report had a limited impact on policy making during the 1980s and much of the 1990s. However, it did stimulate extensive research into health inequalities by social scientists and, increasingly, epidemiologists. It inspired similar research in European countries and kept health inequalities at the forefront of the public health agenda in the UK.

Chapter Two in this part examines the ways in which research on health inequalities has developed in recent years, first looking at the Black Report and its legacy and second at key research developments in the 1990s and 2000s, which include the rise of lifecourse epidemiology. The way in which different explanations for health inequalities give rise to different policy responses is explored during this discussion, with particular reference to the distinction that is commonly drawn between so-called 'upstream' policies that target the underlying determinants of health and 'downstream' interventions that target narrow clinical or behavioural factors, usually at an individual level.

This is examined practically in Chapter Three, which traces the evolution of policy responses to health inequalities research. Focusing in particular on developments since New Labour assumed power, we find a policy rhetoric that is highly responsive to research findings on the causes of health inequalities. However, the level at which theoretically driven policy recommendations have been translated into actual policy mechanisms suggests that current interpretations of the policy implications of health inequalities research tend more towards the conservative than the radical. This in part reflects the strong emphasis that has been placed on the need for *evidence-based* policy that fulfils the quality criteria of medical research. However, the individualising tendency of new social policies is also a product of the ideological shift that has taken place within the Labour Party. For some commentators, the failure of successive policies to respond to wider calls for structural reform is responsible for the fact that inequalities in health are continuing to widen in the first years of the 21st century (Shaw et al, 2005). Chapter Three assesses this contention with reference to evidence of social polarisation in key areas that are often described as the 'underlying determinants of health'. It also examines the role of territorial approaches or area-based initiatives (such as English Health Action Zones or HAZs) that have been identified as an innovative approach to addressing health inequalities (Mackenbach and Bakker, 2003).

References

Black Report (1980) *Inequalities of health*, Report of a Research Working Group, Chair, Sir Douglas Black, London: DHSS.

Mackenbach, J. and Bakker, M. (2003) 'Tackling socio-economic inequalities in health: analysis of European experiences', *The Lancet*, vol 330, pp 1409-14.

Shaw, M., Davey Smith, G. and Dorling, D. (2005) 'Health inequalities and New Labour: how the promises compare with real progress', *British Medical Journal*, vol 330, pp 1016-21.

TWO

Researching health inequalities

Introduction

Since the publication in 1980 of the Black Report there has been a dramatic growth in research undertaken on health inequalities. This partly reflects the fact that variations in health lend themselves to analysis from a range of perspectives – social, geographical and historical (see Chapter One). Health variations are remarkably pervasive, being found at all stages of the lifecourse and pertaining to a very wide range of diseases and conditions, and have become an important focus of policy making. Consequently, research into health inequalities attracts interest from a wide range of disciplines, such as sociology, geography, psychology, epidemiology and medicine. Its interdisciplinary nature has resulted in research that is empirically robust and theoretically innovative. Health inequalities is also an area in which international research collaboration is increasingly being forged, particularly around the identification of effective policies and interventions.

By adopting a lifecourse perspective to structure and organise this book, and examining key lifecourse theories, we have responded to what has been described as one of the most important recent developments in epidemiology and public health. For example, Chapter Four discusses evidence of *latent effects* whereby early life environments affect adult health independently of subsequent experience. Chapter Eight builds on the concept of *pathway effects* in which individuals follow different (often self-reinforcing) trajectories of life experiences which are health damaging or health enhancing, while Chapters Ten and Twelve explore the implications of the model of *cumulative effects*. This suggests that because health-damaging exposures gradually accumulate over time to increase the risk of chronic disease, better circumstances in adulthood and even old age can ameliorate the impact of a poor start in life.

In addition to discussing these models with reference to their significance to different periods of the lifecourse, it is important to place them in their wider research context. To this end, this chapter traces the development of research interest in health inequalities since 1980 noting that, although it is in many ways more sophisticated in its approach to explaining health inequalities, lifecourse epidemiology owes much to the legacy of the original Black Report. A developmental perspective thus illustrates some of the continuities that exist in health inequalities research. It also highlights areas where further progress could be made, such as our understanding of the role played by socio-structural factors in health inequalities.

The Black Report and its legacy

The fact that there is such a large and sophisticated body of UK research on health inequalities owes much to the publication in 1980 of the Black Report. While the Report, which was commissioned by the then Labour government in 1977, was not received well by the newly elected Conservative government of Margaret Thatcher, it proved highly influential in both stimulating subsequent research and in shaping explanatory frameworks for the existence of health inequalities. The Black Report had three components: a *description* of differences between occupational classes in mortality, morbidity and use of health services; an *analysis* of likely explanations for these inequalities; and *recommendations* for further research and for a broad-based strategy to reduce health inequalities (Macintyre, 1997, p 726). The legacy of its descriptive, analytical and policy-related work is considered in this chapter.

Describing health inequalities

Drawing on 1971 mortality statistics, the Black Report revealed wide disparities in health between people at opposite ends of the social spectrum. For example, the risk of death for male infants in families of unskilled manual workers was found to be three times that of professional families, while for female babies the gap was even greater. The death rate for adult men in Social Class V (unskilled workers) was nearly twice that of adult men in Social Class I (professional workers). Social gradients in health were also found to be remarkably pervasive with respect to death rates for specific diseases (Black Report, 1980).

Since 1980, an extensive body of research has documented the extent and magnitude of socio-economic differentials in health. As noted in Chapter One, this moved away from the traditional use of social class to examine associations between health status and alternative measures of socio-economic status such as income, education, housing and car ownership (Moser et al, 1984, 1988; Davey Smith et al, 1990, 1998a; Macintyre and West, 1991; Wannamethee and Shaper, 1997). Alternative indicators of social stratification were used, such as civil servant grade in the well-known Whitehall Studies (Marmot et al, 1984, 1991). The period after 1980 also saw a flowering of small-area studies which, using composite indices of deprivation drawn from Census data, compared differences in mortality and morbidity between more and less deprived wards (Carstairs, 1981; Townsend et al, 1988; Carstairs and Morris, 1989; Eames et al, 1993; Phillimore et al, 1994; Sloggett and Joshi, 1998). A strong tradition has evolved of analysing geographical variations in health such as Shaw et al's work (1999), which we have already described in Chapter One. This work graphically illustrated the health gap between political constituencies containing the one million people with the highest mortality rates with constituencies with the lowest mortality rates, and found that the under 65 Standardised Mortality Ratio (SMR) was 2.6 times higher in the worst health than the best health constituency, the under 65 Standardised Illness Ratio (SIR) was 2.8 times higher, and that infant and child (aged 1-4) mortality rates were 2.0 times higher.

Since the publication of the Black Report, which focused overwhelmingly on mortality indicators, researchers have also used a wider range of health measures (Macintyre, 1997). These include physical fitness (Blaxter, 1987); self-assessed health status (Wannamethee and Shaper, 1991); and years of potential life lost (Blane et al, 1990). With an expansion of the number of health surveys undertaken since the 1980s, the range of measures that are available to health inequalities researchers has increased significantly. For example, although the Health Survey for England (HSE) has specifically targeted different conditions in different survey years, the fact that it regularly reports on a wide range of diseases, health-related conditions and health services use has made it a useful source for health inequalities research (Gibson et al, 2002; Saxena et al, 2002; Grundy and Sloggett, 2003). Local-based surveys have also been useful sources from which to analyse variations in morbidity (Saul and Payne, 1999). For instance, the Avon Longitudinal Study of Parents and Children (ALSPAC) has provided a particularly rich source of information on variations in socio-economic status, health risk factors and health outcomes. Such work confirms that inequalities in mortality are preceded by inequalities in ill health and disability, that a very wide set of diseases and conditions are subject to social gradients, and that variations in key health risk factors and health outcomes occur throughout the lifecourse.

As well as informing subsequent academic work, descriptive information of the kind found in the Black Report has been put to political use. The current Labour government has used 'headline statistics' as a backdrop to successive public health initiatives in which the need to address underlying determinants of ill health has been explicitly acknowledged. For instance, in *Saving lives: Our healthier nation* (DH, 1999), the White Paper that set out the government's public health strategy in 1999, a wide range of indicators of health variations was presented, including infant mortality, birth weight, life expectancy, death rates from circulatory disease and cancer, prevalence of mental illness and injuries, lifestyle factors, use of health services and social variations in the wider determinants of health including education, income and employment. The HM Treasury's 2002 Cross-cutting Review *Tackling health inequalities* (HM Treasury and DH, 2002) similarly reported social and geographical differences in life expectancy, birth weight and educational attainment, for example highlighting the seven-year gap in male life expectancy between Social Classes I and V. By contrast, in the 2004 White Paper, *Choosing health: Making healthy choices easier* (DH, 2004), few statistics are provided about social variations in health and, because they are embedded in the text, they hardly amount to 'headline' figures. This may be as much a reflection of a perceived need for a change in style as a shift in underlying philosophy. However, there is also a strong emphasis in the report on supporting individual behaviour change. Thus, the lack of 'headline statistics' may signal a change from the portrayal of health inequalities in the Black Report as a societal problem that demands state action (a view apparently endorsed by New Labour when it first came to power) to one that perceives the adoption of healthy lifestyles to be primarily a matter of individual freedom. The more muted style in which recent statistics on health inequalities have been published may also be a response to the fact that there has been no narrowing in health inequalities. Indeed, since Labour came to power, socio-economic differences in both life expectancy and infant mortality have widened (DH, 2005).

Explaining health inequalities

While the Black Report supported the link between material deprivation (for example, poor living conditions, unsafe working conditions and pollution) and ill health, it accepted that, in addition to material/structural explanations, observed associations between class and health lent themselves to the artefact explanation, the theory of social selection and cultural/behavioural explanations (see below). Much academic activity on health inequalities has been structured around this four-fold typology (Carr-Hill, 1987) and it continues to be influential today (Singh-Manoux and Marmot, 2005). However, Macintyre (1997) suggests that while each of the Black Report's four explanatory models has a 'soft' version that can be legitimately subjected to empirical analysis, the initial response was to focus on 'hard' caricatured versions that were easy targets for criticism. The resulting health inequalities 'debate' was polarised, politicised, often acrimonious and, during the 1980s and much of the 1990s, elicited an indifferent policy response.

The artefact explanation

It is today generally accepted that the Black Report's four models do not provide a satisfactory framework for explaining how health inequalities are produced, in part because it is so difficult to avoid treating them as mutually exclusive categories. Nevertheless, work based on this typology has made a valuable contribution to the continued evolution of the health inequalities field by stimulating both methodological and theoretical advances. For instance, the search for alternative measures of socio-economic position and health status and the development of longitudinal study designs (Fox et al, 1985; Davey Smith et al, 1990; Goldblatt, 1990; Marmot et al, 1991) was in part a response to the artefact explanation, which argues that observed social gradients in health may be the product of poor-quality data. This work confirmed the existence of health inequalities. Indeed, it suggested that, far from artefacts exaggerating their magnitude, health inequalities have been underestimated by conventional analysis (Bloor et al, 1987). It generated an interest in the presence of health inequalities in groups such as older people, women and adolescents who had been previously neglected because they could not be easily classified on the basis of occupational class (Moser et al, 1988; West, 1988; Ginn and Arber, 1991; Macintyre and West, 1991; Arber and Ginn, 1993; Marmot and Shipley, 1996). It inspired the generation of new hypotheses about the causes of health inequalities. For instance, the observation in the first Whitehall Study that, even among relatively affluent civil servants, mortality from coronary heart disease (CHD) varied significantly according to grade gave rise to an interest in the role of psychosocial factors in the generation of social gradients in health (Marmot and Theorell, 1988). Finally, with the replacement of social class by the National Statistics Socio-economic Classification (NS-SEC) in 2001, work that questioned the relevance of the Registrar General's social class schema (Illsley, 1986) has been officially accepted.

Social selection

In addition to eliminating bias from statistical artefacts, methodological developments such as longitudinal study design were used to challenge the suggestion that inequalities in mortality largely reflected selective social mobility (Goldblatt, 1988, 1989). The social selection hypothesis explains inequalities in health as a process of health-related social mobility (also referred to as health selection), in which people in poor health move down the social class scale while those in good health experience upward social mobility. As with other explanations for health inequalities, there are soft and hard versions of this approach. These relate to the size of the contribution that social selection is purported to make to health inequalities. The soft version accepts that illness can result in downward social mobility – for example, those who are ill or disabled may be excluded from certain types of jobs or from the labour market altogether. However, it suggests that this process is, at most, a very minor contributor to socio-economic differentials in health. The hard version, by contrast, gives greater priority to the selection of unhealthy people into lower social classes (health status determining social status) than to the effect of social position on health. At its most extreme, this version has been depicted as a form of social Darwinism, an approach that suggests that predisposition to ill health, low intelligence, social disadvantage and so on are transmitted over selective generations in a way that is biologically natural and, as such, is neither unfair nor amenable to policy intervention.

The hard version of the social selection hypothesis not surprisingly proved controversial and, although it is not at all clear that this version elicited much support, much of the debate around health inequalities in the period following the publication of the Black Report focused on the role of health selection (Illsley, 1986, 1987; Wilkinson, 1986, 1987). The legacy of this debate has been both methodological and theoretical. Because longitudinal studies (which follow up the same subjects over a period of time) allow the temporal sequence of relationships between health and social position to be disentangled, they were to become an important tool in research investigating the role of selection (for early examples, see Fox et al, 1985; Wadsworth, 1986; Power et al, 1991). Such studies fairly quickly concluded that, while there is some evidence for health-related social mobility, health selection cannot be regarded as a major explanation for health inequalities because any such effects are very small compared to the effects of social causation (Goldblatt, 1989; Blane et al, 1993; Hart et al, 1998; Chandola et al, 2003).

The contribution of this work went beyond refuting the social selection hypothesis. It also highlighted the validity of tracking interactions between health and social position across the lifespan and, challenging the assumption that the concept of selection inevitably had social Darwinist connotations, showed how early adversity (including ill health) could direct individuals onto certain life trajectories or contribute to the accumulation of disadvantage in ways that had important implications for health (Power et al, 1991; West, 1991; Manor et al, 2003). As we discuss during the course of this book, these themes, together with the use of longitudinal study design, have been of central interest in lifecourse research. Thus, research investigating the effects of health selection was arguably an important precursor to what is seen by many as the dominant approach in current social epidemiology.

Cultural/behavioural explanations

While investigation of artefact and social selection explanations has contributed to a paradigm shift in health inequalities research, research relating to the other explanatory models identified in the Black Report has made less impact. The hard and soft versions of the cultural/behavioural explanation remain much the same today as in 1980. Both start with the observation that health-damaging behaviours such as smoking, poor diet and lack of exercise are more prevalent among the poor than the socially advantaged. The hard version explains this in individualistic terms, lower social groups 'choosing' to adopt less healthy lifestyles due to ignorance, recklessness or fatalism. This is essentially a libertarian perspective and one thus associated with the political right. For example, Edwina Currie, a junior Health Minister in the Conservative government of John Major, gave the following explanation for health inequalities: "I honestly don't think that [health] has anything to do with poverty. The problem very often for many people is just ignorance ... and failing to realise that they do have some control over their lives" (quoted in Townsend, 1993, p 383). Of course, this type of explanation separates behaviour from the social context in which it takes place and effectively blames the victims of health inequalities for the poor health that they experience. The soft version of the cultural/behavioural explanation thus suggests that rather than seeing health-related behaviours as a *cause* of health inequalities, they should be seen as an *outcome* of differences in the material circumstances between socio-economic groups. The key challenge is to find out why health-damaging behaviours are persistently more common in poorer groups.

There has been a number of responses to the critique of individualistic explanations of health inequalities. One has been to explore the role of direct material constraints on the choices of those living in poor environments. For example, several authors (for example, Dowler, 2002; Darmon et al 2003) propose that economic constraints contribute to the unhealthy food choices observed among low socio-economic groups in industrialised countries. However, as we discuss in Chapters Four and Ten, empirical evidence of 'food poverty' is contradictory. Another approach has been to examine whether psychosocial factors associated with poverty play a role in unhealthy lifestyles. For example, since Graham's (1993) study on smoking among working-class mothers, several studies suggest that, for women living in disadvantaged circumstances, smoking is perceived as an important mechanism with which to cope with anxiety and stress. This and other work examining relationships between material deprivation, psychosocial health and lifestyle factors are described in more detail in Chapter Ten. We find, however, that the factors that give rise to socio-economic differences in health behaviours are still poorly understood.

This partly reflects the fact that relatively little research effort has been devoted to examining the cultural/behavioural explanation. With a few exceptions, such as the work undertaken by the Health Behaviour Unit of the Department of Epidemiology and Public Health at University College London, the greater part of academic effort within social epidemiology since the 1990s has focused on lifecourse models, work which, as we have noted earlier, evolved from an interest in the role of social selection. The growth of interest in the role of early life circumstances in determining future health status (discussed later) may have also resulted in a swing away from a concern with adult lifestyle factors. Finally, there may have been an implicit assumption that, because the cultural/behavioural explanation raised questions about the ways in which health-related behaviours were embedded within the structures of society, this was the domain of sociology rather than epidemiology. Yet, as Scrambler suggests, compared to the sway of pioneering research within social epidemiology, the research literature on the sociology of health inequalities has been disappointing, displaying a "poverty of sociological imagination and ambition ... and a stultifying lack of interest in generative mechanisms" (Scrambler, 2001, p 35).

The lack of progress that has been made in disentangling the relationships between social disadvantage and health-damaging behaviours has had important consequences for health inequalities policies. In what will become a recurrent theme in this book, it has allowed the conceptualisation of health behaviours and of interventions designed to promote healthier behaviours to remain overwhelmingly focused on the individual. By contrast, although there is recognition that individual choices are constrained by factors beyond their control, there is also uncertainty about how best to address these factors. Such uncertainty

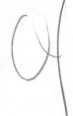

is evident in the failure of the White Paper *Choosing health* (DH, 2004) to resolve philosophical tensions regarding the balance that should be struck between state involvement and individual freedom. While the government is prepared to legislate over the retailing of tobacco to children, it sees the promotion of healthier diets among the young as a matter of choice, leading to the accusation that the logic behind the latest public health strategy is "at best opaque and at worst defeatist and inconsistent" (McKee, 2005, p 370).

Materialist/structural explanations

Like the cultural/behavioural explanation, the materialist explanation stresses the role of the wider social, economic and political context. Indeed, although the hard version of this approach is more economically deterministic, proposing that the physical, material conditions of life, which are determined by occupational class position, are the main influences on health status, the soft version recognises factors other than material inequality (psychosocial influences, for example), and thus shares some common ground with the soft version of the cultural/behavioural approach. Despite widespread support among health inequalities researchers for the role played by material deprivation in health inequalities, research in this area has not advanced greatly since the publication of the Black Report (Shaw et al, 1999, p 102). Epidemiological studies suggest that, individually, factors such as unemployment, poor housing and a lack of education make modest contributions to the total socio-economic gradient in health, leading researchers to suggest that the materialist contribution to social class gradients in health could be explained by the accumulation of multiple factors over the lifecourse (Shaw et al, 1999, p 101). This assumption may well be implicit in the technically excellent work undertaken by lifecourse epidemiologists. However, it is a vague assertion in a policy environment that increasingly demands 'robust evidence' to legitimise political action.

As noted already, the lack of understanding about the role played by socio-structural factors in health inequalities may reflect the relative lack of sociological input in recent research. Important exceptions include the work of David Coburn, Graham Scrambler and, insofar as he explores a socio-structural model, Richard Wilkinson. Arguing that the underlying social, economic and political context of health inequalities has been insufficiently analysed, Coburn (2000) focuses on the ways in which the globalisation of capital has brought about changes in the balance of power (for example, between business and the state), which has important consequences for key intervening variables such as the priority given to welfare. Refining his ideas in a later paper, he proposes that a class/welfare regime model provides a useful approach for exploring how countries with more neo-liberal policies display greater social and health inequalities than social democratic nations (Coburn, 2004). We have considerable sympathy for Coburn's interest in welfare regimes. Indeed, we have drawn on this very concept in setting out our own research agenda for evidence-based public health, one that involves the analysis of public health regimes (see Chapter Fourteen). However, like much work examining the socio-structural context of health inequalities, Coburn's framework fails to offer sufficiently plausible pathways that link wider contextual factors to health outcomes. In this respect, the psychosocial hypothesis concerning the relationship between income inequality, the quality of the social environment and key health outcomes (Wilkinson, 1996, 1999) is more convincing. According to this model, direct psycho-neurological pathways and indirect effects associated with a lack of social cohesion (such as the adoption of unhealthy lifestyles) act as intervening variables linking socio-economic structure and individual health. As we observe later, the psychosocial hypothesis became a conventional wisdom in the late 1990s. However, it has also been subjected to significant criticism.

One criticism that has been levelled at both Coburn and Wilkinson concerns their narrow focus (on the role of welfare and income inequality respectively). Two papers widen the focus of enquiry. The first builds directly on Bourdieu's concept of habitus:

> Bourdieu's basic thesis is that there is a correspondence between social structures (throughout the life course) and mental structures. He advances the concept of 'habitus' to describe the homologous relations between social structure and practices in different domains – economic, political, social, cultural etc of a individual's life. Habitus is thus a generative schema whereby social structures, through the processes of socialization, come to be embodied as schemes of perception that enable individuals to live their lives, leading societies to reproduce existing social structures (Bourdieu, 1984). It provides the individual with class-dependent and predisposed ways of thinking, feeling and acting. (Singh-Manoux and Marmot, 2005, p 2130)

For Singh-Manoux and Marmot, it is through the socialising influence of socio-economic environments on attitudes, belief and behaviours that social class differences in health are produced and maintained. They suggest that health behaviours, psychological resilience, the ability to build social networks and future time perspective are all areas that have a learnt component and that also have clear implications for health inequalities. Thus, for example, children who observe their parents, siblings or friends smoking are more likely to take up the habit. They learn to respond to life events and difficulties from their parents, which shapes their reactions to adversity in adulthood. The resources they have to participate socially are influenced by their family's socio-economic position, as are the social connections they inherit and their ability to learn social skills. A disposition to place high value on long-term planning and goal setting is also in part learned.

Although Singh-Manoux and Marmot deny that their hypothesis negates the importance of material circumstances (2005, p 2131), the concept of socialisation, as outlined earlier, leads to a focus on health-related and psychosocial *behaviours*. By contrast, Scrambler's framework (2001) encompasses social, cultural and material factors. Scrambler proposes that class relations are predominantly responsible for health inequalities in countries like Britain (that is, they are the generative mechanism), but that the impact of unequal class relations (and indeed unequal relations based on gender and ethnicity) takes place through variable *capital flows*. Six types of capital flow are identified: biological, psychological, social, cultural, spatial and material. Working through the pathways that give rise to health inequalities during the course of this book, we find that Scrambler's concept accommodates many of the key areas through which social disadvantage and adverse health outcomes are linked. For example, the flow of biological capital refers to the fact that even before birth, the children of low-income mothers are at higher risk of being disadvantaged with regard to their physical development (see Chapter Four). Support and stimulation in early childhood are good examples of the flow of psychological capital and, as we observe in Chapters Four and Six, there is evidence of socio-economic variation in key factors associated with emotional, behavioural and cognitive development. Through socialisation, there is a link between psychological capital and the flow of cultural capital. However, after the early years, factors outside the household such as formal educational opportunities and peer networks become more influential in determining life chances and the flow of norms and values relating to health behaviours (see Chapter Eight). The concept of social capital is very similar to that explored in Wilkinson's (1996) psychosocial hypothesis. We discuss this in more depth in the next part of this chapter, which also alludes to Scrambler's notion of spatial capital in its discussion of neighbourhood effects on health. In Chapters Ten and Twelve, we explore the impact of material factors more directly, by assessing links between unemployment, income poverty, poor housing and ill health.

As is evident from the way in which Scrambler's schema maps onto our own account of the factors that give rise to health inequalities through the lifecourse, this framework is remarkably comprehensive. Moreover, inequalities in the wider social structure lie at its heart, and this is important. As Graham (2004) points out, many models that describe the 'social determinants of health' draw attention to the factors that promote health in general but not to the social processes that determine the unequal distribution of these factors. Against this, it is not certain that Scrambler's approach does more than restate (albeit in a conceptually attractive way) the links between causal factors at the individual level which, due to epidemiological research, we can be increasingly clear about, and the structure in which they are embedded which, as an essentially conceptual device, is inevitably vague. In other words, this framework brings us no closer to understanding how the wider determinants of health inequalities can be appropriately targeted by policy.

The policy recommendations of the Black Report

The political reaction to the Black Report is well known. Indeed, it has attained almost iconic status as the textbook example of a government cover up (Berridge and Blume, 2002). Its publication was delayed due to the failure of the Working Group's scientific members to reach consensus over the relative role of hospital services in tackling health inequalities, and the Report, commissioned by a Labour government, was received by a new Conservative administration that was particularly hostile to its recommendations for socio-structural change. For Patrick Jenkin, the Secretary of State for Social Services responsible for the release of the Report, it read like "a policy manifesto from a party who do not expect the responsibilities of office" (cited by Berridge, 2003). In order to distance the government from the Report, Jenkin arranged for only 260 typescript copies to be released on an August Bank Holiday and, in his foreword, made it quite clear that he did not endorse the Group's recommendations: "I am making the report available for discussion, but without any commitment by the Government to its proposals" (cited by Berridge, 2003).

Although the government went on to ignore the Report's recommendations for socio-structural change, a number of its proposals for healthcare were to be practically implemented. The Working Group made a detailed case for a change in the way in which NHS resources were distributed and, in 1995, the government introduced a new weighted capitation formula for Hospital and Community Health Services that explicitly reflected the demand for healthcare produced by deprivation. The 1980s and early 1990s also saw a number of policy developments that supported a shift in the roles of inpatient and community care, although not all would agree that key community services were given 'greater priority' as advocated by Black and his colleagues. Similarly, key changes to the organisation of general practitioner services such as the decline in single-handed practices and the introduction of financial incentives for preventive work were motivated by similar concerns to those expressed in the Black Report about the quality of primary healthcare.

The main thrust of the Report, however, was that government action needed to be focused in areas other than the NHS:

> While the health care service can play a significant part in reducing inequalities in health, measures to reduce differences in material standards of living at work, in the home and in everyday social and community life are of even greater importance. (Townsend and Davidson, 1982, p 304)

The lack of clarity noted earlier about how materialist/structural determinants of health inequalities can best be targeted did not prevent the Black Report from making quite specific social policy recommendations. These included the need to abolish child poverty, to achieve a fairer distribution of resources and wealth, to promote fairer employment rights and to raise living standards through better housing. A case was made for prioritising families and children through improved benefits, the statutory provision of preschool education and day care and free nutritional school meals. Disabled people were targeted for attention and support through a comprehensive disablement allowance and the Group called for legislation banning the advertising of tobacco and the sales promotion of tobacco products. The Working Group also provided rough estimates of the cost implications of its proposals, acknowledging that four measures alone (an increase in child benefit, the introduction of an infant care allowance, the expansion of day care provision and free school meals) would require around £1.5 billion.

Concerns about the cost implications of these recommendations contributed to the government's hostile response to the Black Report. As Jenkin suggested in his foreword:

> I must make it clear that additional expenditure on the scale which could result from the report's recommendations – the amount involved could be upwards of £2 billion a year – is quite unrealistic in present or any foreseeable economic circumstances, quite apart from any judgement that may be formed of the effectiveness of such expenditure in dealing with the problems identified. (Jenkin, 1980)

Subsequent analysis by government suggested that funding for three groups of activity – those pertaining to families and children, disabled people and special programmes for the 10 areas with the highest mortality – would amount to £5.5 billion in 1982 prices, the equivalent of 2.2% of the country's Gross Domestic Product (GDP) (Townsend, 1999, p xvi). While Townsend points out that this is a fraction of the amount spent on social security, such an increase in the level of public social expenditure would be significant for any government, let alone one committed to the retrenchment of welfare. Tensions around the economic implications of addressing health inequalities were therefore a strong factor behind the rejection of the Black Report.

Despite this, the legacy of the Black Report for subsequent policy making was substantial. In part because it was so coolly received, the Report came to have enormous symbolism for those committed to social justice. It not only inspired similar research in European countries, but it kept health inequalities at the forefront of the public health agenda in the UK. Indeed, one of the first actions by the incoming Labour government of 1997 was to commission an Independent Inquiry into Health Inequalities. The product of this Inquiry, the Acheson Report (1998), is sometimes referred to as the 'Second Black Report' in the sense that both documented the evidence of health inequalities and made recommendations for action (Exworthy, 2002). Like the Black Report, the Acheson Report supported a socio-economic explanation for health inequalities, recognised that healthcare had a relatively small role to play in addressing social gradients in health and identified broad social policy areas (poverty, income, tax and benefits; education; employment; housing and environment; transport and pollution; nutrition) for policy action. Again, the need to ensure that children had a better start in life was highlighted, as was the case for reducing income inequalities and improving the living standards of poor households.

The policy response to some of the main recommendations of the Acheson Report is considered at length in Chapter Three. At this point, however, it is useful to reflect on ways in which this report and the political response to it were shaped by its predecessor. Unlike the Black Report, the *Independent Inquiry into Inequalities in Health* avoided providing detailed costs for its recommendations. According to Michael Marmot, a member of the Inquiry team:

> We took the view that as a scientific group we were charged, as stated in our terms of reference, with 'identifying priority areas for future development', not with telling the finance minister at which level to set the rate of taxation and benefits. (Marmot, 1999, cited by Exworthy, 2002, p 181)

It is likely that the political reaction to the Black Report shaped this view. However, it was to attract criticism on the grounds that the Working Group's policy proposals were too vague and, in the absence of detailed costs, it was impossible to judge the extent to which the recommendations were affordable and cost-effective or to weigh up the opportunity costs of not investing in other areas (Davey Smith et al, 1998b). This, it was argued, would encourage inactivity on the part of government:

> In the present and foreseeable political climate the best – and maybe the only – hope of serious governmental action to tackle the inequalities in health so fully described in the report is to produce concrete and costed proposals. These, moreover, should engage as much as possible with the government's social agenda. The proposals need to be explicit enough for it to be clear where current policies are inadequate or will work against the government's declared aim of reducing inequality. (Davey Smith et al, 1998c, p 601)

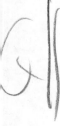

In fact, the lack of concrete and costed proposals did not hold back policy making. As we discuss in Chapter Three, the government can claim to have addressed virtually all of the Acheson Report's 39 recommendations. However, policy responses to the broad areas identified by the Independent Inquiry can be either conventional or radical, a distinction that is linked to the level at which policies are practically implemented, and many would argue that the materialist/structural factors identified in the Report have been translated into individualised policies. The vagueness with which the recommendations were made certainly gave the government large scope for interpretation. Ironically, however, criticisms relating to the lack of costs in the Report may have also influenced the direction that policy has taken. It is difficult to carry out economic evaluations of policies relating to structural reform with as much rigour as clinical and behavioural interventions that give rise to measurable inputs, output and outcomes, usually at the individual level. Thus, demands for better information on cost–effectiveness, together with a wider approach to evidence-based policy that has generally valued 'scientific' rigour above qualitative methods, may have contributed to the tendency to focus on discrete 'downstream' interventions and to neglect 'upstream' initiatives that target the wider determinants of health.

It is clear that the Black Report has had a long arm of influence. In time, however, the number of references to its explanatory framework has gradually decreased and, as media interest in other approaches to researching health inequalities grows, so too are policy makers less likely to invoke the broad social policy areas highlighted by the Working Group. Today, policies relating to health inequalities are more likely to be targeted at key demographic groups such as pregnant women, infants, preschool children, young people and older people. This approach to policy organisation corresponds with the current interest in social epidemiology in factors that give rise to adverse health outcomes during different periods of the lifecourse. It is to this body of research and the other theoretical highlights of the 1990s and 2000s that we now turn.

Health inequalities research since the Black Report: theoretical highlights of the 1990s and 2000s

As we observed at the beginning of this chapter, health inequalities research is an exciting area to work in due to its interdisciplinary nature, the high quality of empirical work that is undertaken in the field and the extent to which research has been theoretically innovative. Next, we describe three important themes that were to provide foci for research and debate in the 1990s: psychosocial effects, contextual effects, and the relative role of risk factors at different periods of the lifecourse. The advancement of all three of these research areas has been underpinned by empirical research. For example, the observation of a stepwise social gradient in health outcomes was one of a number of factors that contributed to the development of the psychosocial hypothesis. Interest in the relative importance of compositional and contextual effects was stimulated by developments in multi-level modelling techniques, which suggested that, over and above the effects of individual socio-economic status, health could be influenced by wider neighbourhood effects; and it is unlikely that lifecourse epidemiology would have developed in the way that it has without the insights afforded by longitudinal study design and analysis. Theoretical developments have also benefited from the judicious targeting of research funding, initiatives such as the Economic and Social Research Council's (ESRC) Health Variations Programme playing an important role in stimulating research of this kind.

Health inequalities and the psychosocial environment

The idea that health inequalities reflect the psychological effects of living in an unequal society is particularly associated with Richard Wilkinson. Examining the relationship between income and health in developed countries, he observed that while there was a positive but weak relationship between the GDP *per capita* of a country and average life expectancy it was not the richest countries that had the highest life expectancy but the most equal and socially cohesive (Quick and Wilkinson, 1991; Wilkinson, 1992, 1996). Thus, once a country had reached the point in epidemiological transition when degenerative diseases took over from infectious diseases as the major cause of death, health appeared to be related less to absolute levels of wealth than to the way in which income was distributed. The explanation for this link, he hypothesised, lay in psychosocial pathways.

At around the same time that Wilkinson was exploring macro-level evidence of links between income and health, the Whitehall Studies of British civil servants were also highlighting the importance of psychosocial factors to health. Social gradients in disease and mortality were found to run across the social hierarchy from the top employment grades to the bottom (Marmot et al, 1991; Marmot and Shipley, 1996). As the Whitehall civil servants were not poor, position in the social hierarchy appeared to be more significant than absolute deprivation. Biochemical and physiological risk factors for CHD in Whitehall II subjects were studied and levels of protective high-density lipoproteins found to be significantly related to employment grades in civil servants. The fact that a similar pattern was observed in the social hierarchy of wild male baboons (Sapolsky and Mott, 1987, cited by Brunner, 1996) suggested that psychosocial effects rather than lifestyle factors were at work. Thus, it was hypothesised, subordinate status contributed to chronic stress in both human and non-human primates, elevating cortisol levels which in turn produced metabolic effects relating to cholesterol levels, central obesity and increased risk for CHD as well as other effects such as depression and poorer immune function (Brunner, 1996, 2001; Brunner and Marmot, 1999).

In a third strand of work, evidence suggested that the quality and type of people's social networks influenced health, as positive social relationships offered a protective effect while negative relationships and social isolation increased vulnerability to ill health (Stansfeld, 1999). Again, neuroendocrine reactivity (particularly relating to the hypothalamic-pituitary-adrenal axis and cortisol secretion) was identified as a possible mechanism linking social support and health with subsequent implications for risk for CHD and depression. Social isolation and high levels of psychosocial stress could also contribute directly to ill health by promoting health-damaging behaviours such as excess alcohol consumption and drug misuse. Significantly, the effects of social support not only operated at the individual level. The role of neighbourhood cohesion emerged as an area of research interest with evidence that in communities with high levels of social cohesion, some health indicators were better than in those with low levels (Ellaway et al, 2001). Factors relevant to perceptions of neighbourhood cohesion included social/cultural composition, the quality of the physical environment, fear of crime, level of communal activity, and so on (a further discussion of contextual effects is included later in this chapter). Wider societal factors were also highlighted. For example, high rates of mortality in Eastern and Central Europe were partly attributed to the psychosocial effects of feelings of relative disadvantage, unfulfilling work, low control over lifestyle, and dealing with food and other shortages (Bobat and Marmot, 1996).

Bringing these various strands together, Wilkinson hypothesised that the significance of income inequality to mortality lay in the psychosocial effects of low social status and in the poorer quality of social relations found in more hierarchical societies (Wilkinson, 1999). Both contribute to poor health outcomes through producing stress and promoting health-damaging behaviours. In addition, an unjust social climate results in little social provision for the well-being of the poor such as adequate access to health services (Kawachi and Kennedy, 1999). While there has been some debate as to whether the mechanisms linking income inequality and health are lagged or instantaneous (Blakely et al, 2000), proponents of the income inequality or psychosocial hypothesis generally agree that the stress and lack of social support associated with poverty combine to produce negative health consequences for the poor themselves (depression, CHD and poorer immune function, for example) and for others (hence the close relationship between income inequality and both homicide and violent crime). In these ways, inequality affects the health of all members of a community, not just the poor.

Within a relatively short time, the psychosocial hypothesis became a conventional wisdom. Despite its popularity, however, it has been attacked on a number of grounds. In 2000, Lynch et al proposed that the psychosocial hypothesis was an essentially conservative model that, by ignoring the fact that the health effects of social hierarchy are contingent on material living conditions, potentially blamed poor and minority ethnic communities for their lack of social and political cohesion. Others have focused on methodological areas of concern. For example, Macleod and Davey Smith (2003) point out that interpreting any association between psychosocial and physical health is difficult due to potential reporting bias. Thus, people who report greater stress may also be prone to reporting poorer health, without any objective evidence of a greater amount of physical disease. The difficulties of establishing which group(s) people compare themselves with in order to gain a sense of relative deprivation have been highlighted (Lynch et al, 2004). It has also been argued that the relationship between income inequality and health at the population level is artefactual, reflecting the curvilinear relation between income and the life expectancy of individuals (Gravelle, 1998).

Due in part to such methodological objections, empirical evidence of an association between psychosocial health and physical health is in dispute. Macleod and Davey Smith (2003) argue that before the spread of 'victim culture' among the working class, higher stress was associated with material advantage and higher rates of unhealthy behaviour, yet lower rates of heart disease. Lynch et al (2004) accuse proponents of the psychosocial hypothesis of selectively citing animal evidence of positive associations between stress and disease even though other studies find lower levels of the stress hormone cortisol in subordinate primates. The very association between income inequality and population health has been called into question (Judge et al, 1998; Lynch et al, 2001, 2004), most international studies using recent data showing null or mixed results. With the possible exception of the US, doubts have also been expressed as to whether a relationship exists between income inequality and mortality at a country level (Lynch et al, 2004), or whether even lagged income inequality is significantly associated with health status (Mellor and Milyo, 2003). Finally, experimental evaluation of psychosocial interventions suggests that they are ineffective in terms of improving physical health (see also Chapter Eleven), which casts doubt on the causal nature of the relationship between psychosocial exposure and health outcomes (Macleod and Davey Smith, 2003).

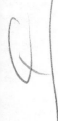

Many of these concerns have been robustly countered (Marmot and Wilkinson, 2001) and there are grounds for proposing that the psychosocial hypothesis has been misrepresented by its critics. First, far from being a conservative model, the psychosocial interpretation supports radical income redistribution. Its proponents cite the example of countries such as Costa Rica that, by adopting broadly socialist/social democratic policies, have achieved high levels of health at relatively low levels of wealth (Marmot, 2004). This is in direct opposition to the neo-liberal model that values economic policy above social policy and assumes that, due to basic welfare provision and the trickledown effect of pursuing economic growth, poverty no longer exists in Western societies.

Second, the causal pathways linking stress and disease in adult life are plausible and have arguably become more so given widespread acceptance of the role of neuroendocrine pathways in other key stages of development (see, for example, Chapter Four). The psychosocial hypothesis also provides a potential explanation for contextual or neighbourhood effects and for the stepwise gradient in health outcomes across the whole social hierarchy. These aspects of health inequalities have been otherwise difficult to explain. Davey Smith (2003) suggests that, with respect to the Whitehall Studies, the grades of civil servants strongly reflect social origin and this is as likely to explain gradients in mortality in this group as psychosocial influences. However, he highlights the fairly large distinctions between administrative, executive and clerical grade civil servants. As noted in

Chapter One, it is the finely tuned nature of social gradients in health that suggest that something more than material deprivation is of significance here.

Third, methodological concerns are being addressed by the use of better-quality data, including more objective indicators of psychosocial health. As a result there is growing empirical support for the psychosocial hypothesis in the behavioural sciences and medicine (Krantz and McCeney, 2002). Reviewing evidence from systematic reviews of independent associations between psychosocial factors and the development and progression of CHD, an Expert Working Group of the National Heart Foundation of Australia concluded that "there is strong and consistent evidence of an independent causal association between depression, social isolation and lack of quality social support and the causes and prognosis of CHD" (Bunker et al, 2003, p 272). As we discuss in Chapter Ten, it is today widely accepted that economic circumstances influence both stress and health. For example, unemployment has been associated with reduced psychological well-being, increasing illness and higher mortality.

In order to make some sense of this conflicting evidence, Mellor and Milyo (2001) point out the distinction between studies that focus on the health consequences of direct economic distress and the income inequality hypothesis because the latter asserts that it is not the level of economic distress that affects health but the variation in economic circumstances within a community. Whitehead and Diderichsen (2001) similarly suggest that one source of confusion about the psychosocial hypothesis has been a failure to separate out the individual from the population effects. Thus, while there is good evidence that individual-level factors such as strong social networks and high control at work are good for a person's health, there are no grounds for extrapolating such evidence to whole populations. Despite claims that empirical evidence for the income inequality/health link is 'slowly dissipating' (Mackenbach, 2002, cited by Subramanian et al, 2003), however, Wilkinson's theory is not without its supporters. Subramanian et al (2003) note that many of the country-level studies that show null results are carried out in societies that are egalitarian and that have far-reaching welfare state protections. This would explain why the strongest evidence for direct health effects of income inequality has come from the US, one of the most unequal of countries in the Western World.

On balance, we conclude that it would be premature to dismiss the psychosocial hypothesis. However, concerns raised by recent epidemiological studies should be taken seriously. Given evidence that the specific mechanisms through which socio-economic disadvantages are expressed in health may differ across context and time, critics are right to question claims that any single mechanism can account for socio-economic gradients in health and mortality (Lynch et al, 2004). Psychosocial mechanisms are likely to work in conjunction with material conditions to increase vulnerability to disease. Questions remain, however, as to whether biological responses to stress constitute a common pathway for a range of diseases or whether psychosocial health contributes to some health outcomes

but not others. As intervention trials have continued to have disappointing r...
(Strike and Steptoe, 2004), there is also debate about the utility of addressing t...
mediating pathways at the individual level (by helping individuals to develop
better ways of coping with stress, for example) as opposed to targeting low
socio–economic status itself through broader social policies (Adler and Snibbe,
2003).

Contextual effects

GLASGOW

As we described in Chapter One, there is a distinct geography to health
inequalities, higher death rates occurring in the North and West of Britain and
in urban and declining industrial areas. To a large extent, the geographical
distribution of mortality in Britain echoes the geographical distribution of poverty.
For example, in Shaw et al's (1999) study, 37% of households in the 15 'worst
health' areas were living in poverty, compared to 13% of households in the 'best
health' areas. For households with children, the difference was even more
pronounced, 53% and 13% living in poverty in the worst and best health areas
respectively.

The strong association between mortality and the spatial concentration of
deprivation suggests that geographical health variation in Britain reflects the
composition of the population in different areas (that is, the aggregated effect of
individual characteristics). However, a purely compositional explanation implies
that similar types of people will have similar health experiences, no matter where
they live, an assumption challenged by evidence of residual area effects once
individual differences have been accounted for. This suggests that the social and
physical environment in which people live has an additional effect on their
health status.

The relative importance of compositional and contextual explanations emerged
as an important theme in health inequalities research in the 1990s (Shaw et al,
1998), largely through the use of multilevel modelling techniques that allowed
the investigation of the way in which contextual effects added to and interacted
with individual-level variables (Duncan and Jones, 1995; Duncan et al, 1998).
Reviews of multilevel studies suggest that compositional effects play the major
role in geographical health variation. However, evidence for modest
neighbourhood effects on health is fairly consistent (Curtis and Jones, 1998;
Pickett and Pearl, 2001). The impact of context appears to vary according to age,
gender, ethnicity and health outcome. For example, contextual effects have been
demonstrated for health behaviours (such as smoking, diet and domestic violence)
and a range of physical health outcomes (such as mortality and CHD). By contrast,
evidence of an association between area of residence and mental health has been
weak (Duncan and Jones, 1995; Pickett and Pearl, 2001; Wainwright and Surtees,
2003; Weich et al, 2003). The relative importance of context and composition
may also vary according to neighbourhood type. For example, living in socially

39

impoverished settings appears to exacerbate health disadvantage
1998, p 622). It has also been proposed that the experience of
enerally affluent area may confer additional risk (Shouls et al,
cent analysis of data from the Whitehall II Study found no
sonal poverty combined with affluent neighbourhood had
nsequences (Stafford and Marmot, 2003).

thways have been proposed to explain neighbourhood effects
on individual health. Macintyre et al (1993) proposed five groups of factors that
may be of relevance: the physical features of the environment; the availability of
healthy environments at home, work and play; the provision of various services;
socio-cultural features; and the reputation of an area. Living in a deprived
neighbourhood may be associated with increased exposure to industrial pollution
and traffic congestion, both of which may pose direct threats to health. Poor
access to facilities such as food outlets, parks, sporting facilities and public transport
may affect health behaviours, as may local community norms and values (such as
pro-smoking attitudes). Indirectly, perceptions of vandalism, crime, drug misuse,
low self-esteem due to the poor physical condition and/or reputation of one's
neighbourhood and isolation from social or community networks may undermine
psychosocial well-being, with implications for lifestyle factors and, perhaps,
immunological status (Halpern, 1995; Sooman and Macintyre, 1995; Kawachi et
al, 1999; Gatrell et al, 2000; Macintyre et al, 2002). Psychosocial mechanisms are
implied in several studies investigating contextual effects. However, it is unclear
why psychosocial well-being should have a greater effect on physical health (for
which studies have found independent area-level variance) than on mental health
(where little evidence has been found of contextual effects). This, together with
the wider critique that has recently been made of psychosocial explanations of
health inequalities (discussed earlier) means that the causal pathways involved in
making context matter remain poorly understood.

Lifecourse epidemiology

When the Black Report was published, epidemiological studies of risk for chronic
disease typically focused on 'lifestyle' factors such as smoking, diet and physical
activity. With few exceptions (Stein et al, 1975; Forsdahl, 1978), the role that
childhood factors could play in increasing risk for disease in adult life received
very little attention. In the 1980s, however, the pendulum began to swing back
again with evidence produced by researchers such as David Barker (Barker and
Osmond, 1986; Barker et al, 1989, 1990; Barker, 1994). This evidence proposed
that biological risk for adult chronic disease was established in early life
(Wadsworth, 1997). Within a remarkably short space of time, the 'early life
experience' paradigm was described as a strong candidate for the replacement of
the 'lifestyle paradigm' of chronic disease aetiology (Robinson, 1992, cited by
Davey Smith and Kuh, 1996). However, concerns about the increasing polarisation

between these two paradigms led to the development of other explanations for continuities between socio-economic circumstances during childhood and health inequalities in adulthood and, by the late 1990s, three distinct lifecourse models had been described (Hertzman et al, 2001).

While the latency model suggests that early life environments affect adult health independently of intervening experience, pathway and accumulation models propose that disadvantage during early and later life operate together, either interactively or additively. Each of these models has important implications for the choice of when and how to intervene to reduce health inequalities (Evans, 2002, p 53). However, as we discuss next, care should be taken in treating them as mutually exclusive categories. It is generally accepted today that all three models have a bearing on adult health, although their relative roles vary according to different health outcomes.

Early life programming

During the first four decades of the 20th century, there was considerable public health interest in the role of nutrition in early life as a determinant of susceptibility to disease. From the 1940s, this gave way to an overwhelming focus on risk factors in adult life (Davey Smith and Kuh, 1996). Thus, by the time the Black Report was published in 1980, very little work examined the significance of development in utero, infancy and childhood to health status in later life. This was to change within a relatively short period of time. In 1986 Barker and Osmond published the first of what was to be an extensive series of studies showing that people who had low birth weights or who were thin or stunted at birth (indicating impaired foetal growth) had high rates of CHD, the related disorders of stroke, diabetes and hypertension and even apparently unrelated disorders such as cancer, depression and schizophrenia (Barker and Osmond, 1986; Barker et al, 1989, 1990; Law et al, 1991; Barker and Martyn, 1992; Barker, 1994; Martyn et al, 1995, 1996; Ravelli et al, 1998; Sayer et al, 1998; Forsen et al, 2000; Thompson et al, 2001; Wahlbeck et al, 2001).

The basis of these observations was proposed to be that of biological programming whereby exposure to undernutrition and other adverse influences at a critical or sensitive period of development results in long-term change in the structure, physiology and metabolism of the developing baby. In the terminology of lifecourse epidemiology, biological programming is also known as a critical period or latency model. These terms encapsulate the idea that there are limited time windows during which an exposure can have adverse or protective effects on development (outside these time windows there is no excess risk associated with exposure). Changes during these critical periods can have long-term effects on disease risk many years later. According to the strict version of the latency model, these are not modified in any dramatic way by later experiences (Kuh et al, 2003). In other words, changes caused by adverse exposures to the developing body are permanent, even though the effects of these changes may not manifest in disease outcomes for many years. The significance of this model for health inequalities stems from the fact that a range of factors that are known to adversely affect foetal development (for example, nutrition deficiencies, smoking in pregnancy and maternal stress) are associated with lower socio-economic status. Consequently, this is a process by which social disadvantage is literally 'embodied' in the developing child (Krieger, 2001; Graham and Power, 2004).

In addition to foetal programming, latent effects of adversity in infancy and early childhood have been postulated (see Chapter Four). For example, breastfeeding in infancy has been linked to long-term benefits with regard to cardiovascular health (Forsyth et al, 2003), while rapid weight gain among toddlers who were thin at birth has been identified as a risk factor for both diabetes and cardiovascular disease (Eriksson et al, 1999). Fruit and vegetable consumption during childhood may have a long-term protective effect on cancer risk in adults (Maynard et al, 2003). Early exposure to *Helicobacter pylori* has been proposed as a key factor in the aetiology of stomach cancer. Similarly, risk for haemorrhagic stroke may be influenced by exposure to infection in childhood (Davey Smith et al, 1998d; Hart and Davey Smith, 2003). A growing body of research is also exploring the interplay between biological and psychological/behavioural influences on early development. Evidence suggests that critical periods for brain development continue up to the age of six (McCain and Mustard, 1999) with long-term consequences not only for cognitive development, socio-emotional health and behaviour, but also for physical health outcomes.

In addition to promoting a shift from the largely descriptive studies of health inequalities in the early 1980s to a more explanatory approach, Barker's work on biological programming is generally seen as the springboard for lifecourse epidemiology. It has received considerable media and policy attention and is an important factor behind the government's strong emphasis on supporting young children. The approach is not without its critics, however. As we discuss in Chapter Four, the way in which the relationship between lifecourse exposures and an individual or family's socio-economic position is conceptualised in epidemiological studies can distort reality. Although such research has highlighted a range of early life factors (from smoking, nutrition and stress in pregnancy to the quality of parenting and family environments) that are linked to adverse health outcomes in the longer term, individual studies tend to focus on one or two risk factors with a view to isolating 'pure effects'. As a result, factors that actively mediate risk may be wrongly treated as confounding factors (Gillman, 2002). At the same time, the demonstration of a pure effect in a controlled study does not mean that the impact of that effect is very strong in real life.

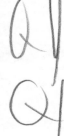

For many social scientists, another criticism of this 'single-risk' approach to epidemiology is that it tends to lead to downstream policy recommendations rather than calls for structural reform. This stems from the fact that studies of this kind spell out *clear* biological and developmental pathways that can be targeted for intervention. For example, responding to the proposal that foetal and infant nutrition play a central role in the programming of susceptibility to adult disease, substantial research effort has been devoted to testing the efficacy of dietary interventions targeting women in pregnancy. Good feeding guidelines have been established with respect to both breastfeeding and weaning practices and a range of breastfeeding promotion projects launched (see Chapter Five). Such initiatives are generally implemented at an individual level and tend to be very singular in approach, nutritional supplementation focusing on individual nutrients rather than diet as a whole. Breastfeeding promotion seeks to improve individual women's awareness and access to practical support, while the Welfare Food Scheme, expanded since 2005 from offering free milk to providing a weekly voucher for 'healthy foods' such as fruits and vegetables and cereal-based foods, targets pregnant women in receipt of Income Support. By narrowly focusing on nutrition and on improving nutrition for individual beneficiaries, important connections are often missed in these schemes, such as the role played by maternal stress in both directly and indirectly shaping foetal development or the extent to which a woman's ability to breastfeed is shaped by wider factors such as the time that she can realistically afford to stay off work. As a result, it is hardly surprising that evidence is lacking that discrete interventions of this kind have substantial effects on desired health outcomes.

In addition to leading to a rather narrow understanding of how to intervene, concerns have been raised about the implications of the biological programming hypothesis for when to intervene. If, as postulated by the model of latency effects, specific biological and developmental factors in early life have a lifelong impact on health and well-being, then interventions to eradicate health inequalities should be strongly focused on maternal and child health. Without such intervention, there may be reduced scope for changing the health prospects of people who have been seriously disadvantaged in their early years. Few deny the importance of supporting the healthy development of babies and young children. However, the emphasis on the need for very early intervention to improve developmental opportunities does raise fears that older children and adults could be 'written off' as beyond help (Selwyn, 2000, p 48).

Concerns that the latency model is overly deterministic have been countered by the development in the 1990s of two alternative models that argue that disadvantage during early and later life operate together, either additively or interactively. Within these accounts, the role of social factors in shaping exposure to risks is of particular interest. Thus, while Barker's work originated in a biomedical epidemiological model and posits biological mechanisms, researchers examining pathway and cumulative effects start with an interest in the way in which exposures to risk are socially patterned. Countering the singular focus of the latency model on mother and child health, they also suggest that there is scope for ameliorating the impact of early disadvantage at later stages of the lifecourse. It is to these lifecourse models that we now turn.

Pathway and accumulation models

Similar to the concept of chain effects that unfold over time (Rutter, 1995, 1999), pathway models are based on the idea that differences in early life environments direct children onto different life trajectories (one bad experience or exposure often leading to another and then another) that in turn affect health status (Hertzman et al, 2001; Kuh et al, 2003). For example, growing up in a family experiencing financial worries or marital conflict exposes young children to stresses that increase risks for cognitive and behavioural difficulties. A lack of readiness to learn, poor behaviour at school, an absence of educational resources at home and attending a school where many other children are struggling with the effects of early childhood deprivation can undermine educational performance. This in turn can increase feelings of alienation and adolescents who are disengaged with school are at higher risk of taking up health-damaging behaviours such as smoking and illicit drug misuse, of having an unplanned pregnancy or of dropping out of school entirely. All of these problems further limit opportunities, making young people more vulnerable to unemployment or employment in low-paid and unskilled or semi-skilled jobs. In turn, financial insecurity in adulthood is linked to factors that impact directly and indirectly on health, such as psychosocial stressors and likelihood of living in an unhealthy physical environment.

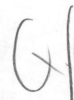

Although pathway models are interested in intergenerational continuities, they should not be confused with work that attributes the transmission of poverty across generations to either genetic inheritance or the cultural attitudes of the so-called underclass. Continuities that exist in disadvantage between parent and child and between childhood and adulthood are seen as probabilistic rather than deterministic. They are also amenable to positive action by publicly funded welfare services (Graham and Power, 2004). Thus, efforts to promote better parenting practices in which conflict is reduced, positive reinforcement encouraged and clear boundaries given, are key to supporting the developmental health of very young children. Experiences at school are important in the transmission of advantage and disadvantage across the generations, teachers' support for and investment in the education of disadvantaged children being critical to escaping the negative long-term effects of early assaults on developmental health. Similarly, wider neighbourhood initiatives can play a role in breaking 'cycles' of deprivation, delinquency and criminality by improving access to neighbourhood peer groups, adults and institutions that encourage pro-social attitudes.

While one version of the pathway model suggests that the effect of early disadvantage on adult health is indirect, influencing social trajectories that eventually trigger increased risk for disease, another postulates an additive effect in which each exposure not only increases the risk of the subsequent exposure but also has an independent effect on disease risk (Kuh et al, 2003). In theory, this version is difficult to distinguish from the accumulation model of health inequalities, which suggests that the adverse health effects of unfavourable environments gradually accumulate over time to increase the risk of chronic disease, poor circumstances throughout life conferring the greatest risk of poor health in adulthood through a type of dose–response relationship (although pathway research tends to focus on social and educational trajectories during childhood and adolescence while research examining cumulative effects is more likely to examine the role of adult circumstances). There are also overlaps between the pathway and accumulation models and the expanded version of the latency model. In contrast to the extreme definition of biological programming, which suggests that an exposure acting during a critical period of development has long-term consequences *irrespective* of later experience, this accepts that the effects of early exposure may be modified by later physiological or psychological stressors.

In addition to overlaps with respect to the way in which causal processes giving rise to health inequalities are hypothesised, methodological difficulties arise in separating out latent, pathway and cumulative effects (Hallqvist et al, 2004). Against this background, there is a strong case for a less polarised and more integrative approach to lifecourse epidemiology that avoids treating these models as mutually exclusive paradigms. Evidence of a broadening in interpretation of specific models of disease causation suggests that this case has been generally accepted (Kuh et al, 2003). Thus, it is generally agreed today that the intrauterine environment, childhood circumstances, the life trajectories of children and young people and adult circumstances can *all* have a bearing on adult health, although the relative strengths of these effects may vary across different cohorts and health outcomes (Graham, 2002). The task for lifecourse research is to tease out these relative strengths. This is, of course, essential for not only understanding disease aetiology but also for informing the targeting of appropriate policies, an observation that informed our decision to use a lifecourse framework to structure this book.

Conclusion

Over the past 25 years, there has been a remarkable growth of interest in the field of health inequalities, and the development of a body of research, much of which is of a very high quality. Several different explanatory frameworks for the persistence of variations in health have been presented, and a range of theories proposed. Some highlight the relationship between health risk factors and socio-economic position at an individual level, lending themselves easily to empirical analysis. Other, more conceptual models, focus on underlying structural factors, the role of which has been more difficult to measure. Indeed, in contrast to the flowering of single-risk studies within epidemiology, we note that the research literature on the role played by socio-structural factors has not advanced greatly. This may partly account for the popularity of the psychosocial hypothesis, which offers a clear and plausible pathway with which to link wider contextual features with individual health outcomes.

The relationship between theory and empirical research has significance for the production of 'evidence' about the causes of health inequalities. By seeking to isolate pure effects, epidemiological research appears to identify clear risk factors that can be readily targeted by interventions with a measurable impact. In comparison, sociological research on the underlying mechanisms that give rise to health inequalities seems vague. However, we cannot fully understand the causes of and potential solutions to health inequalities by focusing on the observable and measurable alone. As Scrambler (2001) suggests, 'beneath the surface' objects of sociological enquiry like relations of class may not be directly measurable. However, the existence of 'enduring and identifiable tendencies' or 'demi-regularities' such as the inverse care law (Lawson, 1997, cited by Scrambler, 2001) can direct social scientific research by providing evidence that potentially identifiable mechanisms are at play. Health inequalities research is an area replete with contrastive demi-regularities (Scrambler, 2001).

We do not recommend an outright rejection of the neo-positivist tradition. As we make clear during the course of this book, the technically excellent and, in some cases theoretically sophisticated work undertaken by social epidemiologists has much to be admired. The challenge, then, is to provide a better balance within health inequalities research, countering the current dominance of neo-positivism with research that helps us to better understand the generative mechanisms that lead to the uneven distribution of factors that impinge on health. This is important because different theoretical frameworks give rise to different policy implications and the current dominance of epidemiological research is one of a number of factors that have given rise to the tendency of policy to focus on the role of specific targeted interventions rather than the 'bigger issues'. The relative emphasis that has been placed on the down- and upstreams is explored in greater detail in Chapter Three.

References

Acheson, D. (Chair) (1998) *Independent Inquiry into Inequalities in Health*, London: The Stationery Office.

Adler, N. and Snibbe, A. (2003) 'The role of psychosocial processes in explaining the gradient between socio-economic status and health', *Current Directions in Psychological Science*, vol 12, pp 119-23.

Arber, S. and Ginn, J. (1993) 'Gender and inequalities in health in later life', *Social Science and Medicine*, vol 36, pp 33-46.

Barker, D.J.P. (1994) *Mothers, babies, and disease in later life*, London: British Medical Journal Publications.

Barker, D.J.P. and Martyn, C. (1992) 'The maternal and fetal origins of cardiovascular disease', *Journal of Epidemiology and Community Health*, vol 46, pp 8-11.

Barker, D.J.P. and Osmond, C. (1986) 'Infant mortality, childhood nutrition, and ischaemic heart disease in England and Wales', *Lancet*, vol 327, pp 1077-81.

Barker, D.J.P., Osmond, C. and Law, C. (1989) 'The intrauterine and early postnatal origins of cardiovascular disease and chronic bronchitis', *Journal of Epidemiology and Community Health*, vol 43, pp 237-40.

Barker, D., Bull, A., Osmond, C. and Simmonds, S. (1990) 'Fetal and placental size and risk of hypertension in adult life', *British Medical Journal*, vol 301, pp 259-62.

Berridge, V. (2003) 'The Black Report: interpreting history', in A. Oliver and M. Exworthy (eds) *Health inequalities: Evidence, policy and implementation, Proceedings from a Meeting of the Health Equity Network*, London: Nuffield Trust.

Berridge, V. and Blume, S. (2002) *Poor health: Social inequality before and after the Black Report*, London: Frank Cass.

Black Report (1980) *Inequalities of health*, Report of a Research Working Group, Chair, Sir Douglas Black, London: DHSS.

Blakely, T., Kennedy, B., Glass, R. and Kawachi, I. (2000) 'What is the time lag between income inequality and health status?', *Journal of Epidemiology and Community Health*, vol 54, pp 318-19.

Blane, D., Davey Smith, G. and Bartley, M. (1990) 'Social class differences in years of potential life lost: size, trends, and principal causes', *British Medical Journal*, vol 301, pp 429-32.

Blane, D., Davey Smith, G. and Bartley, M. (1993) 'Social selection: what does it contribute to social class differences in health?', *Sociology of Health and Illness*, vol 15, pp 1-15.

Blaxter, M. (1987) 'Evidence on inequality in health from a national survey', *Lancet*, vol 330, pp 30-3.

Bloor, M., Samphier, M. and Prior, L. (1987) 'Artefact explanations of inequalities in health: an assessment of the evidence', *Sociology of Health and Illness*, vol 9, pp 231-64.

Bobat, M. and Marmot, M. (1996) 'East–West mortality divide and its potential explanations: proposed research agenda', *British Medical Journal*, vol 312, pp 421-5.

Bourdieu, P. (1984) *Distinction: A social critique of the judgement of taste*, London: Routledge.

Brunner, E. (1996) 'The social and biological basis of cardiovascular disease in office workers', in D. Blane, E. Brunner and R. Wilkinson (eds) *Health and social organisation: Toward a health policy for the 21st century*, London: Routledge, pp 272-99.

Brunner, E. (2001) 'Stress mechanisms in coronary heart disease', in S. Stansfeld and M. Marmot (eds) *Stress and the heart: Psychosocial pathways to coronary heart disease*, London: BMJ Books, pp 181-99.

Brunner, E. and Marmot, M. (1999) 'Social organisation, stress and health', in M. Marmot and R.G. Wilkinson (eds) *Social determinants of health*, Oxford University Press, pp 17-43.

Bunker, S., Colquhoun, D., Esler, M., Hickie, I., Hunt, D., Jelinek,V., Oldenburg, B., Peach, H., Ruth, D., Tennant, C. and Tonkin, A. (2003) '"Stress" and coronary heart disease: psychosocial risk factors', *The Medical Journal of Australia*, vol 178, pp 272-6.

Carr-Hill, R. (1987) 'The inequalities in health debate: a critical review of the issues', *Journal of Social Policy*, vol 16, pp 509-42.

Carstairs, V. (1981) 'Small area analysis and health service research', *Community Medicine*, vol 3, pp 131-9.

Carstairs, V. and Morris, R. (1989) 'Deprivation and mortality: an alternative to social class?', *Community Medicine*, vol 11, pp 210-19.

Chandola, T., Bartley, M., Sacker, A., Jenkinson, C. and Marmot, M. (2003) 'Health selection in the Whitehall II study, UK', *Social Science and Medicine*, vol 56, pp 2059-72.

Coburn, D. (2000) 'Income inequality, social cohesion and the health status of populations: the role of neo-liberalism', *Social Science and Medicine*, vol 51, pp 139-50.

Coburn, D. (2004) 'Beyond the income inequality hypothesis: class, neo-liberalism and health inequalities', *Social Science and Medicine*, vol 58, pp 41-56.

Curtis, S. and Jones, I.R. (1998) 'Is there a place for geography in the analysis of health inequality?', *Sociology of Health and Illness*, vol 20, pp 645-72.

Darmon, N., Ferguson, E. and Briend, A. (2003) 'Do economic constraints encourage the selection of energy dense diets?', *Appetite*, vol 41, pp 315-22.

Davey Smith, G. (1998) letter following the independent inquiry into inequalities in health.

Davey Smith, G. (2003) 'Introduction: lifecourse approaches to health inequalities', in G. Davey Smith (ed) *Health inequalities: Lifecourse approaches*, Bristol: The Policy Press, pp xii-lix.

Davey Smith, G. and Kuh, D. (1996) 'Does early nutrition affect later health? Views from the 1930s and 1980s', in D. Smith (ed) *The history of nutrition in Britain in the twentieth century: Science, scientists and politics*, London: Routledge, pp 214-37 [reproduced in G. Davey Smith (ed) *Health inequalities: Lifecourse approaches*, Bristol: The Policy Press, pp 411-35].

Davey Smith, G., Morris, J. and Shaw, M. (1998b) 'The Independent Inquiry into Inequalities in Health', *British Medical Journal*, vol 317, pp 1465-6.

Davey Smith, G., Morris, J. and Shaw, M. (1998c) 'Independent Inquiry gives detailed recommendations. Authors' reply', *British Medical Journal*, vol 318, p 601.

Davey Smith, G., Shipley, M. and Rose, G. (1990) 'Magnitude and causes of socio-economic differentials in mortality: further evidence from the Whitehall Study', *Journal of Epidemiology and Community Health*, vol 44, pp 265-70.

Davey Smith, G., Hart, C., Blane, D. and Hole, D. (1998d) 'Adverse socio-economic conditions in childhood and cause-specific adult mortality: prospective observational study', *British Medical Journal*, vol 316, pp 1631-5.

Davey Smith, G., Hart, C., Hole, D., MacKinnon, P., Gillis, C., Watt, G., Blane, D. and Hawthorne, V. (1998a) 'Education and occupational social class: which is the more important indicator of mortality risk?', *Journal of Epidemiology and Community Health*, vol 52, pp 153-60.

DH (Department of Health) (1999) *Saving lives: Our healthier nation*, London: The Stationery Office.

DH (2000) *The NHS Plan: A plan for investment, a plan for reform*, Cm 4818-1, London: The Stationery Office.

DH (2004) *Choosing health: Making healthy choices easier*, Cm 6374, London: The Stationery Office.

DH (2005) *Tackling health inequalities: Status report on the Programme for Action*, London: DH.

Dowler, E. (2002) 'Food and poverty in Britain: rights and responsibilities', *Social Policy and Administration*, vol 36, no 6, pp 698-717.

Duncan, C. and Jones, K. (1995) 'Individuals and their ecologies: analysing the geography of chronic illness using a multi-level modeling framework', *Health and Place*, vol 1, pp 27-40.

Duncan, C., Jones, K. and Moon, G. (1998) 'Context, composition and heterogeneity: using multilevel models in health research', *Social Science and Medicine*, vol 46, pp 97-117.

Eames, M., Ben-Shlomo, Y. and Marmot, M. (1993) 'Social deprivation and premature mortality: regional comparison across England', *British Medical Journal*, vol 307, pp 1097-102.

Ellaway, A., Macintyre, S. and Kearns, A. (2001) 'Perceptions of place and health in socially contrasting neighbourhoods', *Urban Studies*, vol 38, pp 2299-316.

Eriksson, J.G., Forsén, T., Tuomilehto, J., Winter, P.D., Osmond, C. and Barker, D.J.P. (1999) 'Catch-up growth in childhood and death from coronary heart disease: longitudinal study', *British Medical Journal*, vol 318, pp 427-31.

Evans, R. (2002) *Interpreting and addressing inequalities in health: From Black to Acheson to Blair to ...?*, London: Office of Health Economics.

Exworthy, M. (2002) 'The "second Black Report"? The Acheson Report as another opportunity to tackle health inequalities', *Contemporary British History*, vol 16, pp 175-97.

Forsdahl, A. (1978) 'Living conditions in childhood and subsequent development of risk factors for arteriosclerotic heart disease: the cardiovascular survey in Finnmark 1974-75', *Journal of Epidemiology and Community Health*, vol 32, pp 34-7.

Forsen, T., Eriksson, J., Tuomilehto, J., Reunanen, A., Osmond, C. and Barker. D. (2000) 'The fetal and childhood growth of persons who develop Type 2 diabetes', *Annals of Internal Medicine*, vol 133, pp 176-82.

Forsyth, J.S., Willatts, P., Agostoni, C., Bissenden, J., Casaer, P. and Boehm, G. (2003) 'Long chain polyunsaturated fatty acid supplementation in infant formula and blood pressure in later childhood: follow up of a randomised control trial', *British Medical Journal*, vol 326, pp 953-8.

Fox, A., Goldblatt, P. and Jones, D. (1985) 'Social class mortality differentials: artefact, selection or life circumstances?', *Journal of Epidemiology and Community Health*, vol 39, pp 1-8.

Gatrell, A., Thomas, C., Bennett, S., Bostock, L., Popay, J., Williams, G. and Shahtahmasebi, S. (2000) 'Understanding health inequalities: locating people in geographical and social spaces', in H. Graham (ed) *Understanding health inequalities*, Buckingham: Open University Press, pp 156-69.

Gibson, A., Asthana, S., Brigham, P., Moon, G. and Dicker, J. (2002) 'Geographies of need and the new NHS: methodological issues in the definition and measurement of the health needs of local populations', *Health and Place*, vol 8, pp 47-60.

Gillman, M. (2002) 'Epidemiological challenges in studying the fetal origins of adult disease', *International Journal of Epidemiology*, vol 31, pp 294-9.

Ginn, J. and Arber, S. (1991) 'Gender, class and income inequalities in later life', *British Journal of Sociology*, vol 42, pp 369-96.

Goldblatt, P. (1988) 'Changes in social class between 1971 and 1981: could these affect mortality differential among men of working age?', *Population Trends*, vol 51, pp 9-17.

Goldblatt, P. (1989) 'Mortality by social class, 1971-85', *Population Trends*, vol 56, pp 6-15.

Goldblatt, P. (1990) 'Mortality and alternative social classification', in P. Goldblatt (ed) *Longitudinal study: Mortality and social organisation 1971-81*, OPCS Series L No 6, London: HMSO, pp 163-92.

Graham, H. (1993) *When life's a drag: Women, smoking and disadvantage*, London: HMSO.

Graham, H. (2002) 'Building an inter-disciplinary science of health inequalities: the example of lifecourse research', *Social Science and Medicine*, vol 55, pp 2005-16.

Graham, H. (2004) 'Social determinants and their unequal distribution: clarifying policy understandings', *The Milbank Quarterly*, vol 82, pp 101-24.

Graham, H. and Power, C. (2004) *Childhood disadvantage and adult health: A lifecourse framework*, London: Health Development Agency.

Gravelle, H. (1998) 'How much of the relation between population mortality and unequal distribution of income is a statistical artefact?', *British Medical Journal*, vol 316, pp 382-5.

Grundy, E. and Sloggett, A. (2003) 'Health inequalities in the older population: the role of personal capital, social resources and socio-economic circumstances', *Social Science and Medicine*, vol 56, pp 935-47.

Hallqvist, J., Lynch, J., Bartley, M., Land, T. and Blane, D. (2004) 'Can we disentangle life course processes of accumulation, critical period and social mobility?: an analysis of disadvantaged socio-economic positions and myocardial infarction in the Stockholm Heart Epidemiology Program', *Social Science and Medicine*, vol 58, pp 1555-62.

Halpern, D. (1995) *Mental health and the built environment*, London: Taylor and Francis.

Hart, C. and Davey Smith, G. (2003) 'Relationship between number of siblings and adult mortality and stroke risk: 25 year follow up of men in the Collaborative Study', *Journal of Epidemiology and Community Health*, vol 57, pp 385-91.

Hart, C., Davey Smith, G. and Blane, D. (1998) 'Social mobility and 21 year mortality in a cohort of Scottish men', *Social Science and Medicine*, vol 47, pp 1121-30.

Hertzman, C., Power, C., Matthews, S. and Manor, O. (2001) 'Using an interactive framework of society and lifecourse to explain self-related health in early adulthood', *Social Science and Medicine*, vol 53, no 12, pp 1575-85.

HM Treasury and DH (Department of Health) (2002) *Tackling health inequalities: Summary of the 2002 Cross Cutting Review*, London: HM Treasury and DH.

Illsley, I. (1986) 'Occupational class, selection and the production of inequalities in health', *Quarterly Journal of Social Affairs*, vol 2, pp 151-60.

Illsley, I. (1987) 'Occupational class, selection and the production of inequalities in health: rejoinder to Richard Wilkinson's reply', *Quarterly Journal of Social Affairs*, vol 3, pp 213-23.

Jenkin, P. (1980) 'Foreword', in Department of Health and Social Security (DHSS) *Inequalities in health: Report of a Research Working Group*, London: DHSS.

Judge, K., Mulligan, J. and Benzeval, M. (1998) 'Income inequality and population health', *Social Science and Medicine*, vol 46, pp 567-79.

Kawachi, I. and Kennedy, B. (1999) 'Income inequality and health: pathways and mechanisms', *Health Services Research*, vol 34, pp 215-27.

Kawachi, I., Colditz, G., Ascherio, A., Rimm, E.B., Giovanucci, E., Stampfer, M.J. and Willett, W.C. (1999) 'A prospective study of social networks in relation to total mortality and cardiovascular disease in men in the US', *Journal of Epidemiology and Community Health*, vol 50, pp 245-51.

Krantz, D. and McCeney, M. (2002) 'Effects of psychological and social factors on organic disease: a critical assessment of research on coronary heart disease', *Annual Review of Psychology*, vol 53, pp 341-69.

Krieger, N. (2001) 'Theories for social epidemiology in the 21st century: an ecosocial perspective', *International Journal of Epidemiology*, vol 39, pp 668-77.

Kuh, D., Ben-Shlomo, Y., Lynch, J., Hallqvist, J. and Power, C. (2003) 'Life course epidemiology', *Journal of Epidemiology and Community Health*, vol 57, pp 778-83.

Law, C., Barker, D., Bull, A. and Osmond, C. (1991) 'Maternal and fetal influences on blood pressure', *Archives of Disease in Childhood*, vol 66, pp 1291-5.

Lawson, T. (1997) *Economics and reality*, London: Routledge.

Lynch, J., Davey Smith, G., Kaplan, G. and House, A. (2000) 'Income inequality and mortality: importance to health of individual income, psychosocial environment, or material conditions', *British Medical Journal*, vol 320, pp 1200-4.

Lynch, J., Davey Smith, G., Hillemeier, M., Shaw, M., Raghunthan, T. and Kaplan, G. (2001) 'Income inequality, the psychosocial environment and health: comparisons of wealthy nations', *Lancet*, vol 358, pp 194-200.

Lynch, J., Davey Smith, G., Harper, S., Hillemeier, M., Ross, N., Kaplan, G. and Wolfson, M. (2004) 'Is income inequality a determinant of population health? Part I. A systematic review', *The Milbank Quarterly*, vol 82, pp 5-99.

McCain, M.N. and Mustard, J.F. (1999) *Early years study: Reversing the real brain drain*, Toronto, Canada: Ontario Children's Secretariat.

Macintyre, S. (1997) 'The Black Report and beyond: what are the issues?', *Social Science and Medicine*, vol 44, pp 723-45.

Macintyre, S. and West, P. (1991) 'Lack of class variation in health in adolescence: an artefact of an occupational measure of social class?', *Social Science and Medicine*, vol 32, pp 395-402.

Macintyre, S., Ellaway, A. and Cummins, S. (2002) 'Place effects on health: how can we conceptualise, operationalise and measure them?', *Social Science and Medicine*, vol 55, pp 125-39.

Macintyre, S., Maciver, S. and Soomans, A. (1993) 'Area, class and health: should we be focusing on places or people?', *Journal of Social Policy*, vol 22, pp 213-34.

McKee, M. (2005) 'Choosing health? First choose your philosophy', *Lancet*, vol 365, pp 369-71.

Mackenbach, J. (2002) 'Income inequality and population health', *British Medical Journal*, vol 324, pp 1-2.

Mackenbach, J. and Bakker, M. (2003) 'Tackling socio-economic inequalities in health: analysis of European experiences', *Lancet*, vol 362, pp 1409-14.

Macleod, J. and Davey Smith, G. (2003) 'Psychosocial factors and public health: a suitable case for treatment?', *Journal of Epidemiology and Community Health*, vol 57, pp 565-70.

Manor, O., Matthews, S. and Power, C. (2003) 'Health selection: the role of inter- and intra-generational mobility on social inequalities in health', *Social Science and Medicine*, vol 57, pp 2217-27.

Marmot, M. (1999) 'Acting on the evidence to reduce inequalities in health', *Health Affairs*, vol 18, pp 42-4.

Marmot, M. (2004) *Status syndrome*, London: Bloomsbury.

Marmot, M. and Shipley, M. (1996) 'Do socio-economic differences in mortality persist after retirement? 25 year follow up of civil servants from the first Whitehall study', *British Medical Journal*, vol 313, pp 1177-80.

Marmot, M. and Theorell, T. (1988) 'Social class and cardiovascular disease: the contribution of work', *International Journal of Health Services*, vol 18, pp 659-74.

Marmot, M. and Wilkinson, R. (2001) 'Psychosocial and material pathways in the relation between income and health: a response to Lynch et al', *British Medical Journal*, vol 322, pp 1233-6.

Marmot, M., Shipley, M. and Rose, G. (1984) 'Inequalities in death – specific explanations of a general pattern?', *Lancet*, vol 323, pp 1003-6.

Marmot, M., Davey Smith, G., Stansfield, S., Patel, C., North, G., Head, J., White, L., Brunner, E. and Feeney, A. (1991) 'Health inequalities among British civil servants: the Whitehall II Study', *Lancet*, vol 337, pp 1387-93.

Martyn, C., Barker, D. and Osmond, C. (1996) 'Mothers' pelvic size, fetal growth, and death from stroke and coronary heart disease in men in the UK', *Lancet*, vol 348, pp 1264-8.

Martyn, C., Barker, D., Jesperen, S., Greenwald, S., Osmond, C. and Berry, C. (1995) 'Growth in-utero, adult blood pressure and arterial compliance', *British Heart Journal*, vol 73, pp 116-21.

Maynard, M., Gunnell, D., Emmett, P., Frankel, S. and Davey Smith, G. (2003) 'Fruit, vegetables, and antioxidants in childhood and risk of adult cancer: the Boyd Orr cohort', *Journal of Epidemiology and Community Health*, vol 57, no 3, pp 218-25.

Mellor, J. and Milyo, J. (2001) 'Income inequality and health', *Journal of Policy Analysis and Management*, vol 20, pp 151-5.

Mellor, J. and Milyo, J. (2003) 'Is exposure to income inequality a public health concern? Lagged effects of income inequality on individual and population health', *Health Services Research*, vol 38, pp 137-51.

Moser, K., Fox, A. and Jones, D. (1984) 'Unemployment and mortality in the OPCS Longitudinal Study', *Lancet*, vol 323, pp 1324-9.

Moser, K., Pugh, H. and Goldblatt, P. (1988) 'Inequalities in women's health: looking at mortality differentials using an alternative approach', *British Medical Journal*, vol 296, pp 1221-4.

Phillimore, P., Beattie, A. and Townsend, P. (1994) 'Widening inequality of health in northern England, 1981-91', *British Medical Journal*, vol 308, pp 1125-8.

Pickett, K.E. and Pearl, M. (2001) 'Multilevel analyses of neighbourhood socioeconomic context and health outcomes: a critical review', *Journal of Epidemiology and Community Health*, vol 55, pp 111-22.

Power, C., Manor, O. and Fox, A. (1991) *Health and class: The early years*, London: Chapman Hall.

Quick, A. and Wilkinson, R. (1991) *Income and health*, London: Socialist Health Association.

Ravelli, A., van der Meulen, J., Michels, R., Osmond, C., Barker, D., Hales, C. and Bleker, O. (1998) 'Glucose tolerance in adults after prenatal exposure to famine', *Lancet*, vol 351, pp 173-7.

Robinson, R. (1992) 'Is the child father of the man?', *British Medical Journal*, vol 304, pp 789-90.

Rutter, M. (1995) 'Causal concepts and their testing', in M. Rutter and D.J. Smith (eds) *Psychosocial disorders in young people: Time trends and their causes*, Chichester: John Wiley, pp 7-34.

Rutter, M. (1999) 'Resilience concepts and findings: implications for family therapy', *Journal of Family Therapy*, vol 21, pp 119-44.

Sapolsky, R. and Mott, G. (1987) 'Social subordinance in wild baboons is associated with suppressed high density lipoprotein–cholesterol concentrations: the possible role of chronic social stress', *Endocrinology*, vol 121, pp 1605-10.

Saul, C. and Payne, N. (1999) 'How does the prevalence of specific morbidities compare with measures of socio-economic status at small area level?', *Journal of Public Health Medicine*, vol 21, pp 340-7.

Saxena, S., Eliahoo, J. and Majeed, A. (2002) 'Socioeconomic and ethnic group differences in self reported health status and use of health services by children and young people in England: cross sectional study', *British Medical Journal*, vol 325, pp 520-6.

Sayer, A., Cooper, C., Evans, J., Rauf, A., Wormald, R., Osmond, C. and Barker, D. (1998) 'Are rates of ageing determined in utero?', *Age and Ageing*, vol 27, pp 579-83.

Scrambler, G. (2001) 'Critical realism, sociology and health inequalities: social class as a generative mechanism and its media of enactment', *Journal of Critical Realism*, vol 4, pp 35-42.

Selwyn, J. (2000) 'Fetal development', in M. Boushel, M. Fawcett and J. Selwyn (eds) *Focus on early childhood: Principles and realities*. Oxford: Blackwell Science, pp 21-34.

Shaw, M., Davey Smith, G. and Dorling, D. (2005) 'Health inequalities and New Labour: how the promises compare with real progress', *British Medical Journal*, vol 330, pp 1016-21.

Shaw, M., Dorling, D. and Brimblecombe, N. (1998) 'Changing the map – health in Britain 1951-91', *Sociology of Health and Illness*, vol 20, pp 694-709.

Shaw, M., Dorling, D., Gordon, D. and Davey Smith, G. (1999) *The widening gap: Health inequalities and policy in Britain*, Bristol: The Policy Press.

Shouls, S., Congdon, P. and Curtis, S. (1996) 'Modelling inequality in reported long term illness in the UK: combining individual and area characteristics', *Journal of Epidemiology and Community Health*, vol 50, pp 366-76.

Singh-Manoux, A. and Marmot, M. (2005) 'Role of socialization in explaining social inequalities in health', *Social Science and Medicine*, vol 60, pp 2129-33.

Sloggett, A. and Joshi, H. (1998) 'Deprivation indicators as predictors of life events 1981-1992 based on the UK ONS Longitudinal Study', *Journal of Epidemiology and Community Health*, vol 52, pp 228-33.

Sooman, A. and Macintyre, S. (1995) 'Health and perceptions of the local environment in socially contrasting neighbourhoods in Glasgow', *Health and Place*, vol 1, pp 15-26.

Stafford, M. and Marmot, M. (2003) 'Neighbourhood deprivation and health: does it affect us all equally?', *International Journal of Epidemiology*, vol 32, pp 357-66.

Stansfeld, S. (1999) 'Social support and social cohesion', in M. Marmot and R.G. Wilkinson (eds) *Social determinants of health*, Oxford University Press, pp 155-78.

Stein, Z., Susser, M., Saenger, G. and Marolla, F. (1975) *Famine and human development: The Dutch hunger winter of 1944-45*, New York, NY: Oxford University Press.

Strike, P. and Steptoe, A. (2004) 'Psychosocial factors in the development of coronary artery disease', *Progress in Cardiovascular Disease*, vol 46, pp 337-47.

Subramanian, S., Blakely, T. and Kawachi, I. (2003) 'Income inequality as a public health concern: when do we stand? Commentary on "is exposure to income inequality a public health concern?"', *Health Services Research*, vol 38, pp 153-67.

Thompson, C., Syddal, H., Rodin, I., Osmond, C. and Barker, D. (2001) 'Birthweight and the risk of depressive disorder in late life', *British Journal of Psychiatry*, vol 179, pp 450-5.

Townsend, P. (1993) *The international analysis of poverty*, Hemel Hempstead: Harvester Wheatsheaf.

Townsend, P. (1999) 'A structural plan needed to reduce inequalities in health', in D. Gordon, M. Shaw, D. Dorling and G. Davey Smith (eds) *Inequalities in health: The evidence presented to the Independent Inquiry into Inequalities in Health, chaired by Sir Donald Acheson*, Bristol: The Policy Press, pp xiv-xxi.

Townsend, P. and Davidson, N. (1982) *Inequalities in health: The Black Report*, Harmondsworth: Penguin Books.

Townsend, P., Phillimore, P. and Beattie, A. (1988) *Health and deprivation: Inequality and the North*, London: Croom Helm.

Wadsworth, M. (1986) 'Serious illness in childhood and its association with later-life achievement', in R. Wilkinson (ed) *Class and health*, London: Tavistock Publications, pp 50-74.

Wadsworth, M. (1997) 'Health inequalities in the life course perspective', *Social Science and Medicine*, vol 44, pp 859-69.

Wahlbeck, K., Forsén, T., Osmond, C., Barker, D. and Eriksson, J. (2001) 'Association of schizophrenia with low maternal body mass index, small size at birth and thinness during childhood', *The Archives of General Psychiatry*, vol 58, pp 48-52.

Wainwright, N. and Surtees, P. (2003) 'Places, people and their physical and mental functional health', *Journal of Epidemiology and Community Health*, vol 58, pp 333-9.

Wannamethee, S. and Shaper, A. (1991) 'Self-assessment of health status and mortality in middle-aged British men', *International Journal of Epidemiology*, vol 20, pp 239-45.

Wannamethee, S. and Shaper, A. (1997) 'Socioeconomic status within social class and mortality: a prospective study in middle-aged British men', *International Journal of Epidemiology*, vol 26, pp 532-41.

Weich, S., Twigg, L., Holt, G., Lewis, G. and Jones, K. (2003) 'Contextual risk factors for the common mental disorders in Britain: a multilevel investigation of the effects of place', *Journal of Epidemiology and Community Health*, vol 57, pp 616-21.

West, P. (1988) 'Inequalities? Social class differentials in health in British youth', *Social Science and Medicine*, vol 27, pp 391-6.

West, P. (1991) 'Rethinking the health selection explanation for health inequalities', *Social Science and Medicine*, vol 32, pp 373-84.

Whitehead, M. and Diderichsen, F. (2001) 'Social capital and health: tip-toeing through the minefield of evidence', *Lancet*, vol 358, pp 165-6.

Wilkinson, R. (1986) 'Occupational class, selection and inequalities in health: a reply to Raymond Illsley', *Quarterly Journal of Social Affairs*, vol 2, pp 415-22.

Wilkinson, R. (1987) 'A rejoinder', *Quarterly Journal of Social Affairs*, vol 3, pp 225-8.

Wilkinson, R. (1992) 'Income distribution and life expectancy', *British Medical Journal*, vol 304, pp 165-8.

Wilkinson, R. (1996) *Unhealthy societies: The afflictions of inequality*, London: Routledge.

Wilkinson, R. (1999) 'Putting the picture together: prosperity, redistribution, health and welfare', in M. Marmot and R.G. Wilkinson (eds) *Social determinants of health*, Oxford University Press, pp 256-74.

THREE

The national policy context

Introduction

Chapter Two described the important academic legacy of the Black Report (1980), and also noted that, although the Report was coolly received by the Conservative government of the time, its recommendations have shaped the subsequent formulation of policy. Ironically, while the Black Report was criticised for the costs that it gave to its proposals, its successor, the Acheson Report, was criticised for not providing detailed costs. This, it was argued, would not provide government with sufficient information about the affordability and cost-effectiveness of proposals to encourage a policy response. In fact, the Labour government can claim to have responded to most of the recommendations made in the Acheson Report (1998). However, policy responses to the broad areas identified by the Independent Inquiry can be either conventional or radical and many would argue that the government's response to the materialist/structural factors identified in the Report has not been radical enough.

As one of the government's responses to the Acheson Report included the commissioning of a Cross-cutting Review to explore how links could be strengthened between government departments to address 'underlying determinants of health inequalities', it seems ungenerous to question its commitment to undertaking the necessary structural reforms. In practice, however, the way in which 'underlying determinants' have been defined has become increasingly narrow over time. For example, the government has set the Department of Health (DH) Public Service Agreement (PSA) targets to reduce variations in mortality and life expectancy between the fifth of areas with the worst health and deprivation indicators (the Spearhead Group) and the population as a whole. This has certainly given an increased profile to tackling inequalities in health. However, the objective of tackling the "underlying determinants of ill health and health inequalities" by reducing adult smoking rates, reducing the year-on-year rise in child obesity and reducing the under-18 conception rate suggests a somewhat narrow interpretation of the causes of variations in health (www.hm-treasury.gov.uk/media/4B9/FE/sr04_psa_ch3.pdf).

Government commitment to addressing what might normally be described as underlying determinants of health inequalities is apparent in other PSAs. In education, for example, more challenging 'floor targets' have been set to drive further improvements in schools in deprived areas, while local authority wards with the worst labour market performance are expected to increase the employment rate on average by 1%. Taken together, these PSAs suggest that, through concerted local action, the wider determinants of health inequalities may be effectively tackled. In practice, however, the very setting of targets works against joined-up working and encourages a tendency for policy to be implemented in 'silos'. For example, 'best practice guidance' designed to support primary care trusts (PCTs) in achieving the PSA targets for health inequalities acknowledges that primary disease prevention and work to reduce the uneven distribution of health determinants will make the largest long-term contribution. However, it also suggests that a service-orientated agenda that focuses on tackling cancer, cardiovascular disease and smoking in disadvantaged groups and areas will be necessary for reaching targets set for 2010. Thus, interventions are highlighted that have a 'high and fast impact on health inequalities', that would help PCTs to achieve a 'strong performance' on relevant local delivery plan lines and that ensure 'delivery', particularly among the 88 PCTs that make up the Spearhead Group. These include the improved management of high blood pressure and cholesterol levels in patients with, or at high risk of, cardiovascular disease; the provision of effective emergency care and treatment for heart attack; improved management of atrial fibrillation; the reduction of smoking; and the prevention and management of other risk factors such as poor diet, physical inactivity and obesity (HIU, 2005).

In addition to responding to the target-setting agenda, local bodies that are charged with addressing health inequalities will look for available evidence of 'what works'. The fact that they are more likely to encounter clear information about the role and potential impact of 'downstream' interventions than 'upstream' policies reinforces the narrow focus of local policy making. As will become clear during the course of this book, most of the 'evidence' available to those concerned with public health and health inequalities refers to individualised behavioural or clinical interventions. By contrast, the evidence base for more holistic interventions, such as housing, crime and employment, is very weak. As well as shifting the focus away from the social to the individual, this kind of evidence places more emphasis on the role of local policies implemented by local agencies than the 'bigger issues' that can only be dealt with at a central level. This has also reinforced the narrow way in which 'upstream' initiatives targeting the 'underlying determinants' of health inequalities have been conceptualised.

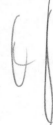

Graham (2004), in a useful discussion about the need to clarify this concept, points out the distinction between the determinants of ill health and the determinants of health inequalities. The tendency to use a single model to describe both phenomena (as in the Acheson Report) can "blur the distinction between the social factors that influence health and the social processes that determine their unequal distribution" (Graham, 2004, p 109). Thus, strategies that seek to improve key social determinants such as education, income and housing quality may result in positive trends in health but make little difference to the distribution of health between more and less advantaged groups. Graham, echoing Scrambler (2001) reminds us that social position is the fundamental cause of health inequality and that the mechanisms that play a role in stratifying health outcomes are the same mechanisms that generate and distribute power and wealth. This means that the focus of interest in the development and evaluation of 'upstream' initiatives to tackle health variations should be the *structural* inequalities in education, the labour market, property and wealth that determine social position.

Against this background, it is important to assess the extent to which the government's mainstream policies have diminished inequalities in social position. We address this in the second part of this chapter, which explores the government's response to the recommendations of the Acheson Report. In the third part we examine what might be referred to as 'mid-stream' policies in the form of area-based initiatives (ABIs). We begin, however, by discussing how commitments to 'evidence-based policy' have shaped the policy response and particularly the relative emphasis placed on 'downstream' interventions.

The role of 'evidence' in shaping the policy response

As a book concerned with 'what works' in addressing health inequalities, the current study responds explicitly to the central importance placed by New Labour on the need for policy to be 'evidence-based'. According to the White Paper *Modernising government*, "Government should regard policy as a continuous, learning process, not as a series of one-off initiatives". It should, therefore, improve its "use of evidence and research so that we understand better the problems we are trying to address" (Cabinet Office, 1999a, p 17). Similarly, *Professional policy making for the twenty-first century* (Cabinet Office, 1999b) established a nine-fold taxonomy of the features of modern policy making, which included the use of the best available evidence from a wide range of sources, systematic evaluation of the effectiveness of policy, ongoing review so that redundant or failing policies are scrapped and the ability to learn lessons (Bullock et al, 2001).

It is, of course, difficult to reject the idea that policy making should be 'evidence-based' rather than founded on unsupported opinion. Nor does evidence have to be based on a narrow scientific model that inevitably focuses on individualised interventions. The growth of interest in evidence-based policy across different academic disciplines and different government sectors suggests scope for a breadth in methodological approach. This has been actively encouraged by government. The *Adding it up* report of the Performance and Innovation Unit (PIU, 2000) made clear reference to the need for policy makers and analysts across departments to work together and to make the best use of a range of external expertise. The government has established cross-cutting units such as the Children and Young People's Unit (Chapter Five), the Teenage Pregnancy Unit (Chapter Nine) and the Neighbourhood Renewal Unit (Chapter Eleven) and commissioned cross-cutting reviews. This effort has encouraged thinking across traditional boundaries, opened up policy thinking to outsiders through the appointment of specialist advisors, contributed to high-quality summaries of available evidence and formed the basis for a series of important policy initiatives. For example, the cross-cutting review on childcare led to the development of the government's Sure Start initiative (see Chapter Five), while the series of Policy Action Team findings comprised the evidence base for neighbourhood renewal (see Chapter Eleven).

Despite good indications that government itself has been receptive to a range of different epistemological and methodological approaches, methodological pluralism has not featured strongly in the collection of evidence pertaining to public health and health inequalities. Instead this tended to reflect the approach taken in evidence-based medicine. Here experimental/quasi-experimental techniques such as randomised controlled trials (RCTs) and observational studies that fulfil robust statistical criteria (for example, in the analysis of associations between risk factors, treatments and outcomes and the testing of confounding and selection bias) have been valued above other knowledge. In order to generate evidence for policy, the results of studies that fulfil such criteria are typically synthesised into systematic reviews. These are carried out to agreed standards including the focus on a specific question, the identification of as much relevant research as possible, the admission of studies to the process of appraisal and synthesis only if they accord to quality standards, and the use of protocols to guide the process and facilitate replication (Boaz et al, 2002). The two best-known techniques used in systematic reviews are meta-analysis and narrative synthesis. Meta-analysis, generally viewed as the superior technique (Davey Smith and Egger, 1998), is a statistical procedure that combines or integrates the results of studies that meet the inclusion criteria to provide an arithmetic summary of the effect of a particular risk factor, treatment or intervention. Narrative synthesis looks at the similarities and differences between studies and their outcomes without calculating an average effect size and makes recommendations not by quantification but by the use of exemplars.

Evidence-based medicine came to prominence in the UK in the early 1990s in parallel with the purchaser/provider split in the National Health Service (NHS). The aim was to improve policy outcomes and accountability and to provide the basis of priority setting for health expenditure, by providing an alternative basis to clinical expertise for health decision making (Elliott and Popay, 2000). Since this period, a significant institutional base has been established, including the National Institute for Clinical Excellence (NICE), the NHS Centre for Reviews and Dissemination, the Health Development Agency (HDA) and the Cochrane Collaboration. All of these centres prepare and disseminate evidence about the impact of medical treatments and health interventions, largely through the use of systematic reviews. The HDA focused in particular on "maintaining an up to date map of the evidence base for public health and health improvement ... and effective and authoritative dissemination of advice to practitioners" (Kelly et al,

2004, p 2). In 2005, it merged with NICE to form the National Institute for Health and Clinical Excellence.

Support for the systematic review as the gold standard for evidence-based policy making is no longer restricted to medicine and public health. The Campbell Collaboration extends the Cochrane Collaboration into the social policy fields of education, criminal justice and social work while the Economic and Social Research Council (ESRC) UK Centre for Evidence-based Policy and Practice (CEBPP) has been funded by the ESRC to promote the concept of evidence-based policy and practice in the social sciences. The Evidence for Policy and Practice Information and Coordination Centre (EPPI-Centre) provides a resource for those wishing to undertake systematic reviews in the field of education and also undertakes systematic reviews on health promotion topics, and the Social Care Institute for Excellence (SCIE) has been set up to promote the quality and consistency of social care practice including the views, experiences and expertise of users and carers.

As it is generally agreed that these and other social policy areas have a key role to play in the promotion of public health, the systematic review has assumed an increasingly central role in establishing 'what works' in addressing health inequalities. This is apparent throughout the policy chapters in the second part of this book. The growing dominance of the hierarchical approach to evidence is not, however, without its problems. Two key areas of contention have arisen. The first relates specifically to the ability to transfer the methods developed for the field of evidence-based medicine to the more complex task of synthesising evidence for wider public policy (Petticrew et al, 2004). The second relates to the wider relation between the evidence base, however defined, and the process of practical policy making, which continues, it has been suggested, for the most part to be "about 'muddling through' rather than a process on which the social or policy sciences have had an influential part to play" (Parsons, 2002, p 43).

Drawbacks to the systematic review

Drawbacks to the extension of the process of systematic review to policies addressing health inequalities can be divided into two broad classes, those that address the hierarchy and logic of the review process (which we consider here), and those that address the quality of its implementation (which we discuss in further detail in Chapter Fourteen).

A key objection to the systematic review is that it underplays the role of theory and the development of theory, placing the stress on which interventions produce statistically significant outcomes rather than the way such interventions achieve this effect, the circumstances in which they are effective or the population groups for whom they work. Two important reservations follow. The first is that "without the theory of what is important we are stuck with trying to duplicate the whole thing" (Pawson and Tilley, 1997, p 191; Haynes, 2003). The second is that with so many potential variables relating to every intervention the outcomes are often not statistically significant and the policy maker is left with an array of inconsistent results rather than an increased understanding of the options available. For example, RCTs which were widely used in the US throughout the 1960s and 1970s in areas as diverse as income maintenance, supported work environments, housing allowance and support for prisoners, have become far less extensive as policy makers reacted to evidence of near zero and sometimes damaging effects (Oakley, 1998; Petticrew, 2001).

Most of the systematic reviews considered in this book have taken the form of narrative review rather than meta-analysis, largely because the very diversity of interventions considered and the multiplicity of outcomes militate against any attempt at numerical abstraction. In Chapter Seven, for example, we consider Towner et al's (2001) narrative review of accidental injuries to children and adolescents. This includes individual and behavioural approaches (ranging from the issue and adoption of safety equipment, such as cycle helmets, to road safety education), environmental modifications such as traffic calming, and legislation, with each category including a range of different approaches. Further variations relate to the age of the children concerned, the nature of the environment (ranging from roads to leisure and sport) and whether the intervention addresses one issue only or is multimodal. In such circumstances it has been suggested that it would be more logical to test the same policy idea in different settings rather than compare variants working through very different programme mechanisms (an idea we return to in Chapter Fourteen). As interventions move from the medical to the social domain, complexity increases and such problems become increasingly pronounced.

Where meta-analysis is conducted the basic problem concerns the nature and number of the simplifications that are necessary to achieve summary statistics. In effect each individual intervention is "boiled down to a single measure of effectiveness, which is then drawn together in an aggregate measure for that sub-class of programmes, which is then compared with the mean effect for other intervention categories" (Pawson, 2001, p 8). In the process the vital explanatory content is lost and the results "are insensitive to differences in programme theories, subjects and circumstances" (Pawson, 2001, p 4) with like rarely compared with like. Narrative review, in contrast, allows for a greater understanding of how programmes work, with interventions typically described by type, objectives, target group, setting and method of implementation. However, it has been criticised as lacking a "formal method of abstracting beyond these specifics of time and place, and so is weak in its ability to deliver transferable lessons" (Pawson, 2001, p 4). Exemplary programmes may be highlighted or an attempt made to define successful components yet, without a causal analysis and reference to the underlying theory, significant components may again be omitted.

A second fundamental objection is that the selection of studies for inclusion in systematic reviews is done on the basis of the quality of the research (defined according to pre-ordained criteria), not on the quality of the intervention (Speller et al, 1997). A hierarchy of evidence that gives prominence to the systematic review because of its assumed methodological strengths (chiefly its reliance on RCTs) may well, therefore, "attenuate public health decisions", favouring "interventions with a medical rather than a social focus, those that target individuals rather than communities or populations, and those that focus on the influence of proximal rather than distal determinants of health" (Rychetnik et al, 2002, p 125).

Certain types of interventions (those sponsored by the pharmaceutical industry, for example) are also more likely to be supported by high-quality evidence, simply because more resources are available to conduct the evaluation and produce that evidence rather than because the interventions are better. Yet, while rigour remains closely identified with RCTs, research using other designs is marginalised (Elliott and Popay, 2000). In consequence, little evidence is available about the effectiveness/cost-effectiveness of public health and preventative policies (Wanless, 2002). This does not necessarily mean that interventions aimed at whole communities are not effective but "rather reflects the paucity of good quality studies of these more 'upstream' interventions" (Macintyre et al, 2001, p 224).

The tendency to conflate high-quality evidence with randomisation also means that insufficient evidence exists on interventions for disadvantaged groups (Rychetnik et al, 2002, p 125). Due to a lack of understanding about the ways in which different segments of the population respond to similar interventions, systematic reviews often have very little to say about inequalities or inequities (Petticrew et al, 2004). An overview of the extent to which academic and research output related to the key public health areas outlined in the White Paper *Saving lives* (DH, 1999a), and *The NHS Plan* (DH, 2000) found work focusing on inequalities to be limited, with no more than 0.4% of the academic and research output examined relating to public health intervention research. Such restrictions were particularly true of the larger review organisations such as Cochrane. This, it was suggested, was accounted for by a combination of the complexity of the issues involved, methodology (with the public health community reluctant to settle for methodological pluralism), timescale/structure (with long-term evidence and hence long-term health gains often neglected) and theory (Millward et al, 2003, p 31).

In summary, there is a dissonance between systematic reviews, which focus largely on individualised behavioural or clinical interventions, and health inequalities, which are not primarily generated by medical causes and require solutions at a different level such as the redistributive effects of national fiscal policies, or economic investment to counter unemployment (Davey Smith et al, 2001, p 185). It has been argued that research designs with fewer requirements of scientific orthodoxy are more likely to accommodate the bigger issues and more likely to lend themselves to policy applications envisaging major socio-political change (McKinlay, 1993). Our own approach to this, a framework for the analysis of *public health regimes*, is presented in the final chapter of this book.

The evidence base and the policy-making process

In addition to concerns about the appropriateness of transferring methods developed for evidence-based medicine to the task of synthesising evidence for wider public policy, evidence-based policy making has been criticised for its positivist stance (which is rooted in a managerialistic and mechanistic way of thinking about policy making that recognises only positive facts and observable phenomena) and its assumption that the relationship between research and policy making is linear. The value of research is then judged only in terms of its impact on policy (Black, 2001) while the normative basis of policy making (that admits power, politics, people and a variety of goals), and requires an understanding of the mechanisms and structures within which policy makers work, is eroded (Sanderson, 2002).

Typically, such research is characterised as ideologically or value-free, based on what works rather than what you believe. "It is about efficiency, effectiveness and economy in delivery, rather than ethics" (Parsons, 2002, p 54). Questions have thus been raised about how to handle the value judgements that inevitably inform the research and policy-making processes, how to manage the process of transferring research into practice and about how to integrate evidence from research, clinicians and healthcare users into decision making (Elliott and Popay, 2000). Perhaps not surprisingly the influence of evidence-based research on health services policy or governance policies has, therefore, been questioned. Studies of social research projects that were initiated by NHS health authority managers or general practitioner (GP) fundholders in one NHS English region found the direct influence of research evidence on decision making was tempered by factors "such as financial constraints, shifting timescales and decision makers' own experiential knowledge" (Elliott and Popay, 2000, p 461). Black (2001), in similar vein, adds the nature of the services available locally, whether the social environment is conducive (staff morale, for example) and the quality of the knowledge purveyors (carrying research evidence into the policy-making forum) to the list. Research was more likely to impact on policy in indirect ways, including shaping the policy debate and mediating the dialogue between service providers and users.

Use also depends on the arena. Some authors suggest that research evidence is "more influential in central policy than local policy, where policymaking is marked by negotiation and uncertainty" (Black, 2001, p 277). Others suggest there is a clearer link at the local level between research, policy and practice (Davis and Howden-Chapman, 1996) and others that it is the type of evidence required that differs at the local and national levels (Petticrew et al, 2004). It also depends on the degree of consensus on the policy goal. The evidence base tends to be used if it supports the consensus but used only selectively if there is a lack of consensus. Some authors have even questioned whether research evidence can and should influence health policy, or whether it should be considered less as a problem-solving tool and more as a process of argument or debate to create concern and set the agenda. One of the most useful roles for research may be to "make people review their beliefs and legitimise unorthodox views" (Black, 2001, p 277). Such arguments rest on a model in which knowledge is considered to be inherently contestable and in which other legitimate influences on policy (social, electoral, ethical, cultural and economic) are accorded prominence. It is also a model that questions whether there is any useful or reliable 'firm ground' in what Schön termed the 'policy swamp', with the problems of the high ground "often relatively unimportant to clients or to the large society" while the problems of greatest human concern lie in the swamp (Schön, 1983, pp 42-3, cited in Parsons, 2002).

For some, such dilemmas signal the need to improve evidence-based policy making, disseminate findings, and ensure the integration of evidence into policy and practice. For others it merely highlights deficiencies in the model. In other words, there are profound epistemological differences between those who believe in evidence-based policy making and those who have doubts as to either its feasibility or the values it embodies. These tensions should be borne in mind when considering the range of public health 'evidence' that is presented during the course of this book.

At this juncture it is necessary to outline briefly our approach to collecting evidence. Given the scope of the book it was not possible to assemble the information on policy and practice in anything that could be described as a 'systematic' way, with a common methodology, defined search criteria for each topic, or a protocol to assess the quality of the research or the intervention. Indeed, there was a concern to admit the 'grey' literature: reports, conference proceedings, local evaluations, case studies, best practice guidance and so on that tends not to be published and is unlikely to be included in review-level publications. Such documentation is, however, increasingly accessible via the web and describes and assesses initiatives on the ground, often placing considerable emphasis on process and providing a counterbalance to the more academic and clinical emphasis of many RCTs. In between lie the hundreds of published academic articles, together with, for example, reports and research papers emanating from government, charities, professional organisations and national evaluations, which we accessed. Many were the product of structured searches of electronic databases, others were more serendipitous and we always knew we were just touching a diverse and eclectic literature in what could ultimately only ever be an idiosyncratic synthesis. Another drawback is obviously that if systematic reviews find their evidence base often to be flawed then this more wide-ranging approach to a more extensive and diverse literature is even more suspect. The advantage is the scope to juxtapose review-level evidence with pragmatic, local commentary.

It is also worth emphasising that each policy-related chapter contains a table summarising the evidence base and these focus on review-level evidence only. This in itself was not an easy process. Neat classifications relating to either target group or focus of intervention are difficult to sustain, systematic reviews overlap and generalisations are limited by the scope and complexity of the area under study. The emphasis thus often remains on what could or might work rather than what does work. Salient areas where review-level evidence is lacking are also highlighted in the tables (see also Chapter Fourteen). The one exception is the inequalities dimension, because this is so pervasive. For every table there is a lack of evaluation focusing on what works for particular socio-economic, minority ethnic or vulnerable groups and those subject to multiple risks. The same applies to cost-effectiveness.

The Acheson Report and the national policy response

The fact that much of the evidence pertaining to public health is located far down the causal chain, focusing on 'downstream' proposals to address health behaviours and clinical issues rather than the broader social determinants of health may go some way towards explaining why, although the government has ostensibly addressed many of the recommendations made by the Acheson Report, commentators believe that its policies are not sufficient to fundamentally tackle health inequalities (Shaw et al, 1999, 2005). Before exploring this in more detail, it is worth briefly outlining the evolution of health inequalities policies under New Labour.

An overview of Labour's policies on health inequalities

As noted in Chapter Two, the policy recommendations of the Black Report were largely ignored by the Conservative administration of 1979-97. However, the Report is generally acknowledged to have been instrumental in keeping health inequalities at the forefront of the public health agenda. While in opposition the Labour Party stated its commitment to addressing health inequalities once it returned to power and, on gaining office, it made a number of important decisions to this end. In less than a year, the first Minister of Public Health had been appointed, the flagship policy of Health Action Zones (HAZs) announced and a major Independent Inquiry into Health Inequalities commissioned. The results of this inquiry, published as the Acheson Report (1998), shaped the subsequent evolution of policies, most particularly the establishment of the Cross-cutting Review. This aimed to explore how health inequalities could be mainstreamed into the work done by other local and national government departments as well as the health service. The Review informed the development of the government's Programme for Action, which, like the Acheson Report, specifically highlighted the importance of supporting families with children and the role of the NHS in preventing illness and providing effective healthcare. However, the other broad areas for future policy development that were identified in the Acheson Report were subsumed into the Programme's remaining two themes: the need to engage communities and individuals, and to address the 'underlying determinants of health', dealing with the "long-term underlying causes of health inequalities" (DH, 2003, pp 4-5).

Table 3.1 demonstrates a substantial investment of policy attention to the problem of health inequalities. However, this effort has not been immune to criticism. As early as 1999, Shaw et al suggested that "subtly, slowly and almost imperceptibly, the priority of reducing inequalities in health [had] dropped down the agenda" (Shaw et al, 1999, p 171). Basing the flagship policy in health inequalities on area-based HAZs ignored widespread evidence of the ineffectiveness of area-based approaches in tackling inequalities in poverty, deprivation and health. Moreover, funding dedicated to HAZs was very modest. The emphasis placed on tackling health inequalities through partnership was criticised for spreading the responsibility too thinly. Finally, there were signs that key policies of redistribution that would reduce the underlying inequalities in income, wealth and poverty that caused health inequalities were giving way to other priorities, such as wealth creation and service modernisation. This appeared to be accompanied by a shift in the underpinning philosophy for addressing health inequalities, with growing interest in the role of individual responsibility (Shaw et al, 1999, pp 171-82).

Many of these criticisms remain salient today. As we discuss later, the 'flagship policy' of HAZs has not only slipped imperceptibly down the agenda, it has disappeared into relative obscurity. The problems associated with tackling health inequalities through partnerships also remain relevant. As already noted, target setting tends to encourage 'silo' management. Consequently, the NHS (which has the responsibility for meeting PSA targets on health inequalities) is advocating a service-orientated agenda to tackle the major causes (heart disease and cancer) of premature death among the poor, while other sectors are presumed to take a lead on addressing the underlying determinants of health. A number of policies are listed on the DH website as areas that address these underlying determinants (see Box 3.1) and *A programme for action* highlights the role played by, among other measures, new Child and Working Tax Credits; improvements in the quality of public and social sector homes; the fall in the number of fuel-poor households; some improvements in public transport; the national adult literacy and numeracy strategy; and programmes such as the New Deal and the introduction of a National Minimum Wage (DH, 2003, pp 20-3). However, there is no joined-up mechanism for assessing the extent to which action in sectors other than the NHS is contributing to the reduction of health inequalities. Moreover, many of these initiatives have been associated with improvements overall but not with a significant change in socio-economic inequality (see later in this chapter).

Finally, a shift away from the politics of centralised redistribution towards an emphasis on the role of individual responsibility has become the hallmark of the government's rhetoric on welfare. According to the Commission on Social Justice, which set out many of the proposals which have come to be identified as the 'Third Way' approach,

Table 3.1: Key reports and policies on health inequalities (1997-2005)

May 1997	Tessa Jowell appointed as first Minister of Public Health
June 1997	Frank Dobson announces Health Action Zone (HAZ) policy
July 1997	Independent Inquiry into Inequalities in Health established, chaired by Sir Donald Acheson
September 1997	Publication of *Health inequalities: Decennial supplement* (Drever and Whitehead, 1997)
April 1998	First 11 HAZs established
August 1998	Second wave of (15) HAZs announced
November 1998	Report of the Acheson Inquiry published (Acheson, 1998)
July 1999	White Paper on public health, *Saving lives: Our healthier nation* (DH, 1999a) and Action Report on *Reducing health inequalities* published (DH, 1999b)
February 2000	NHS Public Health Observatories established at regional level
July 2000	The *NHS Plan* published, announcing the creation of national and local health inequalities targets (DH, 2000)
February 2001	National health inequalities targets announced
June 2002	*Tackling health inequalities: Consultation on a plan for delivery* published (results of a public consultation on the actions needed to tackle health inequalities and meet inequality targets)
November 2002	Results published of HM Treasury and DH's Cross-cutting Review on *Tackling health inequalities* inviting joined-up thinking across government departments
July 2003	*Tacking health inequalities: A programme for action* launched (DH, 2003)
December 2003	*Health equity audit: A guide for the NHS* published identifying Health Equity Audit as a key tool for embedding evidence on inequalities into mainstream NHS activity
July 2004	PSA targets set for health inequalities
November 2004	White Paper on public health, *Choosing health: Making healthier choices easier* published (HM Government and DH, 2004)
February 2005	*Tackling health inequalities: What works* document published to provide best guidance practice for local NHS bodies (HIU, 2005)
March 2005	*Creating healthier communities: A resource pack for local partnerships* published
August 2005	Scientific Reference Group of Health Inequalities chaired by Professor Sir Michael Marmot compiled *Tackling health inequalities: Status report on the Programme for Action*, which reviewed progress towards the 2010 health inequalities PSA target (DH, 2005)

Box 3.1: Addressing the underlying determinants of health

In response to the Acheson Report, which emphasised the need for effective interventions to address the wider influence on health inequalities, the government commissioned a Cross-cutting Review on how links could be strengthened between policies that address these underlying determinants. This stressed that a way to narrow the gap in health outcomes was by taking concerted action through joined-up policy making and implementation across departmental boundaries. The government highlights the following policies as examples of areas in which it is acting in order to tackle the wider causes of health inequalities:

Child Tax Credit and Working Tax Credit
Community Legal Service
Connexions
Crime and Disorder Partnerships
Healthy Living Centres
Hospital Travel Costs Scheme
Jobcentre Plus
Learning and Skills Councils
Low Pay Commission
Making the connections: Final report on transport and social exclusion
Minimum Income Guarantee
National Minimum Wage
Neighbourhood Management
Neighbourhood Renewal Fund
New Deal for Programmes
New Opportunities Fund
NHS Purchasing and Supply Agency
Regional Development Agendas
Renewal.net
Skills for Life
Sustainable communities: Building for the future
Sustainable Development Commission
UK Fuel Poverty Strategy

Source: DH (2003)

We must transform the welfare state from a safety net in times of trouble to a springboard for economic opportunity ... the welfare state must enable people to achieve self-improvement and self-support. It must offer a hand-up, not just a hand-out. (CSJ, 1994, p 8, cited by Baldock et al, 2003, p 21)

Central to this vision is a concern with equality of opportunity and the obligation of individuals to make the best of opportunities provided to them. This individualising stance is evident in the Public Health White Paper *Choosing health: Making healthier choices easier* (HM Government and DH, 2004), the main subject of which is focused interventions that address so-called lifestyle factors. It is also apparent in the way in which the government sets out the problem of and main solutions to poverty. Here, opportunities that allow people to get into paid work and achieve economic self-sufficiency are seen as the key strategy for protecting them against both poverty and social exclusion (Baldock et al, 2003, p 22). These developments suggest that the concepts of universalism and redistribution have been largely replaced by the use of targeting, the promotion of individualism and an acceptance of inequality of outcomes. Against this, the government's Child Poverty Strategy (discussed later) represents a serious commitment to promoting greater equality. The fact that it has been restrained in trumpeting its ambitions for and progress towards the eradication of child poverty leads some to wonder if it is seeking to achieve 'redistribution by stealth' (Dornan, 2005, p 17).

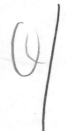

In many respects, then, New Labour's approach to welfare policies suggests an acceptance that inequality is an inevitable characteristic of capitalist societies. Implicit too is the idea that the role of welfare is not to bring about an overall redistribution in power and resources but to help those living under a certain poverty threshold through targeted or means-tested interventions. These ideas are more commonly associated with the political right and the assumption that poverty is an absolute phenomenon. Yet, by using measures of relative poverty (for example, in its approach to monitoring levels of child poverty), the government also acknowledges that minimally acceptable standards of living must relate to the prevailing living standards of society as a whole. It has also stated its commitment to addressing health inequalities – a problem that is fundamentally linked to the concept of relative rather than absolute poverty. In doing so, is it accepting the case for closing the socio–economic gap between the rich and the poor? The need for redistribution is explicit in Graham's (2004) distinction between social determinants of health and social determinants of health inequalities, which suggests that unless the distribution of social position is changed, the worst off in social and economic terms will always have the worst health and the highest risk of premature mortality. Against this background, it is important to examine the extent to which the government's policies have made a difference to the distribution of key resources in society. We do this with reference to the policy areas identified in the Acheson Report.

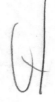

The recommendations of the Acheson Report

The Acheson Report, which was published in 1998, drew on a substantial research base. A total of 19 input papers were submitted as evidence to the Inquiry, covering policy sectors such as education and transport; different periods of the lifecourse;

social groups including minority ethnic groups; and disease categories such as mental and oral health (Gordon et al, 1999). After a descriptive section on health inequalities, the Inquiry summarised this evidence into 12 main areas for future policy development (see Box 3.2). These, together with the general themes of (a) ensuring that all policies likely to have a direct or indirect effect on health underwent a health impact assessment with reference to their impact on health inequalities, and (b) giving a high priority to policies aimed at improving health and reducing health inequalities in women of childbearing age, expectant mothers and young children, formed the basis for 39 recommendations.

Box 3.2: The recommendations of the Acheson Report

- *General recommendations:* ensuring that all policies likely to have a direct or indirect effect on health undergo a health impact assessment with reference to their impact on health inequalities; giving a high priority to policies aimed at improving health and reducing health inequalities in women of childbearing age, expectant mothers and young children.
- *Poverty, income, tax and benefits:* reducing income inequalities; improving the living standards of households receiving benefits; increasing employment opportunities.
- *Education:* providing additional resources for schools serving disadvantaged children; developing high-quality preschool education, particularly for disadvantaged families; developing health-promoting schools; improving nutrition provided in schools.
- *Employment:* improving opportunities for work and ameliorating the health consequences of unemployment through improving the quality of jobs, reducing psychosocial work hazards and increasing the level of control, variety and appropriate use of skills in the workforce; supporting these measures through policies to reduce income inequalities, improve living standards of those in receipt of benefits and provide high-quality day care and preschool education.
- *Housing and environment:* improving the availability of social housing for the less well-off; improving housing provision and access to healthcare for the homeless; improving the quality of housing; reducing the fear of crime and violence; supporting these measures through policies to reduce income inequalities and improve living standards of those in receipt of benefits.
- *Mobility, transport and pollution:* improving public transport; encouraging walking and cycling; reducing the use of motor vehicles; reducing traffic speed; making public transport affordable for pensioners and disadvantaged groups.
- *Nutrition and the Common Agricultural Policy (CAP):* comprehensively reviewing CAP's impact on health and health inequalities; increasing the availability and accessibility of food to reduce food poverty (supporting these measures through policies to reduce income inequalities, improve living standards of those in receipt of benefits and improve public transport); reducing the sodium content of processed foods.

- *Mothers, children and families:* reducing poverty in families with children by promoting their material support, removing barriers to work but also enabling those who wish to devote full time to parenting; developing an integrated policy for the provision of affordable, high-quality childcare and preschool education with extra resources for disadvantaged communities; improving the health and nutrition of women and children by other measures (such as reducing poverty, eliminating food poverty, improving nutrition at school) but also by promoting breastfeeding, fluoridating the water, reducing the prevalence of smoking in pregnancy, and providing social and emotional support of parents.
- *Young people and adults of working age:* improving opportunities to work and the quality of jobs; preventing suicide; promoting sexual health; promoting healthier lifestyles by encouraging physical exercise, reducing tobacco smoking, and reducing alcohol-related harm.
- *Older people:* promoting the material well-being of older people through policies to reduce income inequalities and improve the living standards of those in receipt of benefits; improving the quality of homes; development of policies to promote the maintenance of mobility, independence and social contacts; further developing health and social services for older people so that these services are accessible and distributed according to need.
- *Ethnicity:* specifically considering the needs of minority ethnic groups when reducing socio-economic inequalities, developing services and allocating resources. Of particular relevance here are policies to reduce income inequalities and to improve the living standards of those in receipt of benefits, to improve opportunities to work, improve the availability of social housing, housing quality and environmental safety, and transport policies.
- *Gender:* reducing excess death from accidents and suicides in young men (through employment, housing, transport and policies relating to mental health and alcohol misuse); improving psychosocial ill health in disadvantaged women with young children (through measures to reduce poverty, improve the availability of social housing, improve transport, provide opportunities for work, provide better childcare, promote health and nutrition, offer social and emotional support and promote better sexual health); reducing disability and its consequences among older women (through reductions to poverty, improvements to environments, transport policies and the further development of health and social services).
- *The NHS:* providing equitable access to effective care in relation to need; achieving a more equitable allocation of NHS resources; ensuring that populations are profiled with respect to their public health indicators and progress towards achieving health inequalities objectives is regularly monitored.

Some of the Report's recommendations focused on discrete groups or issues that are considered in more detail during the course of this book. For example, with respect to mothers, children and families, the Report recommended policies that increase the prevalence of breastfeeding; the further development of programmes to help women to give up smoking before or during pregnancy; and policies that promote the social and emotional support for parents and children. The subsequent development of key policy initiatives relating to these areas is described in Chapter Five, together with an assessment of research evidence of 'what works' and the limitations of the existing evidence base. Policies that the Report specifically recommended should be targeted at young people and adults of working age (including the prevention of suicide, the promotion of sexual health and the promotion of healthier lifestyles by encouraging physical exercise, reducing tobacco smoking and reducing alcohol-related harm) are considered in Chapters Nine and Eleven; while the Report's recommendations for policies targeted at older people, including the promotion of material well-being, improvements to the quality of homes, the development of policies to promote the maintenance of mobility, independence and social contacts, and the further development of health and social services for older people so that these services are accessible and distributed according to need, are considered in Chapter Thirteen. Policies relating to nutrition, by contrast, pertain to the whole range of demographic groups and, as such are discussed in several chapters, including Chapter Fourteen.

Other policy recommendations made by the Independent Inquiry are more generic. For example, policies "that will further reduce income inequalities, and improve the living standards of households in receipt of social security benefits" are recommended within the areas of poverty; income, tax and benefits; employment; housing and environment; nutrition and CAP; older people; and ethnicity. Recommendations for developing high-quality preschool education are considered relevant to education, employment, and mothers, children and families. The potential impact of policies to improve opportunities for work, ameliorate the health consequences of unemployment, improve the quality of jobs and reduce psychosocial work hazards is identified, not only in relation to employment, but in the areas of poverty, income, tax and benefits, young people and adults of working age, ethnicity and gender; while the case for housing policies is made in respect to older people, ethnicity and gender. National policy making in these major public policy sectors (fiscal, education, employment and housing policy) is considered next.

Policies relating to poverty, income, tax and benefits

In discussing evidence of the role played by poverty, income, tax and benefits in the production of health inequalities, the Acheson Report drew conclusions about the importance of targeting both absolute and relative poverty. Thus, it called for an increase in benefits (in cash or kind) to raise the standard of living of those who depend on them *and* a narrowing in the gap between their standard of living and average living standards (Acheson, 1998, p 36). Particular attention was paid to the need for policies to benefit families with children and pensioners. These, it was argued, were groups that would not reap the full benefits of the government's work-related reforms.

Child Poverty Strategy

Over the 20 years prior to 1997, children replaced pensioners as the group with the highest incidence of relative income poverty in the UK. Using a poverty level of 60% of the median income, 25% of children were living in poverty in 1997/98 before housing costs (BHC), 33% after housing costs (AHC). The highest incidence of poverty was among lone-parent families (37.5% BHC and 62% AHC in 1996/97) (Sutherland et al, 2003). Poverty is lower when measured BHC rather than AHC because housing costs are a larger proportion of total expenditure of low-income families with children.

In 1999, the government announced its intention to end child poverty within a generation. Its Child Poverty Strategy has since been described as the most significant single development in social security policy under New Labour (Deacon, 2003). The aim was to reduce child poverty by 25% by 2004, to halve it by 2010 and subsequently to eradicate it by 2020 (HM Treasury, 2001). The Child Poverty Strategy is predicated on providing more support for family finances (via major tax and benefit reforms) alongside increased support for parents and increased priority to children's services, especially in health and education. Various indicators are used to monitor its effectiveness, including literacy and numeracy, health outcomes and teenage pregnancy (MacGregor, 2003). It is resource intensive. According to government, financial support for children through tax credits, Child Benefit and other measures had increased by £10.4 billion by 2004/05, a rise of 72% in real terms from its 1997 level (HM Treasury, 2004a, p 33).

In-work credit is a long-established form of support for families on a low income. Family Income Supplement was introduced in 1971 and was replaced by Family Credit in 1988. New Labour then introduced the Working Families' Tax Credit (WFTC) in 1999 to replace Family Credit. This was a tax credit payable to working families (normally paid directly through the pay packet) with the aim of raising the living standards of low-income households, encouraging self-sufficiency and providing an incentive to work. By the time it was abolished, it provided support for 1.34 million low-paid families working 16 hours or more a week (equating to a reduction in the average tax bill of about £20 a week) (Evans and Cerny, 2003). Yet one third of eligible families failed to claim it. Uptake of the Childcare Tax Credit was even lower. It was claimed by only 167,000 families and related to a 2.5% tax cut for the average family – paid to the family's highest rate taxpayer, generally the father.

In 2003 WFTC was replaced by the Working Tax Credit (WTC) and the Child Tax Credit (CTC). The former supports adults with or without children in low-paid work as well as providing subsidies for certain childcare expenditure for some working parents. The latter, also means-tested, provides an allowance for parents and carers of children in full-time education and is made up of two elements, a family element and a child element (paid for each child). The child elements of both credits are payable to the child's main carer. CTC now represents the greater proportion of government financial support for children. Its progressive structure means that the poorest families benefit to the greatest extent. According to the HM Treasury (2004a, p 33), 65% more low- and moderate-income families are reached by CTC than by previous tax credit systems, and, as a result of its tax and credit reforms, families in the poorest fifth of the population were in real terms £3,000 a year better off in 2004 than when Labour first gained office.

Evidence suggests that, even before the introduction of WTC and the CTC, these developments (together with the lowering of National Insurance Contributions and tax levels for lower-paid workers) had had a positive impact on the incomes of the poorest households. Surveys undertaken as part of the Families and Children Study (FAC) show that, between 1999 and 2001, both working and non-working families experienced net gains in their disposable incomes. In this same period, levels of severe hardship in non-working households had also declined (Vegeris and Perry, 2003). Nevertheless, financial difficulties and material deprivation were commonly found in low-income families. The 2000 FAC, which focused on low- and moderate-income families (those whose incomes qualified them for social security benefits and tax credits) found that 56% of all families suffered from either severe or moderate hardship (measured using nine dimensions of material living). Non-working families were particularly vulnerable, 33% experiencing severe hardship and a further 42% moderate hardship. A significant proportion of low-income families suffered from difficulties such as poor-quality and overcrowded housing. Lone parents were particularly vulnerable (with 67% living in hardship). Housing problems, difficulties affording food, clothing, consumer durables and leisure activities and money worries each affected around a quarter of all lone-parent families (Vegeris and McKay, 2002).

The 2001 FAC noted a decline in rates of severe hardship but confirmed the difficulties faced by those on very low incomes. Of families below the low-income threshold (60% of median income), 22% were in severe hardship compared with 4% of families above the threshold. In this representative sample of all British families, one in four families fell under the low-income threshold. A total of 72% of non-working households were officially poor, 47% of lone-parent families and 15% of families with couples (Vegeris and Perry, 2003). The extent to which poor families are struggling with low incomes is also reflected in levels of indebtedness. In mid-2002, 34% of families whose gross incomes were between £7,500 and £15,000 a year were in arrears with their financial commitments. The next highest proportion of indebtedness (26%) was found in the very poorest families with annual incomes below £7,500 (Kempson et al, 2004).

The fact that financial difficulties and material deprivation are commonly found in low-income families suggests that the poverty line may lie above basic Income Support levels. Nevertheless, there is no doubt that the government has taken important steps to increase the absolute incomes of the poorest families with children. The fact that it is broadly on course to meet its PSA targets on child poverty (which are based on a relative income measure) also suggests that the policy has been redistributive. Progress between the 1998/99 baseline and 2003/04 shows a fall from 3.1 to 2.6 million children living in poverty BHC and from 4.1 to 3.5 million AHC (DWP, 2005c). It is worth noting that this reversal of a long-term trend has been achieved against rapidly rising real incomes (and thus a fast-moving poverty target) and that the whole length of the income distribution has moved to the right (Stewart, 2005).

These are very positive trends and go some way towards countering the assumption that, because the government has continued to focus on low Income Tax, it has "no more interest in redistributing income between rich and poor than its Conservative predecessors" (Brehony and Deem, 2003, p 193). When the difference between the incomes of the highest and lowest earners is considered, there *is* evidence of a narrowing in the gap since 1990 when the top 10% of the earnings distribution earned over four times the amount of the bottom 10% (Church and Whyman, 1997). In 2003, the top income decile earned 3.5 times the amount of the bottom income decile (data derived from the Office for National Statistics [ONS]). Within this overall reduction of income polarisation, however, there are a number of negative trends. The national income share of the poorest 10th of the population remained at 2% between 1994/95 and 2001/02 while the share of the richest 10th rose from 27% to 29% (Flaherty et al, 2004). Relative poverty rates for those of working age without children have continued to increase since 1997. Finally, wealth is even less evenly distributed than income, the wealthiest 10% of the population owning 56% of the nation's wealth in 2002 (compared with 52% in 1996, suggesting a trend towards greater polarisation since Labour assumed power). If housing is excluded from the estimates, marketable wealth is even more skewed, the wealthiest 10% of the population in 2002 owning 75% of the national share (data derived from the ONS).

A conflicting picture thus emerges with respect to the government's policies on poverty, income, tax and benefits. On the one hand, it has strongly focused support on the very poorest of families with children and, by improving low income in absolute terms, has contracted the spread of incomes to the left of the distribution. However, due to a host of other factors such as the continued increase in wage inequality (whereby incomes at the upper end have continued to rise rapidly), overall levels of income inequality have remained fairly stable. Moreover, the distribution of wealth has become more unequal since Labour assumed power. These themes (a reduction in absolute poverty but stability or growth in inequality) are also apparent at the other end of the age spectrum.

Pensions policy

The position of pensioners improved relative to the rest of society between 1979 and 1996/97. Nevertheless, old age is a period of significant income poverty. In 2002/03, one fifth of pensioners were living in poverty (on incomes below 60% of the median) and a further 15% were just above this level (Evandrou and Falkingham, 2005). Pensioners are also at greater risk of being persistently poor (spending at least three years in the bottom three tenths of incomes) than working-aged people. Between 1998 and 2001, 18% of pensioners were experiencing persistent poverty, compared with around 7% of the working population (Flaherty et al, 2004).

While the overall position of pensioners improved during the period of Conservative power, the gap between rich and poor pensioners widened substantially. Divisions in wealth are pronounced in older age. According to the Child Poverty Action Group, pensioner couples in the bottom fifth of the income distribution received an average of £136 a week in 2001/02 compared with £498 for the top fifth. Among single pensioners, the bottom fifth received £71 and the top fifth £238. These differences largely reflect received income from occupational pensions. In 2001/02, over half of those in the bottom fifth of the income distribution did not receive any occupational pension, representing 43% of all pensioner couples and 27% of all single pensioners. Certain groups are particularly vulnerable to loss of pension entitlements. Women are more likely than men to have taken time out of the labour market due to caring responsibilities. Older pensioners have lower incomes than the more recently retired, in part because the latter are more likely to have private pensions but also because there are more women in the older age groups. Minority ethnic pensioners are also vulnerable to poverty due to higher rates of unemployment and low pay during working age and because many arrived in the UK in the middle of their working lives and have thus not built up full entitlements (Flaherty et al, 2004).

When wealth (defined as savings and investments, excluding housing) is considered, the gulf that exists between the affluent and poor older people is even more stark. According to analysis of the British Panel Household Survey (BPHS) by the Institute of Fiscal Studies, the net financial wealth of households aged 60+ years in the bottom quintile is barely an eighth of that of those in the top quintile. These statistics are based on mean figures from the BHPS. The median figures reveal a disparity in which the wealthiest fifth have median holdings more than 25 times greater than the poorest fifth (Brook Lyndhurst Ltd, 2004). This degree of polarisation is in marked contrast to the 1970s and early 1980s when, because the vast majority of older people were poor, Britain was characterised by less income inequality among older people than its European counterparts (Victor, 1991, p 38). Since the 1980s, a significant proportion of affluent older people has emerged who are active and enjoy a good quality of life. This growth in socio-economic variation may have important implications for the level of health variation within this age group.

As part of an emphasis on tackling poverty, the Labour government has introduced a number of policies designed to benefit pensioners financially and therefore tackle pensioner poverty. These include a winter fuel allowance, free TV licences for the over-75s and changes to benefits and pensions. In 1999 Income Support for pensioners was re-badged as the Minimum Income Guarantee (MIG) for all pensioners with a full working record and significantly increased. For example, support for a single pensioner who would have received £68.80 in 1997 rose to £100 from April 2003. The government also made a commitment to raise support in line with earnings rather than prices from 2000 onwards. However, efficacy was reduced by limited take-up. Up to 37% of pensioners failed to claim means-tested payments in 2001/02, the majority of whom were 75 or over and living in the bottom fifth of the income distribution (Evandrou and Falkingham, 2005). Because MIG penalised people who had made provisions for their retirement, it also provided a disincentive to save (see Chapter Eleven).

While the Institute for Public Policy Research urged raising the basic state pension to the level of MIG, instead it was replaced by Pension Credit in 2003. This is a further extension of means testing but one that provides some reward for small savings. Thus, the new system increases the number of pensioners who are eligible for Income Support, Housing Benefit and Council Tax Benefit and offers additional income to pensioners who qualify for a full state pension and who have accumulated moderate savings. In April 2004 the guaranteed element of Pension Credit for a single person was £105.45 per week, equivalent to approximately 25% of average earnings and akin to what the basic state pension would have been if the link to earnings had not been broken (Evandrou and Falkingham, 2005).

The introduction of the Pension Credit has also been accompanied by a drive to increase benefit awareness and a more proactive approach to claims. Previously, relative pensioner poverty had not improved significantly, although in absolute terms the number living in poverty had fallen. With Pension Credit, relative poverty has also decreased, although as we noted earlier, pensioner poverty is not insignificant, affecting one fifth of those aged 65 years and over. Significant differences also remain within the pensioner population, female and minority ethnic pensioners facing the greatest risk of poverty. The Department for Work and Pensions (DWP) aims to increase the number of households receiving Pension Credit to at least three million by 2006. However, the implied target take-up rates of 72% would still leave over one million low-income pensioner households without the benefits they are entitled to (Evandrou and Falkingham, 2005).

In summary, the government has taken important steps to reduce levels of absolute poverty among pensioners and the number living in relative income poverty has also declined in recent years. Against this, take-up of new benefit entitlements has been relatively poor (leading some to suggest that universal benefits are more appropriate for this group than means-tested schemes). Some of the new schemes are targeted at less well-off but not the poorest of pensioners and other schemes such as tax relief are weighed in favour of the already wealthy. For example, of the £9 billion spent on tax relief for pensions, over half is received by the wealthiest 10% of the population (Flaherty et al, 2004). It is important to remember that the fundamental cause of growing income polarisation among older people – the shift from public to private sector pension provision – has been accelerated under the Blair Labour government, necessitating reforms to support the poorest pensioners. There has also been a general growth of income, particularly among the better-off in society, so, rather than closing the income gap between pensioners and those of working age, income gains for the poorest pensioners have simply maintained their incomes in line with those of the overall population. Thus, although progress has been made in addressing basic rates of poverty, somewhat less has been done to reduce income inequality in this group.

Education policies

During the 1997 General Election campaign, Tony Blair repeatedly claimed that the top three priorities of a New Labour government would be 'education, education, education'. On gaining office, the government has certainly lived up to its promise that education would be a top priority and there has been a deluge of policies and changes in almost every area of education (Walford, 2005). It has also increased the education budget. However, the proportion of the GDP spent on education is still less than in the majority of OECD (Organisation for Economic Co-operation and Development) countries and, while there are plans to increase this to 5.6% of GDP by 2007/08 (a level last seen in 1980/81), this compares with levels of 8% in Sweden and Denmark (McKnight, 2005).

As is the case for poverty, income, tax and benefits, the government's education strategy comprises a confusing mix of policies with regard to its potential for addressing health inequalities. Some of the government's policies have been explicitly aimed at reducing inequality and providing better educational opportunities for the disadvantaged. However, there are also strong continuities with the educational policy framework of the previous Conservative administration, including an emphasis on choice and competition and the use of new public management accountability processes (Taylor et al, 2005). These suggest a greater concern with differentiation than with equality and with economic competitiveness than social justice (Brehony and Deem, 2003). The tension that exists between the government's choice agenda and its commitment to redressing the effects of poverty and deprivation is therefore a recurrent theme in our assessment of New Labour's education policies.

Early years education and care

As we discuss in Chapter Four, psychological and neurological research has demonstrated the lasting benefits of positive stimulation in the early years. This research is complemented by the findings of several high-profile international studies that show that out-of-home care and preschool education can significantly improve social, behavioural and cognitive outcomes, especially for children from disadvantaged backgrounds (see Chapter Five). Against this background, the New Labour government put the early years high on its agenda for reform. A Treasury-led Cross-cutting Review of services for young children led to the proposals for the development of the Sure Start initiative (see later in this chapter). Financial support for childcare was made available to families on low incomes through the WFTC and, more recently, WTC and CTC. A Foundation Stage has been established for children aged three to five/six with clear curriculum guidance, and free part-time nursery education places introduced for all three- and four-year-olds. These are available in statutory nurseries, nursery classes in primary schools, private and voluntary sector nurseries and playgroups, provided that they meet nationally approved standards (Sylva and Pugh, 2005).

Rather than relying on direct state provision, the government thus encourages a mixed economy of early years education and care within a regulatory framework. Funding also comes from a mixture of sources. Preschool *education* has been provided on a universal basis for 12.5 hours a week across 33 weeks in the year. In 2002/03, £2.5 billion was spent by local authorities on these free nursery education places. Outside this provision, early years support has been treated as *care* and, as such, a largely private matter. In 2002/03, £680 million of Department for Education and Skills (DfES) and Sure Start monies were invested to support the development of childcare services and an additional contribution of £315 million made through Childcare Tax Credit. However, the bulk of funding came from parents, who paid £3 billion towards childcare costs (NAO, 2004).

The government's approach to a mixed economy of funding and provision reflects its belief that public–private partnerships offer the best means of achieving "choice and flexibility, availability, quality and affordability" (HM Treasury, 2004b). However, questions have been raised about the implications of this strategy for affordability, availability and the quality of services, particularly for disadvantaged children. For example, relatively few low-income parents have benefited from support for childcare costs. According to the National Audit Office, only 15% of eligible couples and 24% of lone parents receive the childcare element of WTC (NAO, 2004, cited by Sylva and Pugh, 2005). The average award through the childcare element of WTC (around £50 a week) is also significantly less than the costs of childcare which, in 2004, averaged £128 a week for a full-time nursery place. Even among low-income families, parents are privately responsible for a far higher proportion of childcare costs than in most other European countries. Thus, it is hardly surprising that many rely on informal care.

Affordability problems are being addressed by an increase in the childcare element of the WTC (see Chapter Five), a measure that still fails to help those who do not work or only work limited hours. However, problems remain with the availability of early years facilities. Again, a distinction needs to be drawn between education and care elements. There is no doubt that the government's strategy has encouraged an expansion of preschool education. In 1997, local authorities were providing places for 82% of four-year-olds and 34% of three-year-olds using their own budgets (NAO, 2004, p 21). By 2005, 100% and 98% of four- and three-year-olds were respectively taking up at least one free early education session a week with a maintained, voluntary or private provider (DfES, 2005a). It is important to note, however, that many settings do not extend their provision beyond the free two-and-a-half hour early education places. Thus, important shortfalls remain with respect to the provision of full-time childcare places.

For example, a significant gap exists between provision in deprived and non-deprived areas (NAO, 2004). Although this has narrowed since 2001, problems have been encountered with the government's Neighbourhood Nursery Initiative (which aimed to create 45,000 new childcare places by 2004 in the 20% most deprived wards and pockets of deprivation but which offered 10,700 additional places by October 2003). This has been attributed in part to the complexity of funding arrangements (NAO, 2004). Provided with start–up funding but expected to become self-sustaining within three years, many Neighbourhood Nurseries failed to obtain private sector loans due to concerns about financial sustainability. The tendency of targets to promote new rather than sustainable provision has also been linked to the high levels of closures in the childcare sector, particularly among childminders.

Many of these challenges are acknowledged in the *Ten-year strategy for childcare* (HM Treasury, 2004b). A total of 3,500 Children's Centres are to be established, with a role as integrated provider in the most disadvantaged areas (supported by more direct capital funding) and coordinator in others. Perhaps in recognition of the relative ease with which universal early years education can be expanded as opposed to good–quality targeted childcare, there will also be an increase in the entitlement to free part-time early years education to 15 hours a week from 2005 and to 20 hours per week across 38 weeks by 2008. Provision, however, will continue to rely on a mix of maintained, private and voluntary providers. As we discuss in Chapter Four, questions have been raised about the extent to which this approach has resulted in services of the highest quality. Early years education is a specialised area which, in several continental educational systems, is supported by graduate-level training and professional development. In England, however, less than half of workers in playgroups and only 50% of staff in day nurseries are qualified to National Vocational Qualification (NVQ) level (which is some way below graduate level). Even within reception classes situated in primary schools, fully qualified teachers may not be trained to work with very young children. Thus, the education that preschool children (and particularly disadvantaged children) need to best promote social, behavioural and cognitive outcomes is not necessarily delivered by the choice agenda.

While tremendous progress has been made in the provision of early years education and care, international evidence suggests that high-quality, affordable and accessible services tend to be associated with a higher level of state involvement than achieved by a strategy that relies on public–private partnership. The Nordic welfare states provide a particularly strong contrast to the approach used by the British government to develop early years education and care. Here, generous rights to parental leave, childcare subsidies, an emphasis on developmentally appropriate practice and high levels of public sector provision are strongly embedded into welfare systems.

In Sweden, for example, high-quality childcare has been seen as a universal, public good (Quarmby, 2003). Until 2003, the training of preschool teachers involved an extensive three-year university degree programme, resulting in a highly qualified workforce with particular expertise in the early years (Lohmander, 2004). Practical access to preschool education is high. Care for one- to five-year-olds is provided on a full-time basis for children whose parents are working or studying or who have special needs and for up to 15 hours a week for children whose parents are unemployed. Childcare places are very heavily subsidised and financial access, together with the widely held view that early childcare is an important part of a child's development, has resulted in high uptake of services, even among the under-threes. In 2000, 36% and 67% of one- and two-year-olds respectively attended *förskolar* or preschools, the vast majority using public sector services. A further 6% and 11% of children were cared for by childminders. Children who are cared for at home or by childminders may also attend *öppna förskolar* (open preschools) to take part in educational group programmes (Swedish Institute, 2001). In the UK, under three-year-old children of unemployed parents currently have no entitlement to formal childcare. Nor is there a British equivalent to the Swedish *öppna förskolar*, leading some to question whether the current expansion of early years provision is driven more by the wish to enable parents to return to work than a recognition that early years policy is important in its own right.

Britain, of course, has traditionally spent significantly less on its early childhood services than Sweden – 0.3% of GDP compared to 2% in Sweden (Quarmby, 2003). The new childcare strategy, however, allocates an extra £600 million a year to the current £9.9 billion spent on early years and childcare in order to achieve its goals (Burke, 2005), bringing spending to just over 0.95% of GDP. This is an impressive increase. However, it may not be enough to transform what has been a relatively (in Scandinavian terms) under-funded system. A study commissioned by the Daycare Trust and the Social Market Foundation (PriceWaterhouseCoopers, 2004) suggests that universal, affordable and accessible early education and care could, by increasing parental employment and the future productivity of children, bring long-term benefits to the economy of around 1 to 2% of GDP per annum. However, this would require an increase in government spending of up to £20 billion by 2010 and £30 billion by 2020. On the basis of current proposals, it is unlikely that such a financial investment will be made.

Primary and secondary schooling

The tensions between the desire to counteract the effects of poverty and social disadvantage and the pursuit of a choice agenda have been even more acute with respect to primary and secondary education. As we discuss in Chapter Eight, socio-economic differences in educational performance are pronounced. Moreover, children with similar levels of competency diverge as they progress through school according to their socio-economic background, suggesting that the education system is not successfully promoting greater social justice. The government has recognised the constraints placed by factors such as low community aspirations, high pupil turnover, serious poverty and/or fractured communities on educational outcomes (Barber, 2002, cited by Brehony, 2005). Policies that have been aimed at providing better educational opportunities for the disadvantaged include revisions to the school funding system, so that an increased share goes to local authorities with the most deprived populations, and the introduction of additional grants for secondary schools in challenging circumstances (McKnight, 2005). Two of New Labour's main ABIs have also had an educational focus (see Chapter Nine). In 1998, 73 Education Action Zones (EAZs) were established to bring together schools, community and business influence in order to improve attainment in disadvantaged areas. The following year, EAZs were amalgamated into the Excellence in Cities Programme. This has a more extensive geographical coverage (covering one third of local education authorities [LEAs] and their schools), more substantial funding and a more prescriptive programme, including special programmes for gifted and talented children, the provision of more Learning Support Units for disruptive pupils, and the provision of learning mentors for children. However, although the DfES claimed that these programmes had helped raise achievement in inner cities, other research has been more equivocal about their impact (Tomlinson, 2005).

One factor limiting the potential of targeted initiatives to address educational disadvantage is the fact that continued commitment to the marketisation of education has served to increase social and educational polarisation (Mortimore and Whitty, 1997; Lauder et al, 1999; Thrupp, 1999; Gibson and Asthana, 2000). The thrust of the government's policies in England (Scotland, Wales and Northern Ireland have adopted different approaches) is to promote school improvement through choice and competition. This involves a continuation of the educational project established by the Conservative government, in which a diversity of schools has been created and market competition between schools fuelled by league table publications, school 'choice', the extension of a specialist school programme, and enhanced private funding and influence in education (Tomlinson, 2005, p 156).

The White Paper *Excellence in schools* (DfEE, 1997) supported the continuation of selection (with public schools and grammar schools left alone) and differentiation (with increased designation of specialist colleges) (Brehony and Deem, 2003). This was furthered by the White Paper *Schools: Achieving success* (DfEE, 2001), the 2003 strategy document *A new specialist system: Transforming secondary education* (DfES, 2003a) and the 2005 White Paper *Higher standards, better schools for all: More choice for parents and pupils* (DfES, 2005c). As a result of these and other initiatives, the New Labour government has expanded school diversity well beyond the scope and extent achieved by previous Conservative administrations. Through the course of its administration, the government has created Beacon Schools, Training Schools, Federations, Leading Edge Partnership Schools, specialist schools and City Academies alongside LEA-controlled comprehensive schools, foundation, voluntary-aided, grammar and independent schools. A common feature of this strategy has been a blurring in private and public functions. Thus, the role of LEAs has been reduced and, in some cases (such as City Academies), control of schools passed to commercial and not-for-profit agencies (Taylor et al, 2005). Notwithstanding uncertainty about the impact of this strategy on educational outcomes, this model of diversity and independence from the state is to be extended nationally. Thus, the 2005 White Paper (DfES, 2005) envisages that schools will be set up by parents' groups, charities, universities, faith groups and businesses while the role of the LEA will change from provider to commissioner.

The promotion of diversity has been paralleled by the emphasis placed by government on driving up standards through the introduction of the National Curriculum and the related regime of targets, inspections, testing and the publication of performance statistics. This, it is argued, guides parental choice, which, by introducing an element of competition between schools, is an effective engine for school improvement. However, because school performance largely reflects school catchment characteristics, the system gives schools that serve socially advantaged populations a competitive advantage. By contrast, poorly performing schools in deprived areas tend to be seen as the least desirable by parents who exercise a choice. This system exacerbates socio-economic (and ethnic) segregation in a number of ways (Gewirtz et al, 1994; Tomlinson, 1997, 2005). Although choice has been promoted for parents, the most popular schools are able to select their intake, rather than the other way round, and modes of selection tend to favour children from socially advantaged backgrounds. Where choice systems do operate, better-off parents do more choosing than their lower-income counterparts. Selection by mortgage also remains an important source of differentiation in the social composition of English schools, reflected in the significant premiums attached to house prices within the catchment areas of the most popular schools. Again, the rich are more able to respond to such price differentials than the poor.

Against this background, it is hardly surprising that the increasing marketisation of English education has exacerbated existing differences between schools in terms of the social status of their pupils (Gibson and Asthana, 2000). It is estimated that only 40% of pupils in England go to genuinely non-selective schools (Green, 2003). In Wales, by contrast, where secondary education is largely provided by LEA comprehensive schools, and where there are low numbers of fee-paying, selective or specialist schools, socio-economic segregation is markedly lower (Taylor et al, 2005). Marketisation has also promoted growing polarisation in educational performance as the best-performing schools are able to increasingly attract more able pupils. Between-school variation in educational performance is much higher in England than in most other countries with nominally comprehensive systems, reflecting the high degree of selection that takes place (Green, 2003).

Like other countries that have actively promoted the marketisation of their comprehensive systems, the UK is characterised by relatively high levels of educational inequality (separate figures are not available for each of the home nations). Analysis of international comparative data on educational performance found that the UK ranked 16th out of 24 OECD countries with respect to relative educational disadvantage (a measure of the extent to which low-achieving pupils fall behind the national average). The US and New Zealand, countries that have adopted a similar policy framework, ranked 21st and 23rd (UNICEF, 2002). As we note in Chapter Eight, low levels of educational disadvantage (that is, greater equality) are not incompatible with high absolute standards of achievement. Thus, countries such as Finland, Korea and Japan have contained inequality by not allowing their low achievers to fall too far behind average performance while at the same time producing higher average standards than in the UK.

Even in the most egalitarian education systems, there remain differences in the relative performance of the socially disadvantaged compared to the socially advantaged. In Finland, for example, access to higher education depends strongly on socio-economic background, the children of academically educated parents being nine times more likely to enter a university, polytechnic or college than the children of parents who have completed only basic education (Parjanen and Tuomi, 2003). Evidence from Sweden suggests that, although educational reforms in the 1960s appear to have promoted greater equality, there are limits to the extent to which class inequalities in educational outcomes can be further reduced (Hatcher, 1998). Given the range of factors that influence educational attainment, few would claim that educational *equality* is a realistic goal. Nevertheless, the degree to which social background in Britain determines educational and subsequent occupational trajectories suggests that there is scope for promoting greater *equity*.

Post-compulsory education

Post-compulsory education is important to social inequality because the vast majority of young people continue education past the school leaving age of 16. By the end of 2004, 75.4% of 16- to 18-year-olds were in education or training. A total of 10% were not in education, training or employment, a proportion that has remained broadly level since the mid-1990s (DfES, 2005b). Despite a rhetoric of lifelong learning, most of the policy focus with respect to increasing participation in post-compulsory education is on 16- to 30-year-olds. However, efforts have been made to target young people from disadvantaged backgrounds. For example, the Education Maintenance Allowance (EMA) introduced in 2004 is a weekly cash allowance designed to encourage young people (aged 16-19) from low-income families to remain in full-time education (see Chapter Nine).

A further source of inequity is the continued separation of further education (FE) and higher education (HE). FE is the locus of much of the expanded working-class participation in post-compulsory education. Furthermore, entry to HE for underrepresented groups is supported via two-year foundation degrees at teaching-intensive universities and FE colleges. The 1999 White Paper *Learning to succeed* (DfEE, 1999) (which covered post-16 education) established the Learning and Skills Councils (that replaced the private sector Training and Enterprise Councils and the Further Education Funding Council) with responsibility for distributing and allocating funding for all post-compulsory school-age education. However, HE funding remained separate with a disparity in staff–student ratios and staff qualifications.

In 2001, the government announced that 50% of 18- to 30-year-olds should have the opportunity to benefit from higher education. The main target of widening participation is students from socio-economically disadvantaged backgrounds. However, increases in the proportions of all students have left the participation rate of poorer students relative to other socio-economic groups much the same as a decade ago (Taylor, 2005). Due to the differential emphasis on younger as opposed to older learners, trends in adult participation are even less encouraging. Taylor (2005) reports that, in 2004, the number of adults reporting that they were currently learning was, at 19%, the lowest of any year since 1996. Moreover, since 1996 the learning divide has widened, with participation rates falling among all but the highest socio-economic groups. It is likely that the shift in finance for HE from general taxation to students themselves has contributed to this trend. The change from means-tested maintenance grants to student loans has largely benefited more affluent families (who previously had not had access to grants but now qualify for cheap loans). By contrast, HE has become a more risky investment for those from a poorer background, given their higher tendency to drop out, have poorer employment rates and enjoy lower wages. Although the policy has been described as a way of reducing the level of state subsidy that reaches (largely) middle-class students, the introduction of tuition fees may have further discouraged mature students from socially disadvantaged backgrounds.

Employment policies

The Acheson Report recognised the potentially major risks for health associated not just with unemployment but with stressful and hazardous working environments (the explanations for which we explore in Chapter Ten). One set of recommendations thus focused on providing opportunities for work and ameliorating the effects of unemployment. This included employment generation, the provision of adequate childcare, family-friendly employment policies, increased training and education opportunities for at-risk groups and adequate income levels for those without work. The second focused on the quality of jobs provided and the reduction of psychosocial work hazards. This included recommendations for employer and union-led improvements to management practices, in order to increase the level of control, variety and appropriate use of skills in the workforce, and the assessment of the impact of employment policies on health and health inequalities.

The government response has been to focus on the former by both increasing rates of employment and connecting welfare benefits closely to work incentives (Exworthy et al, 2003). It has also focused specifically on both disadvantaged people and places (for a discussion of the ABIs for employment see Chapters Nine and Eleven). Essentially, it has placed the emphasis on supply-side policies designed not to create jobs but to help people become more employable, search for work and remain in work and to influence who gets the available work (young people and lone parents, for example). It has also made significant changes to the administration of welfare benefits based both on the individualisation of support and an element of compulsion or coercion. This is captured in the government's PSA for employment. This seeks "to promote work as the best form of welfare for people of working age, while protecting the position of those in greatest need", and aims not only to increase the employment rate but also to (a) increase the employment rate of disadvantaged areas and groups (lone parents, minority ethnic groups, people aged 50 and over, those with the lowest qualifications, and those living in the local authority wards with the poorest initial labour market position); and (b) significantly reduce the difference between the employment rates of the disadvantaged groups and the overall rate (HM Treasury, 2004c, p 37).

The largest employment policy initiatives have been the changes to the administration of welfare benefits and the investment in the welfare-to-work programme, by far the government's largest single public spending commitment. Central to this are the national New Deal programmes. Funded originally (£5 billion) from the windfall tax on the privatised utilities (McKnight, 2005) they are now administered by Jobcentre Plus (part of the DWP) with the aim of integrating the job search and benefit payments of over six million people through a focus on personal advisors. The New Deal for Young People (NDYP) covers those aged 18-24 who have been out of work for over six months (see Chapter Nine). It was introduced in April 1998, and was followed between 1998 and April 2000 by five further New Deals: those for the long-term unemployed aged 25 or over (ND25plus); disabled people (NDDP); lone parents (NDLP) (which is voluntary because of the enduring political reluctance to introduce compulsion for lone mothers); those over 50 (ND50plus); and the partners of unemployed people (ND for Partners). Together, they have the two-fold aim of helping people into employment and increasing long-term employability (including the ability to sustain a job and progress within employment). Benefit sanctions apply to those who do not comply with the compulsory programmes, such as NDYP, and the initiative has been criticised for being part of a coercive regime designed to make access to benefits more difficult. The situation is actually more complex because there are multiple if sometimes conflicting objectives: labour market efficiency, controlling benefit payments and enhancing the welfare of the individual unemployed (Finn, 2003).

By the end of 2000 NDYP had reached its initial target of assisting 250,000 young unemployed people to find employment (see Chapter Nine), with the most dramatic impact being on those registered as unemployed for over a year – where a fall of almost 95% was recorded (from 90,700 to 5,100 in the period April 1997-April 2002). The National Audit Office estimated that the *net* additional employment impact was a reduction in levels of youth unemployment by 25,000-45,000 and (because many entered education or training) an increase in youth employment of 8,000-20,000 (NAO, 2002). Unemployment rates for 16- to 17-year-olds, who remain outside this policy envelope, have not fallen (Hills and Stewart, 2005). Evaluations of the ND25plus and NDLP suggest they are also making a net, if modest, impact (Finn, 2003). For example, lone-parent employment rates in 2000 in the UK were among the lowest of the OECD countries, contributing to high rates of poverty, and the government is aiming, therefore, to raise employment rates among lone parents to 70% by 2010 (the employment rate among lone parents with preschool children was only 34% in 2002). It has been estimated that employment rates among lone parents are actually about five percentage points higher than they would have been in the absence of New Labour's policies. In contrast, the take-up of the pilot NDDP was only 3%.

The New Deals have been supplemented by area-based employment initiatives aimed at reducing long-term unemployment in particular localities (see Chapter Eleven). Employment Zones (EZs) were introduced in 13 areas in 2000 with the aim of helping the long-term unemployed (Jobseeker's Allowance claimants aged over 25 out of work for over 18 months) into work and testing the concept of personal job accounts to buy tailored support. They are delivered by private sector contractors who are paid through an output-related funding system. They have been criticised, however, for their differential impact, including poorer outcomes for disabled people and a tendency to categorise claimants into the employable and the unemployable and then to focus resources on the former. Their impact was also strongest in the first year and weak thereafter (McKnight, 2005). Employment Action Teams (a voluntary programme) have been introduced in another 20 areas in order to tackle specific local problems and obstacles to job matching. These initiatives have also been bolstered by the introduction of a National Minimum Wage, in an attempt to raise living standards.

McKnight suggests it would be "difficult to refute the claim that employment has been one of Labour's big success stories" (2005, p 28), with registered unemployment reaching a 30-year low in May 2004, supported by a favourable economic climate. Yet, increases in claims for Incapacity Benefit make this a difficult judgement to make. In February 2005 in Britain the unemployed made up under one fifth of those claiming out-of-work benefits. Then, 4.84 million people of working age were claiming key benefits, with 4.52 million of these claiming out-of-work benefits, 13.5% and 12.6% of the working-age population respectively. The most striking feature of these figures is the significance among this group of sick and disabled claimants. Over 3 million of those claiming key benefits are classified as sick and disabled (8.6% of the population of working age), compared to 700,000 in 1979. This compares with just 816,000 unemployed people (2.3% of the working-age population), 761,000 lone parents (2.1%) and 197,000 'others' (DWP, 2005a, table 3.1, p 9). Moreover, this trend continues. As the overall stock of claimants has increased (by 0.15 million between February 2002 and February 2005) the proportion of the total stock accounted for by sick and disabled people has increased (rising from 60% to 63% of the total in the same period). A second striking feature is the continued regional variations. A total of 18.4% of the working-age population in the North East are claiming key benefits, as are 18.2% of those in Wales and 16.8% in Scotland, dropping to just 8.8% in the South East. A third important dimension is age: only 4.3% of those aged under 18 claim a key benefit but this rises with age (and disability) until 18.5% of those aged 55-59 and 30.2% of those aged 60-65 are claimants.

The Green Paper *Pathways to work* (DWP, 2002) set out to challenge this situation and move people from Incapacity Benefit into employment, with a focus on the most disadvantaged areas. Its underlying premise was that most people entering Incapacity Benefit expected eventually to return to work and did not report severe health conditions. Obstacles additional to poor health then combined to keep them on benefits with a return to employment likely to improve health (see also the White Paper *Choosing health*, HM Government and DH, 2004). Seven Pathways to Work pilots, based on Jobcentre Plus districts, were introduced therefore across Britain from October 2003. These build on the New Deal model with a personal advisor providing contact every month in the first eight months (the period when people can be most readily helped back to work), access to a range of specialist employment programmes (including the NDDP) and financial incentives to seek work and move into employment.

Additionally, they provide work-focused rehabilitation support involving local NHS providers. The initial focus was on new Incapacity Benefit claimants (and existing claimants who volunteered) but was extended from early 2005 to those who have been on Incapacity Benefit for over a year.

Early evaluation (November 2004) suggested that double the number of people were getting jobs through Jobcentre Plus compared to the previous year, with an 8% to 10% increase in the rate of people coming off Incapacity Benefit after four months of their claim compared to non-pilot areas, and five times as many people in pilot areas joining NDDP compared to old-style jobcentres (DWP, 2004). From October 2005 the scheme will therefore be extended to a further 14 Jobcentre Plus districts focusing on the most disadvantaged areas and local authority areas with the greatest concentration of Incapacity Benefit claimants. Related measures include £30 million to support the NDDP, the placing of specialist personal advisors in every Jobcentre Plus district by 2006, all new Incapacity Benefit claimants being required to attend a work-focused interview after eight weeks of their claim from October 2005 and reform of the 'permitted work' rules. It also includes training materials for doctors to help them support patients get back to work effectively, the placing of specialist employment advisors in GP surgeries and a pilot scheme to enable doctors to give patients better advice on fitness for work and rehabilitation. This includes liaison with specialist GPs dealing with mental health (such as anxiety, stress and depression), musculo-skeletal and cardio-respiratory problems – the most common types of both work-related disease (ONS, 2004, table 9.7) and Incapacity Benefit claims (a reflection, perhaps of the government's inability to tackle the quality of jobs provided and to reduce psychosocial work hazards). The DWP's *Five-year strategy* (DWP, 2005b) launched in 2005 will take the process still further with plans to replace Incapacity Benefit with two new benefits. A 'rehabilitation support allowance' will provide a strong work focus for the majority of people deemed to have more manageable conditions while a higher rate 'disability and sickness allowance' will provide for those with the most severe health conditions, acknowledging their vulnerability to prolonged poverty. Debate continues, however, as to whether this policy is truly predicated on a concern for individual health and welfare or a desire to reduce expenditure on welfare benefits.

Housing policies

For much of the post-war period, housing (like health and education) was a social policy sector in which the case for strong state involvement was generally accepted. There was a continued rise in the production of council housing until 1977/78, when it accounted for 32% of the total housing stock. Council housing thus played a broad role rather than catering for a small minority of the poorest households. Between 1979 and 1997, however, there were radical changes to the housing landscape. The Conservative government's 'Right to Buy' (or council house privatisation) policy, together with the dearth of new provision in the local authority sector, saw a significant decline in the size of this sector (which fell to 13% of the total housing stock in 2001) and a growth of owner-occupation (from 56% in 1979 to 69% in 2001). As the council housing sector has shrunk, it has come to play a residual role for the very poorest of households. Thus, in 2001, 69% of households in council housing in England had no earners compared with 7% in 1962 (Pickvance, 2003). The growing incidence of unemployment among social housing tenants and the numbers of households dependent on state support for housing costs was compounded by the poor physical condition of much of the housing stock. By the end of the Conservative administration, the backlog of local authority repairs was estimated to exceed £19 billion (Ford, 2003).

New Labour took some immediate action on gaining office, using the £800 million released from council house sales to address the problems of poor housing stock, followed by an injection of further funds as a result of the 1998 comprehensive spending review. Between 1996 and 2002, the proportion of social units falling below the decency threshold fell from 46% to 33% (Barker, 2004). Homelessness, the housing issue most visibly connected to social exclusion, also became one of the first priorities for the Social Exclusion Unit, resulting in the establishment of the Rough Sleepers Unit (see Chapter Eleven), and an initial target of reducing the numbers of people sleeping rough in England by two thirds by 2002. Under Labour the significance of housing to a wide range of other policy areas has also become more explicit. For example, the government has sought to enhance social inclusion via lettings policy and an embryonic attempt has been made to address the failure of the housing market in the South East through the Sustainable Communities Plan (Lupton and Power, 2005). The link between health and housing has "moved up the UK policy agenda" (Marsh et al, 2000, p 411). The Acheson Report (1998) served to highlight housing and environment as key areas for future policy development if health inequalities were to be reduced and this was furthered by the White Paper *Saving lives* (DH, 1999), which similarly recognised housing as one of the key environmental factors that affects health. The floor target established in support of neighbourhood renewal also aims to bring not only all social housing into decent condition by 2010 but to increase the proportion of private housing in decent condition occupied by vulnerable groups. Of all the national deprivation-related targets this is the target that shows the clearest sign of improvement, with a reduction from 2.3 to 1.6 million homes falling below the decency standard since 1995/96 (Lupton and Power, 2005).

Alongside these developments, the government has continued to rely on the housing market, which raises important questions about the implications of its housing strategy for social inequality. The number of social houses built in the UK has fallen from around 42,700 per year in 1994/95 to around 21,000 in 2002/03 (Barker, 2004). With the purchase of existing dwellings, around 31,000 social housing units are provided every year in total (CPRE, 2004). Yet Shelter suggests that 67,000 units are annually required to meet emerging needs for additional social housing and an additional 22,000 units to overcome the backlog of housing need (Holmans et al, 2004). The Barker Report (2004), using a stricter definition of need, suggests that 48,000 social and affordable houses are required per year. However, this still leaves an annual shortfall of at least 17,000 units. Support for market mechanisms is also evident in other policies. For example, sustainable ownership is a matter of individual responsibility, the government favouring mortgage payment protection insurance rather than assuming responsibility for interest payments for homeowners who lose income. This is despite a take-up rate of only 22.5% in 2002. The transfer of local authority housing to registered social landlords has also continued.

Trends in housing provision for the disadvantaged have also taken place within a broader context of growing inequalities in housing wealth within Britain. Between 1971 and 2002, the value of homes held by the UK population rose fifty-fold in contemporary prices from £44 billion to £2.4 trillion, increasing the share of national wealth held in the form of housing from 22% to 42%. This share has become more socially and geographically polarised, average price rises for the wealthiest areas exceeding those of the worst-off areas. As a result, the wealthiest 10th of households possess over five times the housing wealth of the 10% of households with the least wealth by area (Thomas and Dorling, 2004). It is important to note that these figures do not include those who rent in the private or social sectors, who have no housing wealth and who are therefore excluded from what has become the greatest single repository for wealth held by individuals within the country. According to Thomas and Dorling (2004), this means that the children from the poorest households will be significantly more disadvantaged with respect to their relative access to resources than those of previous generations, making the gulf between the rich and the poor wider than any time since the Victorian era.

Midstream policies addressing health inequalities

Policy making at national level has been somewhat ambiguous in intent, some initiatives focusing strongly on the reduction of poverty while others have promoted the role of the market, although this tends to exacerbate socio-economic polarisation. By contrast, ABIs represent a consistent attempt by government to concentrate resources in the most disadvantaged of areas. Moreover, because they are targeted at communities rather than individuals, they allow for a broader understanding of the causes of and solutions to social exclusion than individualised interventions.

ABIs have a long history in welfare policy (Crawshaw et al, 2004) but are particularly favoured by New Labour, which has introduced a considerable range of such measures including action zones for education, employment, health, and sport, the New Deal for Communities, Sure Start and the Neighbourhood Renewal Fund. Time-limited in nature, the intention has been to tackle the problems of particular areas through a joined-up approach to planning and service delivery that includes local residents. The use of partnerships and community involvement (or community development allied to a bottom-up approach) are thus key themes, so too is a concern to test ideas that could influence mainstream programmes and a growing emphasis on mainstream delivery. Area-based regeneration initiatives are thus increasingly expected to work with and influence the resources of statutory service providers (see Chapter Eleven). The renewed focus on ABIs has also seen their extension beyond their traditional urban and inner-city focus. The three predominantly rural areas of Cornwall, Northumberland and North Cumbria, for example, were among the 26 areas designated as HAZs, while EAZs typically covered two or three secondary schools and their feeder primaries.

The rationale behind such targeting has been usefully summarised (Smith, 1999). A concentration of problems puts mainstream programmes and service delivery under pressure. The introduction of an ABI allows remedial measures to be directed easily at a relatively large number of deprived people. It provides a mechanism for rationing scarce resources, an ability to concentrate resources to potentially greatest impact and the opportunity to experiment. It also allows adequate consideration to be given to local need: the salient factors that operate at the area level such as housing tenure, skills mismatch, racial and postcode discrimination, and limited social networks. This includes the possibility of an area effect – such that interaction of all factors (disadvantaged people, a poor physical environment, poor services and so on) may have cumulatively and qualitatively different effects on individuals, organisations and infrastructure than less concentrated poverty (Tunstall and Lupton, 2003).

The ability of ABIs to generate large-scale improvement is also, however, constrained by definition. Most deprived people do not live in deprived areas and, as we have noted, many of the structural problems faced by such people are generated at a national or international level and not, therefore, amenable to local solution (Oatley, 2000). They have also been criticised for being iniquitous (in that other areas with similar problems will always miss out), for displacing problems to neighbouring areas, for providing only short-term solutions and a time-limited intervention, and for offering an undemocratic partnership base and a vehicle for central control. While improvements in statistics mean that the Index of Multiple Deprivation 2000 is now recognised as "a more complete way of reaching the poor than has been claimed by opponents of area-based targeting in the past" (Tunstall and Lupton, 2003, p iii) it also remains more effective for some subgroups, such as children in poor households and unemployed people, than others such as pensioners, lone parents and disabled people. Area-based measures similarly remain inappropriate for capturing deprivation in rural areas.

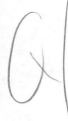

In the context of this book they occupy the mid ground between the overt emphasis on individual responsibility for (and behavioural solutions to) the management of health and national structural solutions relating, for example, to the redistribution of wealth together with access to employment, education and housing. They have, however, also been criticised for effectively shifting "responsibility for regeneration, renewal and the improvement of health, from the state to the community itself" (Crawshaw et al, 2004, p 342) and hence again ultimately to the individual. Despite some early manifestations (such as the World Health Organization [WHO] Healthy Cities Initiative, which dates from 1987) it is also an area where health is only recently emerging as a strategic partner despite its manifest links with place and deprivation.

Health Action Zones

HAZs remain the only ABI in the UK to have been targeted specifically at health. They were the first regeneration-type initiative in which health was the lead agency and in which health issues were paramount rather than an adjunct to economic or physical regeneration (Matka et al, 2002). They were also unusual in being spatially very extensive, a product of the structure of the (then) health authorities and local authorities on which they were based. The 26 zones (areas of deprivation and poor health) thus ranged in population from 200,000 to over 1.4 million people and between them covered one third of the population of England (Bauld et al, 2001), First announced in 1997 and designated in 1998 and 1999, they were also one of the first ABIs to be established by New Labour (Bauld and Judge, 2002). A partnership between the NHS, local authorities, community/voluntary groups and business, their aim was to identify and address public health needs and health inequalities, modernise services (focusing on efficiency, effectiveness and responsiveness) and to create synergy between different agencies by developing partnerships for health.

Approximately one fifth of their effort, as measured by activities, was directed at the root causes of ill health, spanning areas such as education, unemployment, income and improvements to the housing stock (Judge et al, 1999). Other key areas included: reshaping health and social care (the provision of primary and community services and health promotion, for example); addressing lifestyle issues such as smoking (see Chapter Five), sexual behaviour, substance misuse, diet and exercise; community empowerment; and capacity development. What was most noticeable, however, was the sheer breadth of activity, ranging from children and young people through to older people, and from the provision of services to organisational development and community empowerment. What was envisaged as a seven-year programme for change was, however, short-lived. A change of ministers early in their history saw the emphasis shift towards more traditional health service-driven priorities such as tackling waiting lists and addressing cancer, coronary heart disease (CHD) and mental health (Bauld and

Judge, 2002). They were also overtaken by reforms in the health community, which saw PCTs assume responsibility for local healthcare in 2002 and the development of Local Strategic Partnerships (LSPs) charged with, among other things, rationalising the proliferation of partnerships dealing with social exclusion, such as HAZs, that had emerged under New Labour (Johnson and Osborne, 2003). Funding was, therefore, largely returned to the mainstream and much of the work that HAZs had undertaken across their first three or four years was taken forward by the PCTs or LSPs. Significantly, the national HAZ evaluation notes that HAZs were able to pilot locally successful strategies for engaging partners and involving communities but that these were resource intensive and thus likely to lose out to the mainstream. Efficient new systems, they stress, "actually require more resources in the short to medium term, not fewer" (Matka et al, 2002, p 106).

Sure Start

Sure Start, in contrast, is an ABI where the target is a particular subgroup of the population, young children aged 0-4 and their families. Described as "a cornerstone of the Government's drive to tackle child poverty and social exclusion" (Tunstill et al, 2002, p 1), it is significant in that child health is explicitly included and that the intervention is pervasive, embracing a wide spectrum of services for the early years. In addition to children's health, Sure Start aims to influence children's ability to learn and their social and emotional development as well as strengthening families and communities. It thus acknowledges the evidence base concerning health inequalities at this stage in the lifecourse. Not only is it considerably more focused than the HAZs, the geographical area of intervention is also tightly defined, typically comprising neighbourhoods of between 400 and 800 children. It is, however, distributed widely with over 500 programmes in operation by 2004. In common with HAZs there is also a strong emphasis on partnership working and community involvement, with each Sure Start local programme managed by a partnership board, drawn from the mainstream agencies providing services to children and families, national and local voluntary and community organisations, and parents.

The programme operates in the most deprived 20% of wards in England with Scotland, Wales and Northern Ireland having their own Sure Start programmes. It focuses on five core services: support for families and parents; support for good-quality early learning, play and childcare; health services and advice; outreach and home visiting; and support for children and parents with special needs, including help in getting access to specialised services (Stewart, 2005). Local programmes thus typically provide support for breastfeeding and healthy eating alongside parenting education, help with smoking cessation and the provision of new childcare places (see Chapter Five). It also aims to be non-stigmatising (with all families in the selected communities eligible). The initiative is, however, clearly focused on deprived areas, with low incomes, child poverty and unemployment in Sure Start areas more than double the national average (Barnes et al, 2003). Additional focus, lacking in the far more disparate HAZ initiative, is also given by four core Sure Start service targets. These commit Sure Start local programmes to improving the social and emotional development of children, reducing the proportion of parents who smoke during pregnancy, improving children's language and communication skills and, most recently, improving the employability of parents.

All 524 local programmes in England are now operational, encompassing up to 400,000 children living in disadvantaged areas – including a third of under-fours living in poverty (Meadows and Garber, 2004) and providing roughly £1,000 per child over the programme's lifetime (Stewart, 2005). This, however, compares with some 2.9 million children below compulsory school age. For the target children an assessment by the DfES suggests considerable progress has been made in terms of parenting and family support (and hence the children's social and emotional development) (see also NESS, 2004), re-registration on the child protection register and the provision of play and learning opportunities. Child health goals are, however, proving more elusive (DfES, 2003b).

The National Evaluation of Sure Start (NESS) similarly finds support for the recognition given by Sure Start to the interconnected nature and extent of social problems; the provision of a long-term funding strategy; the establishment of new relationships between professionals, parents and other members of the community; the continued focus on issues from the perspective of families; and flexibility in the way in which services are delivered (Myers et al, 2004, p 10). In an echo of the national HAZ evaluation it also reveals, however, some tensions between nationally prescribed targets and locally defined needs (see, for example, Chapter Five around employability targets). More significantly, Sure Start settings are expected to become Sure Start Children's Centres over the next few years and a feature of every community by 2010. In the process, it has been suggested that the autonomy and funding that were central to the initiative have been lost and the earlier child-centred focus and concern for community development principles replaced by an increased emphasis on childcare (Glass, 2005).

Neighbourhood renewal

If Sure Start represents an ABI where the health and well-being of a particular target group is now embedded, New Deal for Communities (NDC) and the National Strategy for Neighbourhood Renewal (NSNR) represent an attempt to include health within the wider regeneration agenda (see Chapter Eleven), for a long time focused largely on employment, housing and the physical environment. The NDC was established as a pathfinder programme for the NSNR in 1998. Seventeen pathfinder areas were designated at the outset, covering communities of up to 4,000 households, with a further 22 designations in April

1999. Health was included as one of five outcome areas, alongside crime, education, worklessness and housing, with interventions designed to close the gaps between the 39 areas and national standards. In order to tackle such a comprehensive array of problems, £2 billion was made available over 10 years. However, even in such a spatially intensive intervention more money was going into most NDCs from mainstream agencies in any one year than the £50 million which NDC designation would bring across the decade and many agencies felt designation had resulted in a corresponding reduction in mainstream funding (Lawless, 2004).

In response, the NSNR established goals for poor neighbourhoods as a whole and set out how policy interventions (and funding) by mainstream agencies would be expected to address these neighbourhood inequalities and reinforce the work of ABIs. The focus of activity was the larger but financially less intensive Neighbourhood Renewal Fund (NRF), introduced in 2001 in the 88 most deprived local authority districts. It initially provided a total funding of £900 million over the next three years to improve core services but was extended for a further three years by the 2002 Comprehensive Spending Review with a further £975 million (Atkinson, 2003). Like the NDC it has a clear ethnic dimension, with circa 70% of minority ethnic groups living in these most deprived neighbourhoods. Like the NDC, its scope also encompasses "the fundamental problems of worklessness, crime and poor public services" (SEU, 2001, p 5) with health forming one of five key outcome areas alongside employment, crime, education and housing.

The implementation of such policies has not, however, been without its critics. There is a tension between the pursuit of local agendas and the government's insistence on minimum national standards, pursued via national indicators and targets (Painter and Clarence, 2001; Powell and Moon, 2001). The need for rapid and demonstrable improvements (and the pressures of partnership) can also distort intervention (see Chapter Eleven). The need for quick wins is also at odds with the "abundant evidence … that it can take years to achieve meaningful and sustainable community involvement" (Foley and Martin, 2000, p 487), while the emphasis on direct public participation sits uneasily with traditions of local representative democracy. Finally, the stress on holistic services remains in opposition with the strongly departmentalised structure of central government. "By seeking to encourage greater local flexibility", it has been argued, "ministers have been able to pass to local policy makers much of the responsibility for resolving the paradoxes within the new regimes" (Foley and Martin, 2000, p 488). Indeed, with the advent of the Regional Coordination Unit and the community cohesion (Cantle) report (Independent Review Team, 2001) it has been argued that the emphasis is now moving away again from a focus on particular geographical areas towards thematic programmes with a more universal approach, or district-level interventions that relate clearly to LSPs (Lawless, 2004). In this context it is perhaps important to note that *The Egan Review – Skills for sustainable communities*, which argues for sustainable communities to become a common governmental goal and the focus for community strategies, does not include health among the seven attributes of a sustainable community (ODPM, 2004).

Conclusion

A common theme in much health inequalities research is the idea that health inequalities can only be addressed through a significant redistribution of income or wealth. As Graham (2004) suggests, this is because the unequal distribution of health outcomes reflects the unequal distribution of the social factors that influence health. Yet, although the government has demonstrated a strong commitment to ensuring that lower-income or disadvantaged groups are protected from poverty and social exclusion, its record on tackling *relative* poverty or inequality has been far more uncertain. With the exception of the child poverty strategy, there has been a stronger emphasis on equality of opportunity than equality of outcome and a tendency to focus on reductions in absolute poverty, often through the targeting of initiatives on an individual (means-tested) or community basis. Indeed, rather than reducing inequality, the government's commitment to promoting a market-based approach to social policy has resulted in a growth in socio-economic polarisation in several sectors.

For several reasons, including the dominance of the systematic review, there is also far more 'evidence' about the role and potential impact of 'downstream' interventions than 'upstream' policies. Thus, responsibility for taking forward the health inequalities agenda has been placed very much at the local level. It is important to establish what difference local policy makers, practitioners and agencies can make in the absence of wider socio-structural change. The government's strategy suggests an implicit assumption that health inequalities can be reduced without changing overall levels of inequality. This is by strongly targeting interventions at the poorest individuals and, through ABIs, communities. This assumption needs to be tested. It is therefore important to assess the evidence that exists about the impact of local and individualised interventions. This, of course, is the focus of the second part of the book.

References

Acheson, D. (Chair) (1998) *Independent Inquiry into Inequalities in Health*, London: The Stationery Office.

Atkinson, R. (2003) 'Urban policy', in N. Ellison and C. Pierson (eds) *Developments in British social policy 2*, Basingstoke: Palgrave Macmillan, pp 160-76.

Baldock, J., Manning, N. and Vickerstaff, S. (2003) 'Social policy, social welfare and the welfare state', in J. Baldock, N. Manning and S. Vickerstaff (eds) *Social policy* (2nd edn), Oxford: Oxford University Press, pp 3-28.

Barber, M. (2002) 'The next stage for large scale reform in England: from good to great' (www.cybertext.net.au/tct2002/disc_papers/organisation/barber.htm).

Barker, K. (2004) *Review of housing supply: Delivering stability: securing our future housing needs, Final report − Recommendations*, London: The Stationery Office.

Barnes, J., Broomfield, K., Frost, M., Harper, G., McLeod, A., Knowles, J. and Leyland, A. (2003) *Characteristics of Sure Start local programme areas: Rounds 1 to 4*, London: NESS.

Bauld, L. and Judge, K. (2002) 'Introduction: the development of Health Action Zones', in L. Bauld and K. Judge (eds) *Learning from Health Action Zones*, Chichester: Aeneas Press, pp 1-13.

Bauld, L., Judge, K., Lawson, L., Mackenzie, M., Mackinnon, J. and Truman, J. (2001) *Health Action Zones in transition: Progress in 2000*, Glasgow: University of Glasgow.

Black Report (1980) *Inequalities of health*, Report of a Research Working Group, Chair, Sir Douglas Black, London: DHSS.

Black, N. (2001) 'Evidence based policy: proceed with care', *British Medical Journal*, vol 323, no 7307, pp 275-9.

Boaz, A., Ashby, D. and Young, K. (2002) *Systematic reviews: What have they got to offer evidence based policy and practice?*, Working Paper 2, London: ESRC UK Centre for Evidence-based Policy and Practice.

Brehony, K. (2005) 'Primary schooling under New Labour: the irresolvable contradiction of excellence and enjoyment', *Oxford Review of Education*, vol 31, pp 29-46.

Brehony, K. and Deem, R. (2003) 'Education policy', in N. Ellison and C. Pierson (eds) *Developments in British Social Policy 2*, Basingstoke: Palgrave Macmillan, pp 177-93.

Brook Lyndhurst Ltd (2004) *Sustainable cities and the ageing society: The role of older people in an urban renaissance*, Report for the Office of the Deputy Prime Minister, London: Brook Lyndhurst Ltd.

Bullock, H., Mountford, J. and Stanley, R. (2001) *Better policy-making*, London: Centre for Management and Policy Studies.

Burke, S. (2005) 'Towards universal childcare', *Poverty 120*, Winter (www.cpag.org.uk/info/Povertyarticles/Poverty%20120/childcare.htm), accessed 11 July.

Cabinet Office (1999a) *Modernising government*, Cm 4310, London: The Stationery Office.

Cabinet Office (1999b) *Professional policy making for the twenty-first century*, London: Cabinet Office.

Church, J. and Whyman, S. (1997) 'A review of recent social and economic trends', in F. Drever and M. Whitehead (eds) *Health inequalities: Decennial Supplement*, London: ONS, pp 29-43.

CPRE (Campaign to Protect Rural England) (2004) *Housing the nation: Meeting the need for affordable housing − Facts, myths, solutions*, London: CPRE.

Crawshaw, P., Bunton, R. and Conway, S. (2004) 'Governing the unhealthy community: some reflections on UK Health Action Zones', *Social Theory and Health*, vol 2, no 4, pp 341-60.

CSJ (Commission on Social Justice) (1994) *Social justice: Strategies for national renewal*, London:Vintage.

Davey Smith, G. and Egger, M. (1998) 'Meta-analysis: unresolved issues and future developments', *British Medical Journal*, vol 316, pp 221-5.

Davey Smith, G., Ebrahim, S. and Frankel, S. (2001) 'How policy informs the evidence', *British Medical Journal*, vol 322, no 7280, pp 184-5.

Davis, P. and Howden-Chapman, P. (1996) 'Translating research findings into health policy', *Social Science and Medicine*, vol 43, no 5, pp 865-72.

Deacon, A. (2003) 'Social security policy', in N. Ellison and C. Pierson (eds) *Developments in British Social Policy 2*, Basingstoke: Palgrave Macmillan, pp 129-42.

DfEE (Department for Education and Employment) (1997) *Excellence in schools*, London:The Stationery Office.

DfEE (1999) *Learning to succeed*, Cm 4392, London: DfEE.

DfEE (2001) *Schools:Achieving success*, London:The Stationery Office.

DfES (Department for Education and Skills) (2003a) *A new specialist system: Transforming secondary education*, London: DfES.

DfES (2003b) *Autumn performance report 2003: Achievements against public service agreement targets*, London: DfES.

DfES (2005a) *Provision for children under five years of age in England: January 2005 (provisional)*, Statistical First Release, London: DfES.

DfES (2005b) *Participation in education, training and employment by 16-18 year olds in England: 2003 and 2004*, Statistical First Release, London: DfES.

DfES (2005c) *Higher standards, better schools for all: More choices for parents and pupils*, London: DfES.

DH (Department of Health) (1999a) *Saving lives: Our healthier nation*, London: The Stationery Office.

DH (1999b) *Reducing health inequalities: An action report: Our healthier nation*, London:The Stationery Office.

DH (2000) *The NHS Plan: A plan for investment, a plan for reform*, Cm 4818-1, London:The Stationery Office.

DH (2003) *Tackling health inequalities: A programme for action*, London: DH.

DH (2005) *Tackling health inequalities: Status report on the Programme for Action*, London: DH.

Dornan, P. (2005) 'Halving child poverty: a truly historic third term?', *Poverty*, vol 121, pp 17-18.

Drever, F. and Whitehad, M. (eds) (1997) *Health inequalities: Decennial supplement*, London: ONS.

DWP (Department for Work and Pensions) (2002) *Pathways to work: Helping people into employment*, Cm 5690, London: DWP.

DWP (2004) '£220 million expansion of successful scheme helping people on incapacity benefits get back to work', DWP (Media Centre Press Release), 2 December.

DWP (2005a) *Client group analysis: Quarterly bulletin on the population of working age on key benefits. February 2005*, London: Information Directorate, DWP.

DWP (2005b) *Department for Work and Pensions five-year strategy: Opportunity and security throughout life*, London: DWP.

DWP (2005c) *Delivering PSA targets: Supporting families and children*, London: DWP.

Elliott, H. and Popay, J. (2000) 'How are policy makers using evidence? Models of research utilisation and local NHS policy making', *Journal of Epidemiology and Community Health*, vol 54, no 6, pp 461-8.

Evandrou, M. and Falkingham, J. (2005) 'A secure retirement for all? Older people and New Labour', in J. Hills and K. Stewart (eds) *A more equal society?*, Bristol: The Policy Press, pp 167-87.

Evans, M. and Cerny, P. (2003) 'Globalization and social policy', in N. Ellison and C. Pierson (eds) *Developments in British social policy 2*, Basingstoke: Palgrave Macmillan, pp 19-40.

Exworthy, M., Stuart, M., Blane, D. and Marmot, M. (2003) *Tackling health inequalities since the Acheson inquiry*, Bristol: The Policy Press.

Finn, D. (2003) 'Employment policy', in N. Ellison and C. Pierson (eds) *Developments in British social policy 2*, Basingstoke: Palgrave Macmillan, pp 111-28.

Flaherty, J., Veit-Wilson, J. and Dornan, P. (2004) *Poverty: The facts* (5th edn), London: Child Poverty Action Group.

Foley, P. and Martin, S. (2000) 'A New Deal for the community? Public participation in regeneration and local service delivery', *Policy & Politics*, vol 28, no 4, pp 479-92.

Ford, J. (2003) 'Housing policy', in N. Ellison and C. Pierson (eds) *Developments in British social policy 2*, Basingstoke: Palgrave Macmillan, pp 143-59.

Gewirtz, S., Ball, S.J. and Bowe, R. (1994) 'Parents, privilege and the education market-place', *Research Papers in Education*, vol 9, pp 3-29.

Gibson, A. and Asthana, S. (2000) 'Local markets and the polarisation of public-sector schools in England and Wales', *Transactions of the Institute of British Geographers*, vol 25, pp 303-19.

Glass, N. (2005) 'Surely some mistake?', *The Guardian*, 5 January.

Gordon, D., Shaw, M., Dorling, D. and Davey Smith, G. (eds) (1999) *Inequalities in health: The evidence presented to the Independent Inquiry into Inequalities in Health, chaired by Sir Donald Acheson*, Bristol: The Policy Press

Graham, H. (2004) 'Social determinants and their unequal distribution: clarifying policy understandings', *The Milbank Quarterly*, vol 82, pp 101-24.

Green, A. (2003) 'Is UK education exceptionally unequal? Evidence from the IALS and PISA surveys', *Forum*, vol 45, pp 67-70.

Hatcher, R. (1998) 'Class differentiation in education: rational choices?', *British Journal of Sociology in Education*, vol 19, pp 5-24.

Haynes, P. (2003) *Managing complexity in the public services*, Maidenhead: Open University Press.

Hills, J. and Stewart, K. (2005) 'A tide turned but mountains yet to climb?', in J. Hills and K. Stewart (eds) *A more equal society?*, Bristol: The Policy Press, pp 325–46.

HIU (Health Inequalities Unit) (2005) *Tackling health inequalities: What works*, London: HIU, DH.

HM Government and DH (2004) *Choosing health: Making healthy choices easier*, London: HM Government and DH.

HM Treasury (2001) *Spending Review 2000: Public Service Agreements 2001-04*, Cm 4808, London: The Stationery Office.

HM Treasury (2004a) *Child poverty review*, London: The Stationery Office.

HM Treasury (2004b) *Choice for parents: The best start for children: A ten-year strategy for childcare*, London: HM Treasury, DfES, DWP and DTI.

HM Treasury (2004c) *2004 Spending Review: Public service agreements 2005-2008*, London: HM Treasury.

Holmans, A., Monk, S. and Whitehead, C. (2004) *Building for the future: 2004 update*, London: Shelter.

Independent Review Team, The (2001) *Community cohesion: A report of The Independent Review Team chaired by Ted Cantle*, London: Home Office.

Johnson, C. and Osborne, S.P. (2003) 'Local strategic partnerships, neighbourhood renewal, and the limits to co-governance', *Public Money & Management*, July, pp 147-54.

Judge, K., Barnes, M., Bauld, L., Benzeval, M., Killoran, A., Robinson, R., Wigglesworth, R. and Zeilig, H. (1999) 'Health Action Zones: learning to make a difference. A report submitted to the Department of Health, June 1999' (www.ukc.ac.uk/pssru), accessed 15 March 2002.

Kelly, M., Speller, V. and Meyrick, J. (2004) *Getting evidence into practice in public health*, London: Health Development Agency.

Kempson, E., McKay, S. and Willitts, M. (2004) *Characteristics of families in debt and the nature of indebtedness*, DWP Research Report No 211, London: The Stationery Office.

Lauder, H., Hughes, D., Watson, S., Waslander, S., Thrupp, M., Strathdee, R., Simiyu, I., Dupuis, A., McGlinn, J. and Hamlin, J. (1999) *Trading in futures.: Why markets in education don't work*, Buckingham: Open University Press.

Lawless, P. (2004) 'Locating and explaining area-based urban initiatives: New Deal for Communities in England', *Environment and Planning C: Government and Policy*, vol 22, no 3, pp 383-99.

Lohmander, M. (2004) 'The fading of a teaching profession? Reforms of early childhood teacher education in Sweden', *Early Years*, vol 24, pp 23-34.

Lupton, R. and Power, A. (2005) 'Disadvantaged by where you live? New Labour and neighbourhood renewal', in J. Hills and K. Stewart (eds) *A more equal society?*, Bristol: The Policy Press, pp 119-42.

MacGregor, S. (2003) 'Social exclusion', in N. Ellison and C. Pierson (eds) *Developments in British social policy 2*, Basingstoke: Palgrave Macmillan, pp 56-74.

Macintyre, S., Chalmers, I., Horton, R. and Smith, R. (2001) 'Using evidence to inform health policy: case study', *British Medical Journal*, vol 322, no 7280, pp 222-5.

McKinlay, J. (1993) 'The promotion of health through planned socio political change: challenges for research and policy', *Social Science and Medicine*, vol 36, no 2, pp 109-17.

McKnight, A. (2005) 'Employment: tackling poverty through "work for those who can"', in J. Hills and K. Stewart (eds) *A more equal society?*, Bristol: The Policy Press, pp 23-46.

Marsh, A., Gordon, D., Heslop, P. and Pantazis, C. (2000) 'Housing deprivation and health: a longitudinal analysis', *Housing Studies*, vol 15, pp 411-28.

Matka, E., Barnes, M. and Sullivan, H. (2002) 'Health Action Zones: "creating alliances to achieve change"', *Policy Studies*, vol 23, no 2, pp 97-106.

Meadows, P. and Garber, C. (2004) *Sure Start local programmes and improving the employability of parents*, London: NESS Institute for the Study of Children, Families and Social Issues, Birkbeck, University of London.

Millward, L., Kelly, M. and Nutbeam, D. (2003) *Public health intervention research: The evidence*, London: Health Development Agency.

Mortimore, P. and Whitty, G. (1997) *Can school improvement overcome the effects of disadvantage*, London: Institute of Education.

Myers, P., Barnes, J. and Brodie, I. (2004) *Partnership working in Sure Start local programmes: Synthesis of early findings from local programme evaluations*, London: NESS Institute for the Study of Children, Families and Social Issues, Birkbeck, University of London.

NAO (National Audit Office) (2002) *The New Deal for Young People*, London: The Stationery Office.

NAO (2004) *Early years: Progress in developing high quality childcare and early education accessible to all*, London: The Stationery Office.

NESS (National Evaluation of Sure Start) (2004) *The impact of Sure Start local programmes on child development and family functioning: A report on preliminary findings*, London: NESS Institute for the Study of Children, Families and Social Issues, Birkbeck, University of London.

Oakley, A. (1998) 'Experimentation and social interventions: a forgotten but important history', *British Medical Journal*, vol 317, no 7167, pp 1239-42.

Oatley, N. (2000) 'New Labour's approach to age-old problems', *Local Economy*, vol 15, no 2, pp 86-97.

ODPM (Office of the Deputy Prime Minister) (2004) *The Egan Review – Skills for sustainable communities*, London: The Stationery Office.

ONS (Office for National Statistics) (2004) *Labour force survey, national statistics*, London: ONS.

Painter, C. and Clarence, E. (2001) 'UK local action zones and changing urban governance', *Urban Studies*, vol 38, no 8, pp 1215-32.

Parjanen, M. and Tuomi, O. (2003) 'Access to higher education – persistent or changing inequality? A case study from Finland', *European Journal of Education*, vol 38, pp 55-70.

Parsons, W. (2002) 'From muddling through to muddling up – evidence based policy making and the modernisation of British government', *Public Policy and Administration*, vol 17, no 3, pp 43-60.

Pawson, R. (2001) *Evidence based policy: I. In search of a method*, Working Paper 3, London: ESRC UK Centre for Evidence-based Policy and Practice.

Pawson, R. and Tilley, N. (1997) *Realistic evaluation*, London: Sage Publications.

Petticrew, M. (2001) 'Systematic reviews from astronomy to zoology: myths and misconceptions', *British Medical Journal*, vol 322, no 7278, pp 98-101.

Petticrew, M., Whitehead, M., Macintyre, S., Graham, H. and Egan, M. (2004) 'Evidence for public health policy on inequalities: 1: the reality according to policymakers', *Journal of Epidemiology and Community Health*, vol 58, no 10, pp 811-16.

Pickvance, C. (2003) 'Housing and housing policy', in J. Baldock, N. Manning and S. Vickerstaff (eds) *Social policy* (2nd edn), Oxford: Oxford University Press, pp 486-518.

PIU (Performance and Innovation Unit) (2000) *Adding it up: Improving analysis and modelling in central government*, London: Cabinet Office.

Powell, M. and Moon, G. (2001) 'Health Action Zones: the "third" way of a new area-based policy?', *Health and Social Care in the Community*, vol 9, no 1, pp 43-50.

PricewaterhouseCoopers (2004) *Universal early education and care in 2020: Costs, benefits and funding options*, A report for the Daycare Trust and the Social Market Foundation, London: PricewaterhouseCoopers.

Quarmby, K. (2003) 'The politics of childcare', *Prospect*, November, pp 50-5.

Rychetnik, L., Frommer, M., Hawe, P. and Shiell, A. (2002) 'Criteria for evaluating evidence on public health interventions', *Journal of Epidemiology and Community Health*, vol 56, no 2, pp 119-27.

Sanderson, I. (2002) 'Making sense of "what works": evidence based policy making as instrumental rationality?', *Public Policy and Administration*, vol 17, no 3, pp 61-75.

Schön, D.A. (1983) *The reflective practitioner*, New York, NY: Basic Books.

Scrambler, G. (2001) 'Critical realism, sociology and health inequalities: social class as a generative mechanism and its media of enactment', *Journal of Critical Realism*, vol 4, pp 35-42.

SEU (Social Exclusion Unit) (2001) *A new commitment to neighbourhood renewal: National strategy action plan*, London: Cabinet Office.

Shaw, M., Davey Smith, G. and Dorling, D. (2005) 'Health inequalities and New Labour: how the promises compare with real progress', *British Medical Journal*, vol 330, pp 1016-21.

Shaw, M., Dorling, D., Gordon, D. and Davey Smith, G. (1999) *The widening gap: Health inequalities and policy in Britain*, Bristol: The Policy Press.

Smith, G.R. (1999) *Area-based initiatives: The rationale and options for area targeting*, CASE Paper 25, London: Centre for Analysis of Social Exclusion, London School of Economics and Political Science.

Speller, V., Learmonth, A. and Harrison, D. (1997) 'The search for evidence of effective health promotion', *British Medical Journal*, vol 315, no 7104, pp 361-3.

Stewart, K. (2005) 'Towards an equal start? Addressing childhood poverty and deprivation', in J. Hills and K. Stewart (eds) *A more equal society?*, Bristol: The Policy Press, pp 143-65.

Sutherland, H., Sefton, T. and Piachaud, D. (2003) *Poverty in Britain: The impact of government policy since 1997*, York: Joseph Rowntree Foundation.

Swedish Institute (2001) *Childcare in Sweden*, Factsheet on Sweden, Stockholm: Swedish Institute.

Sylva, K. and Pugh, G. (2005) 'Transforming the early years in England', *Oxford Review of Education*, vol 31, pp 11-27.

Taylor, C., Fitz, J. and Gorard, S. (2005) 'Diversity, specialisation and equity in education', *Oxford Review of Education*, vol 31, pp 47-69.

Taylor, R. (2005) 'Lifelong learning and the Labour governments, 1997-2004', *Oxford Review of Education*, vol 31, pp 101-18.

Thomas, B. and Dorling, D. (2004) *Know your place: Housing wealth and inequality in Great Britain 1980-2003 and beyond*, London: Shelter.

Thrupp, M. (1999) *Schools making a difference: Let's be realistic!*, Buckingham: Open University Press.

Tomlinson, S. (1997) 'Diversity, choice and ethnicity', *Oxford Review of Education*, vol 23, pp 67-76.

Tomlinson, S. (2005) 'Race, ethnicity and education under New Labour', *Oxford Review of Education*, vol 31, pp 153-71.

Towner, E., Dowswell, T., Mackereth, C. and Jarvis, S. (2001) *What works in preventing unintentional injuries in children and young adolescents? An updated systematic review*, London: Health Development Agency.

Tunstall, R. and Lupton, R. (2003) *Is targeting deprived areas an effective means to reach poor people? An assessment of one rationale for area based funding programmes*, CASE Paper 70, London: Centre for Analysis of Social Exclusion, London School of Economics and Political Science.

Tunstill, J., Allnock, D., Meadows, P. and McLeod, A. (2002) *Early experiences of implementing Sure Start*, London: National Evaluation of Sure Start Implementation Team.

UNICEF (United Nations Children's Fund) (2002) *A league table of educational disadvantage in rich nations*, Florence, Italy: UNICEF Innocenti Research Centre.

Vegeris, S. and McKay, S. (2002) *Low/moderate-income families in Britain: Changes in living standards, 1999-2000*, DWP Research Report No 164, London: The Stationery Office.

Vegeris, S. and Perry, J. (2003) *Families and children 2001: Living standards and the children*, DWP Research Report No 190, London: The Stationery Office.

Victor, C. (1991) *Health and health care in later life*, Milton Keynes: Open University Press.

Walford, G. (2005) 'Introduction: education and the labour government', *Oxford Review of Education*, vol 31, pp 3-9.

Wanless, D. (2002) *Securing our future health: Taking a long-term view: Final report*, London: HM Treasury.

Part 2:
Health inequalities pathways, policies and practice through the lifecourse

In this main part of the book, we examine the pathways, policies and practice of health inequalities throughout the lifecourse. As observed in Chapter One, this structure reflects the theoretical orientation of health inequalities research in recent years. It allows us to explore the links between social determinants of health, mediating biological factors and health outcomes and to assess the role of interventions targeting these linkages. It is also broad enough to accommodate more standard approaches to public health (which focus on the role of different risk factors, population groups, policy sectors and health outcomes).

Four critical periods are examined in this section (early life, childhood and youth, adulthood and older age). For each period, chapters are respectively devoted to evidence of health inequalities and the pathways that give rise to health inequalities and to evidence of 'what works' in tackling such health inequalities. Chapter Four, for example, begins by considering research evidence that links early life factors (during pregnancy, infancy and early childhood) to adverse health outcomes. It then discusses the significance of early life experiences to health inequalities. By linking epidemiological evidence that highlights key risk factors to evidence of the social context of risk, it notes that it is theoretically possible to identify the kinds of policy interventions that could improve the healthy development of young children from disadvantaged backgrounds. Thus, on the basis of the evidence provided, smoking cessation, nutrition (with some qualifications), parenting education and early years education and care emerge as key areas for intervention. Chapter Five focuses on these health behaviours. For each area, research evidence of 'what works' is carefully assessed, the limitations of the existing evidence base examined and the recent development of key policy initiatives described. In what is to become an important theme of the book, the tensions that emerge in translating policy recommendations into actual policy mechanisms are explored and the point made that outcomes vary according to a wide range of factors such as content, process, context and the characteristics of the intervention group. The chapter nevertheless concludes by suggesting that it is possible to identify effective interventions and that these tend to be multifaceted.

Despite earlier evidence that suggested that childhood and youth is a period of relative health equality, more recent research has highlighted clear social gradients in current health status. Chapter Six explores some of the methodological considerations involved in the investigation of health inequalities among children and young people and then examines social variations in current mortality and morbidity. Significant variations are found to exist with respect to accidents, injuries and mental health. Chapter Seven focuses on those areas. As in Chapter Five, research evidence of 'what works' is carefully assessed, the limitations of the existing evidence base examined and the recent development of key policy initiatives described. Again, the uneven typology of evidence, policy and practice is highlighted. For example, intervention and policy do not accord equal emphasis across the wide age range encompassed by childhood and youth. Those focusing on accidents and injuries tend to place more emphasis on childhood, while those that focus on mental health, substance abuse and sexual health tend to place more stress on early youth. Few initiatives, by contrast, take late youth as their focus. Indeed, the lack of appropriate services for children in areas such as mental health has long been a cause of concern without the added complication that young people in late adolescence and beyond might also require a differentiated approach.

In addition to variations in current mortality and morbidity, 'lifestyle patterns' tend to be established during childhood and youth. Thus, inequalities in health behaviours during this age form an important pathway by which health variations in later life develop. Continuities in socio-economic circumstances are also an important reason why childhood disadvantage predicts poor health in adulthood. These issues are explored in Chapter Eight, which finds little evidence to suggest that influences such as youth culture are reversing social class differences in health behaviours, many of which are strongly subject to social gradients. Areas discussed include diet and nutrition, physical exercise, substance misuse and sexual behaviour. The evidence base of interventions targeting these areas and recent developments in policy and practice are discussed in Chapter Nine.

Growing interest in the relationship between childhood disadvantage and adult health has quite rightly addressed the neglect of early life influences in a literature previously dominated by a concentration on adult risk factors for chronic adulthood disease. However, it is important that the pendulum does not swing away from a concern with adult risk factors to an excess concentration on early life influences. As we discuss in Chapter Ten, lifestyle factors, psychosocial health, material living conditions and access to key services during adulthood are still of significance to health variations. These sources of vulnerability are the focus of attention in Chapter Eleven, which explores the evidence base for 'what works' and its relationship to the policy environment. We note, however, that the evidence base for interventions targeting psychosocial health and material deprivation is far more tenuous than for behavioural interventions targeting lifestyle. This dissonance between the existing evidence base for public health, with its focus on individualised interventions, and the continuing requirement for structural solutions to health inequalities is a theme to which we return in the final chapter of the book.

In the last pair of chapters in this section, we turn our attention to health inequalities in older age. Because older people are more likely to be living in poverty, many of the factors that present health risks for younger age groups (for example, nutrition, housing quality and transport) would also be expected to impact on health inequalities among older people. Despite this, with respect to health inequalities research, older age has been a relatively neglected period. Examining evidence of health variations in older age, Chapter Twelve finds little justification for this lack of interest. Although differentials in health status decline after middle age, there is sufficient evidence to suggest that lower socio-economic status is associated with greater mortality, poorer mental health and a higher prevalence of disability among older people. While this in part reflects the lifecourse accumulation of disadvantage, current socio-economic circumstances also appear to shape the health of older people, suggesting that this remains an important period during which to target lifestyle and environmental interventions. Because chronic and degenerative diseases primarily manifest during older age, this is also a stage in the lifecourse when access to healthcare can make a significant difference. Chapter Thirteen considers efforts to improve the health and well-being of older citizens through lifestyle/behavioural interventions, initiatives that target housing and living standards and initiatives designed to improve access to health and social care. In contrast to policy and practice focusing on infants, children and young people, however, we note that relatively little evidence of the kind that lends itself to systematic reviews has been produced on this age group, suggesting that research itself may be subject to problems of ageism.

FOUR

Early life and health inequalities: research evidence

Introduction

As discussed in Chapter Two, early life has become a key focus for both research and policy relating to health inequalities, in part because of the recognition that several risk factors for disease that manifest in later life begin during this earlier stage of the lifecourse. The importance attached to improving health in the early years also reflects the fact that, despite the positive impact of recent changes to the tax and benefit system, rates of child poverty in Britain remain high. Using a poverty line of 60% of median income, an estimated 25% of British children were living in poverty in 2003/04 after housing costs are accounted for (Piachaud and Sutherland, 2002). Thus, it is important to target factors that are associated with poverty and deprivation and that are known to present risks to healthy development.

The strong focus on children may also reflect a perception that there is greater practical scope to design and implement child health interventions than to tackle the processes by which social disadvantage impacts on adult health. At least some of the factors that are known to adversely affect child development appear to lend themselves to medical, behavioural and educational interventions that, compared with the policy implications of tackling problems such as low income, unemployment and poor housing, seem 'contained'. Children's capacity to develop cognitive skills, effective coping strategies and improved self-esteem are believed to be more adaptable than that of adults (Wadsworth, 1999). Insofar as young children and their mothers are already major users of health and other community services, they represent a relatively 'captive' population for certain intervention programmes (although issues of access and non-attendance must be considered). The existing base of community services also provides a springboard from which to launch child development initiatives that may not carry the stigma of new programmes that are specifically targeted at 'excluded' groups.

In assessing the significance of early life experiences to health inequalities, a distinction has been made between latent, pathway and cumulative effects (see Chapter Two). This distinction is important because it has implications for the choice of when and how to intervene to reduce health inequalities (Evans, 2002, p 53). If, as postulated by the model of latency effects, specific biological and developmental factors in early life have a lifelong impact on health and well-being, then interventions to eradicate health inequalities should be strongly focused on maternal and child health. Indeed, if early life programming is the main stimulus for susceptibility to adult disease, there would appear to be little point in intervening later in the lifecourse. Cumulative and pathway models offer a different message. Like the good fairy in the tale of *Sleeping beauty*, they suggest that the impact of early disadvantage can be ameliorated. However, as these models tend to place greater emphasis on the ways in which biological factors are integrated with social risk processes, their policy implications are significantly more challenging.

Notwithstanding the fact that lifecourse researchers themselves are calling for a less polarised approach that avoids treating these models as mutually exclusive paradigms, research that focuses on latency effects (and that appears to spell out *clear* biological and developmental pathways that can be targeted for intervention) has elicited a stronger policy response than other lifecourse models. Such research is the focus of this chapter that begins by considering research evidence that links early life factors to adverse health outcomes. It then discusses the significance of early life experiences to health inequalities. By linking epidemiological evidence that highlights key risk factors to evidence of the social context of risk, we note that it is theoretically possible to identify the kinds of policy interventions that could improve the healthy development of young children from disadvantaged backgrounds. However, as the chapter concludes, it is one thing to derive theoretical policy recommendations and another to translate them into practice.

The biology of risk

Risk factors before birth

There is a large body of evidence that suggests that risk for many chronic conditions is set, at least in part, in very early life (Marmot and Wadsworth, 1997). Barker and colleagues have investigated extensively the relationship between early physical development and later adult outcomes. According to Barker, "undernutrition and other adverse influences arising in foetal life or immediately after birth have a permanent effect on the body's structure, physiology and metabolism" (Barker, 1994, p 21). For example, airway and alveolar growth can be impaired in the lungs of a foetus deprived of calories or oxygen and this may have an important effect on childhood respiratory illness and risk for chronic bronchitis in later life (Dezateux and Stocks, 1997). Low protein intake during pregnancy has been linked to the impaired development of the kidneys that may in turn lead to raised blood pressure in adult life. Although the brain tends to be 'spared' in relation to other organs, early undernutrition also adversely affects healthy brain development. Most of a human's lifetime supply of brain cells is produced between the fourth and seventh months of gestation and although the production of synapses and neural pathways continues after early life, it is particularly active in utero and during the first year (McCain and Mustard, 1999, pp 26-7).

As well as leading to the suboptimal development of vital organs, growth retardation in utero has been linked to important metabolic changes that increase risk for later obesity, cardiovascular disease, hypertension and diabetes (Remacle et al, 2004). For example, Barker has argued that impaired liver development disturbs cholesterol metabolism and blood clotting, both of which are important features of coronary heart disease (CHD) (Barker, 1997, p 100). Poor nutrition during critical periods of foetal life has also been linked with changes in glucose-insulin metabolism (Hales et al, 1991; Hales and Barker, 2001). According to the 'thrifty phenotype' hypothesis, undernutrition gives the foetus a forecast of the nutritional environment into which it will be born. Processes are thus set into motion that lead to a postnatal metabolism adapted to survive under conditions of poor nutrition. Under conditions of plentiful nutrition, however, these adaptations become detrimental, insulin resistance and glucose intolerance leading to accelerated weight gain and the subsequent development of the metabolic syndrome (a constellation of risk factors that includes a propensity to central obesity, hypertension, blood fat disorders and insulin resistance and that significantly increases risk for cardiovascular disease and premature death).

Barker's theory of 'biological programming' (Barker, 1994) has received considerable attention in both the media and policy circles, for instance influencing the recommendation made by the Acheson Inquiry for measures to improve the diets of girls and women (Acheson, 1998, p 70). Research suggests that the balance of particular nutrients such as protein and carbohydrates and levels of micronutrients may have important effects on foetal growth and the programming of later disease risk. For example, there is some evidence to suggest that high carbohydrate intake in early pregnancy suppresses placental growth, especially if combined with a low dairy protein intake in late pregnancy (Godfrey et al, 1996). Poorer foetal growth and an increased placenta-to-birth weight ratio (a factor that predicts adult disorders) have also been reported in women with iron deficiency anaemia (Godfrey et al, 1991). Severe folic acid deficiency has been associated with a range of problems, notably neural tube defects (MRC Vitamin Study Research Group, 1991); and lack of n–3 fatty acids during pregnancy linked with poorer placental function (Nelson, 1999) and reduced brain development in the foetus (Helland et al, 2003; Daniels et al, 2004). A role for selenium and iron intake has also been tentatively proposed in influencing risk for wheezing and eczema in early childhood (Shaheen et al, 2004).

Against this, other studies question the significance of maternal diet to foetal growth in countries such as the UK. Mathews et al (1999) found little association between placental and infant birth weights and maternal diet among a cohort of British women, concluding that, among the relatively well-nourished women in industrialised countries, concern over the impact of maternal diet on the health of the infant had been premature. Similarly, data from the Avon Longitudinal Study of Parents and Children (ALSPAC) found no evidence that maternal diet in pregnancy has an important influence on offspring height, sitting height, leg length (Leary et al, 2005a) or blood pressure (Leary et al, 2005b). Barker himself has proposed that a mother's physiological capacity to nourish her foetus is established when she is in utero (Barker, 1994, p124), which suggests that inequalities in birth weight today may partly reflect poor maternal and infant health in the past.

To reconcile the apparent paradox between the role that nutrition plays in the regulation of foetal growth and the lack of relationship between maternal diet and infant birth weights, Harding (2001) points out the need to distinguish maternal nutrition from foetal nutrition. While factors such as micronutrient deficiencies play a role in biological programming due to unhealthy maternal diets, foetal growth is also influenced by other factors. These include uterine blood flow and the capacity of the placenta to metabolise key nutrients, to transfer nutrients to the growing foetus and to produce hormones that influence foetal and maternal nutritional supply. Intriguingly, maternal stress appears to play a role in a number of these functions. For example, stress-related hormones may constrict blood flow to the placenta, so the baby may not receive the nutrients and oxygen it needs for optimal growth. High levels of stress have been linked to elevated levels of corticotropin-releasing hormone (CRH) that sets the placental clock for early delivery (Hobel et al, 1999; Schulkin, 1999). Babies who are born prematurely are often of low birth weight. However, studies also suggest that babies of women who suffer from elevated levels of CRH are more likely to be of low birth weight even when born at full term (Wadhwa et al, 2004).

In addition to these 'direct' effects, stress may indirectly increase risk of adverse exposures in utero by influencing behaviours such as cigarette smoking. Although more attention has been paid to the direct effects of smoking and alcohol misuse on the developing foetus, there is also evidence of secondary nutritional effects. Nicotine readily crosses the placenta and may compete with nutrients for placental nutrient carriers, thus reducing nutrient transfer and therefore foetal growth (Blackburn, 2003, p 322). Alcohol may also deplete levels of specific nutrients, such as Vitamin A and zinc, by decreasing nutrient intake, altering gastrointestinal absorption and compromising metabolism (Hannigan and Abel, 1996, p 87).

Maternal substance misuse also has a range of direct effects on foetal growth and development. Smoking is associated with low birth weight, intrauterine growth restriction, placental abruption, premature rupture of the membranes and pre-term delivery. Alterations in lung function have been reported with in utero exposure to smoking and an increased risk of asthma, pneumonia and bronchitis reported in children of smokers. Smoking causes direct damage to the blood vessels of the placenta and affects the flow of oxygen to the foetus. Carcinogens are carried across the placenta and individuals exposed to tobacco smoke in the womb may be at increased risk of developing cancers such as non-

Hodgkin lymphoma, acute lymphoblastic leukaemia and central nervous system tumours (Filippini et al, 2000; Blackburn, 2003, p 321). The development of the ovaries and testes also appear to be affected by smoking. A woman whose mother smoked has a greater chance of starting her periods early and of having a miscarriage. Boys are more likely to have undescended testes. Thus, having a mother who smokes has an impact on more than just one generation (Selwyn, 2000, p 27).

Alcohol can also interfere with normal foetal development. Foetal Alcohol Syndrome (FAS), the main features of which are poor growth, abnormal facial features and cognitive impairment, appears only to arise in a small percentage of cases where sustained heavy drinking occurs throughout all three trimesters of pregnancy. However, the foetus is susceptible to alcohol's toxicity throughout its development and exposure to high levels of alcohol (particularly binge drinking) during critical periods has been linked with adverse pregnancy outcomes (Whitty and Sokol, 1996). Drug use during pregnancy has also raised concerns about persistent adverse effects (Arendt et al, 1999; Chiriboga et al, 1999) and these are not limited to the use of illegal substances. For example, research from ALSPAC suggests that maternal use of paracetamol in late pregnancy increases risks of wheezing and elevated Immunoglobulin E in children of school age (Shaheen et al, 2005).

While Barker's biological programming hypothesis and related research has focused in particular on biological risk factors, a growing body of research is exploring the interplay between biological and psychological/behavioural influences on foetal development (Mancuso et al, 2004; Pike, 2005). As noted earlier, maternal stress has been implicated in risk of prematurity and low birth weight. It has also been linked to increased risk of adverse neurodevelopment and chronic degenerative disease in adulthood (Wadhwa et al, 2002; Hobel and Culhane, 2003; Huizink et al, 2003; O'Connor et al, 2003). This is likely to be an important area for future research as it may cast further light on the factors that give rise to growth restraint and physiological change in utero and the relative role that nutritional factors play in shaping foetal development.

Development during infancy

According to Barker, optimal child development is not only determined in utero but remains at risk during the first year of life (Barker, 1994). Several studies suggest that babies who are small or thin at birth but who then show significant 'catch-up' growth in the first one to two years of life have increased risk for disease in adulthood (Bavdekar et al, 1999; Eriksson et al, 1999; Forsén et al, 1999; Ong et al, 2000; Barker et al, 2001). This may be because babies who are thin at birth lack muscle. If they go on to develop a high body mass index in childhood, they may have a disproportionately high fat mass, a factor associated with increased risk for both diabetes and CHD. Alternatively, the link between catch-up growth and CHD may reflect persisting changes in the secretion of hormones which are established in utero in response to undernutrition (or indeed other adverse influences) and which influence both childhood growth and the development of adult disease. As noted earlier, the 'thrifty phenotype' hypothesis suggests that undernutrition in utero sets processes into motion that lead to a postnatal metabolism adapted to survive under conditions of poor nutrition. Good nutrition in the postnatal period thus results in accelerated weight gain (Hales and Barker, 2001).

Increased appetite and nutrition appear to play a role in rapid catch-up growth, which raises questions about the role that appropriate diet in infancy can play in conferring a protective effect. Breast milk is generally described as the ideal source of adequate nutrition for babies as its complex composition includes a wide range of specific nutrients and bioactive substances that enhance optimal growth and development. However, evidence of a protective effect of breastfeeding against rapid catch-up in infancy and later obesity is inconclusive (Parsons et al, 1999). Despite an earlier assumption that prolonged and exclusive breastfeeding is more likely to produce lower infant weight gain than bottle feeding, recent evidence suggests that by 12 months there are no significant differences in weight gain between early and late weaners (Kramer et al, 2002, 2003). Indeed, breastfeeding may promote faster growth in infants compromised by poor growth in utero (Lucas et al, 1998).

In the 1958 British birth cohort, breastfeeding was not associated with body mass index in childhood (Parsons et al, 2003). However, data from the Scottish Child Health Surveillance Programme suggest that breastfeeding is associated with a modest reduction in childhood obesity risk (Armstrong et al, 2002). In the ALSPAC sample, breastfeeding was also found to be associated with reduced risk of child obesity, but only among children of women who did not smoke during pregnancy (Reilly et al, 2005). A recent systematic review concludes that breastfeeding has a small but consistent protective effect against obesity in children (Arenz et al, 2004). Tracking forward to adulthood, however, many studies find no association between breastfeeding and later obesity (Power and Parsons, 2000; Eriksson et al, 2003; Parsons et al, 2003).

If the protective effect of breastfeeding against obesity is subject to debate, breast milk is known to offer a number of other important benefits. It comes in its own hygienic 'container' (thus reducing exposure to external pathogens). It promotes the maturation of the gut and may actively stimulate the infant's immune system, thus offering efficient protection against infection. Breastfeeding may help to prevent respiratory morbidity (Oddy et al, 2003a) and the development of allergic diseases, especially among high-risk infants (Hanson et al, 2002, 2003; van Odijk et al, 2003). Evidence of a relationship between infant feeding method, blood pressure and cholesterol levels has suggested that breastfeeding may have long-term benefits for cardiovascular health (Forsyth et al, 2003; Owen et al, 2003). However, data from ALSPAC questions this (Martin et al, 2005). There is also interest in the role of long chain polyunsaturated fatty acids in breast milk in enhancing visual and cognitive development (Makrides et al, 2000; Oddy et al, 2003b).

In addition to its nutritional benefits, breastfeeding is valued as a way of providing positive sensory stimulation through touch, sight, sound, taste, warmth and smell. The quality of sensory stimulation in early life influences the 'wiring' of the nerve cells (neurons) and neural pathways of the brain, having "a direct and decisive effect on a child's brain development" (McCain and Mustard, 1999, p 26). Accumulating evidence suggests that negative experiences in infancy, including abuse, neglect and social deprivation, produce a cascade of neurobiological events that in turn affect emotional, behavioural, cognitive and physiological development (Glaser, 2000; Bremner and Vermetten, 2001; Sanchez et al, 2001, Teicher et al, 2003; Shea et al, 2005). Neurohumoral changes, especially to the hypothalamic-pituitary-adrenal axis, combined with structural and functional changes in certain midbrain and limbic areas, imply long-lasting effects that are difficult to overcome later (McCain and Mustard, 1999). Early adverse experiences have thus been associated with increased risk of socio-emotional problems and psychiatric disorders such as depression in later life (Mullen et al, 1996; Bremner and Vermetten, 2001). Children deprived of appropriate stimulation are also more likely to have cognitive and behavioural difficulties and are at greater risk of engaging in antisocial and criminal behaviour as young adults (McCain and Mustard, 1999, p 35). Alterations to the functioning of the hypothalamic-pituitary-adrenal axis have also been implicated in metabolic changes that increase risk of cardiovascular disease in later life and that contribute to impaired immune function, diabetes and the development of musculoskeletal disorders (Lundberg, 1999; Charmandari et al, 2003).

Although there is plentiful evidence to suggest that loving care and positive stimulation do make a difference to learning, behaviour and health throughout life, important questions remain about the relationship between early sensory stimulation and brain development. These relate as much to the 'bio' as to the 'social' in biosocial models of early child development (Granger and Kivlighan, 2003). For example, the nearly sole reliance on salivary cortisol to assess the nature and function of the hypothalamic-pituitary-adrenal axis has been questioned, as this may have led researchers to overlook the potentially protective role of other hormones secreted by the adrenal gland. Concern has also been expressed about the use of linear analyses in developmental psychology as the relationships between hormones and behaviour are probably U-shaped rather than linear, moderate amounts of hormones leading to better functioning than either too little or too much (Granger and Kivlighan, 2003).

Turning to social factors, little is known about the relative impacts of chronic stress and acute traumatic experiences, nor about the degree of adversity involved in long-term damage. Some researchers have focused on the relationship between severe forms of maltreatment such as extreme neglect, physical and sexual abuse and later negative outcomes (Rutter et al, 1998; O'Connor et al, 2000). By contrast, others propose that even subtle forms of 'maltreatment', such as emotional withdrawal by mothers (for example, as a consequence of maternal depression), or a failure to respond sensitively to the developing infant, have long-term negative consequences on socio-emotional health, cognitive development and immune disorders (Bugental et al, 2003). There are questions, too, about individual variability in vulnerability and about the brain's capacity to compensate for poor development during the early period. Some studies show that children who have faced such adversities can and do overcome tremendous hardship (Werner and Smith, 1992). Others suggest that as the brain rapidly loses its plasticity with age, the window of opportunity to reverse dysfunction is limited. The subsequent call for very early intervention to improve developmental opportunities raises fears that older children may be 'written off' as beyond help (Selwyn, 2000).

While much of the recent interest in infant care has focused on the social environment, optimal infant development also depends on the provision of a safe physical environment. The risks of exposure to pathogens in unhygienic environments are well known in very low-income countries where a synergistic relationship exists between malnutrition and repeated bouts of infection in highly vulnerable children. Among the relatively well-nourished children of industrial countries, growth retardation due to repeated infection does not appear to be a significant problem. Good hygiene clearly reduces the likelihood of harmful contact with pathogens and has been linked with reduced risk for gastrointestinal disease. In the West, however, more concern has been expressed about the health risks associated with excessive cleanliness. This may lead to a lack of exposure to certain types of infectious agents that stimulate a balanced immune response, leading to a rise in atopic illness such as wheeze and atopic eczema (Rook and Stanford, 1998; Sherriff et al, 2002).

The respiratory health of infants is susceptible to a number of environmental risk factors, including home dampness, low ventilation and exposure to tobacco smoke (Lodrup Carlsen, 2002). The latter has been associated with an increased risk for lower respiratory tract infections, chronic middle ear disease and asthma (Gaffney, 2001; Rushton et al, 2003). Lower respiratory tract infection during infancy may increase risk for chronic bronchitis in adult life (Barker, 1994, p 103). Research suggests that, compared with later childhood, early infancy is a period of increased vulnerability of the airways to tobacco products (Nuesslein et al, 2002).

Air pollutants have also been implicated in respiratory morbidity in children, such as acute respiratory disease, aggravated asthma and lower lung function (Bates, 1995; Pershagen et al, 1995). However, statistical evidence of a relationship between key pollutants (such as nitrogen dioxide) and infant health outcomes has been weak or inconclusive (Farrow et al, 1997; Brauer et al, 2002). There is also little evidence to support earlier concerns that exposure to traffic-related air pollution increases the risk of developing cancer during childhood, with the possible exception of risk for Hodgkin's disease (Raaschou–Nielsen et al, 2001).

Development during early childhood

As in infancy, excessive weight gain in early childhood may signal increased risk of disease in later life because it is underpinned by metabolic changes that occurred in response to growth restraint in utero (Ong and Dunger, 2002; Power and Jefferis, 2002; Singhal et al, 2003). There is some evidence to suggest that, by creating hormonal imbalances, alterations in the functioning of the hypothalamic-pituitary–adrenal axis (caused, for example, by emotional deprivation and psychosocial stress) may predispose individuals to central obesity (Power and Parsons, 2000). Childhood obesity is also understood to have a genetic basis (Kiess et al, 2001). Indeed, one area of current interest is the way in which genetic factors interact with intrauterine growth restraint to create differential risk of impaired glucose tolerance and the metabolic syndrome (Ong and Dunger, 2004).

With growing evidence supporting the role of early life factors in determining risk of later obesity, the role of the usual suspects behind the epidemic of childhood obesity (lack of physical activity and an increased consumption of fast food, sweets, sugary drinks and snacks) has been open to question. There is, however, a general acceptance that diet and activity play a role. Analysis of ALSPAC data found that preschool dietary patterns were generally not significantly associated with risk of obesity at age seven, although there was some relationship with a junk food type dietary pattern at age three. The likelihood of being obese also increased with the amount of television that young children watched and was inversely related to sleep duration. In other respects, however, the study supported the role of the early life environment in programming regulation of energy balance. Infants who experienced catch-up growth between birth and two years and/or who had high rates of weight gain in the first 12 months were at significantly increased risk of being obese in childhood (Reilly et al, 2005). There remains uncertainty about the relative role of different factors in the development of obesity (Power and Parsons, 2000). While low birth weight has traditionally been associated with increased risk for obesity and other risk factors that make up the metabolic syndrome, birth weight in ALSPAC was positively and linearly associated with risk. Wilkin et al (2004) similarly report a dissociation between birth weight and weight at five years of age, suggesting that poor nutrition during gestation, as expressed by low birth weight, may no longer be a clear marker of later disease risk.

Although obesity in childhood has been identified as a major public health problem that is associated with negative consequences in both the short and long term (Reilly et al, 2003), much of the evidence of obesity prevalence in childhood, of its impact on health and of interventions used in its prevention and treatment focuses on *school-aged* children and adolescents. The prevalence of obesity does increase with age (Kinra et al, 2000) and, as evidence suggests that, over time, the distribution of overweight is skewing further to the right (Livingstone, 2001), it is perhaps understandable that those children who are already exhibiting adverse health effects have been targeted as a particular cause for concern (see Chapter Eight, this volume). However, it should not be assumed that obesity is not a significant problem among younger children. Of children aged three to four from the Scottish Child Health Surveillance Programme, 8.5% were found to be obese, and 4.3% severely so (Armstrong et al, 2003). Looking over a 10-year period at weight and body mass index in children aged four years and under in the Wirral, Bundred et al (2001) report a highly significant increasing trend in the proportion of overweight and obese children. Analysis of Health Survey for England (HSE) data similarly found that the proportions of obesity in three-year-old girls had increased from 4.5% in 1995 to 9.1% in 2000 (from 2.9% to 5% in boys) (Nessa and Gallagher, 2004). While the way in which these studies have measured the prevalence of obesity in young children has been subject to criticism (see Chapter Eight), these findings are suggestive of a significant upward trend.

As just noted, the role of diet in the development of childhood obesity is uncertain. However, there is no doubt that the consumption of sugary foods, snacks and fizzy drinks is linked to poor dental health (Watt et al, 2000; Eckersley and Blinkhorn, 2001; Freeman et al, 2001). Dental health problems have been observed in very young children. In one UK study, visible dental plaque was present in 18% and 25% of children at 12 and 18 months of age, respectively (Habibian et al, 2001). In the 2001/02 survey coordinated by the British Association for the Study of Community Dentistry, 40% of five-year-old children in England and Wales had evidence of caries experience (Pitts et al, 2003).

After the age of one, as children become more mobile, risk of injury increases. Under the age of five, children have most accidents at home, as this is where they spend most of their time. In 1999, over one million UK children under 15 visited hospital as a result of an accident that had occurred at home. Of these, 579,000 were aged under five. Falls account for the vast majority of accidents in young children, although in 1999 30,000 attended hospital after a suspected poisoning, 6,500 after a scald and over 2,500 after choking (CAPT, 2002a).

In addition to physical risks, the social environment shapes the health and well-being of young children. As in infancy, early child development requires nurturing or positive stimulation and, although a significant amount of brain development occurs before the age of one, key wiring and sculpting processes continue up to the age of six and particularly in the first three years. There appear to be differences in the plasticity of different brain functions. Thus, while the sensitive period for emotional regulation and arousal wanes between the ages of two and five, the part of the brain that is responsible for abstract cognition and language remains sensitive to positive stimulation throughout and beyond the preschool period (McCain and Mustard, 1999).

Such evidence raises difficult questions about the timing of interventions to minimise the negative impacts of early disadvantage. If a great deal of brain development takes place in the first three years, then questions could be asked about the emphasis in early intervention programmes to date on three- to five-year-old children (see Chapter Five). Neural networks that regulate response to stress and capacity for self-control are in a critical stage of development before the age of three. As a reduced ability to tolerate stress or novel sensory stimulation not only affects cognitive ability, but also mental health, antisocial behaviour, and potentially risks for chronic disease, efforts to promote optimal child development should perhaps begin well before children reach the age of preschool entry (Dawson et al, 2000; DiPietro, 2000).

Questions then arise about the difference that schools can make to educational attainment and other outcomes such as attitudinal and personal qualities and behaviour (see Chapter Eight). Research certainly suggests that non-school factors (such as socio-economic status) are a hugely important source of variation in educational attainment (Gibson and Asthana, 1998a, 1998b). However, recent analysis of the UK British Cohort Study suggests that changes in cognitive performance in middle childhood (ages 5-10) are strongly predictive of adult outcomes (such as income, educational success, unemployment, criminality, teen parenthood, smoking and depression) and often outweigh the effects of cognitive development before the age of five years (Feinstein and Bynner, 2004). This finding is compatible with results that show that schools can make a difference in setting the basis for learning and behaviour throughout life (that is, all is not determined in the preschool years) but that when schools do have an independent effect on performance, this is greater for primary than for secondary-level education (Sparkes, 1999).

Making the links between early child development and health inequalities

Despite the apparent scientific objectivity of studies that link early life experiences to later health outcomes, such research does not lend itself to objective explanations of health inequalities or to precise and uncontroversial policy implications. Part of the problem stems from the methodological difficulties of teasing out the independent effects of different variables that are not only closely associated with each other, but that also appear to contribute to similar health outcomes. For example, a wide range of early life factors has been implicated in risk of CHD in later life. These include maternal smoking, diet and chronic stress; low birth weight, rapid postnatal catch-up growth, method of infant feeding and nutrition during early childhood; and emotional deprivation or absence of appropriate stimulation. Epidemiological studies inevitably focus on the relationship between one or two of these factors and adverse health outcomes and, in so doing, introduce bias regarding the prominence given to both the chosen independent variable and the chosen confounding variable(s). Is it, for instance, significant that research on biological programming often controls for smoking but rarely for psychological status?

By isolating variables of interest by statistical control, epidemiological research also runs the risk of wrongly treating variables that mediate risk as confounding factors (Kramer et al, 2000). For example, recent research has demonstrated that the more time children spent in non-maternal care during the first four-and-a-half years of life, the more problem behaviours they exhibited. In examining the effects of childcare, many potential confounding variables were controlled for, including income and maternal depression (NICHD Early Child Care Research Network, 2003). Newcombe (2003) suggests that, by concentrating on the 'pure effects' of using childcare, the study has eliminated the positive effects that working motherhood may have on children such as higher income and lower maternal depression. In real life, these may well offset any negative effects of non-maternal care.

A third criticism of the 'single-risk' approach is that it focuses attention on to individual-level exposures and behaviours. This may lead in turn to a tendency to individualise failure, provoking feelings of guilt or a belief that irresponsible and/or inadequate mothers are to blame for deficits in their children's growth and neurocognitive performance. This has been denounced as victim blaming and, rather than describing health-damaging behaviours as a *cause* of health inequalities, contemporary researchers are more likely to view factors such as smoking, high fat/sugar diets and poor parenting as *outcomes* of socio-economic disadvantage. However, while a sensitivity to the social context of risk avoids an emphasis on individual culpability, it still introduces the danger of making stigmatising generalisations. For example, it is one thing to suggest that poor parenting skills may be a product of poverty and social exclusion rather than the fault of individual parents. It is quite another to imply that, on average, poor people make worse parents than their middle-class counterparts.

The social context of risk

The social context of risk factors before birth

Bearing these caveats in mind, there is substantial evidence to suggest that a number of specific risk factors are more prevalent among the poor than among the more affluent, that these are implicated in differences in key outcomes such as low birth weight, and that they contribute directly to observed inequalities in health according to socio-economic status. Prevalence of smoking during pregnancy, a risk factor that has been strongly implicated in intrauterine growth retardation, is significantly associated with socio-economic disadvantage. High rates of smoking among the poor have been partly attributed to the 'area effect' of living in a stressful environment with limited opportunities for respite and recreation, where cigarette smoking is the norm and support networks seem to encourage rather than challenge the habit (Jarvis and Wardle, 1999; Stead et al, 2001). At an individual level, too, smoking has been associated with stress and poor psychological health (Graham and Der, 1999; Copeland, 2003). Graham (1994), for example, notes that for poor women, smoking is the one thing they do for themselves, giving them their own time and space from the difficult task of caring for children in poverty.

Echoing this general socio-economic relationship, rates of smoking during pregnancy exhibit a strong class gradient. In the 2002 HSE, 6% of mothers in managerial and professional households smoked during pregnancy, compared with 29% of mothers in semi-routine and routine households. Area deprivation and income were also significantly related to smoking habits. Over a third (36%) of mothers in the bottom income quintile smoked during pregnancy, compared with 6% of those in the top income quintile. Twice as many mothers in the most deprived areas smoked during pregnancy (25%) as in the least deprived areas (12%). Age and family structure were also related to the prevalence of smoking during pregnancy. A total of 42% of mothers in lone-parent households reported they had smoked in pregnancy compared with 13% of mothers in two-parent households (Herrick and Kelly, 2003). Younger mothers were also more likely to smoke, 34% of those aged 16-24 smoking during pregnancy compared with 12% of those aged 35+. Rates are particularly high among teenage mothers, almost half of whom smoke during pregnancy (DH, 2002).

In contrast to smoking, poverty does not appear to be strongly associated with alcohol consumption among British women (Marmot, 1997), although rapid changes in the social and cultural factors that influence drinking behaviours may change this. In studies to date, poorer women have been more likely than affluent women to abstain completely or drink very rarely. Affluent women are more likely to drink above the recommended limits. However, they are also less likely to report being drunk (which may give an indication of binge drinking) or to experience drinking problems (Wardle et al, 1999). As consumption of alcohol during pregnancy tends to be highest among those mothers who are the heaviest drinkers before pregnancy (Waterson and Murray-Lyon, 1989), the relationship between deprivation and maternal alcohol consumption is likely to be inverse. Higher rates of alcohol consumption have certainly been noted among more educated pregnant women in Sweden (Dejin-Karlsson et al, 1997) and New Zealand (McLeod et al, 2002). However, in the 2002 HSE, none of the mothers reported consuming more than 14 units of alcohol per week during pregnancy. Less than 1% reported consuming 7-14 units and 2% reported consuming 2-7 units per week. Thus, 97% of mothers consumed no more than two units per week during pregnancy (Herrick and Kelly, 2003), although these figures may be subject to reporting bias.

As noted earlier, the significance of maternal nutrition to adverse pregnancy outcomes in the industrialised West has been debated (Mathews et al, 1999), in part because of contradictory evidence. A detailed examination of the diets of a population of London women did identify class differences in diet, but only with regard to the intake of certain nutrients during pregnancy (Wynn et al, 1994). Thus, no social class gradient was found for the intake of total energy, or the energy carriers carbohydrate and fat. There were, however, statistically highly significant social class gradients for the intake of protein, seven minerals and six B-vitamins, all of which were also highly significantly correlated with birth weight. Maternal intake of these 14 components of diet fell progressively as birth weight fell, but only for the mothers of smaller babies. Qualitatively, inadequate nutritional status was observed in only a minority of women in the study. These belonged to all social classes, but an increase was found from Social Class I to V, and single mothers were particularly prone to eat foods that did not meet basic maternal needs. The authors suggest that inadequate intake of nutrients present in foods such as whole grains, vegetables, fruit and dairy produce may partly be explained by their high cost.

These findings reflect those of general studies of British adults and older women that suggest that the consumption of 'healthy diets' is significantly associated with higher education, belonging to a higher socio-economic group and being married (Billson et al, 1999; Pollard et al, 2001; Lang et al, 2003). Age and smoking status also emerge as key variables. Young pregnant women are at particular risk of low micronutrient intake. In those who smoke, vitamin C and carotenoid intakes appear to be further depressed (Mathews et al, 2000). Age, socio-economic status, education, marital status and smoking status have also been associated with folic acid supplementation in the periconceptional period, an intervention designed to reduce the risk of neural tube defects (Sen et al, 2001). In the 2002 HSE, women aged 35+ were significantly more likely to have taken folate supplementation before pregnancy than women aged 16-24 (60% and 32% respectively), reflecting a higher proportion of pregnancies that were planned. A total of 65% of women in households in the top income quintile had taken folic acid in the preconception period compared with 25% in the bottom income quintile. Folate supplementation also varied according to family structure, 58% of women in two-parent families taking folic acid compared with 25% of lone parents (Herrick and Kelly, 2003).

In addition to research examining socio-economic differences in risk behaviours, there is growing interest in the role of maternal psychological health in influencing pregnancy outcomes. Drawing largely on American and Canadian studies, Kramer et al (2000) propose that pregnant women of low socio-economic status experience more stressful life events during their pregnancies. Besides the obvious links to the chronic stress caused by financial insecurity, poverty is associated with poor and crowded housing conditions, living without a partner, unsatisfying marital relationships, domestic violence and stressful working conditions.

Unintended, unwanted pregnancies are more common among low socio-economic status women and low pregnancy commitment has been associated with cigarette smoking and the use of alcohol and street drugs. As well as being more exposed to acute and chronic stressors, Kramer et al (2000) suggest that poorer pregnant women have less social resources to moderate the impact of stress. Especially significant is the presence and quality of an intimate relationship that can act as a stress buffer (Kramer et al, 2000).

Although there is evidence that antenatal stress and anxiety has a programming effect on the foetus that results in later behavioural/emotional problems (O'Connor et al, 2003), far less attention has been paid in Britain to antenatal than postnatal depression. Evidence suggests that antenatal depression is more common than generally thought. Indeed, symptoms of depression after childbirth do not appear to be more common or severe than during pregnancy (Evans et al, 2001). While a growing body of research is now monitoring the extent of depressive symptoms during pregnancy, few British studies have examined differences in rates of antenatal depression according to socio-economic status. However, a study of women attending an inner London antenatal clinic reported similar findings to international research (for example, Seguin et al, 1995; Marcus et al, 2003). Depressive symptoms were associated with having no educational qualifications, being unmarried, the woman being unemployed, having poor support from a partner if present, and being in a second or subsequent pregnancy (Bolton et al, 1998). The 2002 HSE did not explicitly seek to measure symptoms of antenatal depression. However, expectant mothers were asked about their feelings about pregnancy and similar risk factors emerged. Of women in households in the bottom income quintile, 14% reported being unhappy or very unhappy about their pregnancy compared with 1% of women in the top income quintile. Lone parents were significantly more likely to report feelings of unhappiness (22%) than women in two-parent families (5%). Feelings about pregnancy also varied by age, 16% of 16- to 24-year-olds expressing unhappiness compared with 6% of women aged 35+ (Herrick and Kelly, 2003). As antenatal (and indeed postnatal depression) is frequently missed during routine consultations (Johanson et al, 2000), this is one area of health variation that could be targeted for future research.

There is a growing critique of the tendency to depict teenage pregnancy as a public health 'problem' (see Chapter Eight). Nevertheless, teenage pregnancy has been associated with prenatal depression and anxiety, risks that reflect both cumulative lifecourse exposure to stressors and current circumstances. ALSPAC data suggest that teenage mothers are more likely to have suffered separation, divorce, step-parents, financial hardship, parental mental health or alcohol abuse in their families; to have regularly moved house and school; to have become sexually active at younger ages; and to describe their childhoods as not being happy (Meadows and Dawson, 1999). Younger mothers in the 2002 HSE were significantly less likely to have planned their pregnancies than older mothers

(43% of 16- to 24-year-olds compared with 75% of 25- to 34-year-olds), and during pregnancy younger mothers reported more negative feelings and were more likely to smoke (Herrick and Kelly, 2003).

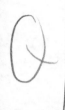

Attempting to tease out the relative importance of different risk factors in producing adverse pregnancy outcomes, Kramer et al (2000) suggest that, on the basis of current evidence, cigarette smoking is probably the most important variable mediating socio-economic disparities in intrauterine growth retardation. Throughout their article, however, the authors emphasise the role of psychosocial factors, not only in producing independent effects, but in influencing behaviours such as cigarette smoking and the use of alcohol and street drugs during pregnancy. For instance, pregnancy commitment (an idea that encompasses both the desire and intention to have a baby) is associated with healthy behaviours during pregnancy. By contrast, depression about one's current state, dissatisfaction with life, a sense of hopelessness and a lack of optimism about the future may promote unhealthy behaviours (Kramer et al, 2000, p 201).

Thus, individual risk factors such as maternal smoking do not exert their influence in isolation, but in interaction with other influences. If simplistic, individually focused, largely ineffective policy recommendations are to be avoided, it is important to contextualise risk and acknowledge the fact that adverse pregnancy outcomes often reflect the accumulation of multiple difficulties. As noted earlier, however, it is also important to avoid stigmatising generalisations. Given the problems experienced by teenage mothers, including poor educational achievement and lack of work opportunities, the current policy focus on teenage pregnancy may well be appropriate. However, it is also important to remember that many young mothers become pregnant intentionally, are happy with their babies, are in stable relationships with young men who share their responsibilities, are not on benefits and are living in their own accommodation (Allen and Bourke Dowling, 1998).

The social context of risk factors during infancy

Many social gradients in risk factors that are observed during pregnancy hold after the birth of a baby. As pregnancy acts as an important trigger for spontaneous smoking cessation for a large number of women, it is unlikely that women who have not responded to smoking cessation advice while expecting their babies will quit once their babies are born. For those who have successfully maintained smoking cessation throughout their pregnancies, the postpartum period presents risks for relapse. It is estimated that over 70% of women who stop smoking during pregnancy return to the habit within six months of delivery and around half within six weeks of giving birth (Bull et al, 2003). Having a partner who smokes is one of the critical components of a woman's smoking behaviour, so socio-economic inequalities in male smoking have a bearing on a mother's ability to quit smoking and to maintain smoking cessation.

Given that the birth of a baby and the changes associated with the transition to parenthood are themselves socially and psychologically stressful (Nicolson, 1998), there is little reason to assume that stress experienced by women living in poverty will reduce during the postnatal period. Women suffering from prenatal anxiety and depression are more likely to go on to suffer from postnatal depression (Johanson et al, 2000; Honey et al, 2003), a relationship that suggests that socio-economic differences in poor psychological health during pregnancy are likely to be carried forward into the postnatal period. Relatively few British studies have examined social inequalities in postnatal psychological health, in part because of the continued tendency to treat postnatal depression as a psychiatric disorder rather than a problem that is located within the broader social context (Lee, 1997). One exception, a study of 701 English women, found maternal depression to be significantly associated with, among other factors, educational, housing and employment status and reliance on state benefit (Sheppard, 1998). However, in the 2002 HSE, which included the Edinburgh Postnatal Depression Scale (EPNDS) to assess levels of postnatal depression, no association was observed between the prevalence of depression and maternal age, income or area deprivation. Family structure was associated with postnatal depression, 41% of lone mothers being classified as depressed, compared with 21% of mothers in two-parent households (Herrick and Kelly, 2003). Lone mothers were also more likely to report a lack of social support (51%) than mothers in two-parent households (23%).

Maternal depression can result in some mothers being withdrawn and disengaged in their interactions with their infants, whereas others are insensitive, intrusive and sometimes angry (Glaser, 2000). As noted earlier, a lack of sensitive interaction during young infancy can have an enduring influence on child psychological adjustment and learning capacity. Exposure to postnatal depression has been identified as a significant predictor of subsequent emotional, behavioural and cognitive difficulties in childhood (Beck, 1998; Murray et al, 1999; Hay et al, 2001). Significantly, the effect of maternal depression appears to be more marked in the presence of socio-economic disadvantage (Kurstjens and Wolke, 2001). The susceptibility of infants may also vary according to gender, boys being more adversely affected (Weinberg et al, 1999).

Of course, postnatal depression (when treated as an acute, time-limited event) is not the only manifestation of poor psychological status, nor the only risk factor for parenting difficulties. Chronic depression and anxiety have also been associated with negative interaction with the child and poor parenting. A parent's own upbringing can also be the basis for poor parenting behaviour, although parents' own difficult childhood experience is frequently counterbalanced by later protective factors such as support from their partner (Bifulco et al, 2002, p 1077).

While many studies have focused on the relationship between individual parental vulnerability (presence of depression, for example) and parenting, some critics argue that relatively little attention has been paid to the social, economic and political context of such vulnerability (Taylor et al, 2000). For example, there is strong empirical evidence suggesting that parents struggling with financial problems are at higher risk of suffering from depression and anxiety (Reading and Reynolds, 2001). In marital relationships, this can increase hostility and lack of supportiveness, both major stressors that negatively influence the quality of parenting (Leinonen et al, 2002). Citing various studies, Taylor et al (2000) suggest that an increase in economic hardship has been linked with a decrease in parental nurturing and an increase in inconsistent and punitive discipline by both parents. UK studies examining the prevalence of severe forms of child maltreatment (by focusing on children placed on child abuse or child protection registers) suggest that male unemployment and council housing accommodation are strongly associated with child abuse (Creighton, 1985; Gillham et al, 1998; Sidebotham et al, 2002).

For lone parents, the stress associated with financial insecurity can be exacerbated by a lack of partner support. Teenage mothers in the ALSPAC commonly had difficulties with their partners including the breaking up of their relationships, and felt they lacked wider support in the community. Many reported having no one to confide in. High rates of depression and anxiety were found in the study, teenagers reporting more negative feelings about parenting and fewer positive feelings. There were also signs that teenage mothers' parenting practices were less child-centred. They were less confident, more intolerant of the mess and disruptiveness of babies, had less developmentally appropriate equipment for the children, engaged them less in developmentally positive activities such as reading, singing and conversation, and were more likely to leave them to watch television unsupervised (Meadows and Dawson, 1999).

While such research throws light on the ways in which the stress of living in poverty can impact on parental well-being and, in turn, on parent–child interaction, socio-economic differences in parenting behaviours are still poorly understood. Part of the problem stems from the fact that parenting involves a complex set of behaviours. While it is plausible to identify a potentially direct effect of socio-economic status on some parenting dimensions, this is not always the case for others. For example, Hoghughi and Speight (1998) suggest that the facilitation of development is one of three components of 'good-enough parenting' (with love, care and commitment and control/consistent limit setting). Poverty (and lack of access to economic, social and educational resources) is likely to undermine families' ability to provide rich and varied stimulation (Taylor et al, 2000), but there are other aspects of parenting (for example, love) where a relationship between 'risk' and socio-economic status is not immediately obvious. Taylor et al (2000) warn against returning to historical concepts such as maternal inefficiency that conflate poverty with poor parenting. However, by emphasising the way in which poor socio-economic conditions undermine positive parenting, the authors could themselves be accused of doing just this and "consigning all the children of economically poor parents to despair" (Speight and Hoghughi, 2000, p 119).

A further problem that arises in teasing out the relationship between socio-economic status and parenting behaviours is that there has been much more focus on parenting in low-income than more affluent families. This bias may stem from the tendency of many studies to only select families from disadvantaged neighbourhoods and (particularly with regard to older children), to recruit cases by referral rather than screening. Thus, it should not be assumed that indicators of 'poor parenting' such as laxity and inconsistency, lack of bonding and attachment and exposure to marital discord are not found in rich households. Inept parenting styles among the rich may have been simply overlooked in the literature. The fact that the more affluent are able to draw on a wider range of social and material resources (including well-qualified substitute carers) may also be significant by modifying the impact of parenting deficits in this group.

In addition to social and emotional interaction, parenting includes physical aspects of infant care such as infant feeding. As noted earlier, there is evidence that shows that breastfeeding has both short- and long-term health benefits. The World Health Organization (WHO) recommends that, where possible, infants should be fed exclusively on breast milk from birth until six months of age. In the UK, however, rates of breastfeeding at birth are relatively low, at 71% in England and Wales, 63% in Scotland and 54% in Northern Ireland. After six weeks, rates fall to around 43% in England and Wales (Hamlyn et al, 2002). There is considerable socio-economic variation in breastfeeding behaviour, older and more educated women being more likely to both initiate and to continue breastfeeding. In the 2002 HSE, breastfeeding in mothers in the top household income quintile was 91% at birth, falling to 65% at two months and 28% at six months. By contrast, breastfeeding rates in the bottom income quintile started at 53%, falling to 28% at two months and 8% at six months (Blake, 2003).

Differences in breastfeeding behaviour may be less indicative of differences in knowledge than cultural attitudes. A qualitative study that examined expectations and experiences across the transition to motherhood found that mothers expressed pre-existing preferences about infant feeding that appeared to have been formed long before they were pregnant. Even women who acknowledged the health benefits of breast milk expressed firm intentions to bottle feed, in part because of a cultural familiarity with infant formula, but also due to a degree of embarrassment. As early as childhood, girls can form opinions of breastfeeding as either 'rude' or 'best for babies' (Gregg, 1989). Such attitudes are shaped in part by the way in which girls' own mothers have fed their babies (White et al, 1992), but also by wider community norms.

The timing of return to paid employment is another factor influencing breastfeeding behaviour (Noble et al, 2001; Galtry, 2003). Although the period during which British women are eligible to receive statutory maternity pay increased in 2003 from 18 weeks to 26 weeks and a further extension to 12 months has been proposed (HM Treasury et al, 2004), the UK's policies regarding paid maternity leave remain among the least generous in the West. Maternity pay only relates to a woman's earnings for six weeks, after which it is paid at a low flat rate (well below average earnings). The period of postnatal maternity leave may also be shortened if a woman is absent from work due to a pregnancy-related illness, or if she takes maternity leave before her due date and the baby is born late. Such factors (particularly the 'six-week trigger') may be key determinants of early cessation of breastfeeding in the UK. However, as statutory maternity pay excludes women who are working for very low wages and/or relatively few hours a week (who may be eligible for a flat-rate maternity allowance), the extent to which low benefit levels cause low-income women to resume employment and cease breastfeeding is debatable.

The social context of risk factors during early childhood

As in infancy, many of the risk factors that influence early child development are in place before a child grows from babyhood to preschool age. Without support and intervention, for example, negative parenting practices that develop during infancy can become ingrained, particularly if, with growing mobility and independence, a child is perceived to be difficult or challenging. Children who have been exposed to physical risks such as accidents will become more vulnerable as they become more mobile toddlers. Risk of accident is strongly associated with socio-economic status (Alwash and McCarthy, 1988; Ramsay et al, 2003), a relationship that reflects the quality and safety of the physical environment in which a child lives or plays. For example, high-rise flats with balconies or communal stairs where stair gates are not permitted, or a lack of access to safe play areas, can increase the likelihood of accidents happening (CAPT, 2002b).

Poor dietary practices that begin during infancy are also likely to continue into childhood. Social class differences in weaning practices have been observed during the first year of a child's life, infants from lower social classes or income groups tending to consume larger amounts of potatoes, biscuits, confectionary and soft drinks and less breast milk, cow's milk and fruit than more privileged babies. By the time they are toddlers and consuming a wider range of foods, socio-economic differences in children's consumption patterns become pronounced. Processed foods (that are high in sugar, salt, fat and starch) are more commonly given to toddlers from poorer families, while they tend to have a lower consumption of high fibre foods, including fruit and vegetables (Nelson, 2000). Socio-economic differences have also been noted in consumption of fizzy drinks (Northstone et al, 2002). Poor dietary practices at this age have been linked to socio-economic variation in key nutrient deficiencies (Watt et al, 2001), although young children of a lower socio-economic status are less likely to receive nutritional supplements than more affluent children (Bristow et al, 1997).

Early food-related experiences of vegetables and fruit appear to influence children's acceptance of these foods at a later age (Skinner et al, 2002).

Although there is uncertainty about the role that diet plays in determining overweight and obesity in young children, socio-economic differences in dietary patterns correspond with socio-economic differences in weight. Analysis of data from the Scottish National Preschool Child Health Surveillance System found that children aged three to four from the most deprived areas had a 30% higher risk of obesity when compared with children in the least deprived group. Undernutrition was also significantly associated with social deprivation, even after adjusting for birth weight (Armstrong et al, 2003). Significant geographical and socio-economic variation in dental health has also been found within national surveys (Pitts et al, 1999, 2003; Nunn et al, 2003). For example, a study of a deprived urban community in Glasgow found that 86% of four-and-a-half- to five-year-olds had dental caries. In some cases lesions were unrestorable (Sweeney and Gelbier, 1999). Differences in dental health reflect social differences in the consumption of sugary foods, snacks and drinks. However, statistical links between diet and dental erosion are somewhat weaker than the association between socio-economic status and dental health (Nunn et al, 2003).

The reasons for socio-economic differences in diet have been debated. Commentators to the right of the political spectrum tend to link patterns of food consumption with individual food preferences and/or good housekeeping, arguing that, as cheap but nutritional food is readily available, low income is not a barrier to improving the dietary health of poor children. Others, by contrast, suggest that "undernutrition is a consequence of inadequate spending on food because of limited money to spend and poor access by many low-income families to a healthy and affordable food supply" (Nelson, 2000, p 314). The concept of the 'food desert' has been proposed to capture the experience of what it is like to live in a deprived inner-city area where, because of the inaccessibility of out-of-town supermarkets and a dependence on corner shops, cheap, nutritious food is unavailable. Several studies that have quantified the costs of typical 'food baskets' suggest that those living on low wages or state benefits cannot afford to purchase sufficient, appropriate food to meet healthy dietary guidelines (Dowler, 2002). However, research findings are contradictory. For example, a large and systematic investigation of the price and availability of foods in Greater Glasgow found that food items showed few differences in price between more or less affluent areas and that foods that did differ in price tended to be cheaper in poorer places. Lower-quality high fat foods were particularly available at cheaper prices, although the prices of a small number of more healthy items (for example, wholemeal bread, carrots and orange juice) were also lower in more deprived areas (Cummins and Macintyre, 2002).

These findings do not necessarily support individualistic explanations for poor dietary practices among low-income groups. However, they suggest a need to guard against equally narrow explanations that focus on poverty alone. Murcott

(2002), for example, suggests that as well as the direct effects of poverty, nutritional inequalities are influenced by lay knowledge and attitudes towards diet and health, and differences in styles of eating according to socio-economic status. The fact that such enduring ideas are embedded in the social organisation of the home is relevant not only to dietary practices, but to other issues that impinge on health. For example, the adoption of hygiene practices appears to be influenced by social factors, mothers from socially disadvantaged backgrounds tending to use chemical household products and to aspire to higher levels of hygiene than their more affluent counterparts (Sherriff and Golding, 2002). Excessive cleanliness has been associated with increased prevalence of diseases of the immune system.

As noted earlier, the stresses of living in poverty and embarking on parenthood at a very young age have been associated with less positive parenting practices that may in turn impair emotional and behavioural adjustment and learning capacity. Social differences in behavioural problems (Galboda-Liyanage et al, 2003; Spencer and Coe, 2003) have been recorded in children as young as three. Social disadvantage has also been linked to poor language development at preschool age, which in turn affects subsequent academic achievement (Locke et al, 2002). In homes where books are readily available and where children are drawn into activities that support their language acquisition, linguistic skills are more likely to develop. Material resources and parental education (and related expectations) shape early linguistic environments. Both factors are, of course, strongly related to socio-economic status.

Against this background, it is argued that out-of-home care (in a nursery or preschool) can contribute positively to children's social and cognitive development. Several randomised trials that have been conducted among disadvantaged populations in the US suggest that day care not only has beneficial effects on children's behavioural development and school achievement. In the long term, attendance at preschool has been associated with increased employment, lower teenage pregnancy rates and decreased criminal behaviour (Zoritch et al, 1998). In the UK, exposure to preschool experience has been found to have a significantly positive effect on seven-year-olds' performance in reading, writing, number and science, as measured by National Curriculum assessment results (Daniels, 1995). The Effective Provision of Pre-School Education Project (EPPE), the first major European longitudinal study of young children's development between the ages of three and seven, similarly demonstrated the positive effects of high-quality preschool provision on children's intellectual and socio-behavioural development, particularly for disadvantaged children (Sylva et al, 2003; Sammons et al, 2004). Most studies agree that children from disadvantaged backgrounds can benefit enormously from early years provision (Melhuish, 2004). As noted earlier, however, recent research by the US NICHD Early Child Care Research Network (2003) found a positive association between the hours spent in non-maternal care over the first four-and-a-half years of life and behavioural/social competence problems.

Love et al (2003) suggest that the NICHD sample may not have comprised a sufficiently wide range of childcare facilities to properly assess the extent to which service *quality* moderates the impact of the amount of time in care. To address this, they consider the NICHD data in conjunction with data from other studies to yield a more diverse sample of children and families and a wider range of childcare settings. With a larger and more diverse sample, the quality of childcare (reflected in high staff–child ratios, the use of appropriately qualified staff and regulatory standards for curricula, space and equipment) becomes more salient than time in care in influencing children's development (Love et al, 2003). The EPPE Project similarly found that the quality of preschool provision was directly related to better intellectual, cognitive and socio-behavioural developmental outcomes in young children (Sylva et al, 2003).

As discussed in Chapter Three, there has been significant investment in early years education and care since 1997, notably through the introduction of free part-time nursery education places for all three- and four-year-olds, the establishment of a Foundation Stage, the development of the Sure Start initiative and the provision of financial support for childcare to families on low incomes through the Child Tax Credit (CTC). With the publication of its 10-year strategy for childcare (HM Treasury et al, 2004), the government remains committed to further expanding provision for the early years. However, rather than increasing the number of state-funded nurseries, its approach to this is to encourage private and voluntary sector involvement within a regulatory framework.

Legitimate concerns can be raised about this strategy. According to the EPPE Project, there are significant differences in the quality of different preschool settings and in the extent to which they can promote positive child outcomes (Sylva and Pugh, 2005). Integrated centres (that combine education with care and have a high proportion of trained teachers) and nursery schools tend to promote the best intellectual outcomes while integrated settings and nursery classes promote better social development. It is no coincidence that these settings, many of which belong to the statutory sector, have the highest proportions of qualified staff. By contrast, less than half of workers in playgroups, the vast majority of which are run by the voluntary sector, and only 50% of staff in day nurseries are qualified to National Vocational Qualification (NVQ) level (which is some way below graduate level). Early years education is a specialised area that, in several continental educational systems, is supported by graduate-level training and professional development. In the UK, however, most preschool settings offer salaries that are too low to attract fully qualified early years specialists (staff in voluntary-run preschools typically earn between £5.50 and £6.50 an hour). Financial difficulties also contribute to high levels of volatility in the system which in turn undermines overall service quality. For example, high staff turnover has been identified as a problem for private nurseries (NAO, 2004).

Even within nursery and reception classes situated in primary schools, fully qualified teachers may not be trained to work with very young children (Aubrey, 2004). This has raised questions about the extent to which early years provision is always developmentally appropriate. Research suggests that supporting socio-emotional and cognitive development (for example, creativity and language development) in early childhood through developmentally appropriate practice produces better outcomes in the long term than focusing on academic work (Locke et al, 2002; Maccoby and Lewis, 2003). Indeed, the introduction of academic work into the early childhood curriculum may be ultimately counterproductive as it can undermine children's confidence and disposition to learn. One risk of introducing young children to formal academic work prematurely is that those who cannot relate to the tasks required are likely to feel incompetent, to label themselves as poor learners and to behave accordingly. Locke et al (2002) suggest that children who are expected to develop reading skills and written language before they have made sufficient progress in the development of their spoken language are at risk of making poor educational progress and even being classed as having special educational needs, although most are likely to have the potential for normal language development. As age of school entry in the UK is already lower than in most of Europe (Sharp, 2002), it is important to ensure that educating three- and four-year-old children within the context of a primary school does not contribute to further polarisation between early and late developers.

The impact of these trends on disadvantaged children is not yet fully known. Some of the best resourced, highest quality and integrated services are based in highly deprived urban communities. Benefiting from targeted funding from the government's Early Excellence Centres and Neighbourhood Nurseries initiatives as well as subsidies from local authorities, these services provide a range of activities, including training and support for parents and nursery care all day throughout the year. There are, however, relatively few of these 'flagship' statutory facilities. As we discussed in Chapter Three, although the gap in provision between deprived and non-deprived areas has narrowed, it has proved difficult to create sustainable full-time places in formal childcare settings in the most deprived areas. There is also a need to tackle pockets of deprivation outside the 20% most deprived wards. For the vast majority of children, care beyond the part-time provision that is freely available for three- and four-year-olds has to be paid for privately, and although support is available through the Working Tax Credit (WTC), current awards are on average significantly lower than average childcare costs. Consequently, low-income families and lone parents still remain heavily reliant on informal childcare.

Because children from deprived backgrounds are more likely to have delayed language and other key skills than socially advantaged children, they have most to gain from the provision of developmentally appropriate education. Settings can fail to provide such education for a range of reasons. They may lack sufficiently qualified staff to provide intensive work on language enrichment for young children who show poor language development on entry to preschool (Sammons et al, 2004). They may encourage too much unstructured play (a criticism that has been levelled at voluntary playgroups). Alternatively, they may emphasise academic development over social development (a problem that tends to be associated with the provision of early years education in primary schools). There has been a long-standing debate about the long-term impact of introducing formal schooling to children from disadvantaged backgrounds, particularly less mature boys. However, by the age of four, 62% of children are entering reception classes in primary schools, where a class of 30 may only have one fully qualified teacher (DfES, 2005).

As noted earlier, concerns have been raised that this will contribute to further polarisation between early and late developers. The UK is already in the bottom third of the league of OECD (Organisation for Economic Co-operation and Development) countries with regard to relative educational disadvantage (the gap between low and middle achievers) in reading, maths and science. Thus, countries such as Finland, France, Sweden and Italy are doing far better than the UK in containing inequality and preventing their low achievers from falling too far behind their nation's average performance (UNICEF Innocenti Research Centre, 2002, p 9). All of these countries defer school entry until six or seven and have developed a strong and universal tradition of kindergarten care, a strategy explicitly rejected by the UK. What this will mean for the reduction of educational inequality remains to be seen.

The policy implications

The evidence presented in this chapter suggests that early life is a critical and vulnerable stage during which poor socio-economic circumstances can have lasting effects on health chances. Research on early life programming has been extremely influential in highlighting the role of such latent effects and in identifying a number of specific biological and development factors that can be targeted by preventive health programmes. Kramer et al (2000), for example, suggest that cigarette smoking is probably the most important variable mediating socio-economic disparities in intrauterine growth retardation. Barker (1994) emphasises the need for nutritional programmes to improve the diets of girls and young women, while others focus on the role of parenting support and preschool provision to improve cognitive and socio-emotional function in children living in poverty or in psychologically stressful family environments.

Insofar as evidence does support a link between some of these factors and adverse health outcomes, there are grounds for singling them out as key foci for health intervention programmes. For example, smoking during pregnancy is associated with increased risk for low birth weight, pre-term delivery and impaired lung function. Exposure to tobacco smoke in utero is suspected to be associated with Attention Deficit/Hyperactivity Disorder (ADHD) and ADHD symptoms in childhood (see Chapter Six). It has also been implicated in increased risk for certain cancers. Between a quarter and a third of women from socially disadvantaged backgrounds continue to smoke during pregnancy and an estimated 70% of women who stop smoking when they become pregnant resume the habit within six months of delivery. As exposure to tobacco smoke during infancy is associated with an increased risk for lower respiratory infections, chronic middle ear disease and asthma, policy initiatives should not be restricted to helping pregnant women quit, but should also focus on how smoking cessation can be subsequently maintained.

Undernutrition in utero has also been implicated in long-term risk for many chronic conditions, including CHD, diabetes and hypertension. Specific nutritional deficiencies during pregnancy increase risk for a range of problems such as neural tube defects and reduced brain development and, during infancy and early childhood, rapid weight gain (particularly among children of low birth weight) indicates increased risk for obesity in childhood and later life and related diseases. There are significant differences according to socio-economic status with respect to a range of nutritional indicators. For example, several studies suggest that young, socially disadvantaged pregnant women are at greater risk of micro-nutrient deficiencies. During infancy, there is significant socio-economic variation in the initiation and duration of breastfeeding. Important social differences in weaning practices have been observed during the first year of a child's life, infants from lower-income groups tending to consume larger amounts of refined foods, starchy carbohydrates and less fruit than more privileged babies and, by the preschool years, differences in children's consumption patterns become even more pronounced. Such evidence has suggested the need to improve nutritional outcomes in lower-income groups across the early years, key areas of intervention including pregnancy, breastfeeding, weaning and diet in early childhood. However, the role that diet during pregnancy and childhood plays in the development of obesity and risk for chronic disease has been subject to debate, some studies highlighting the lack of relationship between maternal diet and infant birth weights and between diet and obesity in early childhood. Much is still unknown about the development of obesity and the metabolic syndrome. Thus, the extent to which nutritional interventions can effectively address the pathways giving rise to disease is debatable.

In addition to biological risk factors, a growing body of research is exploring the interplay between biological and psychological/behavioural influences. This suggests that chronic stress can have long-term consequences on physical and emotional health from the earliest stage of life and may indeed play an important role in foetal growth and altered foetal physiology. Maternal stress, for instance, has been implicated in risk of prematurity, adverse neurodevelopment and chronic degenerative disease in adulthood. During infancy and early childhood, neglect, abuse and social deprivation can also produce a cascade of neurobiological events than in turn affect emotional, behavioural, cognitive and physiological development. Thus, children deprived of appropriate love and stimulation are not only at increased risk of socio-emotional and psychological problems (also see Chapter Six). Key neurobiological changes are also associated with reduced cognitive ability, impaired immune function and increased risk of cardiovascular disease and diabetes.

While care should be taken to avoid conflating poverty with poor parenting, there is strong evidence suggesting that parents struggling with financial problems and a lack of social support are at higher risk of suffering from depression and anxiety. Poor psychosocial health in pregnancy is strongly associated with social disadvantage and while research findings linking depression in the postnatal period with socio-economic status are mixed, lone mothers do appear to be particularly vulnerable. Depression and anxiety have been associated with negative and less developmentally positive interaction with children. Parents' own childhood experiences together with a lack of information and education can shape attitudes to and expectations of child behaviour and development. Poverty also has a direct effect on parenting practices by undermining a family's ability to provide education resources. All of these factors suggest that parents caring for children in disadvantaged circumstances are likely to need additional family support if they are to protect their children from the effects of disadvantage.

Of course, parents are not the only actors who can influence cognitive and socio-emotional functioning in the preschool period. Other adults can provide developmentally appropriate stimulation and positive role models in, for example, a nursery or preschool. Many studies suggest that children from disadvantaged backgrounds can benefit enormously from access to high-quality care, making this a potentially important intervention with regard to reducing future health inequalities. As noted earlier, Britain has recently expanded the provision of preschool facilities. However, some concerns have been expressed about the quality of early years education and care in the country. Much of the early years workforce remains underqualified and underpaid and, even in settings where levels of qualification are high, concerns have been expressed about the emphasis on academic development in the early childhood curriculum. Thus, while few would dispute the claim that education and care in the early years is a key area for intervention, the ideal philosophy and context of such education remains subject to debate.

It is, then, theoretically possible to identify the kinds of policy interventions that could improve the healthy development of young children from disadvantaged backgrounds. Referring to the pathways and sources of vulnerability that have been identified here, Chapter Five examines evidence of the impact of interventions targeting smoking cessation, nutrition, parenting education and early years education and care, and also explores the extent to which current government strategies are commensurate with the 'evidence base'. It is important to note, however, that not all commentators agree with the current emphasis on *evidence-based policy* when this all too often leads to a narrow focus on 'downstream' initiatives; underestimates the role of *context* in shaping health, health-related behaviour and responses to health interventions; and establishes impossibly stringent criteria by which to measure programme success. Some of these issues have been raised in Chapter Three. They are taken up further in Chapter Five, which explores key areas where the current evidence base provides a poor foundation for policy and practice.

References

Acheson, D. (Chair) (1998) *Independent Inquiry into Inequalities in Health*, London: The Stationery Office.

Allen, I. and Bourke Dowling, S. (1998) *Teenage mothers: Decisions and outcomes*, London: Policy Studies Institute.

Alwash, R. and McCarthy, M. (1988) 'Measuring severity of injuries to children from home accidents', *Archives of Disease in Childhood*, vol 63, pp 635-8.

Arendt, R., Angelopoulos, J., Salvator, A. and Singer, L. (1999) 'Motor development of cocaine exposed children at two years', *Pediatrics*, vol 103, pp 86-92.

Arenz, S., Ruckerl, R., Koletzko, B. and von Kries, R. (2004) 'Breast-feeding and childhood obesity – systematic review', *International Journal of Obesity Related Metabolic Disorders*, vol 28, pp 1247-56.

Armstrong, J., Reilly, J. and the Child Health Information Team (2002) 'Breastfeeding and lowering the risk of childhood obesity', *The Lancet*, vol 359, pp 2003-4.

Armstrong, J., Dorosty, A.R., Reilly, J.J., Emmett, P.M. and the Child Health Information Team (2003) 'Coexistence of social inequalities in undernutrition and obesity in preschool children: population based cross sectional study', *Archives of Disease in Childhood*, vol 88, no 8, pp 671-5.

Aubrey, C. (2004) 'Implementing the foundation stage in reception classes', *British Educational Research Journal*, vol 30, pp 633-56.

Barker, D.J.P. (1994) *Mothers, babies, and disease in later life*, London: British Medical Journal Publications.

Barker, D.J.P. (1997) 'Fetal nutrition and cardiovascular disease in later life', in M.G. Marmot and M.E.J. Wadsworth (eds) *Fetal and early childhood environment. British Medical Bulletin*, vol 53, pp 96-108.

Barker, D.J.P., Forsén, T., Utela, A., Osmond, C. and Eriksson, J.G. (2001) 'Size at birth and resilience to effects of poor living conditions in adult life: longitudinal study', *British Medical Journal*, vol 323, pp 1273-6.

Bates, D.V. (1995) 'The effects of air pollution on children', *Environmental Health Perspectives*, vol 103, suppl 6, pp 49-53.

Bavdekar, A., Yajnik, C.S., Fall, C.H., Bapat, S., Pandit, A.N., Deshpande, V., Bhave, S., Kellingray, S.D. and Joglekar, C. (1999) 'Insulin resistance syndrome in 8-year old Indian children: small at birth, big at 8 years, or both?', *Diabetes*, vol 48, pp 2422-9.

Beck, C.T. (1998) 'The effects of postpartum depression on child development: a meta-analysis', *Archives of Psychiatric Nursing*, vol 12, no 1, pp 12-20.

Bifulco, A., Moran, P.M., Ball, C., Jacobs, C., Baines, R., Bunn, A. and Cavagin, J. (2002) 'Childhood adversity, parental vulnerability and disorder: examining inter-generational transmission of risk', *The Journal of Child Psychology and Psychiatry*, vol 43, no 8, pp 1075-86.

Billson, H., Pryer, J.A. and Nichols, R. (1999) 'Variation in fruit and vegetable consumption among adults in Britain: an analysis from the dietary and nutritional survey of British adults', *European Journal of Clinical Nutrition*, vol 53, no 12, pp 946-52.

Blackburn, S.T. (2003) *Maternal, fetal and neonatal physiology: A clinical perspective* (2nd edn), St Louis, MO: Saunders.

Blake, M. (2003) 'Infant health', in K. Sproston and P. Primatesta (eds) *Health survey for England 2002: Maternal and infant health*, London: The Stationery Office.

Bolton, H.L., Hughes, P.M., Turton, P. and Sedgwick, P. (1998) 'Incidence and demographic correlates of depressive symptoms during pregnancy in an inner London population', *Journal of Psychosomatic Obstetrics and Gynaecology*, vol 19, no 4, pp 202-9.

Brauer, M., Hoek, G., van Vliet, P., Meliefste, K., Fischer, P.H., Wijga, A., Koopman, L.P., Neijens, H.J., Gerritsen, J., Kerkhof, M., Heinrich, J., Bellander, T. and Brunekreef, B. (2002) 'Air pollution from traffic and the development of respiratory infections and asthmatic and allergic symptoms in children', *American Journal of Respiratory and Critical Care Medicine*, vol 166, no 8, pp 1092-8.

Bremner, J.D. and Vermetten, E. (2001) 'Stress and development: behavioural and biological consequences', *Development and Psychopathology*, vol 13, pp 473-89.

Bristow, A., Qureshi, S., Rona, R.J. and Chinn, S. (1997) 'The use of nutritional supplements by 4-12 year olds in England and Scotland', *European Journal of Clinical Nutrition*, vol 51, no 6, pp 366-9.

Bugental, D.B., Martorell, G.A. and Barraza, V. (2003) 'The hormonal costs of subtle forms of infant maltreatment', *Hormones and Behaviour*, vol 43, no 1, pp 237-44.

Bull, J., Mulvihill, C. and Quigley, R. (2003) *Prevention of low birth weight: Assessing the effectiveness of smoking cessation and nutritional interventions: Evidence briefing* (1st edn), London: Health Development Agency.

Bundred, P., Kitchiner, D. and Buchan, I. (2001) 'Prevalence of overweight and obese children between 1989 and 1998: population based series of cross sectional studies', *British Medical Journal*, vol 322, pp 1-4.

CAPT (Child Accident Prevention Trust) (2002a) *Child accident facts: Factsheet*, London: Capt.

CAPT (2002b) *Children and accidents: Factsheet*, London: Capt.

Charmandari, E., Kino, T., Souvatzoglou, E. and Chrousos, G.P. (2003) 'Pediatric stress: hormonal mediators and human development', *Hormone Research*, vol 59, no 4, pp 161-79.

Chiriboga, C., Brust, J., Bateman, D. and Hauser, W.A. (1999) 'Dose response of fetal cocaine exposure on newborn neurologic function', *Pediatrics*, vol 103, pp 79-85.

Copeland, L. (2003) 'An exploration of the problems faced by young women living in disadvantaged circumstances if they want to give up smoking: can more be done at general practice level?', *Family Practice*, vol 20, no 4, pp 393-400.

Creighton, S.J. (1985) 'An epidemiological study of abused children and their families in the United Kingdom between 1977 and 1982', *Child Abuse and Neglect*, vol 9, no 4, pp 441-8.

Cummins, S. and Macintyre, S. (2002) 'A systematic study of an urban foodscape: the price and availability of food in Greater Glasgow', *Urban Studies*, vol 39, no 11, pp 2115-30.

Daniels, J.L., Longnecker, M.P., Rowland, A.S., Golding, J. and the ALSPAC Study Team (2004) 'Fish intake during pregnancy and early cognitive development of offspring', *Epidemiology*, vol 15, pp 394-402.

Daniels, S. (1995) 'Can preschool education affect children's achievement in primary school', *Oxford Review of Education*, vol 21, no 2, pp 163-78.

Dawson, G., Ashman, S.B. and Carver, L.J. (2000) 'The role of early experience in shaping behavioral and brain development and its implications for social policy', *Development and Psychopathology*, vol 12, no 4, pp 695-712.

Dejin-Karlsson, E., Hanson, B.S. and Ostergren, P.O. (1997) 'Psychosocial resources and persistent alcohol consumption in early pregnancy – a population study of women in their first pregnancy in Sweden', *Scandinavian Journal of Social Medicine*, vol 25, no 4, pp 280-8.

Dezateux, C. and Stocks, J. (1997) 'Lung development and early origins of childhood respiratory illness', *British Medical Bulletin*, vol 53, pp 40-57.

DfES (Department for Education and Skills) (2005) *Provision for children under five years of age in England: January 2005 (provisional)*, London: DfES.

DH (Department of Health) (2002) *Tackling health inequalities: 2002 Cross Cutting Review*, London: DH.

DiPietro, J.A. (2000) 'Baby and the brain: advances in child development', *Annual Review of Public Health*, vol 21, pp 455-71.

Dowler, E. (2002) 'Food and poverty in Britain: rights and responsibilities', *Social Policy and Administration*, vol 36, no 6, pp 698-717.

Eckersley, A.J. and Blinkhorn, F.A. (2001) 'Dental attendance and dental health behaviour in children from deprived and non-deprived areas of Salford, north-west England', *International Journal of Paediatric Dentistry*, vol 11, no 2, pp 103-9.

Eriksson, J.G., Forsén, T., Osmond, C. and Barker, D.J.P. (2003) 'Obesity from cradle to grave', *International Journal of Obesity Related Metabolic Disorders*, vol 27, no 6, pp 722-7.

Eriksson, J.G., Forsén, T., Tuomilehto, J., Winter, P.D., Osmond, C. and Barker, D.J.P. (1999) 'Catch-up growth in childhood and death from coronary heart disease: longitudinal study', *British Medical Journal*, vol 318, pp 427-31.

Evans, J., Heron, J., Francomb, H., Oke, S. and Golding, J. (2001) 'Cohort study of depressed mood during pregnancy and after childbirth', *British Medical Journal*, vol 323, no 7307, pp 257-60.

Evans, R. (2002) *Interpreting and addressing inequalities in health: From Black to Acheson to Blair to . . .?*, London: Office of Health Economics.

Farrow, A., Greenwood, R., Preece, S. and Golding, J. (1997) 'Nitrogen dioxide, the oxides of nitrogen, and infants' health symptoms. ALSPAC Study Team. Avon Longitudinal Study of Pregnancy and Childhood', *Archives of Environmental Health*, vol 52, no 3, pp 189-94.

Feinstein, L. and Bynner, J. (2004) 'The importance of cognitive development in middle childhood for adulthood socioeconomic status, mental health, and problem behavior', *Child Development*, vol 75, pp 1329-39.

Filippini, G., Farinotti, M. and Ferrarini, M. (2000) 'Active and passive smoking during pregnancy and risk of central nervous system tumours in children', *Paediatric and Perinatal Epidemiology*, vol 14, pp 78-84.

Forsén, T., Eriksson, J.G., Tuomilehto, J., Osmond, C. and Barker, D.J.P. (1999) 'Growth in utero and during childhood among women who develop coronary heart disease: longitudinal study', *British Medical Journal*, vol 319, pp 1403-7.

Forsyth, J.S., Willatts, P., Agostoni, C., Bissenden, J., Casaer, P. and Boehm, G. (2003) 'Long chain polyunsaturated fatty acid supplementation in infant formula and blood pressure in later childhood: follow up of a randomised control trial', *British Medical Journal*, vol 326, pp 953-8.

Freeman, R., Oliver, M., Bunting, G., Kirk, J. and Saunderson, W. (2001) 'Addressing children's oral health inequalities in Northern Ireland: a research–practice–community partnership initiative', *Public Health Reports*, vol 116, no 6, pp 617-25.

Gaffney, K.F. (2001) 'Infant exposure to environmental tobacco smoke', *Journal of Nursing Scholarship*, vol 33, no 4, pp 343-7.

Galboda-Liyanage, K.C., Prince, M.J. and Scott, S. (2003) 'Mother–child joint activity and behaviour problems of pre-school children', *Journal of Child Psychology and Psychiatry and Allied Disciplines*, vol 44, no 7, pp 1037-48.

Galtry, J. (2003) 'The impact on breastfeeding of labour market policy and practice in Ireland, Sweden and the USA', *Social Science and Medicine*, vol 57, no 1, pp 167-77.

Gibson, A. and Asthana, S. (1998a) 'School performance, school effectiveness and the 1997 White Paper', *Oxford Review of Education*, vol 24, no 2, pp 195-210.

Gibson, A. and Asthana, S. (1998b) 'Schools, pupils and exam results: contextualising school performance', *British Educational Research Journal*, vol 24, no 4, pp 269-82.

Gillham, B., Tanner, G., Cheyne, B., Freeman, I., Rooney, M. and Lambie, A. (1998) 'Unemployment rates, single parent density, and indices of child poverty: their relationship to different categories of child abuse and neglect', *Child Abuse and Neglect*, vol 22, no 2, pp 79-90.

Glaser, D. (2000) 'Child abuse and neglect and the brain – a review', *The Journal of Child Psychology and Psychiatry*, vol 41, no 1, pp 97-116.

Godfrey, K.M., Redman, C.W.G., Barker, D.J.P. and Osmond, C. (1991) 'The effect of maternal anaemia and iron deficiency on the ratio of fetal weight to placental weight', *British Journal of Obstetrics and Gynaecology*, vol 98, pp 886-91.

Godfrey, K.M., Robinson, S., Barker, D.J.P., Osmond, C. and Cox, V. (1996) 'Maternal nutrition in early and late pregnancy in relation to placental and fetal growth', *British Medical Journal*, vol 312, pp 410-14.

Graham, H. (1994) 'Gender and class as dimensions of smoking-behaviour in Britain – insights from a survey of mothers', *Social Science and Medicine*, vol 38, no 5, pp 691-18.

Graham, H. and Der, G. (1999) 'Patterns and predictors of tobacco consumption among women', *Health Education Research*, vol 14, no 5, pp 611-8.

Granger, D.A. and Kivlighan, K.T. (2003) 'Integrating biological, behavioural and social levels of analysis in early child development: progress, problems and prospects', *Child Development*, vol 74, no 4, pp 1058-63.

Gregg, J. (1989) 'Attitudes of teenagers in Liverpool to breastfeeding', *British Medical Journal*, vol 299, pp 147-8.

Habibian, M., Roberts, G., Lawson, M., Stevenson, R. and Harris, S. (2001) 'Dietary habits and dental health over the first 18 months of life', *Community Dentistry and Oral Epidemiology*, vol 29, no 4, pp 239-46.

Hales, C. and Barker, D. (2001) 'The thrifty phenotype hypothesis', *British Medical Journal*, vol 60, pp 5-20.

Hales, C.N., Barker, D.J.P., Clark, P.M.S, Cox, L.J., Fall, C., Osmond, C. and Winter, P.D. (1991) 'Fetal and infant growth and impaired glucose intolerance at age 64', in D.J.P. Barker (ed) *Fetal and infant origins of adult disease*, London: British Medical Journal Publications.

Hamlyn, B., Brooker, S., Oleinikova, K. and Wands, S. (2002) *Infant feeding 2000*, A survey conducted on behalf of the DH, the Scottish Executive, the National Assembly of Wales and the Department of Health, Social Services and Public Safety in Northern Ireland, London: The Stationery Office.

Hannigan, J.H. and Abel, E.L. (1996) 'Animal models for alcohol-related birth defects', in H.L. Spohr and H.C. Steinhausen (eds) *Alcohol, pregnancy and the developing child*, Cambridge: Cambridge University Press, pp 77-102.

Hanson, L.A., Korotkova, M. and Telemo, E. (2003) 'Breast-feeding, infant formulas, and the immune system', *Annals of Allergy, Asthma and Immunology*, vol 90, no 6, suppl 3, pp 59-63.

Hanson, L.A., Korotkova, M., Haversen, L., Mattsby-Baltzer, I., Hahn-Zoric, M., Silfverdal, S.A., Strandvik, B. and Telemo, E. (2002) 'Breast-feeding, a complex support system for the offspring', *Pediatrics International*, vol 44, no 4, pp 347-52.

Harding, J. (2001) 'The nutritional basis of the fetal origins of adult disease', *International Journal of Epidemiology*, vol 30, pp 15-23.

Hay, D.F., Pawlby, S., Sharp, D., Asten, P., Mills, A. and Kumar, R. (2001) 'Intellectual problems shown by 11-year-old children whose mothers had postnatal depression', *The Journal of Child Psychology and Psychiatry*, vol 42, no 7, pp 871-89.

Helland, I.B., Smith, L., Saarem, K., Saugstad, O.D. and Drevon, C.A. (2003) 'Maternal supplementation with very-long-chain n-3 fatty acids during pregnancy and lactation augments children's IQ at 4 years of age', *Pediatrics*, vol 111, no 1, pp 39-44.

Herrick, J. and Kelly, Y. (2003) 'Maternal health', in K. Sproston and P. Primatesta (eds) *Health Survey for England 2002: Maternal and infant health*, London: The Stationery Office.

HM Treasury, DfES (Department for Education and Skills), DWP (Department for Work and Pensions) and DTI (Department for Trade and Industry) (2004) *Choice for parents: The best start for children: A ten year strategy for childcare*, London: The Stationery Office.

Hobel, C. and Culhane, J. (2003) 'Role of psychological and nutritional stress on poor pregnancy outcome', *Journal of Nutrition*, vol 133, no 5, suppl 2, pp 1709S-1717S.

Hobel, C., Dunkel-Schetter, C., Roesch, S., Castro, L. and Arora, C. (1999) 'Maternal plasma corticotropin-releasing hormone associated with stress at 20 weeks' gestation in pregnancies ending in preterm delivery', *American Journal of Obstetrics and Gynecology*, vol 180, pp S257–S263.

Hoghughi, M. and Speight, A.N.P. (1998) 'Good enough parenting for all children – a strategy for a healthier society', *Archives of Disease in Childhood*, vol 78, pp 293-6.

Honey, K.L., Bennett, P. and Morgan, M. (2003) 'Predicting postnatal depression', *Journal of Affective Disorders*, vol 76, nos 1-3, pp 201-10.

Huizink, A.C., Robles de Medina, P.G., Mulder, E.J., Visser, G.H. and Buitelaar, J.K. (2003) 'Stress during pregnancy is associated with developmental outcome in infancy', *The Journal of Child Psychology and Psychiatry*, vol 44, no 6, pp 810-18.

Jarvis, M.J. and Wardle, J. (1999) 'The case of cigarette smoking', in M. Marmot and R.G. Wilkinson (eds) *Social determinants of health*, Oxford: Oxford University Press, pp 240-55.

Johanson, R., Chapman, G., Murray, D., Johnson, I. and Cox, J. (2000) 'The North Staffordshire Maternity Hospital prospective study of pregnancy-associated depression', *Journal of Psychosomatic Obstetrics and Gynaecology*, vol 21, no 2, pp 93-7.

Kiess, W., Galler, A., Reich, A., Muller, G., Kapellen, T., Deutscher, J., Raile, K. and Kratzsch, J. (2001) 'Clinical aspects of obesity in childhood and adolescence', *Obesity Reviews*, vol 2, no 1, pp 29-36.

Kinra, S., Nelder, R.P. and Lewenden, G.J. (2000) 'Deprivation and childhood obesity: a cross-sectional study of 20,973 children in Plymouth, United Kingdom', *Epidemiology and Community Health*, vol 54, pp 456-60.

Kramer, M.S., Séguin, L., Lydon, J. and Goulet, L. (2000) 'Socio-economic disparities in pregnancy outcome: why do the poor fare so poorly?', *Paediatric and Perinatal Epidemiology*, vol 14, pp 194-210.

Kramer, M.S., Guo, T., Platt, R.W., Shapiro, S., Collet, J.P., Chalmers, B., Hodnett, E., Sevkovskaya, Z., Dzikovich, I., Vanilovich, I. and the PROBIT Study Group (2002) 'Breastfeeding and infant growth: biology or bias?', *Pediatrics*, vol 110, no 2, pt 1, pp 343-7.

Kramer, M.S., Guo, T., Platt, R.W., Sevkovskaya, Z., Dzikovich, I., Collet, J.P., Shapiro, S., Chalmers, B., Hodnett, E., Vanilovich, I., Mezen, I., Ducruet, T., Shishko, G. and Bogdanovich, N. (2003) 'Infant growth and health outcomes associated with 3 compared with 6 months of exclusive breastfeeding', *American Journal of Clinical Nutrition*, vol 78, no 2, pp 291-5.

Kurstjens, S. and Wolke, D. (2001) 'Effects of maternal depression on cognitive development of children over the first 7 years of life', *The Journal of Child Psychology and Psychiatry*, vol 42, no 5, pp 623-36.

Lang, R., Thane, C.W., Bolton-Smith, C. and Jebb, S.A. (2003) 'Consumption of whole-grain foods by British adults: findings from further analysis of two national dietary surveys', *Public Health Nutrition*, vol 6, no 5, pp 479-84.

Leary, S., Ness, A., Emmett, P., Davey Smith, G. and the ALSPAC Study Team (2005a) 'Maternal diet in pregnancy and offspring height, sitting height, and leg length', *Journal of Epidemiology and Community Health*, vol 59, pp 467-72.

Leary, S., Ness, A., Emmett, P., Davey Smith, G., Headley, J. and the ALSPAC Study Team (2005b) 'Maternal diet in pregnancy and offspring blood pressure', *Archive of Disease in Childhood*, vol 90, pp 492-3.

Lee, C. (1997) 'Social context, depression and the transition to motherhood', *British Journal of Health Psychology*, vol 2, no 2, pp 93-108.

Leinonen, J.A., Solantaus, T.S. and Punamäki, R. (2002) 'The specific mediating paths between economic hardship and the quality of parenting', *International Journal of Behavioural Development*, vol 26, no 5, pp 423-35.

Livingstone, M.B. (2001) 'Childhood obesity in Europe: a growing concern', *Public Health Nutrition*, vol 4, no 1A, pp 109-16.

Locke, A., Ginsborg, J. and Peers, I. (2002) 'Development and disadvantage: implications for the early years and beyond', *International Journal of Language and Communication Disorders*, vol 37, no 1, pp 3-15.

Lodrup Carlsen, K.C. (2002) 'The environment and childhood asthma (ECA) study in Oslo: ECA-1 and ECA-2', *Pediatric Allergy and Immunology*, vol 13, suppl 15, pp 29-31.

Love, J.M., Harrison, L., Sagi-Schwartz, A., van Ijzendoorn, M.H., Ross, C., Ungerer, J.A., Raikes, H., Brady-Smith, C., Bollers, K., Brooks-Gunn, J., Constantine, J., Eliason Kisker, E., Paulsell, D. and Chazan-Cohen, R. (2003) 'Child care quality matters: how conclusions may vary with context', *Child Development*, vol 74, no 4, pp 1021-33.

Lucas, A., Fewtrell, M.S., Davies, P.S., Bishop, N.J., Clough, H. and Cole, T.J. (1998) 'Breastfeeding and catch-up growth in infants born small for gestational age', *Acta Paediatrica*, vol 86, no 6, pp 564-9.

Lundberg, U. (1999) 'Coping with stress: neuroendocrine reactions and implications for health', *Noise Health*, vol 1, no 4, pp 67-74.

McCain, M.N. and Mustard, J.F. (1999) *Early years study: Reversing the real brain drain*, Toronto, Canada: Ontario Children's Secretariat.

Maccoby, E.E. and Lewis, C.C. (2003) 'Less day care or different day care?', *Child Development*, vol 74, no 4, pp 1069-75.

McLeod, D., Pullon, S., Cookson, T. and Cornford, E. (2002) 'Factors influencing alcohol consumption during pregnancy and after giving birth', *New Zealand Medical Journal*, vol 115, no 1157, p U29.

Makrides, M., Neumann, M.A., Simmer, K. and Gibson, R.A. (2000) 'A critical appraisal of the role of dietary long chain polyunsaturated fatty acids on neural indices of term infants: a randomised control trial', *Pediatrics*, vol 105, pp 32-8.

Mancuso, R., Schetter, C., Rini, C., Roesch, S. and Hobel, C. (2004) 'Maternal prenatal anxiety and corticotropin-releasing hormone associated with timing of delivery', *Psychosomatic Medicine*, vol 66, pp 762-9.

Marcus, S.M., Flynn, H.A., Blow, F.C. and Barry, K.L. (2003) 'Depressive symptoms among pregnant women screened in obstetrics settings', *Journal of Women's Health*, vol 12, no 4, pp 373-80.

Marmot, M. (1997) 'Inequality, deprivation and alcohol use', *Addiction*, vol 92, suppl 1, pp s13-20.

Marmot, M. and Wadsworth, M. (eds) (1997) *Fetal and early childhood environment: long term health implications*, British Medical Bulletin, vol 53, no 1.

Martin, R., Ben-Shlomo, Y., Gunnell, D., Elwood, P., Yarnell, J. and Davey Smith, G. (2005) 'Breast feeding and cardiovascular disease risk factors, incidence and mortality: the Caerphilly study', *Journal of Epidemiology and Community Health*, vol 59, pp 121-9.

Mathews, F., Yudkin, P. and Neil, A. (1999) 'Influence of maternal nutrition on outcome of pregnancy: prospective cohort study', *British Medical Journal*, vol 319, pp 339-43.

Mathews, F., Yudkin, P., Smith, R.F. and Neil, A. (2000) 'Nutrient intakes during pregnancy: the influence of smoking status and age', *Journal of Epidemiology and Community Health*, vol 54, pp 17-23.

Meadows, S. and Dawson, N. (1999) *Teenage mothers and their children: Factors affecting their health and development*, Final report to the DH, Bristol: Graduate School of Education, University of Bristol.

Melhuish, E. (2004) *A literature review of the impact of early years provision on young children, with emphasis given to children from disadvantaged backgrounds*, London: Audit Commission.

MRC (Medical Research Council) Vitamin Study Research Group (1991) 'Prevention of neural tube defects: results of the Medical Research Council Vitamin Study', *Lancet*, vol 338, pp 131-7.

Mullen, P., Martin, J., Anderson, J., Romans, S. and Herbison, G. (1996) 'The long-term impact of the physical, emotional, and sexual abuse of children: a community study', *Child Abuse and Neglect*, vol 20, pp 7-21.

Murcott, A. (2002) 'Nutrition and inequalities: a note on sociological approaches', *European Journal of Public Health*, vol 12, no 3, pp 203-7.

Murray, L., Sinclair, D., Cooper, P., Ducournau, P., Turner, P. and Stein, A. (1999) 'The socioemotional development of 5-year-old children of postnatally depressed mothers', *The Journal of Child Psychology and Psychiatry*, vol 40, no 8, pp 1259-71.

NAO (National Audit Office) (2004) *Early years: Progress in developing high quality childcare and early education accessible to all*, London: The Stationery Office.

Nelson, M. (1999) 'Nutrition and health inequalities', in D. Gordon, M. Shaw, D. Dorling and G. Davey Smith (eds) *Inequalities in health: The evidence presented to the Independent Inquiry into Inequalities in Health, chaired by Sir Donald Acheson*, Bristol: The Policy Press, pp 118-37.

Nelson, M. (2000) 'Childhood nutrition and poverty', *Proceedings of the Nutrition Society*, vol 59, pp 307-15.

Nessa, N. and Gallagher, J. (2004) 'Diet, nutrition, dental health and exercise', in ONS, *The health of children and young people*, London: ONS.

Newcombe, N.S. (2003) 'Some controls control too much', *Child Development*, vol 74, no 4, pp 1050-2.

NICHD (National Institute for Child Health and Human Development) Early Child Care Research Network (2003) 'Does amount of time in child care predict socioemotional adjustment during the transition to kindergarten?', *Child Development*, vol 74, no 4, pp 976-1005.

Nicolson, P. (1998) *Post-natal depression: Psychology, science and the transition to motherhood*, London: Routledge.

Noble, S. and the ALSPAC Study Team (2001) 'Maternal employment and the initiation of breastfeeding', *Acta Paediatrica*, vol 90, pp 423-8.

Northstone, K., Rogers, I., Emmett, P. and the ALSPAC Team Study (2002) 'Drinks consumed by 18-month-old children: are current recommendations being followed?', *European Journal of Clinical Nutrition*, vol 56, no 3, pp 236-44.

Nuesslein, T.G., Fischer, H., Welsing, E., Riedel, F. and Rieger, C.H. (2002) 'Early rather than recent exposure to tobacco increases bronchial reactivity', *Klinische Padiatrie*, vol 214, no 6, pp 365-70.

Nunn, J.H., Gordon, P.H., Morris, A.J., Pine, C.M. and Walker, A. (2003) 'Dental erosion – changing prevalence? A review of British national children's surveys', *International Journal of Paediatric Dentistry*, vol 13, no 2, pp 98-105.

O'Connor, T.G., Heron, J., Golding, J., Glover, V. and the ALSPAC Study Team (2003) 'Maternal antenatal anxiety and behavioural/emotional problems in children: a test of a programming hypothesis', *The Journal of Child Psychology and Psychiatry*, vol 44, no 7, pp 1025-36.

O'Connor, T.G., Rutter, M., Beckett, C., Keaveney, L., Kreppner, J.M. and the English and Romanian Adoptees (ERA) Study Team (2000) 'The effects of global severe privation on cognitive competence: extension and longitudinal follow-up', *Child Development*, vol 71, no 2, pp 376-90.

Oddy, W.H., Sly, P.D., de Klerk, N.H., Landau, L.I., Kendall, G.E., Holt, P.G. and Stanley, F.J. (2003a) 'Breast feeding and respiratory morbidity in infancy: a birth cohort study', *Archives of Disease in Childhood*, vol 88, no 3, pp 224-8.

Oddy, W.H., Kendall, G.E., Blair, E., de Klerk, N.H., Stanley, F.J., Landau, L.I., Silburn, S. and Zubrick, S. (2003b) 'Breast feeding and cognitive development in childhood: a prospective birth cohort study', *Paediatric and Perinatal Epidemiology*, vol 17, no 1, pp 81-90.

Ong, K.K. and Dunger, D.B. (2002) 'Perinatal growth failure: the road to obesity, insulin resistance and cardiovascular disease in adults', *Best Practice and Research Clinical Endocrinology and Metabolism*, vol 16, no 2, pp 191-207.

Ong, K.K. and Dunger, D.B. (2004) 'Birth weight, infant growth and insulin resistance', *European Journal of Endocrinology*, vol 151, pp U131-9.

Ong, K.K.L., Ahmed, M.L., Emmett, P.M., Preece, M.A., Dunger, D.B. and the ALSPAC Study Team (2000) 'Association between postnatal catch-up growth and obesity in childhood: prospective cohort study', *British Medical Journal*, vol 320, pp 967-71.

Owen, C.G., Whincup, P.H., Odoki, K., Gilg, J.A. and Cook, D.G. (2003) 'Infant feeding and blood cholesterol: a study in adolescents and a systematic review', *Pediatrics*, vol 110, no 3, pp 597-608.

Parsons, T., Power, C., Logan, S. and Summerbell, C. (1999) 'Childhood predictors of adult obesity: a systematic review', *International Journal of Obesity Related Metabolic Disorders*, vol 23, suppl 8, pp 1-107.

Parsons, T.J., Power, C. and Manor, O. (2003) 'Infant feeding and obesity through the lifecourse', *Archives of Disease in Childhood*, vol 88, no 9, pp 793-4.

Pershagen, G., Rylander, E., Norberg, S., Eriksson, M. and Nordvall, S.L. (1995) 'Air pollution involving nitrogen dioxide exposure and wheezing bronchitis in children', *International Journal of Epidemiology*, vol 24, no 6, pp 1147-53.

Piachaud, D. and Sutherland, H. (2002) *Changing poverty post-1997*, CASE Paper 63, London: Centre for Analysis of Social Exclusion, London School of Economics and Political Science.

Pike, I. (2005) 'Maternal stress and fetal responses: evolutionary perspectives on preterm delivery', *American Journal of Human Biology*, vol 17, pp 55-65.

Pitts, N.B., Evans, D.J. and Nugent, Z.J. (1999) 'The dental caries experience of 5-year-old children in the United Kingdom: surveys co-ordinated by the British Association for the Study of Community Dentistry in 1997/98', *Community Dental Health*, vol 16, no 1, pp 50-6.

Pitts, N.B., Boyles, J., Nugent, Z.J., Thomas, N. and Pine, C. (2003) 'The dental caries experience of 5-year-old children in England and Wales: surveys co-ordinated by the British Association for the Study of Community Dentistry in 2001/2002', *Community Dental Health*, vol 20, no 1, pp 45-54.

Pollard, J., Greenwood, D., Kirk, S. and Cade, J. (2001) 'Lifestyle factors affecting fruit and vegetable consumption in the UK Women's Cohort Study', *Appetite*, vol 37, no 1, pp 71-9.

Power, C. and Jefferis, B.J. (2002) 'Fetal environment and subsequent obesity: a study of maternal smoking', *International Journal of Epidemiology*, vol 31, no 2, pp 413-19.

Power, C. and Parsons, T. (2000) 'Nutritional and other influences in childhood as predictors of adult obesity', *Proceedings of the Nutrition Society*, vol 59, pp 267-72.

Raaschou-Nielsen, O., Hertel, O., Thomsen, B.L. and Olsen, J.H. (2001) 'Air pollution from traffic at the residence of children with cancer', *American Journal of Epidemiology*, vol 153, no 5, pp 433-43.

Ramsay, L.J., Moreton, G., Gorman, D.R., Blake, E., Goh, D., Elton, R.A. and Beattie, T.F. (2003) 'Unintentional home injury in preschool-aged children: looking for the key – an exploration of the inter-relationship and relative importance of potential risk factors', *Public Health*, vol 117, no 6, pp 404-11.

Reading, R. and Reynolds, S. (2001) 'Debt, social disadvantage and maternal depression', *Social Science and Medicine*, vol 53, no 4, pp 441-53.

Reilly, J.J., Methven, E., McDowell, Z.C., Hacking, B., Alexander, D., Stewart, L. and Kelnar, C.J.H. (2003) 'Health consequences of obesity', *Archives of Disease in Childhood*, vol 88, pp 748-52.

Reilly, J.J., Armstrong, J., Dorosty, A., Emmett, P., Ness, A., Rogers, I., Steer, C., Sherriff, A. and the ALSPAC Study Team (2005) 'Early life risk factors for obesity in childhood: cohort study', *British Medical Journal*, vol 330, pp 1357-63.

Remacle, C., Bieswal, F. and Reusens, B. (2004) 'Programming of obesity and cardiovascular disease', *International Journal of Obesity Related Metabolic Disorders*, vol 28, suppl 3, pp S46-53.

Rook, G.A.W. and Stanford, J.L. (1998) 'Give us this day our daily germs', *Immunology Today*, vol 19, pp 113-16.

Rushton, L., Courage, C. and Green, E. (2003) 'Estimation of the impact on children's health of environmental tobacco smoke in England and Wales', *Journal of the Royal Society of Health*, vol 123, no 3, pp 175-80.

Rutter, M. and the English and Romanian Adoptees (ERA) Study Team (1998) 'Developmental catch-up and deficit, following adoption and severe global early privation', *The Journal of Child Psychology and Psychiatry*, vol 39, no 4, pp 465-76.

Sammons, P., Eliot, K., Sylva, K., Melhuish, E., Siraj-Blatchford, R. and Taggart, B. (2004) 'The impact of pre-school on young children's cognitive achievements on entry to reception', *British Educational Research Journal*, vol 30, pp 691-712.

Sanchez, M.M., Ladd, C.O. and Plotsky, P.M. (2001) 'Early adverse experience as a developmental risk factor for later psychopathology: evidence from rodent and primate models', *Development and Psychopathology*, vol 13, pp 419-49.

Schulkin, J. (1999) 'Corticotropin-releasing hormone signals adversity in both the placenta and the brain: regulation by glucocorticoids and allostatic overload', *Journal of Endocrinology*, vol 161, pp 349-56.

Seguin, L., Potvin, L., St-Denis, M. and Loiselle, J. (1995) 'Chronic stressors, social support, and depression during pregnancy', *Obstetrics and Gynecology*, vol 85, no 4, pp 583-9.

Selwyn, J. (2000) 'Fetal development', in M. Boushel, M. Fawcett and J. Selwyn (eds) *Focus on early childhood: Principles and realities*, Oxford: Blackwell Science, pp 21-34.

Sen, S., Manzoor, A., Deviasumathy, M. and Newton, C. (2001) 'Maternal knowledge, attitude and practice regarding folic acid intake during the periconceptional period', *Public Health Nutrition*, vol 4, no 4, pp 909-12.

Shaheen, S., Newson, R., Henderson, A., Emmett, P., Sherriff, A., Cooke, M. and the ALSPAC Study Team (2004) 'Umbilical cord trace elements and minerals and risk of early childhood wheezing and eczema', *European Respiratory Journal*, vol 24, pp 292-7.

Shaheen, S., Newson, R., Henderson, A., Headley, J., Stratton, F., Jones, R., Strachan, D. and the ALSPAC Study Team (2005) 'Prenatal paracetamol exposure and risk of asthma and elevated immunoglobulin E in childhood', *Clinical and Experimental Allergy*, vol 35, pp 18-25.

Sharp, C. (2002) 'School starting age: European policy and recent research', Paper presented to the Local Government Association Seminar 'When should our children start school?', LGA Conference Centre, Smith Square, London, 1 November.

Shea, A., Walsh, C., Macmillan, H. and Steiner, M. (2005) 'Child maltreatment and HPA axis dysregulation: relationship to major depressive disorder and post traumatic stress disorder in females', *Psychoneuroendocrinology*, vol 30, pp 162-78.

Sheppard, M. (1998) 'Depression in female health visitor consulters: social and demographic facets', *Journal of Advanced Nursing*, vol 26, no 5, pp 921-9.

Sherriff, A. and Golding, J. (2002) 'Factors associated with different hygiene practices in the homes of 15 month old infants', *Archives of Disease in Childhood*, vol 87, no 1, pp 30-5.

Sherriff, A., Golding, J. and the ALSPAC Study Team (2002) 'Hygiene levels in a contemporary population cohort are associated with wheezing and atopic eczema in preschool infants', *Archives of Disease in Childhood*, vol 87, no 1, pp 26-9.

Sidebotham, P., Heron, J., Golding, J. and the ALSPAC Study Team (2002) 'Child maltreatment in the "Children of the Nineties": deprivation, class, and social networks in a UK sample', *Child Abuse and Neglect*, vol 26, no 12, pp 1243-59.

Singhal, A., Wells, J., Cole, T.J., Fewtrell, M. and Lucas, A. (2003) 'Programming of lean body mass: a link between birth weight, obesity, and cardiovascular disease?', *American Journal of Clinical Nutrition*, vol 77, no 3, pp 726-30.

Skinner, J.D., Carruth, B.R., Bounds, W., Ziegler, P. and Reidy, K. (2002) 'Do food-related experiences in the first 2 years of life predict dietary variety in school-aged children?', *Journal of Nutrition, Education and Behaviour*, vol 34, no 6, pp 310-15.

Sparkes, J. (1999) *Schools, education and social exclusion*, CASE Paper 29, London: Centre for Analysis of Social Exclusion, London School of Economics and Political Science.

Speight, A.N.P. and Hoghughi, M. (2000) 'Commentary on Taylor, J., Spencer, N. and Baldwin, N.: social, economic and political context of parenting', *Archives of Disease in Childhood*, vol 82, pp 119-20.

Spencer, N. and Coe, C. (2003) 'Social patterning and prediction of parent-reported behaviour problems at 3 years in a cohort study', *Child: Care, Health and Development*, vol 29, no 5, pp 329-36

Stead, M., MacAskill, S., MacKintosh, A.M., Reece, J. and Eadie, D. (2001) '"It's as if you're locked in": qualitative explanations for area effects on smoking in disadvantaged communities', *Health and Place*, vol 7, no 4, pp 333-43.

Sweeney, P.C. and Gelbier, S. (1999) 'The dental health of pre-school children in a deprived urban community in Glasgow', *Community Dental Health*, vol 16, no 1, pp 22-5.

Sylva, K. and Pugh, G. (2005) 'Transforming the early years in England', *Oxford Review of Education*, vol 31, pp 11-27.

Sylva, K., Melhuish, E., Sammons, P., Siraj-Blatchford, I., Taggart, B. and Elliot, K. (2003) *The Effective Provision of Pre-school Education (EPPE) Project: Findings from the pre-school period*, London: Institute of Education/Sure Start.

Taylor, J., Spencer, N. and Baldwin, N. (2000) 'Social, economic and political context of parenting', *Archives of Disease in Childhood*, vol 82, pp 113-17.

Teicher, M.H., Andersen, S.L., Polcari, A., Anderson, C.M., Navalta, C.P. and Kim, D.M. (2003) 'The neurobiological consequences of early stress and childhood maltreatment', *Neuroscience and Biobehavioral Reviews*, vol 27, nos 1-2, pp 33-44.

UNICEF (United Nations Children's Fund) Innocenti Research Centre (2002) *A league table of educational disadvantage in rich nations*, Florence, Italy: UNICEF Innocenti Research Centre.

van Odijk, J., Kull, I., Borres, M.P., Brandtzaeg, P., Edberg, U., Hanson, L.A., Host, A., Kuitunen, M., Olsen, S.F., Skerfving, S., Sundell, J. and Wille, S. (2003) 'Breastfeeding and allergic disease: a multidisciplinary review of the literature (1966-2001) on the mode of early feeding in infancy and its impact on later atopic manifestations', *Allergy*, vol 58, no 9, pp 833-43.

Wadhwa, P., Garite, T., Porto, M., Glynn, L., Chicz-DeMet, A., Dunkel-Schetter, C. and Sandman, C. (2004) 'Placental corticotropin-releasing hormone (CRH), spontaneous preterm birth, and fetal growth restriction: a prospective investigation', *American Journal of Obstetrics and Gynecology*, vol 191, pp 1063-9.

Wadhwa, P.D., Glynn, L., Hobel, C.J., Garite, T.J., Porto, M., Chicz-DeMet, A., Wiglesworth, A.K. and Sandman, C.A. (2002) 'Behavioral perinatology: biobehavioral processes in human fetal development', *Regulatory Peptides*, vol 108, nos 2-3, pp 149-57.

Wadsworth, M. (1999) 'Early life', in M. Marmot and R.G. Wilkinson (eds) *Social determinants of health*, Oxford: Oxford University Press, pp 44-63.

Wardle, J., Farrell, M., Hillsdon, M., Jarvis, M., Sutton, S. and Thorogood, M. (1999) 'Smoking, drinking, physical activity and screening uptake and health inequalities', in D. Gordon, M. Shaw, D. Dorling and G. Davey Smith (eds) *Inequalities in health: The evidence presented to the Independent Inquiry into Inequalities in Health, chaired by Sir Donald Acheson*, Bristol: The Policy Press, pp 213-39.

Waterson, E.J. and Murray-Lyon, I.M. (1989) 'Drinking and smoking patterns amongst women attending an antenatal clinic during pregnancy', *Alcohol*, vol 24, no 2, pp 163-73.

Watt, R.G., Dykes, J. and Sheiham, A. (2000) 'Preschool children's consumption of drinks: implications for dental health', *Community Dental Health*, vol 17, no 1, pp 8-13.

Watt, R.G., Dykes, J. and Sheiham, A. (2001) 'Socio-economic determinants of selected dietary indicators in British pre-school children', *Public Health Nutrition*, vol 4, no 6, pp 1229-33.

Weinberg, M.K., Tronick, E.Z., Cohn, J.F. and Olson, K.L. (1999) 'Gender differences in emotional expressivity and self-regulation during early infancy', *Developmental Psychology*, 35, pp 175-88.

Werner, E.E. and Smith, R.S. (1992) *Overcoming the odds: High risk children from birth to adulthood*, Ithaca, NY: Cornell University Press.

White, A., Freeth, S. and O'Brien, M. (1992) *Infant feeding 1990*, London: HMSO.

Whitty, J.E. and Sokol, R.J. (1996) 'Alcohol teratogenicity in humans', in H.L. Spohr and H.C. Steinhausen (eds) *Alcohol, pregnancy and the developing child*, Cambridge: Cambridge University Press, pp 3-13.

Wilkin, T., Voss, L., Metcalf, B., Mallam, K., Jeffery, A., Alba, S. and Murphy, M. (2004) 'Metabolic risk in early childhood: the EarlyBird Study', *International Journal of Obesity Related Metabolic Disorders*, vol 28, suppl 3, pp s64-9.

Wynn, S., Wynn, A., Doyle, W. and Crawford, M. (1994) 'The association of maternal social class with maternal diet and the dimensions of babies in a population of London women', *Nutrition and Health*, vol 9, pp 202-15.

Zoritch, B., Roberts, I. and Oakley, A. (1998) 'The health and welfare effects of day care: a systematic review of randomised controlled trials', *Social Science and Medicine*, vol 47, no 3, pp 317-27.

FIVE

Early life: policy and practice

Introduction

As Chapter Four noted, the early years represent a critical period for interventions designed to reduce health inequalities. Inequalities themselves are manifest, exposure to disadvantage is recognised as having lasting effects on health and socio-economic status in later life, and there is strong evidence that childhood health inequalities can be reduced (Mielck et al, 2002). This strategic importance was underlined by the *Independent Inquiry into Inequalities in Health* (Acheson, 1998). This identified improvements in early years support for children and families as one of five actions likely to have the greatest impact over time. This emphasis has been maintained. The national targets for health inequalities, prefigured by the *NHS Plan* (DH, 2000), thus focused, for example, on reducing the difference in infant mortality across social classes by 2010 (alongside inequalities in life expectancy), while the White Paper *Tackling health inequalities* (DH, 2003a) took support for families, mothers and children as one of its four central themes. The government's long-term goal of first halving, then eradicating child poverty altogether has also ensured scrutiny of the key public services that contribute "to improving poor children's life chances and breaking cycles of deprivation", including early years services, parenting support and education, as well as welfare reforms (HM Treasury et al, 2004, p 12).

This chapter focuses first on the health behaviours that the research evidence in Chapter Four suggests are the key targets for intervention: smoking cessation, nutrition and parenting education. It outlines the range of effective interventions at our disposal and considers the political and practical response. Consideration is then given to the local delivery of two important structural targets: early years education and childcare. The significant issue of childhood poverty underpins the discussion. The enduring tensions between policies that aim, for example, to increase maternal participation in the workforce and those that stress the importance of parental input in early life are recognised, despite the creation of a Minister for Children, Young People and Families. This has led to calls for a politics of parenthood (Moss, 1999), capable of debating the contested domain between employment and caring, including the salient issues of time and gender. Recognition is also accorded to the difficulties in assessing the effectiveness of interventions or the adequacy of the policy response given the different evaluative traditions and challenges of medical as opposed to social models of intervention.

A considerable range of innovative activities remain confined to the periphery of policy and practice because it fails to meet the stringent criteria for inclusion in systematic reviews. This is a theme we return to in Chapter Fourteen.

Organisation is a challenge. It is increasingly recognised that strategies designed to reduce disadvantage in the early years cannot focus solely on the young child but must consider the family as a whole in its various manifestations. The early years agenda thus ranges from preparation for pregnancy and family life in school, through healthy behaviour in pregnancy to parental support across the postnatal and preschool period. Interventions focusing specifically on the baby or young child tend, therefore, to be outweighed by those aimed at informing, educating and supporting families. It is also increasingly accepted that child-rearing is a complex and multifaceted task and that policy approaches need to be similarly multidimensional (Einzig, 1999). Stress is thus placed on joined-up working and the delivery of seamless services in an attempt to address the so-called 'wicked issues'. Recent initiatives such as Sure Start are thus typically wide-ranging, potentially embracing the spectrum of services for the early years and aiming to produce outcomes that span education, health, social inclusion and community development. In consequence, neat classifications relating to either target group or focus of intervention are difficult to sustain.

Smoking cessation

As Chapter Four has shown, the use of tobacco in pregnancy is one of the most important risk factors for foetal growth and development. A considerable number of women quit smoking without assistance during pregnancy, with the largest group (up to one quarter) stopping before their first antenatal visit (Lumley et al, 2001). However, these tend to be light and moderate smokers (Jane et al, 2000), and the proportion of pregnant women who smoke not only remains substantial but is also significantly associated with socio-economic disadvantage. Relapse rates in the postpartum period are also high (Dolan-Mullen, 1999). Estimates suggest that approximately one third of infants are exposed to smoking in their own homes (Hofhuis et al, 2003) rising to 50% of children (Hovell et al, 2000, cited in Taylor et al, 2005). Again, an inequalities dimension is evident. A detailed study of lone parents living in rented accommodation and relying on social security benefits, for example, found smoking levels in excess of 75% (Dorsett and Marsh, 1998). Parental smoking in early life has been estimated to be the cause of hospital admission for 17,000 children under the age of five each year in England and Wales (RCoP, 1992).

What works? Evidence and practice

Advice and support tailored for pregnant women has been shown to have only a modest effect on cessation rates and a tendency not to reach those at highest risk (potentially exacerbating the inequalities dimension). A systematic review suggested that 10% of women still smoking at the time of their first antenatal visit are likely to stop with usual care but that formal interventions can result in an additional 6% to 7% quitting (Lumley et al, 2001). Prenatal counselling, combined with at least 10 minutes personal contact and written material tailored to pregnancy has, for example, been shown to double cessation rates (NHS CRD, 1998), although self-help literature on its own tends to be ineffectual (Moore et al, 2002).

The frequency of contact with health professionals in the prenatal period obviously offers increased opportunities for such interventions. Historically at least, this potential has been under-utilised. General practitioner (GP) surgeries have not been a routine source of advice on the subject (Dawe and Goddard, 1997), and this has extended to the primary care professionals in closest contact with expectant mothers. A study in New Zealand, for example (see Box 5.1), found that while most midwives regarded smoking cessation as an integral part of their job, only half gave such advice to all pregnant smokers. Key constraints were a lack of time and perceptions of patient resistance (McLeod et al, 2003).

Box 5.1: Smoking cessation – training for primary care

The Midwifery Education for Women who Smoke (MEWS) study in New Zealand randomly allocated over 60 midwives to one of four groups, including a smoking education group (trained to support smoking cessation or reduction) and a combined group (trained to implement both smoking and breastfeeding support programmes). This established that midwives often found it difficult to ask women about their smoking, to identify those who would be receptive to change and to support women in making the necessary changes. They were also concerned as to whether advice on smoking cessation would interfere with their central relationship with the patient and whether it would add unnecessarily to existing feelings of guilt (McLeod et al, 2003). Training increased competency and confidence.

Frequent brief interventions were found to help women move from contemplative stages towards action. Realistic goals were set for what each woman could achieve rather than focusing on cessation alone. This included establishing smoke-free rooms in the house and reducing the number of cigarettes smoked. The use of pregnancy-specific resources played an important part in helping midwives deliver their health promotion messages effectively, as did their involvement in the development of these resources (Pullon et al, 2003).

Recent large-scale studies also suggest that results in real-life settings are often less favourable than those conducted in clinical trials (Bull et al, 2003). Attrition rates are highest among those on a low income and among the most mobile

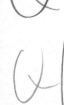

(Lumley et al, 2001). As noted in Chapter Four, contributory factors are likely to include stress (Ludman et al, 2000), with over 60% of women smokers experiencing one or more forms of disadvantage (Graham, 1998) and a culture where cigarette smoking is still seen as the norm. The importance of this social context suggests that smoking cessation should not be tackled in isolation but within the wider context of strategies to address poverty, disadvantage and health, including wide-ranging health promotion initiatives designed to promote parental self-confidence and self-esteem and increase family and community support.

The smoking cessation component of the Health Action Zone (HAZ) programme should theoretically have done just this. Funds for smoking cessation strategies (discussed later) were channelled initially through this wide-ranging programme designed to address health inequalities in communities suffering from low income and multiple deprivation (see Chapter Three). However, the imperative for early results and the requirement to meet government targets militated against HAZs' capacity to think strategically about the best way to reach those groups most at risk, as opposed to reaching as many smokers as possible (Adams et al, 2000). Despite a quit profile heavily weighted towards women, it therefore proved very difficult to target pregnant women effectively. It also proved difficult to integrate the late-funded (and often even later staffed) smoking cessation programmes with the wider work of the HAZ. Additionally, despite high-quality review-level evidence that facilitators needed to be trained (Dolan-Mullen, 1999), most services were able to employ only a minority of counsellors with previous experience of clinical smoking cessation work, and training to address this shortfall was in short supply (Coleman et al, 2002, 2005). There were, however, reported successes. The You Two Can Quit initiative, originating in the North Staffordshire HAZ, for example, employed a full-time midwife to provide a high-profile contact, receiving referrals at booking and providing six to eight weeks' support for pregnant women, their partners and families (West et al, 2003).

A central component of the policy was the provision of one week's free nicotine replacement therapy (NRT) (a feature that was supplemented by many HAZs), and which, subsequent to *The NHS Plan* (DH, 2000), became available on the NHS and thus available free to those in receipt of welfare benefits. While it is recognised that addiction to nicotine prevents many pregnant women from quitting, the safety and efficacy of NRT for smoking cessation during pregnancy has not been well studied (Bull et al, 2003). Some reservations, therefore, remained about this component of the policy, with the National Institute for Clinical Excellence (NICE) recommending that "smokers who are under the age of 18 years, who are pregnant or breastfeeding ... should discuss the use of NRT with a relevant healthcare professional before it is prescribed" (NICE, 2002, para 1.3). Dempsey and Benowitz (2001) suggest further research should focus on intermittent use formulations of NRT (gum, spray, inhaler) in order to reduce the total dose of nicotine delivered to the foetus. One potential advantage, they suggest, is that assault on the unborn child is limited to nicotine rather than the thousands of chemicals contained in cigarettes, many of which are also toxins.

There is consensus that the transition from pregnancy to the postpartum period is critical in preventing relapse, as is the absence of a partner who continues to smoke. It is estimated that half of all mothers who cease smoking during pregnancy resume within six weeks, with over 70% returning within six months (Dolan-Mullen, 1999). Despite this, less emphasis has been given to either the continuation of cessation or cessation by other family members and there is a lack of review-level evidence in either area (Bull et al, 2003; Park et al, 2004).

Research also suggests that increasing support for smoking cessation during pregnancy and its subsequent maintenance could affect breastfeeding rates and thus be a legitimate component of breastfeeding support programmes. Amir and Donath (2002), reviewing evidence from a number of studies, found that women who smoke are less likely than non-smokers either to intend to breastfeed or to initiate breastfeeding and more likely to breastfeed for a shorter period. They may also be less likely than non-smokers to seek help with breastfeeding difficulties. Ratner et al (1999), for example, found not only a strong association between daily smoking and early weaning, but also that women who smoke were more likely to perceive that they had an insufficient milk supply or to question its quality. Contributory factors, they suggested, might be nicotine-induced fretfulness in the infant, which the mother might interpret as a sign of underfeeding, or changes in the taste of milk consequent on a resumption of smoking, causing the infant to refuse to feed.

A synthesis of published interventions designed to reduce children's exposure to passive smoking suggested that the most effective strategies concentrate on strengthening the parents' faith in their ability to create a smoke-free environment and on behavioural strategies to achieve this goal (such as smoking outside) rather than focusing merely on stopping smoking altogether (Arborelius et al, 2000). This is supported by a recent meta-review, which also finds evidence in favour of interventions delivered by clinicians in both the home and the clinic (including information, advice and counselling). The significance of the results tends, however, to vary depending on whether the intervention relies on self-reported behaviour or biochemical measures (cotinine levels or levels of nicotine in the air) (Taylor et al, 2005). A degree of support for intensive counselling as a possible mechanism is also offered by a recent Cochrane Review, although only a minority of the studies produced a statistically significant intervention effect in terms of attitudes and behaviour (and hence exposure to environmental tobacco smoke [ETS]) as opposed to changes in knowledge (Roseby et al, 2004). There was, however, a generally observable reduction in child ETS for participants. Two possible explanations were the widespread use of comparison groups, rather than control groups, so all participants were responding to at least a limited intervention, and the natural history of smoking of parents. Action on Smoking and Health (ASH) stress the importance of public opinion in this respect, suggesting that smoking bans with widespread public support are a prerequisite for the adoption of smoking restrictions at home. Again this is supported by review-level evidence (albeit from the US), which suggests that interventions to decrease exposure to second-hand smoke "can act as a method to 'de-normalise' tobacco use ... and that smoking prevalence will fall as a result" (Taylor et al, 2005, p 2). Education, while limited in effect as a standalone tool, is thus critical to the wider agenda.

Limitations to the evidence base

Bull et al (2003) outline a number of key areas where the current evidence base provides a poor foundation for policy and practice. These include the efficacy of the individual components of a programme (including the effectiveness of interventions when delivered by different medical staff in different settings), features that might increase cessation among particular risk groups (such as heavy smokers and women of lower socio-economic class), strategies that are effective against relapse, interventions that include the family as a whole and cultural appropriateness. Evidence about the unreliability of self-report in healthcare settings, especially during maternity care itself, is very strong in recent trials, reducing the potential contribution of studies that do not validate smoking status (Lumley et al, 2001). A review of smoking cessation and its influence on breastfeeding also found that many studies failed to take into account confounding variables such as age and socio-economic status and tended to treat smoking as a dichotomous variable, failing to consider the often very different experiences of heavy and light smokers (Amir and Donath, 2002).

Policy

Two broad types of policy initiative intended to tackle smoking can be identified: those relating to the supply of tobacco products, such as restrictions on young people buying tobacco, and those relating to demand, such as taxes on tobacco, bans on advertising and promotion, and smoking restrictions (Platt et al, 2002). The 1998 White Paper, *Smoking kills* (DH, 1998), responded directly to the evidence of the harmful effects of smoking by introducing, for the first time, a comprehensive national tobacco control strategy spanning both these areas and ranging from controls on advertising and smuggling, through clean air initiatives, health education and media campaigns.

The focus of the White Paper on health inequalities was furthered by the inclusion of smoking cessation strategies that were aimed particularly at disadvantaged adults and two key risk groups: young people and pregnant women. Over £60 million was thus made available to health authorities between 1999 and 2002 to establish new smoking cessation services. This represented both the development of a new clinical service and the availability for the first time of

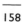

treatment for patients addicted to nicotine (Coleman et al, 2005). In the first year (from April 1999) these funds were made available only to HAZs, areas where smoking prevalence was among the highest in England, and to which £10 million was targeted for the most disadvantaged smokers. Drawing on the evidence base, these services focused on a combination of behavioural support and medication (NRT) (with guidelines proposing opportunistic interventions alongside smoking cessation services) (McNeill et al, 2005). 2000 and 2001 then saw funds more widely distributed across the country to enable health professionals similarly to refer smokers for specialist counselling, advice and support.

This policy has been reinforced by a series of group-specific targets, the most recent being contained in the *Priorities and planning framework 2003-2006* (DH, 2002), which set the targets for the delivery of *The NHS Plan* and made health inequalities a priority for the NHS. Here reducing smoking in pregnancy was identified as one of the key NHS interventions required to deliver the national health inequalities target. This requires both a one percentage point reduction per year in the proportion of women continuing to smoke throughout pregnancy and a special focus on smokers from disadvantaged groups. Arguably, however, the centrality of smoking cessation policies to the government's plans to reduce deaths from coronary heart disease (CHD) and cancer has overshadowed its importance in pregnancy and early life. At the same time, the difficulties evidenced in giving up smoking during pregnancy bear witness to the need to adopt support strategies for the whole community, including actions to reduce initiation by young people (Lumley et al, 2001).

In April 2003 responsibility for the newly established smoking cessation services was transferred from the health authorities to primary care trusts (PCTs), with a further large-scale injection of funds and a performance indicator relating to the overall smoking cessation rate. The accompanying recommendations continue to reflect the evidence base, including the HAZ evaluation, with the PCT-level (or larger) service expected to deliver group and individual-based interventions, be funded on a permanent basis, headed by a full-time equivalent (FTE) coordinator with a core staff of three FTEs in an average sized PCT and linked to both primary care teams and tertiary services (West et al, 2003). The strategy is also expected to reach all smokers while maintaining the focus on those with a low income and pregnant women. However, drawing on research, it also admits that the latter continue to prove difficult to reach and therefore costly on a per capita basis (Taylor and Hajek, 2001). The Health Development Agency (HDA), in highlighting public health interventions where success is likely, stress nevertheless that "formal smoking cessation must be a constituent part of ante-natal care to prevent low birth weight" (Kelly, 2004, p 2), and this is reinforced by the maternity standard within the National Service Framework (NSF) for Children, Young People and Maternity Services, which includes services for women and their partners who request support to stop smoking as one of the markers of good practice (DH, 2004b, p 5).

Sure Start could also have had a potentially important role to play here, as it does in nearly every aspect of early years policy. One of its (four) Public Service Agreement (PSA) targets relates to child health and originally (2000) demanded a 10% reduction in the proportion of mothers who continue to smoke during pregnancy, revised downwards to six percentage points in 2002. However, progress is uncertain. Programmes reported an increase in mothers smoking from 40% to 42% between 2000-01 and 2001-02 (DfES, 2003a) but baseline data for 2002-03 suggested that the mothers of only 29% of babies in Sure Start Local Programme (SSLP) areas smoked during pregnancy, and programmes had reported a six percentage point reduction in women smoking in pregnancy for the period 2000-01 to 2002-03. Official progress against the 2002 target has not, however, been assessed yet (DfES, 2004).

Meanwhile, the fact that most interventions continue to be aimed at the prenatal period represents a wider lost opportunity to use primary care and a failure to address the issues of relapse and family smoking. As Hall and Elliman (2003) note, a child's respiratory or ear, nose and throat illness offers an ideal opportunity to address the issue surrounding smoking, yet the opportunity is under-utilised (see also Winickoff et al, 2003a, 2003b) and the importance to early life of both the preconception and postpartum periods remains tacit in policy terms. One potential lever may be the Public Health White Paper *Choosing health*, which not only includes reducing the number of people who smoke as one of its six overarching priorities but aims to shift the balance significantly in favour of smoke-free environments, with bans on smoking in all enclosed public places and work places expected by 2008 (HM Government and DH, 2004).

Nutritional interventions

The Welfare Food Scheme was introduced in 1940 and nutritional interventions for early life have tended to focus since on the health of the pregnant mother and the subsequent adequacy of the diet, measured primarily through infant weight gain. With greater acknowledgement of the lifecourse approach, there is now, however, increasing interest in the effects of nutritional status on long-term health. The National Heart Foundation, for example, places considerable stress on the dietary status of pregnant women, breastfeeding and healthy weaning as part of a proposed national strategy to ensure children born today remain free from avoidable CHD until old age (National Heart Forum, 2002). This has been compounded by the debate, outlined in Chapter Four, as to the relative significance of diet and activity on weight gain as opposed to biological programming in early life. The key areas for intervention outlined next illustrate both this progression and uncertainty.

What works? Evidence and practice

Maternal nutritional supplements

Nutritional interventions in pregnant women (along with, as we have already seen, smoking cessation) have long been seen as leading candidates for the prevention of low birth weight and, given the general adequacy of diet, attention has focused on the effectiveness of nutrient supplements. There is, however, a paucity of high-quality systematic reviews relating to nutrition and low birth weight, leading one reviewer to suggest that calcium is the only nutritional intervention for which good evidence exists for a reduction in preterm birth and the incidence of low birth weight (Bull et al, 2003), especially among women at risk of hypertensive disorders (Atallah et al, 2001). De Onis et al (1998) find a similar confusion of evidence emerging from systematic reviews, but conclude that only dietary supplementation based on balanced protein and energy content consistently improves foetal growth. Other supplements are found to be either the subject of conflicting evidence (such as vitamin D, fish oils and folate supplementation), or a lack of evidence (for example, magnesium, iron, combined iron and folate, and zinc), despite the fact that, for example, maternal anaemia during early pregnancy has been found to be associated with a 32% increased risk of preterm birth (Xiong et al, 2000). There is also a suggestion that some interventions may not only be ineffective in preventing low birth weight but may indeed be harmful. Not surprisingly, therefore, question marks remain over the effectiveness of nutritional advice in pregnancy.

As Bull et al (2003) stress, there are a number of very persuasive reasons why these low levels of confidence and conflicting results continue. One is the lack of targeted evaluation focusing on particular socio-economic, ethnic or vulnerable groups, those subject to multiple risks from smoking, poor diet and negative psychosocial factors. While there is a lack of evidence for the *routine* use of, for example, iron supplementation as part of a population-based policy, this is not to say that iron supplementation is ineffective in addressing the association between maternal anaemia during early pregnancy and preterm birth (Kramer, 1987; Xiong et al, 2000). Half of all 15- to 18-year-old girls, for example, as Chapter Eight later shows, have iron intakes lower than the Lower Reference Nutrient Intake (LRNI), suggesting supplementation may be potentially important for teenage mothers. Dietary calcium intakes in the female UK population, the area where research finds intervention to be effective, are in contrast notably low across the population. Again, however, Chapter Eight shows the shortfall to be particularly pronounced for young women with one in five 15- to 18-year-olds having lower than the recommended intakes. Jackson and Robinson (2001) argue that there is an allied need to consider metabolic differences between women if the effects of supplementation are to be accurately assessed.

A second limitation concerns the stage of intervention. Most trials have been conducted in mid to late pregnancy, which may be too late to compensate for long-standing nutritional deprivation. In contrast, changes to maternal nutrition before conception and in early pregnancy may have a greater influence on foetal growth. Indeed, following a lifecycle approach, Osrin and de L. Costello (2000) suggest dietary change at a number of stages, starting with infancy. A third obstacle is the focus on single interventions which are unlikely to reduce the rate of a multicausal outcome such as intrauterine growth retardation and which ignore the potential for nutrient-on-nutrient interactions. Instead, a combination of interventions are suggested (de Onis et al, 1998) together with food-based rather than nutrient-based interventions (discussed later in this chapter).

A fourth confounding dimension is the recent debate introduced in Chapter Four between maternal and foetal nutrition. This suggests that while under-nutrition and micronutrient deficiencies are critical in terms of body structure, physiology and metabolism, and hence a range of risk factors for later life, including obesity, it may be other factors such as stress and stress behaviours that have a more pronounced effect on foetal nutrition and hence birth weight. In this context (and given a broadly adequate diet) the link between maternal nutritional supplements and improved health outcomes as measured by birth weight might only be expected to be tenuous.

Breastfeeding initiation and duration

Breastfeeding, as Chapter Four stressed, is a key public health issue for both child and mother. Current healthy eating guidelines issued by the Department of Health (DH) for infants up to one year, recommend that mothers breastfeed exclusively for four to six months, with the World Health Organization (WHO) recommending that, wherever possible, infants should be fed exclusively on breast milk until six months of age (WHO, 2002). In practice, however, only around 70% of babies in the UK are breastfed at all, and the duration of breastfeeding is low, with only one in five infants being breastfed at six months of age (Hamlyn et al, 2002).

Five key types of intervention designed to promote the initiation of breastfeeding can be identified: health education interventions; health sector initiatives; peer support programmes; media campaigns; and multifaceted interventions (NHS CRD, 2000; Protheroe et al, 2003). Most women decide what method of feeding to adopt pre-birth and prior to contact with health professionals. This decision is shaped not just by knowledge but by informal networks, family experience, exposure to infant feeding and factors such as a desire for shared parenting or an identity beyond motherhood (Earle, 2002). The review evidence for health education suggests, nevertheless, that small, informal discussion classes led by health professionals, that emphasise the benefits of breastfeeding and provide practical advice, can increase initiation rates, although one-to-one education sessions may be necessary to persuade women who have decided to feed infant formula to breastfeed instead (Tedstone et al, 1998; Fairbank et al, 2000). Such interventions appear most likely to have a positive effect if they are broad-based, combining advice, education and staff training, span the ante- and postnatal period and draw on repeated contacts with either a professional or peer educator.

Health sector initiatives aim instead to change the organisational nature of health services in favour of promoting breastfeeding. They cover a range of practices that are supported by the evidence base, such as avoiding separating the mother and baby on the first night or offering supplementary fluids, encouraging unrestricted breastfeeding, skin-to-skin contact and the early initiation of breastfeeding consequent on a caesarean section, and offering advice and treatment to prevent mastitis or sore nipples (Rowe-Murray and Fisher, 2002; Renfrew et al, 2004), together with the training of health professionals. Few breastfeeding training courses for health professionals have yet been formally evaluated. Current evidence (Protheroe et al, 2003) suggests that training alone tends to be ineffective (although intensive targeted lactation training may increase initiation rates particularly if it has mandatory status and a minimum duration of 18 hours [Vallenas and Savage, 1999]). Training is more likely to have an effect as part of a package, as in the Baby Friendly Hospital Initiative (BFHI) (Box 5.2).

Box 5.2: Breastfeeding: a health sector initiative

The BFHI is a global programme of the United Nations Children's Fund (UNICEF) and the WHO. It works with health services to improve practices so that parents can "make informed choices about how they feed and care for their babies" (www.babyfriendly.org.uk). The UK BFHI was launched in 1994 and there are now 53 fully accredited Baby Friendly Hospitals and community facilities and 68 maternity units or community services with a Certificate of Commitment. Accredited units have to have a written policy on breastfeeding, provide training for staff, offer information to women and provide a supportive environment. They also collect statistics on breastfeeding rates.

As part of a randomised cluster trial, maternity hospitals were randomly allocated to receive the BFHI, with 16,491 mother–baby pairs followed up for 12 months. Those born in intervention hospitals were significantly more likely to be exclusively breastfed at three and six months of age. They also had significantly reduced incidence of gastrointestinal infection and atopic eczema (Kramer et al, 2001). Some of the largest increments were found in inner-city hospitals where initiation rates have traditionally been low (UNICEF UK BFI, 2000). A review of the evidence base for the initiative found effectiveness most clearly established in terms of the delivery of antenatal education, practical instruction in breastfeeding and continuing support after discharge from hospital (Vallenas and Savage, 1999).

The Women, Infants and Children (WIC) Program of special supplemental nutrition suggests more specifically that initiation rates can be increased among low-income women, particularly if they include a peer support component (NHS CRD, 2000). The inclusion of peers as facilitators and advocates is a significant component of many such multifaceted programmes and appears to be effective because it offers contact over time with women who have successfully breastfed, role models that are often lacking in deprived communities (Hoddinott and Pill, 1999; Taylor et al, 2000; Raine, 2003). It also counters problems non-professional women may have in seeking advice from professionals. Standalone effectiveness is restricted, however, to those who wish to breastfeed, not those wishing to bottle feed (Protheroe et al, 2003). Box 5.3 suggests it may also help compensate for the low priority accorded to breastfeeding among healthcare professionals in deprived areas and the fact that many midwives and health visitors have limited time to support women wishing to breastfeed or to influence initiation rates.

Box 5.3: The Breastfeeding is Best Supporters (BIBS) Project

BIBS is a breastfeeding peer support programme. Based in North Sheffield, it is funded by Social Regeneration Budget (SRB) 5 and Sure Start and was able to build on the work of two earlier DH infant feeding projects. Its aims were to increase initiation and duration rates, consolidate local support networks and develop local role models. The intervention was based around the work of paid support workers and volunteers who provided a 'hands-on approach' via antenatal clinics and postnatal home visits, as well as facilitating the breastfeeding groups. An allied programme aimed to promote breastfeeding awareness by both running awareness days (aimed at groups such as school nurses, crèche workers, nurseries and playgroups) and delivering training for health professionals at the local health centres.

Evaluation of initiation and duration rates had to focus on the Sure Start area alone because of the lack of more generally available infant feeding statistics and thus related to fewer than 200 women. This showed initiation rates more than doubling from 22% in 1998 to 47% in 2002. Continuation rates rose from 2.5% at four months (based on health visitor caseloads) to 19% at three months and 11% at six months. The number of breastfeeding support networks also increased from two to six and 23 women undertook the La Lèche League breastfeeding peer support programme, providing the foundation for a network of role models.

The programme found it harder to attract interest in the breastfeeding awareness days, with many organisations failing to respond. Similarly, none of the local health centres took up the offered training places and progress was only made via training delivered within three of the local health centres. This uncovered a degree of scepticism about the benefits of breastfeeding among health visitors and GPs (Battersby, 2002a, 2002b).

Media campaigns also have the potential to raise awareness and promote breastfeeding, but evaluative evidence is scarce and dated (Kirk, 1980). Again, research suggests that its role is as part of a package, with the majority of effective multifaceted interventions including media campaigns.

In Scandinavia, where initiation rates stand at around 98%, such multifaceted interventions have been standard for the past 20 years. Four elements are key to this strategy, although evaluation does not isolate which elements are the most effective or whether the combined package is necessary (Protheroe et al, 2003). Three of these elements largely mirror the issues considered earlier: health education; maternity ward practice; and peer support groups (combined with increasing collective experience of breastfeeding and hence professional sensitivity). The fourth element is distinct, however: an increase in paid maternity leave and guaranteed return to previous employment. Bailey and Pain (2001) note, for example, that Norway has increased maintenance rates from 30% at 12 weeks in 1968 to 75% at six months, drawing on policy measures such as a year's maternity break, breastfeeding breaks and facilities for expressing at work, together with strict controls on the marketing of formula milk. Indeed, a report for the WHO finds that discontinuing the provision of formula in maternity facilities is one of the most cost-effective health interventions known (Vallenas and Savage, 1999; Renfrew et al, 2004).

The most successful breastfeeding promotions tend, as noted earlier, to be long term, spanning both pre- and postnatal periods; intensive, involving multiple contacts with a professional breastfeeding promoter or peer counsellor; and combine a number of related elements. Their impact thus relates both to initiation and *duration*. Sikorski et al (2004) found clear evidence for the effectiveness of professional support on the duration of (any) breastfeeding and for the effectiveness of lay support in promoting exclusive breastfeeding. Short-term health benefits were also well demonstrated, in particular the effectiveness of exclusive breastfeeding in the management of diarrhoeal illnesses in infants. Studies focusing predominantly on face-to-face contact produced the strongest effects. The authors thus recommended breastfeeding support as part of routine health service provision (see also Renfrew et al, 2004).

Obstacles to continuation are significant, however. The National Infant Feeding Survey found that over 80% of women who stop breastfeeding before four months would have liked to have continued for longer (Hamlyn et al, 2002). Issues such as engorgement and the (generally perceptual) problem of insufficient milk supply can be overcome with support, but the psychosocial factors of a supportive personal (Scott and Binns, 1999) and social environment and the ability to combine motherhood with work require more far-reaching changes. Italy, Portugal, Spain and France, for example, all offer new mothers rest periods during the day or options to use this time to shorten the working day (UNICEF UK BFI, 1999).

Nutrition in the weaning and post-weaning period

Current healthy eating guidelines produced by the DH for infants up to one year suggest that weaning to a solid diet should not begin before four months, with non-wheat cereals, vegetables and some fruit to which no salt or sugar have been added suitable as first weaning foods. The majority of babies, however, are introduced to solids earlier than this, with allied concerns surrounding low iron intakes, the use of unmodified cows' milk, high levels of non-milk extrinsic sugars and the variety of weaning foods.

There is limited review-level evidence in support of promoting good feeding practice in the weaning and post-weaning period, despite the potential importance of catch-up growth in this period (see Chapter Four). Tedstone et al (1998) found just six studies, the focus of which were the diets of minority ethnic or low-income family infants. Only two reported successful interventions. One found delayed introduction of solid foods following a lactation counselling programme, the other showed delayed introduction of cows' milk and improved diet resulting from a peer support programme throughout the first year of an infant's life. Three interventions that focused on infant anaemia failed to produce any significant effects. Modification of the contents of commercial packs given to women on hospital discharge also delayed the introduction of daily solids.

Food-based interventions for mother and child

Poverty is associated with food insecurity, hunger and poor diets, with the poorest 10% of households spending a higher proportion of their income on food but consuming less in real terms (Dowler et al, 2001). Children living in households on Income Support appear at particular risk, although research suggests that parents in such circumstances frequently forsake food themselves in order to feed their children (Dowler, 1998). Not all agree that unhealthy diets can be attributed to a simple lack of money. However, income measures, improvements in accessibility and the movement to promote cheap food in the community, and community cafes, are still more generally considered to be of greater relevance to improving nutrition than nutritional education through didactic means.

Food projects in the UK are subject to both the traditional health driver and the more recent imperative of community regeneration. Many of the former, most notably Breakfast Clubs, the National Fruit Pilot Scheme and Five a Day are focused primarily on school children (and are thus considered in Chapter Nine), while the latter most commonly target women with families. In contrast to the two large-scale US programmes described in Box 5.4, therefore, there is a paucity of nutritional interventions aimed specifically at families with young children.

Box 5.4: Food-based interventions

The WIC Program has been run by the US Department of Agriculture since 1972. It provides food supplements for low-income pregnant and postpartum women, and children under five years of age, who are considered to be at nutritional risk. Findings from evaluations of WIC have shown improved birth and diet-related outcomes such as a reduction in rates of low and very low birth weights of 25% and 44% respectively (Owen and Owen, 1997). They also suggest that the community health nursing practice of teaching nutrition and childcare via home visits can address child growth deficiency rates (Reifsnider, 1998). There are estimated savings in healthcare costs of $1.77 to $3.13 for every dollar spent on WIC.

A parallel programme, the Expanded Food and Nutrition Education Program (EFNEP), provides nutritional advice and education to low-income families and young people, delivered by paraprofessionals and volunteers. Data from the EFNEP Evaluation/ Reporting System show that 87% of participants improved in one or more nutritional practices (for example, making healthy food choices, planning meals or reading nutrition labels). A recent cost-benefit analysis of the Virginia EFNEP found that for every dollar spent in implementing the programme, there was a $10.64 benefit due to reduced healthcare costs (Rajgopal et al, 2002).

Limitations to the evidence base

In what is to become a common theme, there are difficulties in assessing exactly what works because of a lack of structured evaluation, a multiplicity of variables and a paucity of baseline data. With respect to breastfeeding there has been, for example, no commonly accepted definition for either initiation or continuation. The ethical problems associated with randomising mothers' feeding choices also mean that case–control and cohort study experimental designs tend to be the only practical methodological option (Nicoll and Williams, 2002). Scientific reviews, with their emphasis on randomised controlled trials (RCTs), thus admit only a portion of the available research. They also draw heavily on US experience. Messages for policy nevertheless crystallise around the importance of early intervention, the need to promote breastfeeding as an integral part of a much wider nutritional agenda, the need for innovative work with key target groups such as low-income and minority ethnic families, and the need to consider the relationship between early nutrition, income and work.

Policy

The *Independent Inquiry into Inequalities in Health* states that "a baby's long-term health is related to the nutrition and physique of its mother" and recommended "policies which improve the health and nutrition of women of childbearing age and their children" (Acheson, 1998, p 70). This has been reinforced strategically, as noted earlier, by the creation of a headline national target on health inequality, which aims to reduce the gap in infant mortality between manual groups and the population as a whole. Low birth weight is a key element in this equation, being a major cause of infant mortality in developed countries, including the UK. Improving nutrition in women of child-bearing age was thus one of the key National Health Service (NHS) interventions identified in support of the national health inequalities target, as was increasing breastfeeding initiation and duration rates.

Of the four possible intervention areas outlined earlier, it is the promotion of breastfeeding that has received the most political attention. This is also the area for which research evidence is the strongest, yet where initiation rates have remained largely static in England and Wales since 1980 (NHS CRD, 2000). There appear to be three key practical barriers to increasing initiation and duration rates for breastfeeding. The first is a need to change public attitudes towards breastfeeding so that it is seen as normal, health-promoting behaviour, acceptable and practicable outside the home (Acheson, 1998). The second is an improvement in healthcare practices and the third, a key 'upstream' intervention, the issue of maternity leave, which militates against both initiation and continuation.

The White Paper *Saving lives: Our healthier nation* (DH, 1999) recommended policies to increase the prevalence of breastfeeding as a means of both improving health and (given the marked class differences in initiation rates) reducing health inequalities. This included raising awareness of the benefits of breastfeeding, financial support for the annual National Breastfeeding Awareness Week and the appointment of two part-time national infant feeding advisors in England. The potential impact of increasing breastfeeding rates on public health was also recognised in the government's *NHS Plan*, where a commitment to increase support for breastfeeding by 2004 formed part of the proposed strategy to improve diet and nutrition (DH, 2000). This has been translated into national targets, with the DH's *Priorities and planning framework 2003-2006* requiring all PCTs to "deliver an increase of 2 percentage points per year in breastfeeding initiation rate, focussing especially on women from disadvantaged groups" (DH, 2002, p 20), and consolidated by the emphasis within the maternity standard on services that promote breastfeeding (DH, 2004a).

This should give a significant impetus to one of the most stridently criticised aspects of breastfeeding policy, the lack of accurate statistics (Roberts, 2000). As noted earlier, neither initiation nor duration are simple concepts, and there is a marked difference in health and policy terms between a single feed, mixed feeding and prolonged exclusive feeding. The DH has, however, clarified data collection procedures for the calculation of initiation rates in order that local delivery plans can monitor their contribution to this new national target, whereas previously there was no agreed method for monitoring the prevalence of breastfeeding at various ages in England and Wales (DH, 2003b). This situation contrasted starkly with other (admittedly much less complicated) child health promotion strategies such as immunisation (Nicoll and Williams, 2002). It also contrasted with the situation in Scotland where national targets for breastfeeding were established in 1994 and data are routinely collected at the end of the first week of life, allowing calculation of at least initial breastfeeding prevalence by postcode and maternity unit.

This difference may partially explain the increase in breastfeeding prevalence in Scotland from 50% to 63% between 1990 and 2000 compared to the lack of significant change in England and Wales (when adjusted for maternal age and education). Other contributory factors could similarly include the earlier appointment of a part-time national breastfeeding advisor with responsibility for assisting health boards to develop breastfeeding strategies and to reach breastfeeding targets and the formation of the Scottish Breastfeeding Group in 1995. Figures from the five-yearly Infant Feeding Survey do show, however, that practices recommended by the Baby Friendly Initiative (BFI), such as a full discussion of infant feeding during antenatal checks and not giving breastfed babies formula in hospital, are gaining ground, and there has been a 7% rise in breastfeeding rates among mothers from Social Class V (Hamlyn et al, 2002).

The DH's Infant Feeding Initiative (IFI) sought specifically to increase the initiation and duration of breastfeeding among those groups of the population least likely to breastfeed. Between 1999 and 2002 it funded and evaluated 79 best practice projects. The largest number of these, linking closely with the research base, focused on breastfeeding support centres, peer support programmes, antenatal workshops/educational programmes and education and training for health professional (Dykes, 2003). They also offered an opportunity for the involvement of the four key voluntary organisations supporting breastfeeding women: the Association of Breastfeeding Mothers, the Breastfeeding Network, La Lèche League and the National Childbirth Trust. The HDA Collaborating Centre for Maternal and Child Nutrition also now intends to act in support of the evidence base by supporting capacity building among practitioners working with child-bearing women. It recognises, however, that it has to overcome practices that have become embedded in the thinking and behaviour of several generations of practitioners (Renfrew et al, 2004). The same applies to current media representations. One study of breast and bottle feeding images within British television and newspapers found that bottle feeding was normalised and represented as the obvious choice, the subject not only of more frequent references but also of more visual and less problematic references (Henderson et al, 2000).

Similarly, employment policy does not act strongly to support public health policy. Changes in maternity leave could, as the Norwegian figures suggest, increase both initiation and duration of breastfeeding by enabling women to afford longer periods outside the workforce. Changes made by the government in April 2003 represent a move in the right direction, increasing the length of

Statutory Maternity Pay and Maternity Allowance to 26 weeks, raising the rates at which it is paid and reducing the sickness trigger to four weeks before expected childbirth. This still falls short, however, of recommendations to link maternity pay to women's normal earnings (UNICEF UK BFI, 1999), offering a standard rate of £106 per week (from April 2005) for most women after the first six weeks' leave, and tends to reinforce health inequalities by acting as a disincentive to other than the more financially secure. Paid maternity leave will, however, be extended further to nine months from April 2007, with the aim of providing 12 months' paid leave by the end of the next Parliament, together with the ability to transfer a proportion of both maternity pay and leave to the father (HM Treasury et al, 2004). Still, the impact on women outside the labour market or those only marginally engaged is, as Chapter Four discussed, likely to remain minimal. The lowest initiation rates in the UK (52%) are among those women who have never worked. Support on return to work is often also tokenistic. The Health and Safety Executive, for example, recommends the provision of a private, healthy, safe environment for nursing mothers to express and store milk as good employment practice, but it is not a legal requirement and the incidence of such facilities in practice is unknown.

In common with other nutritional interventions, the promotion and support of breastfeeding is also compromised by commercial interests and the lack of political support to challenge these vested interests. The WHO's International Code of Marketing of Breast-milk Substitutes states that such products should not be advertised or promoted, although accurate information should be available. The UK government has, however, only translated one part of this code into law (UNICEF UK BFI, 1999), preventing the promotion of infant formula. Advertising of breast milk substitutes continues therefore to be widespread, although restricted to follow-on milks, as is the existence of sponsored 'carelines' and branded gifts in hospital welcome packs (Baby Feeding Law Group, 2004). One estimate has suggested that if all babies were breastfed, the NHS would save £35 million per year in England and Wales in treating gastroenteritis in bottle-fed infants (DH, 1995).

The Acheson Report (1998) argued for priority to be given to the elimination of food poverty. However, beyond breastfeeding, recent policy changes relating to nutrition at the national level have been aimed primarily at school children (see Chapter Nine). Nutrition appears a neglected policy area at the local level too; a National Society for the Prevention of Cruelty to Children (NSPCC) survey of Health Improvement Programmes produced by 88 health authorities in the UK found only three that included specific nutrition activities (NSPCC, cited in Watt et al, 1999). There is a paradox, therefore, between the potential immediacy of actions that improve maternal and infant nutrition and a paucity of policy. One response has been calls to strengthen the child health component of Sure Start, with particular emphasis on breastfeeding and weaning. As noted earlier, however, there is currently only one Sure Start PSA target for child health and this relates to smoking during pregnancy. Earlier (and unmet) targets similarly neglected infant nutrition, focusing on low birth weight and emergency admissions during the first year of life (DfES, 2003a). In a performance-driven environment, such an omission can be critical in determining the focus of the programme and with Sure Start now accountable to the Department for Education and Skills (DfES) and the Department for Work and Pensions (DWP) rather than the DH, an increased emphasis on child health seems unlikely.

There have also been calls for a review of the Welfare Food Scheme in the UK along the lines of the WIC Program (Nicoll and Williams, 2002). The existing scheme, which provides support primarily for families on a very low income, was the subject of limited review in 2003, resulting in a broadening of the nutritional base to include fruit, vegetables and a variety of other weaning foods, rather than just liquid milk or infant formula. It also aims to increase access, remove the disincentives to breastfeeding by introducing a fixed-value food voucher exchangeable at retail outlets, and provide a choice of milk or fruit to children at nursery school. A third change is the shift in emphasis from welfare to health with the scheme renamed Healthy Start and beneficiaries required to register via a health professional so as to gain access to advice on nutrition and breastfeeding (DH, 2004b). Formula milk will also no longer be available from health centres (HM Government and DH, 2004), ending a major contradiction between official policy and practice. The desire to restrict scheme expenditure to the previous levels of expenditure (£142 million across Britain) means, however, that the scope for real change is limited. Given that one in four children under five live in households qualifying for benefits, the potential for a broader public health programme remains considerable. The growing concern with obesity may provide the imperative for a more holistic approach to nutrition in the early years.

Parenting education and support

"Publicly funded health services have been provided to advise, educate, and support mothers for over a century" in the UK (Patterson et al, 2002a, p 468). However, while this advice has traditionally focused on the physical aspects of parenting (Taylor et al, 2000), attention is now also being directed towards the socio-emotional aspects, with parenting recognised as a risk factor for mental illness and antisocial behaviour in childhood and beyond (Oakley-Browne et al, 1995; Patterson et al, 2002b). The early manifestation of behavioural problems (typically beginning at two or three years) is now known to be linked to conduct disorder in later life, including the likelihood of rejection by peers, truancy from school, juvenile offending and an increased chance of unemployment (Farrington, 1996; Moffit et al, 1996; Rutter et al, 1998).

The prevalence of such behavioural problems in early life is high (see Chapter Six). Studies suggest between 7% and 20% of young children meet the clinical criteria for externalising conduct problems such as Attention Deficit/ Hyperactivity Disorder (ADHD) (Campbell, 1995; Webster-Stratton, 1999; Zwi et al, 2003). The highest rates are found in families who are on a low income or unemployed, among lone-parent families, those without educational qualifications and those living in social sector housing (Meltzer et al, 2000). However, although certain childcare problems may be more prevalent in lower-income groups, the total number of children and parents in need of help is far greater in middle-income groups (Newman and Roberts, 1999), while other risk factors, such as parental isolation and depression, are increasing.

Costs to the individual and society can be considerable. A study following 142 10-year-old children into adulthood identified the long-term costs of conduct problems across six domains: special educational provision; foster and residential care; relationship breakdown; health; crime; and state benefits in adulthood. The average costs by the age of 28 varied tenfold, from £7,423 for children classified as having no problems, to £24,324 for those classified as having conduct problems and £70,019 for those with conduct disorders (Scott et al, 2001a). Parenting and family interaction factors are estimated to account for as much as 30% to 40% of the variation in child antisocial behaviour (Gibbs et al, 2003). There is a growing recognition, therefore, that parenting is an important educational, social and public health issue (Hoghughi and Speight, 1998). Evidence as to what works does not necessarily follow the early years divide, extending often from the young child to the pre-adolescent.

What works? Evidence and practice

An appropriate definition of parenting education is one that acknowledges the breadth of the possible interventions, that is the: "range of educational and supportive activities which help parents and prospective parents to understand their own social, emotional, psychological and physical needs and those of their children and enhances the relationship between them" (Pugh et al, 1994, p 66). These activities, Pugh et al continue, create both a supportive network of services within local communities and help families take advantage of them.

Behavioural interventions

Lloyd (1999), drawing on both a systematic review of quantitative overviews and RCTs with children aged three to 10 years (Barlow, 1997), and a wider-ranging review of evidence-based research (Newman and Roberts, 1999), concludes that parent education programmes *can* improve the behaviour of pre-adolescent children who have behavioural problems. By definition, however, the report emphasises the efficacy of behaviourally orientated interventions. These typically focus on rectifying problems in specific 'problem' groups, such as children with a conduct disorder or families where child abuse has occurred, and have tended to be implemented and evaluated in a primarily medical environment (Webster-Stratton, 1999; Sanders et al, 2000; Bor et al, 2002). Much of the quantitative research in this field has also been conducted in the US, posing questions as to transferability across national boundaries (Barlow and Stewart-Brown, 2000). However, local applications of the Webster-Stratton programmes (see Box 5.5) represent important departures in this respect.

Effects are sustained but not universal. One third of parents typically continue to experience difficulties (Barlow, 1997). A disproportionate number of these are likely to be single parents, those suffering from maternal depression, alcoholism or drug misuse and of a low socio-economic status (Webster-Stratton and Hammond, 1990). Similar attributes, including poverty, high levels of stress, high levels of child conduct disorder and minority ethnic status, apply to attrition from parenting programmes (Danoff et al, 1994; Katz et al, 2001; Mielck et al, 2002; Gibbs et al, 2003), and, indeed, may depress initial uptake. This suggests that even when initiatives target the disadvantaged it remains most difficult to reach those in most need. It may also suggest too narrow an approach in response to complex problems (Macdonald and Roberts, 1995).

Box 5.5: A group-based behavioural intervention

The series of group-based programmes, developed by Webster-Stratton at the University of Washington's Parenting Clinic in Seattle, uses videos to prompt discussions of a wide range of parenting techniques. Topics include play, praise, incentives, setting limits and discipline. The initial goals of improving children's conduct problems and social competence have been extended to strengthen parents' social support and involve schools and the community (Webster-Stratton, 1999).

Related programmes are now becoming available in the UK. Two key applications here have focused on their potential within regular clinical practice – delivered by health visitors in primary care (Patterson et al, 2002b), and clinic staff within child mental health services (Scott et al, 2001b). Targeting parents with children aged between two/three and eight years, the programmes varied between 10 and 13-16 weeks, and required both group attendance and consolidation at home.

Both found significant positive differences between intervention and control groups in terms of a reduction in antisocial behaviour among children and an improvement in the incidence of positive parenting. The cost was approximately £600 per child (Scott et al, 2001b). Reservations remain, however, about low participation, high drop-out rates and differential social uptake (Spencer, 2003). Importantly the optimum age for invitation onto this programme is considered to be between two and three years of age (Stewart-Brown et al, 2004). The programmes do not focus explicitly on parents' mental health and the ways in which this could be improved.

The effects for participants can, however, be quantified in terms of benefits to the individual and society. A longitudinal study of the High/Scope programme across 30 years (which included parental involvement and home visits as well as preschool education) found, for example, a sevenfold return on investment measured in terms of savings in health costs, reduced criminality and drug misuse, lower demand for special education, welfare and other public services (Schweinhart et al, 1993), while the Elmira home visiting study was estimated to be cost-neutral within four years as a result of reduced use of healthcare and welfare services (Olds et al, 1993; Leventhal, 1997). Significantly, the role of health savings in such longitudinal studies tends to be very small compared, for example, to the reduced costs to the criminal justice system, education and welfare services (Karoly et al, 1998; Scott et al, 2001a). Hence, the need for an integrated policy framework capable of taking the wider context into account (Vimpani, 2002).

The indications are that programmes where both parents are involved are also more successful than those where only the mothers take part, and that parenting programmes that include direct work with the child are likely to be more effective than those that do not (Lloyd, 1999). Group-based programmes may also produce more changes in children's behaviour and be more cost-effective and user-friendly than individual programmes, providing a source of non-stigmatising support (Cunningham et al, 1995). Evaluations suggest that parents feel listened to, understood and valued through the group process alone, independent of any discrete skills taught. However, there is not necessarily a strong correlation between the strength of client approval and the impact of the intervention when measured by third parties (Macdonald et al, 1992).

A more recent review focused just on the effectiveness of group-based programmes for improving the emotional and behavioural adjustment of children under three (Barlow and Parsons, 2003). This found the interventions produced significant improvements as measured by independent observations, but evidence for the maintenance of this improvement over time was not significant, with only limited follow-up data.

Relational programmes

Relational programmes emphasise emotional understanding as a requisite to behavioural change and are typically implemented in the community. They tend, as Box 5.6 illustrates, to promote more universal access, seeing problems as part of a spectrum of normal behaviour and family functioning (Stewart-Brown, 1998), address public health issues, involve social welfare practitioners and volunteers and place considerable emphasis on process rather than outcomes. However, the distinction is not clear cut. The Systematic Training for Effective Parenting (STEP) programme has, for example, been used with abusive or potentially abusive parents (Fennell and Fishel, 1998).

Critically, given the risk factors associated with the antenatal period and infancy outlined in Chapter Four, relational programmes such as Parents in Partnership–Parent Infant Network (PIPPIN) are also able to intervene before the presentation of behavioural problems, starting with the transition to parenthood. Bryan (2000), for example, reports on a supplement to antenatal classes where couples received three extra sessions covering roles and relations in the transition to parenthood, including infant communication. Participants were found to be more sensitive to infant needs and cues, facilitating secure attachment and parental confidence/involvement (see also Abegglen and Schwartz, 1995).

Box 5.6: A group-based relational intervention

Parenting Matters (formerly called Parent Link) aims to improve the quality of family life by helping parents improve their relationship with their children. It is based on a 30-hour open access course typically delivered through adult and community education or family centres (that is, in a non-health-related environment) over 12 weeks. Trained facilitators include parents. Participants are encouraged to develop communication and listening skills, develop assertiveness and set appropriate behavioural boundaries. Workshops are available on specific issues such as tantrums and sibling rivalry and parents are encouraged to continue with mutual support groups after the course (Sure Start Unit, 2002).

An evaluation (where the average age of the child was six) found short-term improvements in parental self-esteem, levels of stress and family relationships, including lower levels of parental/child conflict. Children's behaviour also improved relative to a comparison group. Parents themselves reported a reduction in authoritarian attitudes and the acquisition of new skills and ideas (Davis and Hester, 1996). In contrast to the targeted behavioural interventions described in Box 5.5, those participating in the evaluation were, however, predominantly middle-class mothers, living with a partner. Applicability to other social, ethnic and cultural backgrounds thus remains to be established, as does long-term efficacy (Lloyd, 1999).

There is, however, a paucity of rigorously evaluated research in this second field (Pugh et al, 1994; Smith and Pugh, 1996), and a suggestion that such interventions may take longer to have an impact on children's behaviour. Relationally orientated parent education programmes appear, therefore, to produce fewer subsequent changes in children's behaviour than behaviourally orientated programmes (Barlow, 1997), and there is insufficient evidence yet to presuppose a preventative effect for the more serious types of parent/child interaction (Lloyd, 1999). Current indicators for the efficacy of relational work include the fact that support from neighbours, friends and families living locally is protective (Pugh, 1999). The best programmes will, therefore, encourage relationships between parents, support the wider family and help build more cohesive communities. They will also encourage collaboration between community-based services and partnership between parents and practitioners, with the most effective facilitation seeming to be an interactive model of learning. Such increasing involvement of parents can also be justified on moral, educational and economic grounds (Wolfendale, 1999), while there is evidence from a number of widely varying studies that befriending and social support increases mothers' perceptions of their emotional well-being and ability to cope (Frost et al, 1996; Davis and Spurr, 1998; Kilgour and Fleming, 2000). Other key factors associated with success are cultural appropriateness and the adoption of a non-stigmatising approach (Eisenstadt, 2000).

Prior to the advent of Sure Start, the main parenting programmes in the UK had emerged in response to demands from parents for a peer-led community-based approach to support child-rearing. In some instances the immediate beneficiaries were the parents/children, while in others the focus was on enhancing professional/support skills so that families could then benefit. Many, like Sure Start, include a central role for volunteers (most notably volunteer mothers) and draw on parents in various guises (from befrienders, home visitors, trained coordinators and project workers), to provide information, support play and early learning and deliver community health and social care. Initiatives such as these continue to be widely distributed and, while often drawing on small studies, provide "at least some positive evidence concerning their effectiveness" (Sure Start Unit, 2002, p 3). Themes running throughout these reviews include an emphasis on the family as a whole and parental well-being rather than just children's behaviour; the development of the role of 'interested friends' rather than experts; enhanced training for practitioners in new roles; and the identification of a positive correlation between sustained involvement and functional improvement. Critically, they also suggest that those on a low income are less likely to believe in or seek out help with parenting (Keller and McDade, 2000).

An integrated approach

Given that the need for education and support is not confined to a particular sector of society, policy and practice need to draw on both relational and behavioural approaches, universal and indicative interventions. There is evidence that targeted approaches are increasingly admitting the importance of the wider context (Webster-Stratton and Hammond, 1998; Park, 1999; Webster-Stratton, 1999; Sanders, 2002) with Park (1999) suggesting that focused parenting programmes can have a more powerful impact if complemented by a broader strategy for enabling individuals through emotional literacy. The Head Start programme, for example, has advocated embedding targeted interventions in universal strategies, having found that home visiting achieved higher participation rates and more sustained improvements in parenting skills than parallel parenting programmes (Stormshak et al, 2002).

Box 5.7 illustrates a tiered approach to child mental health. Tier one (the first point of contact between the family and health agencies) is made more accessible by a combination of home visiting and in-service training of non-specialists, from a diversity of backgrounds, who provide support for families. At tier two child mental health specialists support both front-line staff and parents in the community. Tiers three and four (not described) provide access to increasing practitioner specialisation for the most complex cases.

Box 5.7: A tiered approach to mental health in the community

In Lewisham and Guy's Mental Health NHS Trust local health visitors and paediatric community doctors are trained in parent counselling, parenting and child behaviour management. Once trained, these 'Parent Advisors' (supported by child mental health specialists based in the community) work at home with parents with preschool children. Referred families tend to have multiple problems including emotional/behavioural problems in the children, psychosocial problems in the parents and relationship difficulties in the family (Day and Davis, 1999).

The scheme has increased the knowledge, expertise and confidence of the parent advisors, making expertise more accessible and less stigmatised (Davis et al, 1997). It has also led, at least in the short term, to improvements in maternal self-esteem; reduced levels of stress, depression and anxiety; improvements in the home environment for children; and reductions in their behavioural and emotional problems as measured against a waiting-list control (Davis and Spurr, 1998). Positive results mean training and supervision of a similar nature has been extended to other professional groups in the community, including school nurses and early years centre staff. This will increasingly enable cultural and ethnic differences to be reflected in the Parent Advisor resource. The scheme is also being modified in an attempt to increase the availability of social support to parents. Parent groups are being planned and the Parent Advisor training programme modified so that it addresses relationship issues.

In conjunction with the Parent Advisor Service, the Community Child and Family Service has also developed a specialist early intervention service based in local GP surgeries. Here, the child mental health specialists spend half a day per week in each of the GP practices in the locality, running clinics for parents and children of all ages with emotional and behavioural difficulties. The aim is to provide an accessible and effective service for early identification and intervention. Initial findings suggest significant beneficial changes in parenting and childhood difficulties, and high levels of satisfaction with the service (Day and Davis, 1999). Drawbacks to the evaluation include the lack of random assignment and blind assessment, the degree of reliance on maternal self-report and the absence of a longer-term follow-up assessment.

Supporting families at home

Home visiting has been identified as an important intervention for tackling health inequalities from an intergenerational perspective, capable of producing improvements in parenting, child behavioural problems, cognitive development in high-risk groups, a reduction in accidental injuries to children (see Chapter Seven), and improved detection and management of postnatal depression (Bull et al, 2004). Its potential is further reinforced by evidence from a number of health-based programmes aimed at improving antenatal and postnatal health and child-rearing strategies that have also proved capable of empowering families (Butz et al, 2001; El-Mohandes et al, 2003). The Community Mothers' Programme, for example, trained experienced mothers to support first-time mothers from the same disadvantaged area by visiting at least monthly for the first year of the child's life. Intervention children were more likely than a control group to receive immunisations, appropriate nutrition and better stimulation via, for example, reading and cognitive games (Johnson et al, 1993; Johnson and Molloy, 1995). Mothers reported more positive feelings and a reduction in tiredness and stress. Key attributes include the availability of friendship and support alongside information, often drawing on community educators with similar backgrounds, including experience of parenting (Perkins and MacFarlane, 2001).

A wide-ranging evaluation of the Home Start programme extending across three years (Box 5.8) found volunteer support in the home could usefully extend and complement statutory provision, assisting with parenting difficulties, health problems, isolation and the problems of coping under stress (Frost et al, 1996). However, there is also a significant problem of non-use, which means that many families may fall through the statutory–voluntary sector gap (Oakley et al, 1998). Not all evaluations are positive, however. Goodson et al (2000) followed over 4,000 families participating in the Comprehensive Child Development Program (a home visiting programme for multi-risk low-income children) across a five-year period and found no significant difference in either child outcomes or parent outcomes between the intervention families and the control families. Gray et al (2001) meanwhile found lay therapy unable to address issues of family conflict or stability/meeting basic needs.

Improvements in maternal psychosocial health

Antenatal depression is a significant risk factor for postpartum depression and, as Chapter Four outlined, is higher in situations where the mothers are subject to chronic stressors, such as poverty, housing problems and inadequate social support. In such instances individual psychotherapy can be an effective method of antidepressant treatment during pregnancy with subsequent benefits for mother–infant interaction (Spinelli and Endicott, 2003).

Box 5.8: Home Start

Home Start is a voluntary organisation in which volunteers offer regular support, friendship and practical help to young families under stress in their own home. The majority of families supported in an evaluation of the Wakefield Schemes, for example, were economically vulnerable lone-parent families, unemployed and living in rented accommodation. Nearly two thirds were suffering from ill health and parenting difficulties were identified in a similar proportion of cases.

Evaluation found that key attributes for referrers were the flexible and responsive nature of the service, while the mothers appreciated having someone to befriend them and listen to them as well as a source of support that was neither stigmatising nor threatening. All the surveyed families valued the input of Home Start, with 70% of families satisfied with the support they received and 64% seeing an improvement in their emotional well-being. Home Start was credited as influential in half of these cases (an improvement that was related to regular support from the organisation and improvements in informal support networks).

Reservations concerned the involvement of fathers (which was minimal), a tendency not to refer families where there were concerns about child protection or domestic violence and an unwillingness to accept the service because of perceived stigma. A large proportion of families, therefore, remain vulnerable (Frost et al, 1996). A second study of Home Start also suggested 42% of referrals either did not use the service or did so only briefly. Low users were again more likely to be the most vulnerable (from socially disadvantaged backgrounds, with a history of depression, larger families and children at risk) (Oakley et al, 1998).

A Cochrane Review of group-based parenting programmes suggests that parenting programmes can also make a significant contribution to the short-term psychosocial health of mothers, although it was not obvious which factors contributed to successful outcomes (Barlow and Parsons, 2003). Levels of depression, anxiety/stress, self-esteem and relationship with partner all showed statistically significant improvements, but levels of social support were not affected (Barlow et al, 2002). There was also a paucity of evidence concerning the maintenance of these results over time, although it was suggested that improvements in depression, self-esteem and relationships with partners could be sustained. Stewart-Brown et al (2004) point to the importance of the qualitative dimension in illuminating how such programmes may help parents, including enabling them to feel more able to cope, confident, supported and skilled in dealing with their children's problem behaviour.

Limitations to the evidence base

Despite the existence of an extensive evidence base on parenting and an established research focus on the young child, it is not easy for policy makers to extract clear messages from such a diffuse subject area. The beneficiaries can be the child, the parent, or society as a whole, while within any one dimension the range of positive outcomes is considerable, as is the potential classification of the intervention. Overviews do not tend to isolate effectiveness specifically for the infant or preschool child and confounding dimensions such as gender, ethnicity, family status and race are often neglected (see, for example, Forehand and Kotchik, 1996; Dosnajh and Ghuman, 1998). Studies also often fail to discriminate between the contribution of different programme elements such as format, method of intervention, group support or therapists'/facilitators' skills (Newman and Roberts, 1999; Barlow and Coren, 2003), while the lack of long-term evidence is a constant theme irrespective of target group (Feldman, 1994). There is a bias too in the research focus and hence in the potential messages for policy makers. Most effort, despite the sources of vulnerability outlined in Chapter Four, is focused on behavioural problems in early life and relationship and parenting skills for parents and carers, rather than on preparation for parenthood and family life, whether for school-age children or young people and adults (Lloyd, 1999).

Policy

The potential of parenting education across the spectrum means that it is subject to a number of policy drivers. Support for parents is recognised, for example, as an important element of public health policy (it is another of the NHS interventions identified as key to meeting the national health inequalities target). It was identified as one of four key strands in the government's policy to tackle child poverty (HM Treasury, 2001), and is similarly one of the four main areas that structures the Green Paper *Every child matters*, which aims to reform service delivery for children and protect children at risk (DfES, 2003b). Other imperatives include mental health (also a national priority), antisocial behaviour and social exclusion, particularly in high-risk areas.

One of the main delivery mechanisms is Sure Start. It is delivered (see Chapter Three) via community-based local programmes and grounded in evidence that early intervention and support can help reduce family breakdown, strengthen children's readiness for school and benefit society by preventing social exclusion, regenerating communities and reducing crime (Sure Start Unit, 2002). It focuses on five core services including family support, with perhaps the most direct initiative under this heading being the Community Parental Support Project. This will build on the NSF for Children, Young People and Maternity Services to promote greater parental involvement in children's early learning and development in the most disadvantaged areas and involves training four lead

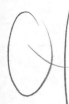

workers in each of the 500 communities supporting every Sure Start local programme, Early Excellence Centre and Children's Centre in England (DH, 2004c). The funds directed into the Sure Start programme also suggest that the rhetoric of support for parenthood may now actually be being matched by resources (for earlier criticism see, for example, Oakley et al, 1998). A total of £540 million was allocated to the programme just for the period 1998-2002 (Pickstone et al, 2002), and a large-scale national evaluation is assessing the impact of the first 260 programmes approved between 1999 and early 2002 (Anning et al, 2004).

Joined-up working (including working in multidisciplinary teams) is, however, as in many area-based initiatives (ABIs), proving challenging. Most programmes operate in an extremely complex policy arena alongside, on average, 10 other government initiatives (Tunstill et al, 2002). The programmes have taken longer to set up than expected, partnership formation has been problematic (including the involvement of parents and the demands placed on voluntary agencies) and attendance at partnership meetings poor (Myers et al, 2004). Sure Start programmes often find themselves in competition with local statutory providers. Staff are often recruited from among local partner agencies, increasing problems for mainstream delivery in areas of staff shortage, while the maintenance of expenditure on mainstream services in Sure Start areas is often under pressure (NESS, 2002). It has also proved difficult to encourage all groups to make use of services and, despite the importance attached, both in the programme and in the evidence base, to 'parenting', there are low levels of father involvement and a paucity of male staff (Lloyd et al, 2003). The move from planning to implementation has also proved problematical, with evaluation challenged by the fact that this is not a single unified programme; spend per child on an annual basis varies sixfold between the highest and lowest spending programmes (Tunstill et al, 2002). A further drawback relates to reach, with the fully operational programme encompassing some 400,000 children, approximately one third of under fours living in poverty (Meadows and Garber, 2004), and early targets aiming for comprehensive contact with young families failing to be met (DfES, 2003a).

Despite these challenges, evaluation suggests that Sure Start is having some measurable impact on a range of child, parenting and family measures. In a preliminary survey of 150 SSLPs and 50 comparison areas, the National Evaluation of Sure Start (NESS) found that on average SSLP mothers/primary carers treated their children in a warmer and more accepting manner than in the comparison areas. At the individual community level, SSLP areas were more than twice as likely as comparison communities to show evidence of better-than-expected functioning across a set of 20 different outcomes related to child development and parenting (NESS, 2004). However, the results also suggested that programmes in less deprived disadvantaged communities might be the more effective, potentially exacerbating health inequalities, and offering no further insights at present into the characteristics of successful interventions.

Outside Sure Start areas there are also increasing levels of activity by providers from both statutory and voluntary sectors in providing services for preschool children with behaviour problems. There are a number of health visitor-facilitated parenting programmes, for example, offering practical and emotional support via group-based parenting programmes that have achieved reductions in clinical anxiety and depression among parents alongside more problem-focused coping strategies (Kilgour and Fleming, 2000; Long et al, 2001). The scope for greater work within primary practice has been recognised (Schultz and Vaughn, 1999), and increased funding is being directed to Home Start which is expected to operate in 90% of local authorities by 2006/07 (DH, 2004c). Not surprisingly, however, there is evidence to suggest that some of the main providers of services are not being adequately prepared and supported in the role, that evidence-based programmes are being modified and used in an ad hoc manner and that coordination within and between services remains poor (Coe et al, 2003).

There are indications, nevertheless, as with Sure Start, of a shift towards a more holistic approach in accordance both with the research base and, more recently, in response to the Laming Inquiry and *Every child matters* (DfES, 2003b). Children's Services Plans required social services to work with health and education in planning services for all children, but with a particular stress on those in greatest need. Children and Young People's Plans now extend this focus to all children, with responsibility falling to the newly appointed local authority Directors of Children's Services (who are accountable for local authority education and children's social services). At the same time, the 2004 Children Act also established a duty to cooperate and a leadership role for local authorities to bring together local partners through Children's Trust arrangements. By 2008 Children's Trusts, led by the Directors of Children's Services, will then assume a key role in coordinating and integrating the planning, commissioning and delivery of children's social services, education, some children's health services, Connexions and optionally other services such as Youth Offending Teams. Thirty-five pathfinders were established in 2003. Additionally, the government aims to establish up to 2,500 Children's Centres also by 2008. These will offer integrated early years education, family and parenting support and health support as well as links to employment and education (DfES, 2003b).

This move towards improved integration at local level is being reinforced at national level. In November 2000 the government announced that it was to set up the Children and Young People's Unit in the DfES in a first attempt to create a cross-cutting departmental unit for children and young people, complete with a £380 million preventative budget for the next three years – the Children's Fund (see Chapter Seven). This process was consolidated (and the Unit superseded) by the transfer of responsibilities for policies on children and families to the DfES in 2003. This included responsibility for children's social services, family policy, teenage pregnancy, family law, and the Children and Family Court Advisory and Support Service. A new Minister for Children, Young People and Families was also created to coordinate policies across government and the post of Children's Commissioner created to promote awareness of the views and interests of children in England (Children's Commissioners for Wales, Scotland and Northern Ireland were already in existence). Policy has also drawn on research in acknowledging the importance of primary prevention. This was one of five themes embodied in the Green Paper *Supporting families* which established the National Family and Parenting Institute (NFPI) in 1999 as a source of advice and support and launched Sure Start (Home Office, 1998). It is also reflected in, for example, the renewed emphasis on a family-centred public health role for health visitors, midwives and nurses (DH, 1999, 2004a) and the emphasis in *Every child matters* on shifting from intervention to prevention.

Tensions are evident, however. Resource constraints mean that practice often continues to focus on crisis, with parenting policy focusing on secondary prevention (targeting high-risk families) or tertiary prevention (helping those already in trouble). The 1989 Children Act, for example, allows courts to prescribe parenting programmes in child protection cases (Macdonald, nd), while later in the lifecycle, they are now a key element of the 1998 Crime and Disorder Act (requiring parents of juveniles in trouble with the law to attend parenting classes). Universal policies thus coexist, sometimes uneasily, alongside high-profile strategies for 'problem families' and debate continues as to whether such programmes have a real and direct value or are merely tools for ensuring children conform (Smith, 1997; Gewirtz, 2001). Sure Start in many ways internalises such tensions, offering a policy of universal access delivered in tightly circumscribed areas and an agenda that ranges from child protection, language development and low birth weight through high-quality play and early education.

Perhaps the most significant policy development, however, is the acknowledgement of context. As Lloyd (1999) points out, parenting education cannot address factors that adversely affect parenting such as poverty, unemployment and poor housing. When a primary healthcare component was introduced into Head Start in Alberta, for example, participants' ability to enhance their children's health and manage their children's illnesses was found to be limited as much by low incomes, inadequate healthcare coverage, and lack of transportation as it was by a lack of knowledge (Williamson and Drummond, 2000). Significantly, there is now a Sure Start PSA target (see the later discussion of childhood poverty) directed at reducing the percentage of children living in households where there is no one working and increasing the amount of registered childcare (HM Treasury, 2004).

Early years education and childcare

It is difficult to distinguish categorically between childcare and education for young children with good care always having an educational value. Definitions based on the tripartite emphasis of the provision – the needs of children with their carers, the needs of children while their parents work, and the provision of developmental and educational opportunities for children (DfEE, 1998) – are also increasingly blurred although they have left their marks in terms of policy and practice (Penn, 2000).

What works? Evidence and practice

With a range of imperatives, a diversity of perspectives and a complex mosaic of provision, (ranging from informal to formal care, individual to group-based provision, open access to specialist referred provision and services that are free at the point of delivery or command the market price), it is also difficult, as with parental support, to establish categorically what works and for whom. The most influential programme in public policy terms has been the US High/Scope Perry Preschool Study (see Box 5.9), which was initiated in Michigan in 1962 in order to assist children born in poverty or otherwise at risk of school failure. In the four decades since its inception, many other studies, primarily US in origin, have addressed the effects of preschool programmes on disadvantaged children, but most have been quasi-experimental and only able to follow the intervention group across a few years. These have similarly shown immediate effects on the intellectual and social development of young children.

Criticism has focused on the fact that this improvement in intellectual performance tends only to persist for a few years. However, following High/Scope, attention has now moved forward and recognised the potential importance of more sustained behavioural and attitudinal changes. Effects on subsequent grades have thus been established, with intervention children being less likely to be retained in grade or placed in special education. A few studies have also produced evidence of long-term effects similar to those shown by the High/Scope studies including reduced criminality and increased high school graduation. Given that the total cost of crime to England and Wales in 1999/2000 was estimated at around £60 billion, even a modest percentage reduction would have a large impact (Inter-Departmental Childcare Review, 2002). It has also been pointed out that results still do not match the achievements of children from better-off homes with no preschool intervention programme, suggesting the need for a more comprehensive policy programme to reduce the range of socio-economic inequalities (Graham and Power, 2004).

The amount of time a child spends in education and childcare is also an important determinant of outcomes. Evidence from the first major European longitudinal study, the UK Effective Provision of Pre-School Education (EPPE)

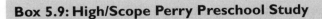

Box 5.9: High/Scope Perry Preschool Study

The long-term success of this holistic preschool programme has been attributed to the fact that it focuses not just on improving language and literacy levels among young children but also on enhancing their social relations, motivation and logical abilities. A wide-ranging evaluation has followed an initial randomised cohort through from the age of three to 27, and demonstrates the effects of high-quality preschool provision across the lifecourse.

Participants were found to be more ready for school than the parallel control group, recording significantly higher IQ scores on school entry. This translated into continued success at school measured, for example, in higher rates of mainstream placement, improved test scores and better high school grades, through to better on-time high school graduation rates and raised literacy levels at the age of 19. This in turn translated into greater economic productivity and social responsibility as adults, captured by higher adult earnings, less reliance on social services, higher rates of home ownership and fewer criminal convictions (Schweinhart, 2001).

The study was also cost-effective, returning 716% of its costs. The evaluators stress that the life-changing properties relate to the quality of the programme. This in turn relates to an adult:child ratio of 1:10, teachers who are trained for early years, a curriculum which draws on validated research, partnership with parents and attention to the educational needs of children and their families. In the US the intervention was institutionalised in the form of the federal Head Start Program, which was introduced in 1964/65.

Project (see Chapter Four), which followed over 3,000 children and their parents, suggests that increased exposure to education between the ages of three and five (as opposed to short or inconsistent exposure), leads to better intellectual development, together with improved independence, concentration and sociability. The same study also found that the optimal time for starting early years education was between the ages of two and three, with group provision conferring no added advantage prior to this age (Sylva et al, 2003).

As with other studies, the nature and quality of the provision was significant. The most positive outcomes were associated with local education authority nurseries, nursery classes or, most notably, combined centres (primarily Early Excellence Centres developed since 1997 to provide an integrated approach to nursery education, childcare, family support and health), settings where education and social development were seen as complementary and where staff had higher qualifications. It also found that children with disadvantages did better in settings with a mixture of children. One in three children were at risk of developing learning difficulties at the start of preschool, but this risk had fallen to one in five by the time they started primary school, suggesting preschool can be an effective intervention for reducing special educational needs, especially for the most disadvantaged and vulnerable children. Overall, the effect of attending or not attending preschool was a more effective predictor of outcome than variations in social disadvantage.

Childcare also enables parents, particularly mothers, to go out to work, or increase their hours in work, thereby potentially lifting their families out of poverty. A systematic review of day care for preschool children reported positive effects on mothers' education, employment and interaction with children, although all the contributory studies were conducted in the US and tended to focus just on socially disadvantaged families (Zoritch et al, 2000).

Policy

The historical reluctance of UK governments to develop an explicit policy on childcare, for long deemed a private responsibility, is well established (Lewis, 2003). However, both childcare and early years education have come to play a central role in antipoverty strategies and family support, being seen as routes to reducing welfare dependency, overcoming educational disadvantage and combating inequalities and social exclusion (Rahilly and Johnston, 2002). Demand for childcare has also risen, chiefly as a consequence of changes in the structure of the UK economy, most particularly the role of women in the labour force, changing family patterns and society's views of working mothers. Between 1984 and 2002, while the employment rate for women in the UK increased from 59% to 70%, the employment rate for women with a child under five nearly doubled, from 27% to 53% (Duffield, 2002).

For most of this period, the resultant demand for childcare has been countered either informally or by the independent sector in the form of day nurseries and childminders, but the response has been recognised as being insufficient, of variable quality and high cost. The need to address this deficit was furthered by recognition of the economic role of childcare, both as part of *A new contract for welfare* (DSS, 1998), with its emphasis on an income from wages rather than benefits, and as a source of employment in itself (Campbell et al, 2003). Demand for childcare will be increased still further if the UK government's target of 70% labour market participation rate among lone parents by 2010 is achieved, together with its target of eradicating child poverty by 2020 (the employment rate for lone mothers with preschool children in 2002 standing at only 34% compared to 58% for partnered mothers [Duffield, 2002]).

The introduction of the National Childcare Strategy in 1998 was considered a watershed, not only because it aimed to address this situation by providing accessible, affordable and high-quality childcare services but also because it aimed simultaneously to expand early years education in the UK (DfEE, 1998).

Specifically it set out, via targets announced in the subsequent Spending Review to:

- create 900,000 new childcare places catering for 1.6 million children by 2004; and
- provide a free part-time nursery education place for every four-year-old whose parents wanted one from September 1998, extended to every three-year-old by 2004.

Key to delivery were the Early Years Development and Childcare Partnerships, attached to local authorities and consisting of representatives from the public, private and voluntary sectors. Their role was to design a childcare strategy that met the needs of the local area, based essentially on provision by the private and voluntary providers, with the public sector acting as regulator, ensuring appropriate standards of care, training and workforce development.

Specific programmes such as Sure Start and Neighbourhood Nurseries were subsequently introduced to target disadvantaged areas. The objective of the Neighbourhood Nurseries, for example, was to provide at least 45,000 full day care places in the 20% most disadvantaged wards by 2004, enabling parents to return to work or to access education. The aim was thus both to address child poverty and to offer high standards of childcare and early learning. Three of Sure Start's four PSAs similarly impact on this policy arena: an improvement in children's ability to learn, an improvement in their social and emotional development and the strengthening of families and communities (DfES, 2003a), although progress has not yet been assessed (DfES, 2004). In addition, the cost of childcare for lower-income families was subsidised through the Childcare Tax Credit element of the Working Families' Tax Credit (WFTC). This provided a maximum of 70% of the costs of formal childcare (up to a maximum of £100 for one child and £150 for two), and was expected to account for an additional £725 million for low-income families between 2001 and 2004.

Targets for free early years education were achieved nationally by 2003, although gaps remain in some localities (NAO, 2004). However, as the Inter-Departmental Childcare Review (2002) found, other parts of the strategy have not worked as well. The provision of pump-priming money to encourage childcare businesses in deprived areas has not produced the number of childcare places needed if the government is to meet its antipoverty and employment targets and, as Chapter Three noted, the Neighbourhood Nurseries initiative failed to meet its target. Deprived wards in England still, therefore, have only approximately half the national average of childcare places (Inter-Departmental Childcare Review, 2002), with levels of provision overall having changed remarkably little – they increased from just one registered childcare place per nine children under the age of eight in 1997 to one registered childcare place per seven children under the age of eight in 2001 (Lewis, 2003). Shortages also remain in most local childcare markets.

There is also a question mark over the sustainability of some childcare provision in the absence of public subsidy. The Early Excellence Centres, based primarily on pre-existing nursery schools in areas of severe economic deprivation, proved successful in reaching people not in paid employment and minority ethnic groups. However, they faced pressures sustaining funding as well as recruiting and developing multidisciplinary staff teams and managing organisational change (Bertram et al, 2002), while the Standard Spending Assessment, which now covers all four-year-olds, was insufficient to support such settings (Lewis, 2003). Short-term 'pump-priming' funding for new ventures also poses problems, giving them little time to establish and develop services (Statham and Mooney, 2003).

The childcare workforce, which expanded substantially (6.6% pa between 1998 and 2001), also needed to increase yet faster to enable targets to be met, with the DfES suggesting a growth rate of between 8-10% per annum between 2003 and 2006. This equates to 175,000 to 180,000 new recruits (NAO, 2004) yet the number of childminders in England, a major component of this workforce, grew by only 900 in this period (www.ofsted.gov.uk) and their numbers overall have declined since 1997 (Mooney et al, 2001). One contributory factor may have been the improvements required by inspections together with the development of National Standards for Under Eights Day Care and Childminding (DfES, 2001) and the *Curriculum guidance for the foundation stage* requirements (DfEE and QCA, 2000), which may have diverted some childminding activity into the unofficial sector. Finally, the take-up rate of Childcare Tax Credit was very low. At the end of 2000, only 12% of those receiving WFTC claimed Childcare Tax Credit although nine out of ten of these were lone parents (Lewis, 2003), while the average payment was only £39.66 per week, about one third of typical nursery fees (Campbell et al, 2003). It also excluded the 20% of women with children under five who work 15 hours or less a week.

In an attempt to address these issues, responsibility and funding for childcare, early years education and Sure Start have been brought together under one integrated (and increased) budget and with a single minister, with the aim of creating an additional 250,000 childcare places by 2005-06 and a further 120,000 by 2008. The *Ten-year strategy for childcare* also introduced an annual Transformation Fund of £125 million each year from April 2006 to support local authority investment in sustainable provision, including issues such as training and business planning (HM Treasury et al, 2004). The focus on disadvantaged areas has also been intensified with Neighbourhood Nurseries, Early Excellence Centres and SSLPs to be developed and rebranded as Children's Centres. A target of 2,500 such centres has now been set (increasing coverage from the 20% to the 30% most disadvantaged wards). These centres (188 had been designated by January 2005) are expected to bring together not just childcare and early years education for the majority of children in these areas but also health services and family support. They will also offer a base for childminder networks and a link to other day care provision and out-of-school clubs, together with local training and education providers. Links to the evidence base are clear, with services that aim to be flexible at the point of delivery, start very early (from the first antenatal visit), that are community driven and professionally coordinated and involve parents as partners. For Sure Start projects this also means the ability to extend their work to include children over the age of three and to integrate their work more closely with other local agencies.

In addition, CTC and Working Tax Credit (WTC) replaced Childcare Tax Credit (and the WFTC) in April 2003. This raised the earnings threshold for help with childcare from £22,000 per annum to £27,000 per annum for families with one child and from £28,000 per annum to £42,000 for families with two or more children (Campbell et al, 2003). The expectation is that these changes will increase the take-up rate and provide more financial help for lower and middle-income families. Indeed, by October 2003, 236,000 families were claiming the childcare element of the WTC, a 58% increase on the highest levels achieved under WFTC (NAO, 2004). The maximum benefit payable has since increased to £175 per week for one child and £300 per week for two or more, with the maximum proportion of costs that can be claimed increasing from 70% to 80% in April 2006. An additional £5 million is also being directed at affordability issues in London (HM Treasury et al, 2004).

Overall, expenditure by government on these early years services (excluding education) now totals £3.6 billion per annum (2002-03) with the largest element accounted for by local government, while parents spend another £3 billion per annum (NAO, 2004). However, as the Child Poverty Action Group (CPAG) stress, the poorest and most disadvantaged children are unlikely to benefit because their parents do not qualify for the childcare element of the WTC (because they are either not in work or work only limited hours), and are unable to finance any additional childcare themselves (CPAG, 2005a). There are some further fundamental tensions within the strategy, too, or as Campbell et al (2003) suggest, the series of strategies. First, most of the money (£5.9 billion out of the £8.2 billion designated to early years education, childcare and Sure Start under the National Childcare Strategy) is actually used to fund the provision of free part-time early education for three- and four-year-olds. Drawing on the evidence base many would argue that this is appropriate, particularly given the fact that only 0.4% of the Gross Domestic Product (GDP) was spent on pre-primary education in 1999. However, the fact that the element of state education provision to have increased most is the proportion of four-year-olds in reception classes is a cause for concern to many (see Chapter Three). So too is the fact that the supporting Foundation Stage and Early Learning Goals (which cover children aged three to the end of their reception year at age five/six) take a largely instrumental view of the curriculum, favouring educational goals (such as speaking, literacy and numeracy) over social skills, informal learning and the role of play (Lewis, 2003; Soler and Miller, 2003).

Second, question marks remain over the nature, sustainability and location of the childcare provision being created. Targets have acted to encourage the creation of new places as opposed to sustainable places. While the government created 626,000 childcare places in England to spring 2003, 301,000 places closed in the same period, undermining the importance of stability in childcare arrangements. Targets also fail to distinguish between full-time, part-time and out-of-school places, all of which fill very different roles in the childcare market. Most of the places created have in fact been out-of-school or holiday places for older children, with only some 96,000 preschool places created in the same period. This figure also masks considerable regional and local variations (unsurprisingly given the order of parental spend). Provision thus ranges from 11-58 places per 100 preschool children at the local authority level with levels remaining highest in the affluent South East. The vulnerability of certain types of provision also continues, with childminder places (the main providers of formal childcare) declining by 24% and playgroup and preschool places declining by 22% (NAO, 2004). Voluntary sector provision in particular, traditionally the main source of affordable childcare and playgroups in the community, is threatened by reductions in grants and a statutory agenda that prioritises work-related childcare and early years education (Rahilly and Johnston, 2002).

Third, there is a conflict between childcare and parenting policies and the objectives of reducing welfare dependency and welfare costs. Gray (2001) points out, for example, that while the heavy expenditure on WFTC/childcare provisions suggests the emphasis is on drawing women into work, rather than merely saving public money, there is a lack of attention to training for other than entry-level jobs. Policy thus fails to contribute to either an up-skilling of the labour force or equal opportunities (see also Rake, 2001). Meanwhile, the means-tested benefits system, with its emphasis on household income, provides a disincentive to re-partnering, despite the advantages of two-parent families for child-rearing outlined in *Supporting families*. There is also evidence that parents' views tend to run contrary to government policy, with many wishing to work fewer rather than more hours, particularly when their child is young, and to avoid weekend working. Over half of all employed lone mothers work atypical times, while in most two-parent families one or both parents frequently workers atypical hours (La Valle et al, 2002). A shortage of childcare remains a contributory factor but so too does a desire to retain responsibility for this care within the family. NESS, for instance, found only a minority of the programmes surveyed actually provided childcare for working parents as demand is low (Meadows and Garber, 2004).

Gray suggests following the Scandinavian model instead, with its emphasis on family-friendly employment policies (enforced by legislation). This includes opportunities for job sharing and extended part-time working, more generous provisions for paid parental and municipal childcare, together with increases in skills training and the National Minimum Wage (which has benefited around three women for every man) (Gray, 2001). In Finland, France and Germany, a home care allowance also supports parents caring for young children at home and affords an explicit value to the role.

Childhood poverty

This chapter has addressed the health behaviours that the research evidence in Chapter Four suggests are the key targets for intervention. While most of the emphasis has been on local or downstream initiatives, care has also been taken to place these in the context of national policy. With respect to nutrition, for example, we have examined the significance of upstream policies concerning maternity leave, paid benefits, the implementation of the WHO code on the marketing of breastmilk substitutes and the reshaping of the Welfare Food Scheme. We have also looked specifically at the upstream policies relating to early years education and childcare. As Chapter Three has stressed, recent policy for the early years has also been influenced by the very considerable emphasis placed on reducing childhood poverty. This has taken the form of encouraging parental employment, providing family support and the increased provision of children's services, most notably education and health. It has therefore been a constant, underpinning many of the discussions in this chapter, such as Sure Start and the National Childcare Strategy.

What works? Evidence, practice and policy

The number of children living in poverty in the UK tripled between 1979 and 1997/98, the result of an increase in both the number living in workless households and the number living in work-poor households (Sutherland and Piachaud, 2001). By the time the government came to power in 1997 one in every three or four children (depending on whether income was measured before or after housing costs [BHC or AHC]) lived in households with less than 60% of the average (median) income (Stewart, 2005).

In 1999 the government introduced the long-term aim of halving childhood poverty by 2010 and eradicating it by 2020. Its strategy was founded, in part, on measures to tackle long-term disadvantage. It thus underpins many of the downstream initiatives relating not just to early life but also to childhood and youth (such as the Children's Fund, Connexions and On Track), together with public health interventions that disproportionately affect children from lower socio-economic groups, such as childhood accidents, obesity and teenage pregnancy (see Chapters Seven and Nine, this volume). With respect to early life it similarly provides a foundation for the range of policies discussed in this chapter, from infant mortality and nutrition to smoking cessation and parenting support. It is particularly evident within Sure Start. In April 2003, for example, 43% of children aged 0-4 in SSLP areas lived in households dependent on Income Support or workless benefits (DfES, 2004). One of Sure Start's four PSA targets thus aims to reduce the number of children aged under four who live in workless households by 12%. The reconciliation of national policy with local programmes is often not straightforward, however. As NESS notes, Sure Start's employability target was introduced after most Round One/Two programmes had established their services. It was introduced into communities where a mother's main role is seen to be that of homemaker and incorporated into a programme where, as noted earlier, it has proved difficult to reach men. Consequently, the proportion of parents who take part in employment and training activities, even in the most active and encouraging programmes, is low. Meanwhile, the emphasis on targets means no credit is given to programmes that increase skills levels or raise confidence and aspirations, approaches that are key to reconciling the conflict between promoting good parenting and employability (Meadows and Garber, 2004). It is also a target where progress has yet to be assessed (DfES, 2004).

Action to eliminate child poverty is also based on direct, upstream intervention, enhancing family finances via major tax and benefit reforms and the promotion of paid work. Chapter Three described the role of the New Deals for employment in increasing access to work (with Chapter Nine discussing further the New Deals for Young People and Lone Parents). It also described the major tax and benefit reforms – the WFTC and WTC – policies that have been considered again in this chapter with respect to childcare. Essentially the WFTC, introduced in 1999, provided support for low-income families working 16 hours or more a week while the Childcare Tax Credit provided additional support for childcare-related costs. These measures were criticised, however, because one third of eligible families (some 600,000 in total) failed to claim WFTC and, as already noted, uptake of the Childcare Tax Credit was very limited (extending to only 167,000 families). As a consequence over 1.2 million children were estimated to be living in poverty in households that did not receive means-tested benefits (Brewer et al, 2003). In 2003 WFTC was, therefore, replaced by the WTC (which supports adults with or without children in low-paid work as well as providing subsidies for certain childcare expenditure for some working parents), and CTC, the two child elements being payable to the child's main carer. The latter now represents the majority of government financial support for children. By April 2005, despite numerous administrative problems, 5.8 million families were in receipt of the benefit (HMR&C, 2005). The structure of the credit also means that it is the per child element that will have the largest direct impact on poverty and this is to be increased in line with average earnings (meaning, however, only a small increase in income for the poorest households) (Brewer and Kaplan, 2003).

As Chapter Three noted, this is a resource-intensive policy. In real terms, for example, figures for 2001-02 suggest an extra spend of £6,000 million on increased benefits and tax credits aimed at low-income families versus £900 million New Deal expenditure (Finn, 2003). Child contingent support now, therefore, comprises a greater proportion of the GDP than at any time since 1975, despite the fall in numbers of children across the same period with, as noted above, the tax system now the main delivery vehicle (Joseph Rowntree Foundation, 2004). Despite this investment, however, the child poverty targets have proved hard to attain. One contributory factor has been the focus on relative not absolute incomes (with median incomes rising considerably in real terms). Others include the assumed extent of benefit uptake, the failure to address the lack of employment opportunities and the tensions for many, particularly lone parents, between providing care for their children (a right enshrined by the UN Convention on the Rights of the Child and central to policies to support child development and the quality of parenting) and entering employment.

Nevertheless, the policy has had a generally redistributive effect, aided by the growth in employment among parents with children (see Chapter Three). The number of children in poverty has fallen from 4.1 million (1998/99) to 3.5 million (2003/04) AHC. Given that these figures do not fully capture the latest tax credit reforms or increases in CTC, "child poverty is likely to have fallen further" (CPAG, 2005b, p 8) and the target of reducing child poverty by 25% by 2004 may still be met at least on a BHC basis. Labour's pledge to end child poverty has now, however, been qualified so that eradication will not mean a zero rate of poverty. Instead the target is a child poverty rate that approaches zero (measured by low income and material deprivation) and a pledge that the UK is ranked among the best in Europe (DWP, 2003). This would suggest an income poverty rate of between and 6% and 9%, or almost one in ten children continuing to live in poverty (Horgan, 2005).

Its impact on the incentive to work has been more mixed, a result of increased support to non-working families and increased support to low-earning parents followed by withdrawal of benefit or tax credits at higher earnings. Blundell et al (2004), for example, estimate tax and benefit reform to have been responsible for increasing the labour supply of lone mothers by an estimated 3.38% or 50,000 in the period 2000-03 while at the same time suggesting that it has allowed some mothers (with and without partners) to reduce the hours they work. There is also a stronger incentive to be a single-earner couple than either a no-earner or dual-earner couple and reduced incentives to progress in the labour market (Brewer and Shephard, 2004). The upstream interventions, as we noted in Chapter Three, are typically not the subject of systematic reviews and childhood poverty does not therefore feature in Table 5.1, which summarises the evidence base relating to interventions in early life.

Conclusion

This chapter has outlined the evidence base as it relates to five key interventions for the early years, and examined the way this evidence base is reflected in policy and practice. The story has not unfolded neatly. As interventions move from clinical practice to complex reality the messages become ever more diffuse and, even in the most controlled settings, vary according to factors such as content, process, culture, time and characteristics of the intervention group. Nevertheless, the premise from which we started in Chapter Four, the notion that health inequalities can be challenged by action in the early years, has gained support.

Table 5.1 summarises the review-level evidence that relates to the key policy areas dealt with in this chapter (a procedure we repeat for each stage in the lifecourse). As noted in Chapter Three, this was not an easy process. Smoking cessation and nutrition in pregnancy and early life and, to a lesser degree, parenting education and support, are the only areas where the evidence base appears extensive (with consideration given to at least 50 trials). Even here, once one starts disaggregating by topic areas, it soon becomes apparent how small the specific evidence base often is. With reference to breastfeeding, for example, most training courses for health professionals have not been formally evaluated, with research identifying only one RCT alongside two UK 'before and after' studies (NHS CRD, 2000). Indeed, a recent systematic review of what works in breastfeeding suggested there was actually "very little research" even in this relatively high-profile area "to inform any aspect of public policy" (Renfrew et al, 2005, p 2).

Salient areas where review-level evidence is lacking are also highlighted in Table 5.1. There are two pervasive exceptions both already outlined in Chapter Three: the inequalities dimension and cost-effectiveness. To use the example of breastfeeding: initiation and duration are known to be lower among disadvantaged groups. Yet, a systematic review that prioritised studies supporting breastfeeding among such groups found only 80 eligible studies, only one fifth of which (17) actually focused on disadvantaged groups. Moreover, only 10 of the studies related to the UK. This underlined, the authors suggested, "the great evidence gap relating to disadvantaged groups" (Renfrew et al, 2005, p 2). Similarly, Taylor et al's review of second-hand smoke is typical in stating that "the majority of Evidence Base papers did not include any cost-related data" and "little is currently known about the cost-effective differential across social gradients or within targets groups of different interventions designs" (Taylor et al, 2005, p 7).

Other factors cannot so readily be captured in tabular form. The family has emerged as a key locus of effective intervention and the relationship has been explored between scope for action at the individual level and collective responsibility at the community and strategic levels. Irrespective of whether one is talking, for instance, about smoking cessation or the decision to breastfeed, individual choice is thus mediated by a range of political and practical variables. These range from community support structures, prevailing attitudes, media representation and legislation to access to the labour market. Not surprisingly, the most effective interventions tend to be multifaceted, ranging from education and health through to social inclusion and community development. Education emerges as key, whether as a precursor to behavioural change for the individual, the practitioner or the policy maker or as a protective resource for the lifecourse. The role of performance management has also been highlighted. Targets provide

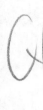

a considerable focus for intervention, yet are often ephemeral and sit in uneasy representation of programme priorities, locally defined need or the evidence base. Sure Start, for example, no longer has a national target relating to maternal mental health or parenting support and its focus on child health is not reflected in a national target relating to breastfeeding. These are themes that are developed further as we move into childhood and youth. *copy*

Table 5.1: Interventions during early life: summary of the evidence base

	Source
SMOKING	
Smoking cessation in pregnancy	
Advice and support tailored for pregnant women has a modest effect on cessation rates, increasing mean birth weight and reducing low birth weight). It tends not to reach those at highest risk	Cochrane Review
Ten per cent of women still smoking at the time of their first antenatal visit will stop with usual care. Formal interventions typically result in an additional 6% to 7% quitting	Cochrane Review
Prenatal counselling, combined with at least 10 minutes person-to-person contact and written material tailored to pregnancy can double cessation rates	Overview
Even reducing smoking in pregnancy can increase health outcomes	Systematic review
Exposure to passive smoking in early life	
Both home-based and clinic-based interventions by a clinician (for example, information, advice and counselling) can be effective in reducing children's exposure to second-hand smoke. But studies tend to rely on self-reported health rather than biochemical measures	Review of reviews
Intensive counselling increases knowledge but few studies show a statistically significant intervention effect in terms of attitudes and behaviour (and hence exposure to environmental tobacco smoke)	Cochrane Review
Lack of review-level evidence	
Safety and efficacy of NRT for smoking cessation during pregnancy	
Strategies that are effective against relapse in the postpartum period	
Interventions that include the family as a whole	
Holistic interventions that address poverty, disadvantage and increase smoking control and support in the wider community	

(continued)

Table 5.1: Interventions during early life: summary of the evidence base (continued)

	Source
NUTRITION	
Maternal nutritional supplements	
Calcium supplements reduce preterm birth and the incidence of low birth weight, especially among women at risk of hypertensive disorders	Cochrane Review
Dietary supplementation based on balanced protein and energy content consistently improves foetal growth	Systematic review
Lack of review-level evidence	
Appropriate combinations of interventions	
Food-based as opposed to nutrient-based interventions	
Interventions relating to maternal nutrition before pregnancy and in early pregnancy	
Breastfeeding initiation and duration	
Initiation rates can be increased by:	
Multifaceted interventions, including, for example, health education, changes to maternity ward practice, such as unrestricted mother–baby contact and feeding and the prevention of discharge packs containing formula feeding information and samples, the use of peer facilitators and advocates	Systematic review
Education – small, informal discussion classes led by health professionals that emphasise the benefits of breastfeeding and provide practical advice But one-to-one education sessions may be necessary to persuade women who have decided to feed infant formula to breastfeed	Other review
Training – intensive targeted lactation training for health professionals (particularly if accorded mandatory status)	Review of reviews
A peer support component (particularly important for low-income women). But only effective as a standalone component with women intending to breastfeed	Cochrane Review
Professional support increases the duration of (any) breastfeeding	Cochrane Review
Lay support is effective in promoting exclusive breastfeeding	Review of reviews
Efficacy is increased if sessions are broad-based, span the ante and postnatal period and draw on repeated contacts with either a professional or peer educator	Systematic review
Lack of review-level evidence	
Evaluation of public policy, for example, provision of maternity leave	
Provision of supportive environment (public acceptability and social barriers to breastfeeding)	
Inclusion of issues that are important to mothers and their partners and families	

(continued)

Table 5.1: Interventions during early life: summary of the evidence base (continued)

	Source
PARENTING EDUCATION AND SUPPORT	
Group-based behavioural interventions can improve the emotional and behavioural adjustment of children under the age of three	Cochrane Review
Parenting programmes can improve behavioural problems in children aged 3-10	Systematic review
Parenting programmes can make a significant contribution to the short-term psychosocial health of mothers	Cochrane Review
Home visiting can produce improvements in parenting, child behavioural problems, cognitive development in high-risk groups, a reduction in accidental injuries to children and improved detection and management of postnatal depression	Review of reviews
The involvement of both parents and direct work with the child increases efficacy	Overview

Lack of review-level evidence

Role of parenting programmes in primary prevention as opposed to treatment

Long-term effectiveness on both maternal mental health and children's adjustment

Efficacy of relational interventions

Ability to isolate the effective components

EARLY YEARS EDUCATION AND CHILDCARE	
Day care has a beneficial effect on children's development and school achievement	Cochrane Review
Limited long-term follow-up suggests increased employment, lower teenage pregnancy rates, higher socio-economic status and decreased criminal behaviour	Cochrane Review
There are positive effects on mothers' education, employment and interaction with children	Cochrane Review

Lack of review-level evidence

Absence of UK-based studies

Disaggregated studies allowing the effects of non-parental day care to be isolated from parental training and education

References

Abegglen, J.A. and Schwartz, R. (1995) 'Enhancing self-care parenting', *Advanced Practice Nursing Quarterly*, vol 1, no 3, pp 74-83.

Acheson, D. (1998) *Independent Inquiry into Inequalities in Health*, London: The Stationery Office.

Adams, C., Bauld, L. and Judge, K. (2000) *Leading the way: Smoking cessation services in Health Action Zones*, Glasgow: Report submitted to the DH, November, by the University of Glasgow.

Amir, L. and Donath, S. (2002) 'Does maternal smoking have a physiological effect on breastfeeding? The epidemiological evidence', *Birth*, vol 29, no 2, pp 112-23.

Anning, A., Ball, M., Barnes, J., Belsky, J., Botting, B., Frost, M., Kurtz, Z., Leyland, A., Meadows, P., Melhuish, E. and Tunstill, J. (2004) 'The national evaluation of Sure Start Local Programmes in England', *Child and Adolescent Mental Health*, vol 9, no 1, pp 2-8.

Arborelius, E., Hallberg, A.C. and Hakansson, A. (2000) 'How to prevent exposure to tobacco smoke among small children: a literature review', *Acta Paediatrica*, vol 89, pp 65-70.

Atallah, A.N., Hofmeyr, G.J. and Duley, L. (2001) 'Calcium supplementation during pregnancy for preventing hypertensive disorders and related problems (Cochrane Review)', *The Cochrane Library, issue 3*, Oxford: Update Software.

Baby Feeding Law Group (2004) *United Kingdom code violations: A survey of the international code of marketing of breastmilk substitutes and subsequent WHA resolutions*, Cambridge: Baby Milk Action.

Bailey, C. and Pain, R. (2001) 'Geographies of infant feeding and access to primary health-care', *Health and Social Care in the Community*, vol 9, no 5, pp 309-17.

Barlow, J. (1997) *Systematic review of the effectiveness of parent-training programmes in improving behaviour problems in children aged 3-10 years*, Oxford: University of Oxford.

Barlow, J. and Coren, E. (2003) 'Parent-training programmes for improving maternal psychosocial health (Cochrane Methodology Review)', *The Cochrane Library*, Chichester: John Wiley & Sons Ltd.

Barlow, J. and Parsons, J. (2003) 'Group-based parent-training programmes for improving emotional and behavioural adjustment in 0-3 year old children', *The Cochrane Database of Systematic Reviews 2003, issue 2*, Art. No. CD003680.

Barlow, J. and Stewart-Brown, S. (2000) 'Behaviour problems and group based parenting education programmes', *Developmental and Behavioral Pediatrics*, vol 21, no 5, pp 356-70.

Barlow, J., Coren, E. and Stewart-Brown, S. (2002) 'Meta-analysis of the effectiveness of parenting programmes in improving maternal psychosocial health', *British Journal of General Practice*, vol 52, no 476, pp 223-33.

Battersby, S. (2002a) *The Breastfeeding Is Best Supporters Project (BIBS): Spreading the word: A community initiative to promote breastfeeding awareness: A research and evaluation report for the Foxhill and Parson Cross Sure Start*, Sheffield: University of Sheffield.

Battersby, S. (2002b) *The Breastfeeding Is Best Supporters Project: An evaluation of the merged breastfeeding peer support programmes: A research and evaluation report for the Foxhill and Parson Cross Sure Start*, Sheffield: University of Sheffield.

Bertram, P., Pascal, C., Bokhari, S., Gasper, M. and Holtermann, S. (2002) *Early Excellence Centre pilot programme: Second evaluation report 2000-2001*, Research Report RR361, London: DfES.

Blundell, R., Brewer, M. and Shephard, A. (2004) *The impact of tax and benefit changes between April 2000 and April 2003 on parent's labour supply*, Briefing Note No 52, London: Institute for Fiscal Studies.

Bor, W., Sanders, M.R. and Markie-Dadds, C. (2002) 'The effects of the triple p-positive parenting program on preschool children with co-occurring disruptive behavior and attentional/hyperactive difficulties', *Journal of Abnormal Child Psychology*, vol 30, no 6, pp 571-87.

Brewer, M. and Kaplan, G. (2003) 'What do the child poverty targets mean for the child tax credit?', in R. Chote, C. Emmerson and H. Simpson (eds) *The IFS green budget: January 2003*, London: Institute for Fiscal Studies, pp 42-53.

Brewer, M. and Shephard, A. (2004) 'Has labour made work pay?' (www.jrf.org.uk/bookshop), accessed 4 May 2005.

Brewer, M., Clark, T. and Goodman, A. (2003) 'What really happened to child poverty in the UK under Labour's first term?', *The Economic Journal*, vol 113, no 488, pp F240-F257.

Bryan, A.A. (2000) 'Enhancing parent–child interaction with a prenatal couple intervention', *American Journal of Maternal/Child Nursing*, vol 25, no 3, pp 139-44.

Bull, J., Mulvihull, C. and Quigley, R. (2003) *Prevention of low birth weight: Assessing the effectiveness of smoking cessation and nutritional interventions*, London: Health Development Agency.

Bull, J., McCormick, G., Swann, C. and Mulvihill, C. (2004) *Ante- and post-natal home-visiting programmes: A review of reviews*, London: Health Development Agency.

Butz, A.M., Pulsifer, M., Marano, N., Belcher, H., Lears, M.K. and Royall, R. (2001) 'Effectiveness of a home intervention for perceived child behavioral problems and parenting stress in children with in utero drug exposure', *Archives of Pediatrics and Adolescent Medicine*, vol 155, no 9, pp 1029-37.

Campbell, J., Scott, G. and Thomson, E. (2003) 'Childcare: an investigation of labour market issues', *Regional Studies*, vol 37, no 9, pp 957-67.

Campbell, S. (1995) 'Behaviour problems in pre-school children: a review of recent research', *Journal of Child Psychology and Psychiatry*, vol 36, no 1, pp 113-49.

Coe, C., Spencer, N., Barlow, J., Vostanis, P. and Laine, L. (2003) 'Services for pre-school children with behaviour problems in a midlands city', *Child: Care, Health and Development*, vol 29, no 6, pp 417-24.

Coleman, T., Pound, E. and Cheater, F. (2002) *National survey of the new smoking cessation services: Implementing the smoking kills White Paper*, Nottingham: University of Nottingham.

Coleman, T., Pound, E., Adams, C., Bauld, L., Ferguson, J. and Cheater, F. (2005) 'Implementing a national treatment service for dependant smokers: initial challenges and solutions', *Addiction*, vol 100, suppl 2, pp 12-18.

CPAG (Child Poverty Action Group) (2005a) *Child Poverty Action Group's response to choice for parents, the best start for children: A ten-year strategy for childcare*, London: CPAG.

CPAG (2005b) *Ten steps to a society free of child poverty. Child Poverty Action Group's manifesto to eradicate child poverty 1965-2005*, London: CPAG.

Cunningham, C.E., Bremner, R. and Boyle, M. (1995) 'Large group community-based parenting programs for families of preschoolers at risk for disruptive behaviour disorders: utilisation, cost effectiveness and outcome', *Journal of Child Psychology and Psychiatry and Allied Disciplines*, vol 36, no 7, pp 1141-59.

Danoff, N.L., Kemper, K.J. and Sherry, B. (1994) 'Risk-factors for dropping out of a parenting education-program', *Child Abuse and Neglect*, vol 18, no 7, pp 599-606.

Davis, H. and Hester, P. (1996) *An independent evaluation of Parent-Link: A parenting education programme*, London: Parent Network.

Davis, H. and Spurr, P. (1998) 'Parent counselling: an evaluation of a community child mental health service', *Journal of Child Psychology and Psychiatry*, vol 39, no 3, pp 365-76.

Davis, H., Spurr, P., Cox, A., Lynch, M., von Roenne, A. and Hahn, K. (1997) 'A description and evaluation of a community child mental health service', *Clinical Child Psychology and Psychiatry*, vol 2, no 2, pp 221-38.

Dawe, F. and Goddard, E. (1997) *Smoking-related behaviours and attitudes: A report on research using the ONS omnibus survey produced on behalf of the Department of Health*, London: The Stationery Office.

Day, C. and Davis, H. (1999) 'Community child mental health services: a framework for the development of parenting initiatives', *Clinical Child Psychology and Psychiatry*, vol 4, no 4, pp 475-81.

De Onis, M., Villar, J. and Gülmezoglu, M. (1998) 'Nutritional interventions to prevent intrauterine growth retardation: evidence from randomised controlled trials', *European Journal of Clinical Nutrition*, vol 52, suppl 1, pp S83-S93.

Dempsey, D.A. and Benowitz, N.L. (2001) 'Risks and benefits of nicotine to aid smoking cessation in pregnancy', *Drug Safety*, vol 24, no 4, pp 277-322.

DfEE (Department for Education and Employment) (1998) *Meeting the childcare challenge: A framework and consultation document*, Cm 3959, London: The Stationery Office.

DfEE and QCA (Qualifications and Curriculum Authority) (2000) *Curriculum guidance for the foundation stage*, Ref Qca/00/587, London: QCA.

DfES (Department for Education and Skills) (2001) *National standards for under eights day care and childminding*, London: DfES.

DfES (2003a) *Autumn performance report 2003: Achievements against Public Service Agreement targets*, Cm 6006, London: DfES.

DfES (2003b) *Every child matters*, Cm 5860, London: The Stationery Office.

DfES (2004) *Autumn performance report 2004: Achievement against Public Service Agreement targets, 2000-2004*, Cm 6399, London: DfES.

DH (Department of Health) (1995) 'Breastfeeding: good practice guidance to the NHS' (www.babyfriendly.org.uk/finance.asp), accessed 26 January 2004.

DH (1998) *Smoking kills*, London: The Stationery Office.

DH (1999) *Saving lives: Our healthier nation*, London: The Stationery Office.

DH (2000) *The NHS Plan*, London: The Stationery Office.

DH (2002) *Improvement, expansion and reform: The next 3 years: Priorities and planning framework 2003-2006*, London: DH.

DH (2003a) *Tackling health inequalities: A programme for action*, London: DH.

DH (2003b) *Clarification of breastfeeding initiation data collection*, London: DH.

DH (2004a) *Maternity standard, National Service Framework for Children, Young People and Maternity Services*, London: DfES and DH.

DH (2004b) *Healthy Start: Government response to the consultation exercise*, London: DH.

DH (2004c) *National Service Framework for Children, Young People and Maternity Services: Supporting local delivery*, London: DfES, DH.

Dolan-Mullen, P. (1999) 'Maternal smoking during pregnancy and evidence based interventions to promote cessation', *Primary Care*, vol 26, pp 577-89.

Dorsett, R. and Marsh, A. (1998) *The health trap: Poverty, smoking and lone parenthood*, London: Policy Studies Institute.

Dosnajh, J. and Ghuman, P. (1998) 'Child-rearing practices of two generations of Punjabis: development of personality and independence', *Children and Society*, vol 12, no 1, pp 25-37.

Dowler, E. (1998) 'Families and food poverty', in N. Donovan and C. Street (eds) *Fit for school: How breakfast clubs meet health, education and childcare needs*, London: New Policy Institute, pp 23-7.

Dowler, E., Turner, S. and Dobson, B. (2001) *Poverty bites – Food, health and poor families*, London: CPAG.

DSS (Department of Social Security) (1998) *New ambitions for our country: A new contract for welfare*, Cm 3895, London: DSS.

Duffield, M. (2002) 'Trends in female employment', *Labour Market Trends*, vol 110, no 11, pp 605-16.

DWP (Department for Work and Pensions) (2003) *Measuring child poverty*, London: DWP.

Dykes, F. (2003) *Infant feeding initiative: A report evaluating the breastfeeding practice projects 1999-2002*, London: DH.

Earle, S. (2002) 'Factors affecting the initiation of breastfeeding: implications for breastfeeding promotion', *Health Promotion International*, vol 17, no 3, pp 205-14.

Einzig, H. (1999) 'Review of the field: current trends, concepts and issues', in S. Wolfendale and H. Einzig (eds) *Parenting education and support*, London: David Fulton Publishers Ltd, pp 13-32.

Eisenstadt, N. (2000) 'Sure Start: research into practice, practice into research', *Public Money and Management*, vol 4, October-December, pp 6-8.

El-Mohandes, A.A., Katz, K.S., El-Khorazaty, M.N., McNeely-Johnson, D., Sharps, P.W., Jarrett, M.H., Rose, A., White, D.M., Young, M., Grylack, L., Murray, K.D., Katta, P.S., Burroughs, M., Atiyeh, G., Wingrove, B.K. and Herman, A.A. (2003) 'The effect of a parenting education program on the use of preventive pediatric health care services among low-income, minority mothers: a randomized, controlled study', *Pediatrics*, vol 111, no 6, pt 1, pp 1324-32.

Fairbank, L., O'Meara, S., Renfrew, M.J., Woolridge, M., Sowden, A.J. and Lister-Sharp, D. (2000) 'A systematic review to evaluate the effectiveness of interventions to promote the initiation of breastfeeding', *Health Technology Assessment 2000*, vol 4, no 25.

Farrington, D. (1996) *Understanding and preventing youth crime*, York: Joseph Rowntree Foundation.

Feldman, M.A. (1994) 'Parenting education for parents with intellectual disabilities – a review of outcome studies', *Research in Developmental Disabilities*, vol 15, no 4, pp 299-332.

Fennell, D.C. and Fishel, A.H. (1998) 'Parent education: an evaluation of STEP on abusive parents' perceptions and abuse potential', *Journal of Child and Adolescent Psychiatric Nursing*, vol 11, no 3, pp 107-20.

Finn, D. (2003) 'Employment policy', in N. Ellison and C. Pierson (eds) *Developments in British social policy 2*, Basingstoke: Palgrave Macmillan, pp 111-28.

Forehand, R. and Kotchik, B.A. (1996) 'Cultural diversity: a wake-up call for parent training', *Behavior Therapy*, vol 27, pp 187-206.

Frost, N., Johnson, L., Stein, M. and Wallis, L. (1996) *Negotiated friendship: Home Start and the delivery of family support*, Leicester: Home Start UK.

Gewirtz, S. (2001) 'Cloning the Blairs: New Labour's programme for the re-socialization of working-class parents', *Journal of Education Policy*, vol 16, no 4, pp 365-78.

Gibbs, J., Underdown, A. and Liabo, K. (2003) 'Group-based parenting programmes can reduce behavioural problems of children aged 3-10 years' (www.whatworksforchildren.org.uk: What Works for Children Group Evidence Nugget).

Goodson, B.D., Layzer, J.I., St Pierre, R.G., Bernstein, R.S. and Lopez, M. (2000) 'Effectiveness of a comprehensive, five-year family support program for low-income children and their families: findings from the comprehensive child development program', *Early Childhood Research Quarterly*, vol 15, no 1, pp 5-39.

Graham, H. (1998) 'Promoting health against inequality: using research to identify targets for intervention – a case study of women and smoking', *Health Education Journal*, vol 57, pp 292-302.

Graham, H. and Power, C. (2004) *Childhood disadvantage and adult health: A lifecourse framework*, London: Health Development Agency.

Gray, A. (2001) '"Making work pay" – devising the best strategy for lone parents in Britain', *Journal of Social Policy*, vol 30, no 2, pp 189-207.

Gray, J., Spurway, P. and McClatchey, M. (2001) 'Lay therapy intervention with families at risk for parenting difficulties: the Kempe Community Caring Program', *Child Abuse and Neglect*, vol 25, no 5, pp 641-55.

Hall, D. and Elliman, D. (eds) (2003) *Health for all children* (4th edn), Oxford: Oxford University Press.

Hamlyn, B., Brooker, S., Oleinikova, K. and Wands, S. (2002) *Infant feeding 2000: A survey conducted on behalf of the Department of Health, the Scottish Executive, the National Assembly of Wales and the Department of Health, Social Services and Public Safety in Northern Ireland*, London: The Stationery Office.

Henderson, L., Kitzinger, J. and Green, J. (2000) 'Representing infant feeding: content analysis of British media portrayals of bottle feeding and breast feeding', *British Medical Journal*, vol 321, no 7270, pp 1196-8.

HM Government and DH (Department of Health) (2004) *Choosing health: Making healthy choices easier*, London: HM Government and DH.

HM Treasury (2001) *Tackling child poverty: Giving every child the best possible start in life*, London: HM Treasury.

HM Treasury (2004) *Child poverty review*, London: The Stationery Office.

HM Treasury, DfES (Department for Education and Skills), DWP (Department for Work and Pensions) and DTI (Department for Trade and Industry) (2004) *Choice for parents, the best start for children: A ten-year strategy for childcare*, London: The Stationery Office.

HMR&C (HM Revenue & Customs Analysis Team) (2005) *Child and working tax credits statistics: April 2005*, London: ONS.

Hoddinott, P. and Pill, R. (1999) 'Qualitative study of decisions about infant feeding among women in east end of London', *British Medical Journal*, vol 318, no 7175, pp 30-4.

Hofhuis, W., de Jongste, J. and Merkus, P. (2003) 'Adverse health effects of prenatal and postnatal tobacco smoke exposure on children', *Archives of Disease in Childhood*, vol 88, no 12, pp 1086-90.

Hoghughi, M. and Speight, A.N. (1998) 'Good enough parenting for all children – a strategy for a healthier society', *Archives of Disease in Childhood*, vol 78, no 4, pp 293-300.

Home Office (1998) *Supporting families: A consultation document*, London: Home Office.

Horgan, G. (2005) 'Child poverty in Northern Ireland: the limits of welfare-to-work policies', *Social Policy and Administration*, vol 39, no 1, pp 49-64.

Hovell, M.F., Zakarian, J.M., Matt, G.E., Hofstetter, R., Bernert, J.T. and Pirkle, J. (2000) 'Effect of counselling mothers on their children's exposure to environmental tobacco smoke: a randomised trial', *British Medical Journal*, vol 321, pp 337-42.

Inter-Departmental Childcare Review (2002) *Delivering for children and families*, London: The Stationery Office.

Jackson, A. and Robinson, S. (2001) 'Dietary guidelines for pregnancy: a review of current evidence', *Public Health Nutrition*, vol 4, no 2B, pp 625-30.

Jane, M., Nebot, M., Badi, M., Berjano, B., Munoz, M., Rodriguez, M.C., Querol, A. and Cabero, L. (2000) 'Determinant factors of smoking cessation during pregnancy', *Medicina Clinica*, vol 114, no 4, pp 132-5.

Johnson, Z. and Molloy, B. (1995) 'The community mothers' programme – empowerment of parents by parents', *Children and Society*, vol 9, pp 73-85.

Johnson, Z., Howell, F. and Molloy, B. (1993) 'Community mothers' programme: randomised controlled trial of a non-professional intervention in parenting', *British Medical Journal*, vol 306, pp 1449-52.

Joseph Rowntree Foundation (2004) *Findings: The financial costs and benefits of supporting children since 1975*, York: Joseph Rowntree Foundation.

Karoly, L.A., Greenwood, P.W., Everingham, S.S., Houbé, J., Kilburn, M.R., Rydell, C.P., Sanders, M. and Chiesa, J.R. (1998) *Investing in our children: What we know and don't know about the costs and benefits of early childhood interventions*, Santa Monica, CA: Rand Corporation.

Katz, K.S., El-Mohandes, P.A., Johnson, D.M., Jarrett, P.M., Rose, A. and Cober, M. (2001) 'Retention of low income mothers in a parenting intervention study', *Journal of Community Health*, vol 26, no 3, pp 203-18.

Keller, J. and McDade, K. (2000) 'Attitudes of low-income parents toward seeking help with parenting: implications for practice', *Child Welfare*, vol 79, no 3, pp 285-312.

Kelly, M. (2004) *The evidence of effectiveness of public health interventions – and the implications*, London: Health Development Agency.

Kilgour, C. and Fleming, V. (2000) 'An action research inquiry into a health visitor parenting programme for parents of pre-school children with behaviour problems', *Journal of Advanced Nursing*, vol 32, no 3, pp 682-8.

Kirk, T. (1980) 'Appraisal of the effectiveness of nutrition education in the context of infant feeding', *Journal of Human Nutrition*, vol 34, pp 429-38.

Kramer, M.S. (1987) 'Determinants of low birth weight: methodological assessment and meta-analysis', *Bulletin of the World Health Organization*, vol 65, pp 663-737.

Kramer, M.S., Chalmers, B., Hodnett, E., Sevkovskaya, Z., Dzikovich, I., Shapiro, S., Collet, J.-P., Vanilovich, I., Mezen, I., Ducruet, T., Shishko, G., Zubovich, V., Mknuik, D., Gluchanina, E., Dombrovskiy, V., Ustinovitch, A.T.K., Bogdanovich, N., Ovchinikova, L. and Helsing, E. (2001) 'Promotion of breastfeeding intervention trial (PROBIT): a randomised trial in the Republic of Belarus', *Journal of the American Medical Association*, vol 285, no 4, pp 413-20.

La Valle, I., Arthur, S., Millward, C., Scott, J. and Clayden, M. (2002) *Happy families? Atypical work and its influence on family life*, Bristol/York: The Policy Press/Joseph Rowntree Foundation.

Leventhal, J. (1997) 'The prevention of child abuse and neglect: pipe dreams or possibilities', *Clinical Child Psychology and Psychiatry*, vol 2, no 4, pp 489-500.

Lewis, J. (2003) 'Developing early years childcare in England, 1997-2002: the choices for (working) mothers', *Social Policy and Administration*, vol 37, no 3, pp 219-38.

Lloyd, E. (1999) *Parenting matters: What works in parenting education?*, Barkingside: Barnardo's.

Lloyd, N., O'Brien, M. and Lewis, C. (2003) *Fathers in Sure Start local programmes*, Nottingham: DfES.

Long, A., McCarney, S., Smyth, G., Magorrian, N. and Dillon, A. (2001) 'The effectiveness of parenting programmes facilitated by health visitors', *Journal of Advanced Nursing*, vol 34, no 5, pp 611-20.

Ludman, E.J., McBride, C.M., Nelson, J.C., Curry, S.J., Grothaus, L.C., Lando, H.A. and Pirie, P.L. (2000) 'Stress, depressive symptoms, and smoking cessation among pregnant women', *Health Psychology*, vol 19, no 1, pp 21-7.

Lumley, J., Oliver, S. and Waters, E. (2001) 'Interventions for promoting smoking cessation during pregnancy (Cochrane Review)', *The Cochrane Library*, Oxford: Update Software.

Macdonald, G. (nd) *What works in child protection?*, Barkingside: Barnardo's.

Macdonald, G. and Roberts, H. (1995) *What works in the early years: Effective interventions for children and their families in health, social welfare, education and child protection*, Barkingside: Barnardo's.

Macdonald, G., Sheldon, B. and Gillespie, J. (1992) 'Contemporary studies of the effectiveness of social work', *British Journal of Social Work*, vol 22, no 6, pp 614-43.

McLeod, D., Benn, C., Pullon, S., Viccars, A., White, S., Cookson, T. and Dowell, A. (2003) 'The midwife's role in facilitating smoking behaviour change during pregnancy', *Midwifery*, vol 19, no 4, pp 285-97.

McNeill, A., Raw, M., Whybrow, J. and Bailey, P. (2005) 'A national strategy for smoking cessation treatment in England', *Addiction*, vol 100, suppl 2, pp 1-11.

Meadows, P. and Garber, C. (2004) *Sure Start local programmes and improving the employability of parents*, London: NESS Institute for the Study of Children, Families and Social Issues, Birkbeck, University of London.

Meltzer, H., Gatward, R., Goodman, R. and Ford, T. (2000) *Mental health of children and adolescents in Great Britain*, London: ONS.

Mielck, A., Graham, H. and Bremburg, S. (2002) 'Children, an important target group for the reduction of socioeconomic inequalities in health', in J. Mackenbach and M. Bakker (eds) *Reducing inequalities in health: A European perspective*, London: Routledge, pp 144-68.

Moffit, T.E., Caspi, A., Dickson, N.P.S. and Stanton, W. (1996) 'Childhood-onset versus adolescent antisocial conduct problems in males: natural history from ages 3 to 18 years', *Development and Psychopathology*, vol 8, no 2, pp 399-424.

Mooney, A., Knight, A., Moss, P. and Owen, C. (2001) *Who cares? Childminding in the 1990s*, York: Family Policy Studies Centre in association with the Industrial Society.

Moore, L., Campbell, R., Whelan, A., Mills, N., Lupton, P., Misselbrook, E. and Frohlich, J. (2002) 'Self help smoking cessation in pregnancy: cluster randomised controlled trial', *British Medical Journal*, vol 325, no 7377, pp 1383-6A.

Moss, P. (1999) 'Going critical: childhood, parenthood and the labour market', in S. Wolfendale and H. Einzig (eds) *Parenting education and support*, London: David Fulton Publishers Ltd, pp 75-89.

Myers, P., Barnes, J. and Brodie, I. (2004) *Partnership working in Sure Start local programmes: Synthesis of early findings from local programme evaluations*, London: NESS Institute for the Study of Children, Families and Social Issues, Birkbeck, University of London.

NAO (National Audit Office) (2004) *Early years: Progress in developing high quality childcare and early education accessible to all*, London: The Stationery Office.

National Heart Forum (2002) *Towards a generation free from coronary heart disease: Policy action for children's and young people's health and well-being*, London: National Heart Forum.

NESS (National Evaluation of Sure Start) (2002) *Getting Sure Start started*, Nottingham: DfES.

NESS (2004) *The impact of Sure Start local programmes on child development and family functioning: A report on preliminary findings*, London: NESS Institute for the Study of Children, Families and Social Issues, Birkbeck, University of London.

Newman, T. and Roberts, H. (1999) 'Assessing effectiveness', in E. Lloyd (ed) *Parenting matters: What works in parenting education?*, Barkingside: Barnardo's, pp 39-63.

NHS CRD (Centre for Reviews and Dissemination) (1998) 'Smoking cessation: what the health service can do', *Effectiveness Matters*, vol 3, no 1, pp 1-4.

NHS CRD (2000) 'Promoting the initiation of breastfeeding', *Effective Health Care*, vol 6, no 2, pp 1-12.

NICE (National Institute for Clinical Excellence) (2002) *Guidance on the use of nicotine replacement therapy (NRT) and bupropion for smoking cessation*, London: NICE.

Nicoll, A. and Williams, A. (2002) 'Breastfeeding', *Archives of Disease in Childhood*, vol 87, no 2, pp 91-2.

Oakley, A., Rajan, L. and Turner, H. (1998) 'Evaluating parent support initiatives: lessons from two case studies', *Health and Social Care in the Community*, vol 6, no 5, pp 318-30.

Oakley-Browne, M.A., Joyce, P.R., Wells, J.E., Bushnell, J.A. and Hornblow, A.R. (1995) 'Adverse parenting and other childhood experience as risk factors for depression in women aged 18-44 years', *Journal of Affective Disorders*, vol 34, pp 13-23.

Olds, D., Eckenrode, J., Henderson, C., Phelps, C., Kitzman, H. and Hanks, C. (1993) 'Effect of prenatal and infancy nurse home visitation on government spending', *Medical Care*, vol 31, pp 155-74.

Osrin, D. and de L. Costello, A.M. (2000) 'Maternal nutrition and fetal growth: practical issues in international health', *Seminars in Neonatology*, vol 5, pp 209-19.

Owen, A.L. and Owen, G.M. (1997) 'Twenty years of WIC: a review of some effects of the program', *Journal of the American Dietetic Association*, vol 97, pp 777-82.

Park, E.-W., Schultz, J., Tudiver, F., Campbell, T. and Becker, L. (2004) 'Enhancing partner support to improve smoking cessation (Cochrane Review)', *The Cochrane Library*, Chichester: John Wiley & Sons Ltd.

Park, J. (1999) 'The emotional education of parents: attachment theory and emotional literacy', in S. Wolfendale and H. Einzig (eds) *Parenting education and support*, London: David Fulton Publishers Ltd, pp 90-103.

Patterson, J., Mockford, C., Barlow, J., Pyper, C. and Stewart-Brown, S. (2002a) 'Need and demand for parenting programmes in general practice', *Archives of Disease in Childhood*, vol 87, no 6, pp 468-71.

Patterson, J., Barlow, J. and Mockford, C. (2002b) 'Improving mental health through parenting programmes: block randomised controlled trial', *Archives of Disease in Childhood*, vol 87, no 6, pp 472-77.

Penn, H. (2000) 'Policy and practice in childcare and nursery education', *Journal of Social Policy*, vol 29, no 1, pp 37-54.

Perkins, E.R. and MacFarlane, J. (2001) 'Family support by lay workers: a health visiting initiative', *British Journal of Community Nursing*, vol 6, no 1, pp 26-32.

Pickstone, C., Hannon, P. and Fox, L. (2002) 'Surveying and screening preschool language development in community-focused intervention programmes: a review of instruments', *Child: Care, Health and Development*, vol 28, no 3, pp 251-64.

Platt, S., Amos, A., Gnich, W. and Parry, O. (2002) 'Smoking policies', in J. Mackenbach and M. Bakker (eds) *Reducing inequalities in health: A European perspective*, London: Routledge, pp 125-43.

Protheroe, L., Dyson, L., Renfrew, M., Bull, B. and Mulvihill, C. (2003) *The effectiveness of public health interventions to promote the initiation of breastfeeding*, London: Health Development Agency.

Pugh, G. (1999) 'Parenting education and the social policy agenda', in S. Wolfendale and H. Einzig (eds) *Parenting education and support*, London: David Fulton Publishers Ltd, pp 3-12.

Pugh, G., De'Ath, E. and Smith, C. (1994) *Confident parents, confident children: Policy and practice in parent education and support*, London: NCB.

Pullon, S., McLeod, D., Benn, C., Viccars, A., White, S., Cookson, T., Dowell, A. and Green, R. (2003) 'Smoking cessation in New Zealand: education and resources for use by midwives for women who smoke during pregnancy', *Health Promotion International*, vol 18, no 4, pp 315-25.

Rahilly, S. and Johnston, E. (2002) 'Opportunity for childcare: the impact of government initiatives in England upon childcare provision', *Social Policy and Administration*, vol 36, no 5, pp 482-95.

Raine, P. (2003) 'Promoting breast-feeding in a deprived area', *Health and Social Care in the Community*, vol 11, no 6, pp 463-9.

Rajgopal, R., Cox, R.H., Lambur, M. and Lewis, E.C. (2002) 'Cost-benefit analysis indicates the positive economic benefits of the EFNEP related to chronic disease prevention', *Journal of Nutrition Education and Behavior*, vol 34, pp 26-37.

Rake, K. (2001) 'Gender and New Labour's social policy', *Journal of Social Policy*, vol 30, no 2, pp 209-31.

Ratner, P., Johnson, R. and Bottorff, J. (1999) 'Smoking relapse and early weaning among postpartum women: is there an association?', *Birth*, vol 26, no 1, pp 76-82.

RCoP (Royal College of Physicians) (1992) *Smoking and the young*, London: RCoP of London.

Reifsnider, E. (1998) 'Reversing growth deficiency in children: the effect of a community-based intervention', *Journal of Pediatric Health Care*, vol 12, no 6, pt 1, pp 305-12.

Renfrew, M., Dyson, L., Wallace, L., D'Souza, L., McCormick, F. and Spiby, H. (2004) *Breastfeeding for longer – what works? Summary paper*, London: Health Development Agency.

Renfrew, M., Dyson, L., Wallace, L., D'Souza, L., McCormick, F. and Spiby, H. (2005) *Breastfeeding for longer – what works? Systematic review summary*, London: National Institute for Health and Clinical Excellence.

Roberts, H. (2000) *What works in reducing inequalities in child health?*, Barkingside: Barnardo's.

Roseby, R., Waters, E., Polnay, A., Campbell, R., Webster, P. and Spencer, N. (2004) 'Family and carer smoking control programmes for reducing children's exposure to environmental tobacco smoke', *The Cochrane Library*, Chichester: John Wiley & Sons Ltd.

Rowe-Murray, H. and Fisher, J. (2002) 'Baby friendly hospital practices: caesarean section is a persistent barrier to early initiation of breastfeeding', *Birth*, vol 29, no 2, pp 124-31.

Rutter, M., Giller, H. and Hagler, A. (1998) *Antisocial behaviour by young people*, New York, NY: Cambridge University Press.

Sanders, M.R. (2002) 'Parenting interventions and the prevention of serious mental health problems in children', *The Medical Journal of Australia*, vol 177, pp S87-92.

Sanders, M.R., Markie-Dadds, C., Tully, L.A. and Bor, W. (2000) 'The triple p-positive parenting program: a comparison of enhanced, standard, and self-directed behavioral family intervention for parents of children with early onset conduct problems', *Journal of Consulting and Clinical Psychology*, vol 68, no 4, pp 624-40.

Schultz, J.R. and Vaughn, L.M. (1999) 'Brief report: learning to parent: a survey of parents in an urban pediatric primary care clinic', *Journal of Pediatric Psychology*, vol 24, no 5, pp 441-5.

Schweinhart, L.J. (2001) 'How the High/Scope Perry preschool study has influenced public policy', Evidence-Based Policies and Indicator Systems, Third International Inter-disciplinary Biennial Conference, University of Durham, 4-7 July, 2001.

Schweinhart, L.J., Barnes, H.V. and Weikart, D.P. (1993) *Significant benefits: The High/Scope Perry preschool study through age 27*, Ypsilanti, MI: High/Scope Press.

Scott, J. and Binns, C. (1999) 'Factors associated with the initiation and duration of breastfeeding: a review of the literature', *Breastfeeding Review*, vol 7, pp 5-16.

Scott, S., Knapp, M., Henderson, J. and Maughan, B. (2001a) 'Financial cost of social exclusion: follow up study of antisocial children into adulthood', *British Medical Journal*, vol 323, no 7306, pp 191-4.

Scott, S., Spender, Q., Doolan, M., Jacobs, B. and Aspland, H. (2001b) 'Multicentre controlled trial of parenting groups for childhood antisocial behaviour in clinical practice', *British Medical Journal*, vol 323, no 7306, pp 194-7.

Sikorski, J., Renfrew, M.J., Pindoria, S. and Wade, A. (2004) 'Support for breastfeeding mothers (Cochrane Review)', *The Cochrane Library*, Chichester: John Wiley & Sons Ltd.

Smith, C. and Pugh, G. (1996) *Learning to be a parent*, London: Family Policy Studies Centre.

Smith, R. (1997) 'Parent education: empowerment or control?', *Children and Society*, vol 11, no 2, pp 108-16.

Soler, J. and Miller, L. (2003) 'The struggle for early childhood curricula: a comparison of the English foundation stage curriculum, Te Whāriki and Reggio Emilia', *International Journal of Early Years Education*, vol 11, no 1, pp 57-67.

Spencer, N. (2003) 'Parenting programmes', *Archives of Disease in Childhood*, vol 88, no 2, pp 99-100.

Spinelli, M.G. and Endicott, J. (2003) 'Controlled clinical trial of interpersonal psychotherapy versus parenting education program for depressed pregnant women', *American Journal of Psychiatry*, vol 160, no 3, pp 555-62.

Statham, J. and Mooney, A. (2003) *Around the clock: Childcare services at atypical times*, Bristol/York: The Policy Press/Joseph Rowntree Foundation.

Stewart, K. (2005) 'Towards an equal start? Addressing childhood poverty and deprivation', in J. Hills and K. Stewart (eds) *A more equal society?*, Bristol: The Policy Press, pp 143-65.

Stewart-Brown, S. (1998) 'Public health implications of childhood behaviour problems and parenting programmes', in A. Buchanan and B. Nudson (eds) *Parenting, schooling and children's behaviour*, Aldershot: Ashgate, pp 21-33.

Stewart-Brown, S., Patterson, J., Mockford, C., Barlow, J., Klimes, I. and Pyper, C. (2004) 'Impact of a general practice based group parenting programme: quantitative and qualitative results from a controlled trial at twelve months', *Archives of Disease in Childhood*, vol 89, no 6, pp 519-25.

Stormshak, E.A., Kaminski, R.A. and Goodman, M.R. (2002) 'Enhancing the parenting skills of head start families during the transition to kindergarten', *Prevention Science*, vol 3, no 3, pp 223-34.

Sure Start Unit (2002) *A guide to evidence-based practice*, Nottingham: DfEE.

Sutherland, H. and Piachaud, D. (2001) 'Reducing child poverty in Britain: an assessment of government policy 1997-2001', *The Economic Journal*, vol 111, no 111, pp F85-F101.

Sylva, K., Melhuish, E., Sammons, P., Siraj-Blatchford, I., Taggart, B. and Elliot, K. (2003) *The Effective Provision of Pre-school Education (EPPE) Project: Findings from the pre-school period*, London: University of London.

Taylor, J., Spencer, N. and Baldwin, N. (2000) 'Social, economic, and political context of parenting', *Archives of Disease in Childhood*, vol 82, no 2, pp 113-20.

Taylor, L., Wohlgemuth, C., Warm, D., Taske, N., Naidoo, B. and Millward, L. (2005) *Public health interventions for the prevention and reduction of exposure to second-hand smoke: A review of reviews*, London: NICE.

Taylor, T. and Hajek, P. (2001) *Smoking cessation services for pregnant women*, London: Health Development Agency.

Tedstone, A., Dunce, N., Aviles, M., Shetty, P. and Daniels, L. (1998) *Effectiveness of interventions to promote healthy feeding in infants under one year of age: A review*, London: Health Education Authority.

Tunstill, J., Allnock, D., Meadows, P. and McLeod, A. (2002) *Early experiences of implementing Sure Start*, London: NESS Implementation Team.

UNICEF (United Nations Children's Fund) UK (United Kingdom) BFI (Baby Friendly Initiative) (1999) *Towards national, regional and local strategies for breastfeeding*, London: UNICEF UK BFI.

UNICEF UK BFI (2000) 'Baby friendly news', July (www.babyfriendly.org.uk/july00.asp), accessed 26 January 2004.

Vallenas, C. and Savage, F. (1999) *Evidence for the ten steps to successful breastfeeding*, Geneva: WHO.

Vimpani, G. (2002) 'Sure Start: reflections from Down Under (editorial)', *Child: Care, Health and Development*, vol 28, no 4, pp 281-7.

Watt, R., Dykes, J. and Sheiham, A. (1999) 'Socio-economic determinants of selected dietary indicators in British pre-school children', *Public Health Nutrition*, vol 4, no 6, pp 1229-1233.

Webster-Stratton, C. (1999) 'Researching the impact of parent training programmes on child conduct problems', in E. Lloyd (ed) *Parenting matters: What works in parenting education?*, Barkingside: Barnardo's, pp 85-114.

Webster-Stratton, C. and Hammond, M. (1990) 'Predictors of treatment outcome in parent training for families with conduct problem children', *Behavior Therapy*, vol 21, pp 319-37.

Webster-Stratton, C. and Hammond, M. (1998) 'Conduct problems and level of social competence in Head Start children: prevalence, pervasiveness, and associated risk factors', *Clinical Child and Family Psychology Review*, vol 1, no 2, pp 101-24.

West, R., McNeill, A. and Raw, M. (2003) *Meeting Department of Health smoking cessation targets: Recommendations for primary care trusts*, London: Health Development Agency.

WHO (World Health Organization) (2002) *Infant and young child nutrition: Global strategy for infant and young child feeding. Executive Board paper EB 109/12*, Geneva: WHO.

Williamson, D.L. and Drummond, J. (2000) 'Enhancing low-income parents' capacities to promote their children's health: education is not enough', *Public Health Nursing*, vol 17, no 2, pp 121-31.

Winickoff, J.P., Buckley, V.J., Palfrey, J.S., Perrin, J.M. and Rigotti, N.A. (2003a) 'Intervention with parental smokers in an outpatient pediatric clinic using counseling and nicotine replacement', *Pediatrics*, vol 112, no 5, pp 1127-33.

Winickoff, J.P., McMillen, R.C., Carroll, B.C., Klein, J.D., Rigotti, N.A., Tanski, S.E. and Weitzman, M. (2003b) 'Addressing parental smoking in pediatrics and family practice: a national survey of parents', *Pediatrics*, vol 112, no 5, pp 1146-51.

Wolfendale, S. (1999) 'Parents as key determinants in planning and delivering parenting education and support programmes: an inclusive ideology', in S. Wolfendale and H. Einzig (eds) *Parenting education and support*, London: David Fulton Publishers Ltd, pp 48-58.

Xiong, X., Buekens, P., Alexander, S., Demianczuk, N. and Wollast, E. (2000) 'Anemia during pregnancy and birth outcome: a meta-analysis', *American Journal of Perinatology*, vol 17, pp 137-46.

Zoritch, B., Roberts, I. and Oakley, A. (2000) 'Day care for preschool children', *The Cochrane Library*, Chichester: John Wiley & Sons Ltd.

Zwi, M., Pindoria, S. and Joughin, C. (2003) 'Parent training interventions in attention-deficit/hyperactivity disorder (Protocol for a Cochrane Review)', *The Cochrane Library*, Chichester: John Wiley and Sons Ltd.

SIX

Health inequalities during childhood and youth: research evidence

Introduction

As noted in Chapter Four, much research on the way in which very early life environments affect adult health implies the presence of latency effects, whereby adverse biological or developmental influences at sensitive periods have a lifelong impact on health and well-being, regardless of subsequent living conditions (Hertzman et al, 2001). Because young people are still developing, latency effects may still be at work during childhood and adolescence. For example, evidence suggests that fruit consumption during childhood may have a long-term protective effect on cancer risk in adults (Maynard et al, 2003). Psychological ill health during later life can also be rooted in adverse childhood experiences such as family conflict. During this period of the lifecourse, however, the difficulties of disentangling latency effects from other processes become very apparent. This is because early life environments are both strongly associated with and likely to influence the subsequent trajectories of life circumstances and opportunities experienced by individuals.

Taking the example of fruit consumption, the extent to which early diet influences cancer risk *independently* of subsequent dietary habits is subject to debate. Adult diet is also associated with cancer risk and, as the dietary preferences of adults may in part be established in childhood, it is as plausible to suggest that early dietary habits direct children onto certain nutritional pathways and that diet acts cumulatively on cancer risk as to propose latency effects. Similarly, the fact that early childhood stimulation programmes for disadvantaged children have yielded significant improvements in adult outcomes without additional help during the intervening years is consistent with a latency effect. However, stimulation in early childhood may also modify subsequent readiness to learn, behaviour at school and educational performance (Hertzman et al, 2001). These factors may in turn influence risk of low self-esteem, criminality, drug misuse, teenage pregnancy and employment status. Thus, early socio-emotional development may also be conceived as part of a pathway leading to later adult characteristics that are known to affect health.

The implication of the pathway and cumulative models is that initiatives designed to reduce inequalities in health should not be limited to early life but should continue throughout the lifecourse. As the chances of reducing inequalities for any given generation are likely to be greater, the earlier that attempts at reduction are begun, early life remains a critical period for intervention. However, there are a number of good reasons for proposing that childhood and youth is also an appropriate period at which to target interventions.

First, despite earlier evidence that suggested that childhood and youth is a period of relative health equality (West, 1988, 1997), more recent research has highlighted clear social gradients in current health status. Thus, while social class gradients appear to be absent in the prevalence of major chronic diseases (in part because of the general absence within this age group of diseases that take time to develop), a number of important causes of ill health and, in some cases death in young people, have been shown to be associated with poverty. There is also significant social variation in a range of behaviours and exposures that are strongly related to health outcomes in adulthood (Dennehy et al, 1997; Starfield et al, 2002). Even if childhood is a relatively 'healthy age', socio-economic differences in health behaviours form an important pathway by which socio-economic differences in later health develop.

In addition to responding to new evidence that supports the existence of social inequalities in both current health status and factors that influence health in adulthood, there is a moral case for focusing more attention on children and young people. While parental circumstances and decisions influence the provision of resources that can lead to heightened risk to health or, conversely, to greater resilience, children's everyday lives are also highly institutionalised (Nasman, 1994). Children in the UK spend most of their waking hours in formal education, suggesting that the state has a strong responsibility to address developmental disadvantage among children of school age. Yet the extent to which the education system in the UK, and particularly England, helps children who have been seriously disadvantaged in early life to move onto more favourable life trajectories is open to question.

Education is, of course, but one of a number of wider contextual factors that influence current and subsequent health. However, there are good grounds for singling out this issue for detailed consideration. Level of education is strongly associated with a range of socio-economic circumstances that in turn influence the risk of poor health in adulthood. In itself, education may also shape propensity to adopt and maintain healthy lifestyles. We therefore propose that education forms a critical pathway by which children and young people are set onto health-damaging or health-enhancing life trajectories.

Another powerful predictor of social exclusion in later life is the experience of being in care. Many of the 60,000 or so children in care in the UK have already experienced significant adversity in early life. Instability within care can further exacerbate their sense of emotional disruption. Given generally poorer educational qualifications and a lack of adequate ongoing support, the transition into adulthood is also fraught with problems for many young people in care, for whom risks of low self-esteem, substance misuse, mental health problems, teenage pregnancy, criminality and unemployment are particularly high. Disadvantaged with regard to latent, pathway and cumulative effects, looked-after children should be a key target group for health inequalities policies.

Over the course of the next four chapters, we examine research evidence of inequalities in health, health behaviours and the socio-economic trajectories of children and young people, and explore the range of interventions that have been designed to address factors associated with health exclusion during this period of the lifecourse. This chapter begins by discussing some of the methodological considerations involved in the investigation of health inequalities among children and young people. Then, in the second part of the chapter, we examine social variations in current mortality and morbidity in this age group. Acknowledging the difficulties of teasing out social class effects, particularly where findings have been inconsistent or contradictory, we nevertheless find persuasive evidence of health inequalities with respect to accidents and injuries and mental health. Policy interventions targeting these two main areas of health inequality during childhood and youth, are considered in Chapter Seven.

In Chapter Eight, we move beyond current mortality and morbidity to consider social variations in key behaviours and exposures that are known to have implications for health in the longer term: diet and physical exercise, substance misuse and sexual behaviour. We note, however, that concerns about health-damaging behaviours during childhood should not be confined to what they portend for the future. Given the links, for example, between substance misuse and risk of suicide and between child obesity and comorbidity, social class variations in child and youth health behaviours also impact on current health status. Policy interventions targeting nutrition, substance misuse and sexual behaviour during this period of the lifecourse are considered in Chapter Nine.

Continuity in health and health risk factors is, of course, only one mechanism by which childhood circumstances are linked to health inequalities in later life. A second mechanism is the continuity experienced by many children in their socio-economic circumstances, social disadvantage in childhood predicting social position in adult life, which in turn influences adult health. As noted above, education and the experience of being in care are key determinants of adult socio-economic position. The extent to which mainstream policies in these two areas are improving the prospects of children who have been seriously disadvantaged are also considered in Chapter Eight.

Measuring health inequalities in children and young people

Measuring health

In contrast to the substantial body of health inequalities research on infants, very young children and adults, there has been a dearth of literature on the relationship between poverty and health during childhood and youth (Dennehy et al, 1997, p 3). In part, this may have reflected an assumption that this is a relatively 'healthy' age. After infancy and early childhood, mortality rates fall, making 5-14 the period at which death is least likely to occur. Mortality rates gradually increase with age thereafter. In 2000, male and female mortality rates in the age group 15-19 exceeded those of one- to four-year-old children. However, at 50 and 30 per 100,000 respectively, they remained significantly lower than infant mortality rates (610 and 510 per 100,000) and mortality rates in adulthood and older age (data derived from the Office for National Statistics [ONS]).

Lower levels of mortality among children and young people are underpinned by significantly lower rates in the prevalence of major chronic diseases, many of which require time and sufficient exposure to causal vectors to develop (Starfield et al, 2002). In 2000, the rate of newly diagnosed cases of cancer among 5- to 14- and 15- to 24-year-olds stood respectively at 9.5 and 23.5 per 100,000, compared with rates per 100,000 of 349.7 aged 45-54, 781.6 aged 55-64, 1,502 aged 65-74 and 2,269 among the over-75s. Rates of diabetes similarly rise rapidly with age. Less than 150 per 100,000 children under the age of 15 had been diagnosed with this condition in 1998. This rose to between 360 and 370 per 100,000 among young people aged 16-24. By contrast, rates of diabetes per 100,000 among males rose from 2,580 aged 45-54 to 5,590 aged 55-64 to over 8,000 per 100,000 in the 65-84 age group (data derived from the ONS).

Because certain chronic conditions are relatively rare among children and young people, it is difficult to establish statistically significant social variations in many key health indicators. However, it is misleading to portray childhood and youth as a period characterised by an absence of health risks. In 1999, the prevalence of psychiatric disorders (including emotional and conduct disorders) among 5- to 15-year-olds was 11.4% for boys and 7.6% for girls (Meltzer et al, 2000). Prevalence of respiratory symptoms is also high in this age group. The 1995-97 Health Survey for England (HSE) found prevalence rates of doctor-diagnosed asthma of 23% and 18% among males and females aged 2-15. Over a third of respondents reported a history of wheezing (Primatesta et al, 1998, p 151). According to the 2000 General Household Survey (GHS), 19% of males and 17% of females aged under 20 years reported a long-standing illness or disability that limited their activity in some way. By the late teenage years, accidental death, suicide and violent crime emerge as important health risks, together with sexual disease, the consequences of early pregnancy and drug abuse (Furlong and Cartmel, 1997, p 66). All of these health outcomes lend themselves to statistical analysis of social variation by virtue of their higher prevalence.

Problems remain, however, in obtaining valid health information on children. Until relatively recently, epidemiological surveys have relied on parents to report on their children's health. While serious disorders are likely to be better reported, symptoms or conditions that are less visible, less persistent or ill defined, or that may be subject to censorship on the basis of perceived ideas about medical relevance and social desirability may be underreported (Sweeting and West, 1998, p 428). The longitudinal West of Scotland 11 to 16 Study found that parents were generally less likely to report both conditions and symptoms than children themselves. Particular discrepancies occurred between parent and child accounts of symptoms of malaise – irritability, anxiety and unhappiness – suggesting that psychological distress is an important area of low reportage (Sweeting and West, 1998).

Like the West of Scotland 11 to 16 Study, a growing number of surveys are now making provisions for children to report on their own general health, conditions and symptoms. The Child Health Questionnaire (CHQ), developed in the US but also applied in the Netherlands, is a wide-ranging instrument that measures the physical health, mental health, self-esteem, satisfaction and behaviour of children (Raat et al, 2002; Drukker et al, 2003). Within the UK, the 1995-97 HSE has been an important source of data. In 1997 this over-sampled children aged 2-15 relative to adults in order to provide a sample large enough for detailed analysis. For the main survey (which comprised questions on general health, height, weight, respiratory health, accidents, and physical activity), information was obtained directly from those aged 13 and over. Information about children aged 2-12 was obtained from a parent, with the child present. In addition, informants aged eight and over were asked to complete a self-completion booklet comprising questions on smoking, drinking, perceived current weight status and, in the case of 13- to 15-year-olds, psychological status. A number of physical measures (blood pressure, lung function and cotinine levels in saliva) were also taken by means of a nurse visit (Prescott-Clarke and Primatesta, 1998). In 2002, the HSE again boosted the sample of children, and aggregated findings from the 2001 HSE to permit a more detailed analysis of subgroups. The 2002 HSE also focused on the health of young adults aged 16-24 (Sproston and Primatesta, 2003).

As well as targeting formal survey instruments at children and young people, there has been a growing appreciation of the role of qualitative research in seeking to obtain children's own views and experiences of their health (Ireland and Holloway, 1996; Armstrong et al, 2000; Morrow, 2001; Backett-Milburn et al, 2003). While such research does not lend itself to the statistical analysis of health inequalities, it does help to highlight those elements of a child's life (for example, a safe environment, self-image, relationship with peers) that may mediate the impact of material disadvantage on physical and emotional well-being. There is also growing interest in capturing and defining child health in a broader way that emphasises child *development* (Graham and Power, 2004). The concept of 'developmental health' not only comprises physical health indicators, but also cognitive (such as readiness to learn), emotional (such as self-esteem) and behavioural dimensions (such as smoking and sexual behaviour).

In seeking to evaluate evidence of the presence of social gradients in health during childhood and youth, care should also be taken in treating this period in an undifferentiated way. As Sweeting and West (1998) point out, a child aged five is very different from a 15-year-old teenager, and there is no reason to believe that their health problems will be the same. Yet, in many publications, data on child morbidity is presented using wide age bands, possibly obscuring age-based changes in health or in the determinants of health. An additional problem arises from the use by different surveys of different age thresholds, making the comparison of results difficult. There is, for example, little agreement about when early life ends and childhood begins. Studies drawing on data from the 1958 British birth cohort (for example, Power and Matthews, 1997; Hertzman et al, 2001) use indicators at birth and age seven to capture early life factors because seven was the age at which children born within the cohort were first followed up. By contrast, other statistical sources distinguish between under and over five years of age. We have adopted this threshold in this and the following three chapters as, in the UK context, five marks the transition from preschool to school age.

The definition of 'youth' presents further difficulties. Age 11-12 is commonly used to define the beginning of this period, to correspond with entry into secondary school. However, there is less agreement about what marks the end of youth. With the trend towards continuing education and extended dependency on parents, many commentators suggest that young people do not reach the full citizenship rights of adulthood until they are 25. 'Youth' is thus increasingly understood to extend from the age of 12 to 25 (West, 1999). Given the considerable differences in the circumstances and characteristics of young people at the extremes of this age band, West (1999) suggests that any interpretation of health variations during this period should distinguish between 'early' (aged 12-16) and 'later' (aged 17-25) youth, a convention that informs our own discussion. It is important, however to point out that today the transition from child to adult varies according to socio-economic background (Graham and Power, 2004). While children from advantaged families are more likely to benefit from continuing education and to defer cohabitation and parenthood, children from poorer families are more likely to follow the pattern that predominated 40 years ago – to leave school at the age of 16 and to become parents by their early twenties.

Finally, any attempt to delineate social gradients in the health of children and young people should be sensitive to health differences according to gender. Aside from the obvious areas where the health experiences of young men and women differ according to biological sex (for example, pregnancy), there appear to be important differences in the ways in which males and females experience and express psychological distress. In other areas, too, there are gender differences in health risk (for example, accidents and injuries). Such differences have important implications for the relationship between health outcome and social status.

Measuring socio-economic status

As well as choice of health outcome, evidence of social gradients in the health status of children and young people is shaped by the way in which socio-economic status itself is characterised. In many studies, the socio-economic status of children is represented by the socio-economic status (for example, the occupational social class, income or education) of their parents. Aside from the well-rehearsed criticisms of using traditional measures such as social class, there are a number of problems with this approach. First, it assumes that the intra-household distribution of resources is equal, an assumption challenged by anecdotal evidence that, within poor households, parents may go without items or activities in order to shift resources towards their children (Micklewright, 2002, p 13). The relationship between parental socio-economic status and that of children may also be weakened by the fact that, particularly when they reach adolescence, influences outside the family (for example, the school, the peer group and youth culture) may reduce differences according to household circumstances (West, 1997; Williams et al, 1997). Thus, class of origin may not correspond to class of destination (West et al, 2001). These limitations, together with the development of a more fundamental critique about the need to represent children's own views about the problems and issues that arise in their lives (Christensen and Prout, 2002; Prout and Hallett, 2003), have led to calls for the inclusion of more appropriate, child-centred indicators of socio-economic status.

The methodological debate about the difficulties of capturing children's socio-economic status is, in part, underpinned by epistemological differences between postmodern and structuralist interpretations about the determinants of individual life trajectories (Karvonen et al, 2001). Proponents of the postmodern thesis argue that, with the growth of a global commercial youth culture, structural divisions based on class have diminished in importance (Miles, 2000). Examining determinants of young people's health behaviours (smoking, drinking and drug misuse) in Glasgow and Helsinki, Karvonen et al (2001) found that the influence of youth lifestyles far outweighed that of social class, lending weight to the postmodern thesis.

Against this, others propose that parental socio-economic status remains a major determinant of young people's life chances. For example, educational and labour market outcomes can still be largely predicted on the basis of social class (Furlong and Cartmel, 1997, p 110). As we discuss in Chapter Eight, young people from 'middle-class' families are significantly more likely to achieve good educational qualifications, enter into higher education, obtain well-paid employment and enjoy good living standards. By contrast, children from poorer backgrounds are more likely to achieve few or poor qualifications and to leave school only to gain insecure and low-paid jobs (Coles, 1995, p 14). Similarly, while not all health risks in childhood are strongly associated with social class, social variations have been observed in key indicators of mortality and morbidity, as well as characteristics (such as height) and behaviours that have important implications for health in later life. We therefore conclude that, while it is important to take account of the potentially homogenising effects of globalisation on young people, the outright rejection of more traditional measures of socio-economic status would be premature.

Inequalities in mortality and morbidity

Notwithstanding the methodological difficulties just outlined, research suggests that a number of important causes of ill health and indeed death are subject to significant social gradients. The main health problems during childhood and youth that have been associated with poverty are accidents, injuries, mental illness and limiting long-standing illness. Social differences in certain physical characteristics (for example, height) have also been noted, that may have important implications for health in later life.

Mortality

In 2000 there were 841 deaths among children aged 5-14 in England and Wales, and 3,133 deaths in the 15- to 24-year-old age group. The biggest single cause of death in both age groups was 'injuries and poisoning'. This accounts for 30% of all deaths of children aged 5-14 and 58% of deaths of children and young people aged 15-24. In both age groups, numbers and rates of death by injury are significantly higher among males than females. Of all child and youth deaths by injury and poisoning, 44% are due to transport accidents (and 95% of these involve motor vehicles). However, the number of children killed in road accidents has been steadily declining (DfT, 2003). By contrast, rates of suicide, purposely inflicted injury and injury of undetermined cause have increased over the past two decades, and accounted for 40% of all deaths of children and young people aged 15-24 in 2000. As we discuss later in this chapter, the rise in suicides among young men has been a particular source of public health concern. In 2002, 13.3 per 100,000 men aged 15-24 in the UK died as a result of suicide, compared to 9.8 per 100,000 in 1976 (data derived from the ONS). At 3.7 per 100,000, the rate of female suicide aged 15-24 in 2002 was actually lower than the 1976 figure (4.6 per 100,000), and significantly lower than that of young men. It is important to note that these figures may underestimate the scale of the problem as deaths recorded as of undetermined cause or from methods similar to suicide may in reality have been suicides (Maughan et al, 2004a).

As noted in Chapter One, social differences in risk of death during childhood and youth were highlighted in the 1997 Decennial Supplement on health inequalities (Botting, 1997). Throughout childhood and youth, class gradients in mortality are predominantly attributable to accidents and injuries, a pattern that, in later youth, also applies to suicides (West, 1999). Mortality due to other causes shows much less class variation. As many analyses have not included children of parents outside paid employment (thereby excluding the most disadvantaged group), some commentators have proposed that the extent of social variation in disease prevalence during childhood may have been underestimated (Judge and Benzeval, 1993). However, there is little evidence to suggest that risk of cancer in childhood (the second highest cause of death after injuries) is strongly related to poverty. Indeed, the incidence of acute lymphoblastic leukaemia, one of the most common forms of childhood cancer, is higher in areas of higher socio-economic status (Stiller et al, 2004). Thus, with the exception of deaths from accidents/injuries (including suicide), there is support for the assumption that, as far as risk of death is concerned, childhood and youth is not only a relatively 'healthy' age, but an age characterised by relative health equality.

Accidents and injuries

As noted, accidents and injuries are the biggest single cause of death in both childhood and youth. Over half of deaths by injury among 5- to 14-year-olds involve transport accidents, which are also responsible for a significant burden of childhood morbidity. In 2002, 179 children aged 0-15 were killed in road accidents; 4,417 were seriously injured and 30,093 slightly injured (DfT, 2003). Of those who died or who were seriously injured, 62% were child pedestrians and a further 13% pedal cyclists.

The association between socio-economic status and child mortality due to road-related accidents has been well established (Dougherty et al, 1990; Roberts and Power, 1996; Morrison et al, 1999; Hjern and Bremberg, 2002). A relationship has also been identified between social deprivation and non-fatal road injuries among children (Laing and Logan, 1999; Laflamme and Engström, 2002; Coupland et al, 2003; Lyons et al, 2003). A combination of factors appears to put children from deprived backgrounds at greater risk, including neighbourhood characteristics, housing design, family circumstances and individual behavioural and emotional factors. Urban deprived areas tend to have higher volumes of traffic than more affluent areas, increasing exposure to risk. Living in a home with insufficient space to play or in housing that opens directly onto the street also increases the risk of child pedestrian accidents (Dowswell and Towner, 2002). Evidence suggests that poorer children are more likely to walk to school and to be unaccompanied by an adult than children from more affluent backgrounds (Towner et al, 1994). Marital status (particularly lone motherhood) may also be related to risk, through the ability of parents to supervise children (Roberts and Pless, 1996). Finally, children with hyperactivity (a symptom that is itself associated with lower social status) appear to be at increased risk of accidents involving moving vehicles (Lalloo et al, 2003).

In addition to road traffic accidents, over a million UK children under the age of 15 are injured every year within the home (CAPT, 2002a). While the under-fives are most at risk (accounting for 71% of deaths and around 60% of hospitalisations from home accidents in 1999), over 400,000 5- to 15-year-olds in the UK were admitted to hospital in 1999 following an accident at home (CAPT, 2002b). Again, the relationship between deprivation status and home injuries in children is pronounced across a range of categories, including falls, burns/scalds and poisoning (Hippisley-Cox et al, 2002; Lyons et al, 2003). The mechanisms by which disadvantage increases risk of home accidents are not well understood, although parental knowledge (of, for example, the potential for accidents and effective safety measures), behaviour (for example, drug and alcohol misuse, smoking) and circumstances (such as insufficient income to purchase home safety equipment) have been suggested as factors (Dowswell and Towner, 2002). For example, the steep social gradient in child deaths and injuries in house fires has been attributed in part to higher rates of smoking among parents of lower socio-economic status, but also to the fact that parents living in poverty neither identify buying a smoke alarm nor maintaining its battery as a high priority (DiGuiseppi et al, 1999, p 402). Other studies suggest that, while the prohibitive cost of safety equipment may play a role, differences in knowledge and attitudes do not explain social inequalities in accident risk. For example, Roberts et al (1993) found poorer parents to be very aware of the risks their children faced.

While younger children tend to be more at risk of injury at home, rates of non-traffic-related injuries taking place outside the home (for example, at school, at a playground, sports or leisure facility or on the street) increase with age. The vast majority of these injuries are non-fatal. Evidence of a socio-economic gradient in their occurrence in early youth is equivocal, some studies suggesting that, if anything, risk of injury decreases with lower socio-economic status (West, 1997; Williams et al, 1997; Lyons et al, 2000; Pickett et al, 2002). This may reflect the fact that adolescents of higher socio-economic status have more opportunity to participate in sports and leisure activities. Violence-related injury provides an exception to this pattern, higher rates occurring in 10- to 14-year-old boys from lower socio-economic groups. However, since violence-related injury is relatively rare in this age group, absolute socio-economic differences are small (Engström et al, 2002).

By later youth (aged 15-24), road traffic accidents still account for a significant burden of deaths by injury (41%). Indeed, in absolute terms, greater numbers of older youth are killed or seriously injured on the roads than under-15-year-olds. Risk factors for traffic injury change with increasing age. As noted earlier, nearly two thirds of 0- to 15-year-olds who died or were seriously injured in road accidents in 2002 were pedestrians. By contrast, around 60% of road casualties aged 16/17-24 in 2001 were car occupants and a further 20% were motor cycle/ moped riders (data derived from the DfT, 2002). Young males are at significantly higher risk than young females, accounting for 74% and 62% respectively of the car driver and car passenger casualties in this age group.

A social class gradient exists for fatal road traffic accidents during later youth, although the reasons for this are not well understood. Differences in the nature and volume of traffic between deprived and more affluent areas may play a role. Speeding is more common in low socio-economic than affluent areas (Stevenson et al, 1995, cited by MacGibbon, 1999). Socio-economic differences in drink driving may also play a role. For around 12% of serious road accident casualties aged 16-24 in 2001, at least one of the drivers or riders involved was over the legal blood alcohol limit. Male drivers under the age of 30 had the highest incidence of failing a breath test after being involved in a personal injury road accident, unlicensed drivers (that is those under the age of 17) being at greatest risk (DfT, 2002). Little is known about the socio-economic characteristics of young drink drivers in the UK. However, factors such as unemployment have been associated with hazardous behaviour, including problem drinking, in young men (Montgomery et al, 1998). Lower socio-economic status is also associated with the tendency to binge drink (Casswell et al, 2003). Thus, it is possible that the social class gradient that is known to exist among older drink-drivers (PACTS, 2003) is preceded in youth.

As well as road traffic accidents, alcohol has been attributed to increased risk of assault during youth (Richardson and Budd, 2003; Stanistreet and Jeffrey, 2003). According to the 2002/03 British Crime Survey, 15.1% of young men aged 16-24 experienced a violent crime of some sort in the year prior to interview, compared to only 2.7% of 45- to 64-year-old men and only 0.4% of men aged 75 and over. Between a third and a quarter of all violent crimes are alcohol-related and rates of alcohol-related victimisation are highest among young men aged 16-19. Unemployment is a key factor associated with heightened risk, as is a high level of alcohol consumption (Budd, 2003). Thus, in terms of age, sex and socio-economic status, assault victims have similar profiles to offenders.

Most alcohol attributable deaths in youth are due to road traffic accidents, suicides (discussed later in this chapter) and assaults (Britton and McPherson, 2001). Diseases that are directly related to alcohol take years to develop and are comparatively rare in young people. Despite this, a pronounced social gradient has been observed in directly related alcohol mortality in young men (Harrison and Gardiner, 1999). Such deaths are more likely to be due to acute causes such as alcohol poisoning than chronic alcoholic disease (for example, liver cirrhosis). Excess alcohol consumption has also been linked with death due to ischaemic heart disease (IHD) and cancers of the colon, oesophagus and breast (Britton and McPherson, 2001). Again, such diseases require time and sufficient exposure to risk factors to develop. However, as patterns of problem drinking are often established in youth, the long-term implications of the rise of heavy drinking among young people have become a focus of policy concern. We return to this issue in Chapter Eight, which examines social variations in health behaviours.

Mental health

Mental health has become a key focus of research on the health of children and young people, due to the increasing relative importance of mental illness in this age group. Evidence suggests that there has been a significant increase in rates of psychological disorders among young people since the Second World War (Rutter and Smith, 1995). While this may in part reflect measurement problems and changes in the way in which mental health and illness are conceptualised (see Coppock, 1997, and Kutchins and Kirk, 1997 for critiques of the medicalisation of children's behaviour), the rise in suicides among young males (an objective indicator of mental illness) is suggestive of a worrying trend.

The three most common groups of mental health problems in children and young teenagers are conduct disorders characterised by awkward, troublesome, aggressive and antisocial behaviours; emotional disorders such as anxiety, depression and obsessions; and hyperactivity disorders involving inattention and overactivity (Meltzer et al, 2000, p 12). Eating disorders are a less common but well-known problem affecting this age group. By the late teens and early twenties, schizophrenia and suicide also emerge as relatively rare, although important health problems. Risk of experiencing most psychological disorders varies according to age and sex. Prevalence is higher among older children and youth than young children and, with the exception of emotional and eating disorders, higher in boys than girls. The 1999 ONS Survey on the Mental Health of Children and Adolescents in Britain also suggests that there are ethnic differences in risk, Indian children (particularly girls) having lower rates of mental disorder than both white or black children (Meltzer et al, 2000, p 27). In later youth, however, young Asian women appear to be vulnerable to increased rates of attempted self-harm (Bhugra et al, 1999).

Comorbidity between psychiatric disorders is common during childhood and youth, so that young people with one disorder are at greater risk of having others. The association between hyperactivity and conduct disorders is particularly strong, although children with conduct disorders are also at higher risk of suffering from depression (Maughan et al, 2004b). There are links too between children's mental and physical health. In the 1999 ONS Survey, having a physical condition (for example, epilepsy, difficulties with coordination, muscle disease, speech or language difficulties) increased the odds of having a mental disorder by 82% (Meltzer et al, 2000, p 74). Psychiatric disorders also show strong overlaps with educational difficulties and needs, 49% of children with a mental disorder in the ONS Survey having officially recognised special educational needs (SEN), compared with 15% of children with no disorder (Meltzer et al, 2000, p 95).

For many young people, mental health problems in childhood mark the early stages of difficulties that continue into adult life (Maughan et al, 2004a). In addition to being at increased risk for adult psychiatric disorders, their long-term physical health may be compromised. A follow-up study of former students whose mental health state was assessed during early adulthood found that anxiety was positively associated with increased risk of death from cancer, and that young men labelled as hypomanic had increased cardiovascular mortality risk (McCarron et al, 2003). Rates of substance misuse are significantly higher among young people with mental health problems, as is the risk of getting involved in crime. In the 1997 ONS Survey of Psychiatric Morbidity among young offenders, 81% of sentenced male prisoners aged 16-20 were assessed as having an antisocial personality disorder, compared to between 3% and 7% in the community. Functional psychoses (for example, schizophrenic or delusional disorder) was identified in 10% of young male prisoners, compared to 0.2% of 16- to 19-year-olds living in private households (Lader et al, 2000).

Although mental illness in young people has significant consequences for individuals, families, communities and the wider society, the aetiology of mental and behavioural disorders is still not fully understood. A range of biological, psychological and social factors has been associated with mental illness, including genetic predisposition, physical illness, educational difficulties, abuse/neglect, family breakdown, large family size, parental mental illness, parental criminality, socio-economic disadvantage, unemployment, housing and homelessness and school environment (Wallace et al, 1997). For years, researchers have argued over the relative importance of genetic and environmental factors. Recent developments in genetic research suggest that most childhood disorders do involve a heritable component. However, this does not mean that genetic factors cause mental and behavioural disorders in a direct, deterministic way. Multiple risk genes contribute (with other factors) to variations in *susceptibility* to environmental risks. Exposure to key environmental stresses determines whether or not a particular mental or behavioural disorder will *manifest* (Simonoff et al, 1994; Caprara and Rutter, 1995). Even in strongly genetic disorders such as schizophrenia, environmental risk factors are important. This is even more the case with the range of disorders (for example, conduct problems and anxiety) that more commonly affect children and young people.

Conduct disorders

Conduct disorders are the most common form of childhood psychological disorder, affecting 4.6% of 5- to 10-year-olds and 6.2% of 11- to 15-year-olds in the 1999 ONS Survey (Meltzer et al, 2000). Boys are significantly more likely to be affected (7.4% of all 5- to 15-year-old boys had a conduct disorder, compared with 3.2% of girls). The manifestations of antisocial behaviour change over time, reflecting changes both within the individual and opportunities in the environment. Thus, Farrington (1995, p 83) notes that while the "antisocial child may be troublesome and disruptive at school, the antisocial teenager may steal cars and burgle houses, and the antisocial adult male may beat up his wife and neglect his children". Evidence suggests that antisocial behaviours rise to a peak in the teenage years, then fall in the twenties. Thus, the vast majority of adolescent offenders desist from crime in adulthood (Smith, 1995, p 428).

A distinction has been made between children who display an early onset conduct disorder (before the age of 10) and those whose antisocial behaviour begins around puberty. The former are more likely to be boys, show more aggressive symptoms, account for a disproportionate amount of illegal activity, and persist in their antisocial behaviour into adulthood. These are the subgroup of teenagers most likely to commit violent crimes, drop out of school and abuse drugs, which further limits their opportunities. Children with adolescent-onset conduct disorder are as likely to be girls as boys, display less extreme and less consistent antisocial behaviour and tend to desist from crime and delinquency once they reach adulthood, although factors such as dropping out of school, having an unplanned pregnancy, addiction to drugs and alcohol and unemployment may cause antisocial behaviours to persist for longer (Mash and Wolfe, 2002, pp 144-5). Research supports a significant genetic contribution to lifecourse-persistent antisocial behaviour, but not to antisocial behaviour that occurs in the adolescent years only (Smith, 1995, p 434). Even among the former group, however, differences influenced by heredity are the product of a complex gene–environment interaction.

Most of the environmental risk factors that are associated with conduct disorders in childhood and adolescence are also strongly related to social disadvantage. Children with conduct disorders in the ONS Survey were more likely to be living in a lone-parent or reconstituted family, in social sector housing, in a low-income household, and in a household where the interviewed parent had no educational qualifications and where neither parent was working (Meltzer et al, 2000, p 63). At the household level, the relationship between social disadvantage and conduct problems is mediated, at least in part, by family processes such as marital discord and parenting deficits (Hill, 2002, p 153). Effects of marital conflict may include exposure to violence and negativity, loss of contact with one parent due to divorce, financial hardship and family isolation. Aspects of parenting that have been implicated include poor supervision, inconsistent discipline, authoritarianism, permissiveness and a lack of positive reinforcement.

Having two antisocial parents is a strong predictor of conduct problems, although the extent to which this reflects continuities in biological or genetic factors, peer and partner choices, parenting and socialisation practices or deprivation is subject to debate (Smith and Farrington, 2004, p 231). Virtually all adults with antisocial disorder first developed conduct problems in childhood. They are more likely to have experienced educational failure, unemployment or sporadic employment and criminal convictions. They are also more likely to form relationships with antisocial peers and partners, are at increased risk of entering and contributing to violent marriages and, as antisocial parents, expose their children to behaviours and attitudes that in turn produce risks for conduct problems (Fergusson and Lynsky, 1998; Hill, 2002; Healey et al, 2004; Simonoff et al, 2004). Disentangling the precise mechanisms that result in such pathways is difficult, in part because of the high degree of interrelation between different factors, but also because such pathways do not involve only direct and immediate risk factors, but also a set of chain effects that unfold over time (Rutter, 1995, 1999). Thus, although aggressive and antisocial tendencies run in families, this does not mean that such families are locked into a cycle of delinquency and criminality from which they cannot escape.

Evidence suggests, for example, that behavioural problems can be exacerbated or ameliorated by changes in material circumstances. Using data from a national (US) longitudinal survey, Macmillan et al (2004) found that while long-term exposure to poverty intensified behavioural problems in young children, children whose mothers were initially poor but who escaped from poverty for the majority of the study period were no more likely to develop behavioural problems than children whose mothers had never been poor. Thus, changes in material circumstances that accompany successful escapes from poverty may limit the development of behavioural problems in children (Macmillan et al, 2004, p 215).

Although contested, there is also evidence that, independently of individual and family attributes, neighbourhood conditions influence the development of conduct problems in children. Dutch research suggests that living in a deprived neighbourhood presents risks for children from high as well as low socio-economic backgrounds and for girls as well as boys, although girls are more likely to report internalising problems such as anxiety than to develop conduct disorders (Schneiders et al, 2003). Neighbourhood effects have been demonstrated in children as young as two years of age (Caspi et al, 2000). For very young children, the impact of neighbourhood socio-economic disadvantage may be mediated through parental stress (and the way in which this influences parenting), and by reducing access to the social support and services that parents need to promote their children's welfare. As children become increasingly independent outside the home and have more contact with neighbourhood peer groups, adults and institutions, direct exposure to neighbourhood effects is likely to take on more significance (Leventhal and Brooks-Gunn, 2000; Schneiders et al, 2003). Neighbourhood design may play a role here. Freeman and Stansfeld (1998, p 167) suggest that children playing outside their homes in older established neighbourhoods are constantly seen by passing neighbours or relatives who provide informal supervision and regular contact with adults. By contrast, young people living in high-rise housing estates gather away from adults and thus have fewer opportunities to be influenced by adult role models in the process of socialisation.

Such factors may play a role in the striking rise in conduct disorders among black British children once they reach secondary school age. The 1999 ONS Survey found that although rates of conduct disorder among black and white boys of primary school age are comparable, among 11- to 15-year-olds 17.8% of black boys are affected, compared with 8.6% of white boys, 4.6% of Pakistani and Bangladeshi boys and 2.3% of Indian boys (Meltzer et al, 2000, p 34). Reasons for these ethnic differences are poorly understood. Freeman and Stansfeld (1998, p 152) propose that residential segregation, coupled with the spatial concentration of social disadvantage, can contribute to a loss of positive identification with one's neighbourhood and of communal norms and sanctions among low-income black communities. However, this does not explain why, among similarly segregated and disadvantaged Pakistani and Bangladeshi communities, rates of conduct disorders remain low. Others propose that ethnicity itself is a significant factor, for instance in shaping the way in which psychological response to environmental stresses is expressed. It is worth noting that, although they have lower rates of conduct disorder, teenage Pakistani and Bangladeshi boys exhibit higher than average rates of emotional disorder (see below).

In the US, a positive sense of ethnic identity has been associated with the development of prosocial attitudes among young adolescents (Smith et al, 1999), and one that may buffer the effects of experiencing racial discrimination, a strong predictor of violent behaviour among young African-American adults (Caldwell et al, 2004). Within the British context, the lack of cultural appropriateness in teaching and exposure to discrimination and racism (reflected, for example, in higher rates of school exclusion and police attention) have been linked to disaffection, school failure and poor employment opportunities among African-Caribbean pupils (Bourne et al, 1994; Patel and Fatimilehin, 1999; London Development Agency, 2004; Tomlinson, 2005), although evidence linking institutional racism with the mental health of young black people is lacking. The high rate of conduct problems among this group may thus reflect the way in which multiple stresses or adversities (poverty, neighbourhood conditions and discrimination, for example) combine to increase psychosocial risk.

Emotional disorders

Emotional disorders are the second most prevalent mental health problem affecting children and young teenagers. In the 1999 ONS Survey, 4.3% of children were assessed as having an emotional disorder (3.3% of 5- to 10-year-olds and 5.6% of 11- to 15-year-olds). The vast majority of these suffered from some kind of anxiety disorder (for example, separation anxiety, social anxiety, specific phobia), and less than 1% were assessed as having depression. However, there is a strong relationship between anxiety and depression in children and adolescents and longitudinal evidence suggests that anxiety disorders are often antecedents of depressive conditions (Fombonne, 1995a, p 572).

In contrast to conduct disorders, rates of emotional disorders are generally higher among teenage girls (6.1% compared to 5.1% among boys in the ONS Survey), although Pakistani and Bangladeshi boys aged 11-15 are particularly affected (12.4%). The fact that girls exhibit a tendency towards internalising disorders, whereas boys generally express their problems in a more external way, has been variously attributed to genetic influences and gender role orientation. Cross-cultural research into anxiety disorders is limited, although cultures that favour inhibition, compliance and obedience may affect the expression and developmental course of fear in children (Mash and Wolfe, 2002, p 187).

Like conduct disorders, emotional disorders in childhood and adolescence are strongly associated with social disadvantage. Risk factors identified in the 1999 ONS Survey included living with a lone parent, in a household where the interviewed parent had no educational qualifications and where neither parent was working, in a low-income household and in social sector housing (Meltzer et al, 2000, p 63). Little is known about the relation between family factors and anxiety disorders, although anxiety in children who have a genetic vulnerability may be triggered by the stressful conditions that are often present in socially disadvantaged families. Such children may be particularly sensitive to critical, controlling and punitive parenting. Insecure early attachment may also be a risk factor (Mash and Wolfe, 2002, pp 190-1). As noted in Chapter Four, this has been associated with maternal anxiety and depression.

While anxiety *disorder* affects a small though significant proportion of adolescents, a far larger percentage exhibit emotional *symptoms*. Using the 12-item version of the General Health Questionnaire (GHQ), research carried out in the West of Scotland found that in 1999 15% of boys and 33% of girls aged 15 indicated a level of psychological distress of potential clinical significance. As rates were respectively 13% and 19% in 1987, the mental health of young girls in the study area had deteriorated substantially over time. In contrast to more severe emotional disorder, girls from middle-class and skilled manual backgrounds were found to be at significantly higher risk. No social class differences in psychological distress were observed in boys. Analysis suggests that an increase in educational expectations, together with more traditional concerns about personal identity, are elevating levels of stress among middle-class females, with adverse consequences for their mental health. It is particularly among this group that the pressure to be both clever and attractive at the same time is most strongly felt (Sweeting and West, 2003).

Although rare before puberty, depression occurs quite frequently among adolescents and young adults. Again, a distinction should be made between mild and more severe forms. Depressive *symptoms*, which are usually temporary, occur in 30% to 50% of adolescents and are related to events in the environment rather than being part of any disorder. As a *syndrome*, depression involves a group of observable symptoms and is less common than isolated depressive symptoms. Persistence and impairment distinguish this form from depressive *disorder* (Fombonne, 1995a). Depressive disorders rarely start before the age of 13 and are more common in young adults than children and adolescents. In the ONS Survey 0.2% of 5- to 10-year-olds were assessed as having depression, compared with 1.8% of 11- to 15-year-olds (Meltzer et al, 2000, p 33). As depression is episodic, prevalence rates vary with the length of time in which symptoms are assessed.

When taken at a single point of time (like the ONS Survey), the prevalence of depressive disorder in 14- to 18-year-olds is around 3% (Mash and Wolfe, 2002, p 204). Over a one-year period, the Finnish Health Care Survey found rates of 5.3% for adolescents aged 15- to 19-years and 9.4% for young adults aged 20- to 24-years (Haarasilta et al, 2001), while lifetime prevalence (which reflects whether a young person has ever had a depressive disorder) may be as high as 15% to 20% (Kessler and Walters, 1998; Wittchen et al, 1998).

Young women are significantly more likely to suffer from depression than young men, although the extent to which this reflects genetic vulnerability, normal female hormonal maturational processes or gender socialisation is subject to debate. Problems within the family (for example, economic hardship, marital discord, parental distress) are strongly associated with the development of depressive symptoms in adolescent girls. This may reflect heightened sensitivity to interpersonal stress or gender differences in coping styles. Alternatively, the lower risk that adolescent boys face for internalising symptoms may reflect the fact that, for cultural reasons, they are able to disengage from their families earlier (Crawford et al, 2001). Cultural values have also been linked to risk of developing a negative body image among girls, the recent promotion of a prepubertal body shape meaning that body changes brought about by puberty are not welcomed. In contrast, boys see their increased height and strength as positive attributes (Fombonne, 1995a, p 580). Finally, gender differences in risk of depression may simply stem from the fact that girls and boys respond to similar environmental stressors in different ways, girls developing internalising symptoms while boys develop conduct problems instead.

The most alarming consequence of depression in adolescents and young adults is suicide. As noted earlier, official statistics show that there has been a substantial increase in suicide rates among young men since the 1970s. In 2000, 376 young people in England and Wales lost their lives due to suicide or self-inflicted injuries. While these figures are likely to conceal the real scale of suicide which, it is estimated, may be up to three times the official recorded level (Madge and Harvey, 1999), it is worth noting that youth suicide rates in Britain are lower than in a number of other countries. In 2002, 13.3 per 100,000 men aged 15-24 died as a result of suicide in the UK. By contrast, the male youth suicide rate in New Zealand (1996) was 39.5 per 100,000 (Beautrais, 2000a) and in Australia (in 1997) 30.9 per 100,000 (Lynsky et al, 2000).

In contrast to suicide, which occurs more frequently in young males, rates of deliberate self-harm (DSH) are higher among young women than young men. As the term DSH encompasses both attempted suicide and self-injury where suicide may not be the real intention (Anderson, 1999), the extent to which these gender differences reflect differences in method used, seriousness of intent or the way in which young people express distress is not fully understood. For example, Webb (2002) suggests that the medical recording of DSH is biased towards female overdose hospital admissions, while the way in which DSH is expressed in adolescent boys and young men (for example, through recklessness and self-battery) is often undetected. Thus, gender differences in potential and actual DSH may not be as profound as studies suggest.

Although there are important differences between suicide and DSH, indeed, in some cases, self-mutilation may be a coping strategy against anxiety and a protective factor against suicide (Webb, 2002), similar risk factors appear to increase vulnerability to both attempted and completed suicide. These include mental health factors; individual and personality factors; social and family risk factors; stressful life events and adverse life circumstances; and environmental and contextual factors (Beautrais, 2000b).

Suicidal behaviour in youth is strongly correlated with depression, substance misuse disorders and antisocial behaviours. Depression in childhood and adolescence is a particularly strong risk factor, evidence suggesting that up to 15% of young people with a depressive illness will ultimately die from suicide (Fombonne, 1995a, p 574). Various personality traits have also been suggested as predisposing factors, including low self-esteem, feelings of hopelessness, poor problem solving and a tendency towards social withdrawal and isolation, although research evidence linking such traits with suicidal behaviour is lacking. A wide range of family-level factors have been implicated in increased risk for suicide and DSH (Beautrais, 2000b), including parental psychopathology, family history of suicidal behaviour, marital discord, the absence or breakdown of parental support and exposure to sexual and physical abuse (Diekstra et al, 1995; Anderson, 1999; Sauvola et al, 2001; Webb, 2002). Adverse life events (for example, being arrested, charged or sentenced) frequently precede suicide in young people with and without severe mental illness (Cooper et al, 2002). As risk of mental disorders, exposure to adverse family circumstances and exposure to adverse life events are strongly related to social disadvantage, suicidal behaviour can be portrayed as an outcome of social exclusion, higher rates of suicide and DSH being found among lower social class groups (Hawton et al, 1999, 2001), the unemployed (Gunnell et al, 1999; Hawton et al, 2000), young offenders and drug addicts (Christoffersen et al, 2003). Finally, links between environmental/contextual factors and suicidal behaviour have been explored, including the role of the media in 'normalising' the concept of suicide and of declines in religious beliefs in removing taboos about suicide. Neighbourhood context may also be important. For example, the relative risk of being unemployed may be greater in areas where rates of unemployment are lower or falling due to increased pressure and stigma (Crawford and Prince, 1999).

Attention Deficit/Hyperactivity Disorder

Hyperkinetic disorders are the third most common group reported in the ONS Survey on the Mental Health of Children and Adolescents in Britain, affecting 2.4% of boys and 0.4% of girls aged 5-15 (Meltzer et al, 2000). This prevalence rate is at the lower end of international estimates, recent reviews reporting prevalence estimates of Attention Deficit/Hyperactivity Disorder (ADHD) of between 3% and 5% (Doggett, 2004) and between 5% and 10% of school-age children (Willoughby, 2003). Characterised by persistent, age-inappropriate symptoms of inattention, overactivity and impulsiveness, childhood hyperactivity is associated with increased risk for antisocial behaviour, drug and alcohol problems, peer and self-esteem problems and poor academic performance (Willoughby, 2003). However, there has been debate as to whether ADHD is a legitimate concept, or a scapegoat for individual and societal problems (Sava, 2000). This partly reflects concerns that treating the symptoms that make up ADHD as a pathology has resulted in the inappropriate medication of children and the failure to recognise their need for wider behavioural and social support. Prescribing rates are particularly high in Australia and the US, where evidence of the use of psychostimulant medication on preschool-age children (Zito et al, 2000) has been particularly controversial, although other studies suggest that relatively few US children who meet the full ADHD diagnostic criteria are receiving medication (Jensen et al, 1999). In the UK, concerns have centred less on the medicalisation of ADHD-type symptoms than on the reluctance of doctors to respond to parents' demands to diagnose ADHD and prescribe drugs (Norris and Lloyd, 2000). However, recent evidence suggests a dramatic rise in the use of methylphenidate (Ritalin) for ADHD in the UK (Bramble, 2003).

Notwithstanding the controversy surrounding the diagnosis and management of ADHD, children displaying the symptoms of hyperkinetic disorder are more likely to be socially disadvantaged. Compared with children who did not have any mental disorder, children with a hyperkinetic disorder in the 1999 ONS Survey were more likely to be living in social sector housing, in a lower-income household and in a household where the interviewed parent had no educational qualifications. They were less likely to be living in Social Class I or II households and with parents who were working (Meltzer et al, 2000, p 64). As with other childhood mental disorders, a mixture of genetic and environmental factors has been implicated in the aetiology of ADHD (Biederman and Faraone, 2002). Environmental factors include psychosocial adversity such as early problems in parental attachment and maternal anxiety/depression (Nigg and Hinshaw, 1998). Exposure to tobacco smoke in utero is also suspected to be associated with ADHD and ADHD symptoms in children (Linnet et al, 2003; Thapar et al, 2003).

Eating disorders

Perhaps because of the recent dramatic rise in childhood obesity (see Chapter Eight) somewhat less attention seems to be paid in the current literature to eating disorders such as anorexia nervosa and bulimia nervosa. Eating disorders are also comparatively rare, affecting 0.4% of girls and 0.1% of boys aged 11-15 in the 1999 ONS Survey (Meltzer et al, 2000), although rates are higher for late adolescent girls (Fombonne, 1995b). As with other mental disorders, a distinction can be made between eating *disorders* and eating *disturbances*, such as binge eating, self-induced vomiting and laxative misuse. The latter are significantly more prevalent. For example, a Canadian study found that 13% of 12- to 14-year-old girls and 16% of those aged 15-18 displayed eating attitude scores above the recommended cut-off (Jones et al, 2001).

Risk factors that have been associated with eating disorders include genetic factors, psychological factors such as a tendency towards perfectionism and anxiety in the case of anorexia and family factors such as over-protectiveness. Risk is higher among the higher social classes. Adolescents who have migrated from less industrialised to more industrialised countries appear to be more at risk than those who stay in their country of origin (Fombonne, 1995b), although evidence suggests that risk is also higher in second generation migrants. In Britain, for example, abnormal eating attitudes and behaviours have been found to be higher among Asian schoolgirls, particularly those with Bengali backgrounds (Furnham and Adam-Saib, 2001).

Schizophrenia

Schizophrenia is one of the most chronic and disabling of the mental illnesses. Affecting around 1% of the population, schizophrenia usually manifests in late youth. Early onset (that is, before 25 years of age) tends to be associated with worse symptomatic and social outcomes than onset in later life (Hollis, 2000). Thus, young people living with schizophrenia are more likely to experience educational failure, unemployment, homelessness and unhealthy lifestyles. There is a strong association between schizophrenia and poverty (Koppel and McGuffin, 1999), although the extent to which this reflects social causation or social drift (downward social mobility) has been debated. While Harrison et al (2001) found that subjects whose fathers were in Social Class IV-V, or who were born in deprived areas, were at increased risk of schizophrenia, other studies provide equivocal evidence of a relationship between risk for schizophrenia and socio-economic background. For example, a slight excess risk was found for people from the highest social classes in an Irish study (Mulvany et al, 2001). In a national Danish study, increased risk was associated with parental unemployment and parental lower income, but also with higher education in parents (Byrne et al, 2004). Data from a Swedish cohort born in 1953 also support the drift explanation for social inequalities in the prevalence of schizophrenia, providing some evidence of heightened risk for schizophrenia among the children of higher-status parents (Timms, 1998).

Ethnic differences have been reported in the prevalence of schizophrenia, a disproportionately high number of young African-Caribbean men in Britain receiving this diagnosis. There is debate, however, as to whether these differences are real or result from bias in the diagnosis and management of schizophrenia. The Fourth National Survey (FNS) of Ethnic Minorities, a large representative survey covering white people and the main minority ethnic groups living in Britain in 1993/94, found no evidence to support work based on hospital admissions that first onset schizophrenia is particularly high among young African-Caribbean men. Although treatment rates for psychosis were higher among African-Caribbean men, community prevalence rates were similar to those for white men. These results could themselves be affected by methodological limitations such as non-response. However, they may also suggest that African-Caribbean men are over-represented in psychiatric hospitals due to misdiagnosis, differences in treatment, poor access to general practitioner (GP) services and so on (Nazroo, 1999).

Physical health

In contrast to mental health, evidence of socio-economic variation in physical health has been equivocal. With respect to a number of indicators, the 1995-97 HSE found that differences in physical health were more marked between ethnic groups than social class groups. For example, children of Asian origin were half as likely to report a long-standing illness (Boreham and Prior, 1998). Wheezing and asthma were also less common among minority ethnic children (Primatesta et al, 1998). By contrast, no consistent relationship was found between long-standing illness and socio-economic status and, although prevalence of limiting long-standing illness was higher in the bottom quintile of household income, social class differences were not marked. No clear relationship emerged in the Survey between systolic blood pressure and either social class or household income (McMunn et al, 1998), nor were any significant social class differences observed for wheezing symptoms and doctor-diagnosed asthma, although prevalence was higher among children living in social housing, in a flat and, with the exception of doctor-diagnosed asthma in males, in the lowest household income quintile (Primatesta et al, 1998).

Over time, socio-economic differences in many measures of physical health have become more pronounced. In the 2002 HSE, the prevalence of limiting long-standing illness and long-standing illness was significantly higher in the bottom household income quartile for males and females aged 0-15 and 16-24. The relationship between socio-economic status and respiratory symptoms was more consistent in the 2002 HSE than in the 1995-97 Survey, the prevalence of both wheezing and doctor-diagnosed asthma increasing as household income group decreased, with the exception of doctor-diagnosed asthma among young men (Primatesta, 2003). The latest survey also yielded evidence of social gradients in cardiovascular risk factors among children and young people. Males aged 7-9 and 13-15 and all females, except those aged 20-24 from managerial and professional households, had a significantly lower systolic blood pressure than those in semi-routine and routine households. However, no clear pattern emerged for other indicators of socio-economic status (Falaschetti and Hirani, 2003).

Evidence of health inequalities has also been mixed for other health indicators. A West Midlands Study found that deprivation was associated with increased hospital admission rates for respiratory infection across all age groups (Hawker et al, 2003). An association has also been noted between the prevalence of adult or type II diabetes mellitus in young people and deprivation (Feltbower et al, 2003). By contrast, the prevalence of type I diabetes, which usually starts in childhood or adolescence, does not appear to relate to socio-economic status (Baumer et al, 1998; Connolly et al, 2000). As noted earlier, there is also little evidence to suggest that the risk of cancer in childhood is strongly related to poverty.

Patterns of health during childhood and youth have thus been contrasted with those of early life and adulthood where there is substantial and consistent variation in physical health outcomes by social status. Some researchers suggest that, with the exception of the most severe chronic illness, the transition from childhood to youth is associated with a process of equalisation, class gradients in health status disappearing in youth (West and Sweeting, 2004). This, it is argued, reflects the growing influence of factors outside the family (the school, peer group or youth culture) that reduce the impact of family and neighbourhood influences to equalise social class differences (West, 1997). Evidence of and explanations for the pattern of 'relative equality' have, however, been debated.

First, it should be noted that some, but not all, evidence supports the description of 'relative equality'. Second, some authors propose that young people from lower social classes may be more likely to under-report morbidity (Dennehy et al, 1997, p 50). Finally, demographic differences in disease distribution across the lifecourse may account for the relative weakness of socio-economic gradients in physical health during childhood and youth. Young people enjoy relatively high levels of health. Asthma is the most common chronic disease of childhood and factors that have been implicated in the development of this disease are not strongly associated with social disadvantage (Helms and Christie, 1999). By contrast, the risk factors for the major chronic diseases of late adulthood (heart disease, cancers, type II diabetes) are strongly related to socio-economic status. Equalisation in health in youth may thus be less a reflection of the equalising effects of youth culture than of the way in which health and ill health manifest in this age group. Two observations support this conclusion. First, when the aetiology of a particular disease suggests a role for social causation (as in type II diabetes), strong social variations in prevalence have been observed during youth. Second, although heart disease, cancers and type II diabetes rarely manifest at a young age, exposures that are known to present risks for the development of these diseases are prevalent in young people and, as we discuss in Chapter Eight, these risk factors do vary according to socio-economic status. Thus, with respect to key health behaviours, there is little evidence to suggest that influences such as youth culture are reversing social class differences.

The policy implications

Considerably less attention has been paid to the relationship between poverty and health during childhood and youth than in infancy and adulthood. The evidence in this chapter suggests that the relative neglect of childhood and youth is unfortunate as this is a critical period of the lifecourse at which to target interventions that could have implications for the reduction of health inequalities in both the short and long term. Sadly, the lack of epidemiological research has been accompanied by a lack of service development and evaluation. Thus, as we discuss in Chapter Seven, in some cases policy has failed to target younger age groups. In others, it has focused on either children or young people but has yielded insufficient information to assess the effectiveness of interventions across the age range.

As noted in Chapter Four, research evidence of the kind presented earlier does make it possible to identify key issues, pathways and sources of vulnerability that should be put high on the policy agenda. Accidents/injuries and mental health emerge as the main health issues that are associated with poverty during childhood and youth. Injury is not only the most important cause of child death in the UK. It also has a steeper social class gradient than any other cause of death for this group. A relationship has also been identified between social deprivation and non-fatal injuries on the road and within the home. By contrast, risk of non-traffic-related injury taking place outside the home may decrease with lower socio-economic status. A range of individual, household and neighbourhood factors put children from deprived backgrounds at greater risk, suggesting the need for interventions that operate at a number of levels. Chapter Seven considers the extent to which multilevel programmes have been successfully designed and evaluated; it describes research evidence of what works, for whom and in what context, and identifies key gaps in current research and evaluation findings.

The second area that is characterised by significant health inequality during childhood and youth is mental health. Increases in the rate of psychological disorders among young people and growing concern about the impact of mental health problems on poor educational attainment, limited employment prospects, insecure relationships, early parenting, involvement in crime and adult psychiatric disorders has drawn the spotlight onto mental health problems in childhood and youth. However, as we suggest in Chapter Seven, there has been a preoccupation with symptoms rather than causes, with crime, delinquency and drug use rather than mental health per se. This is unfortunate as evidence suggests that young people suffering from mental health problems are among the most vulnerable in society. The prevalence of the most common disorders in childhood and adolescence are strongly related to social disadvantage, children who have experienced significant adversity in early life being at particularly increased risk (also see Chapter Eight). The presence of a mental health problem in childhood also marks the early stages of difficulties that continue well into adult life. Mental and behavioural disorders can thus be seen as both a product of and a factor for reinforcing social exclusion.

As noted earlier, a range of individual, family and wider environmental influences have been implicated in risk for mental illness, again suggesting the need for a multifaceted approach. Chapter Seven outlines several areas of intervention that address different loci of vulnerability, including individually focused therapy and treatment, family therapy and parenting programmes (also see Chapter Five), school-based interventions and community-based programmes. Despite evidence that suggests that material circumstances and neighbourhood conditions influence the development of mental health problems in children, surprisingly little research has been undertaken to examine the effectiveness of poverty reduction and neighbourhood change on young people's mental health. We note, however, that certain policy developments, notably neighbourhood renewal, may address the role of social and physical context. Neighbourhood renewal policies, together with other area-based initiatives (ABIs) and policies that address the wider influences of health exclusion are considered in Chapter Eleven. As noted in Chapter Four, however, tensions remain between the demand for 'evidence-based policy' that meets stringent evaluation criteria and the growing recognition that the eradication of health inequalities requires both a down- and an upstream focus.

References

Anderson, M. (1999) 'Waiting for harm: deliberate self harm and suicide in young people: a review of the literature', *Journal of Psychiatric and Mental Health Nursing*, vol 6, pp 91-100.

Armstrong, C., Hill, M. and Secker, J. (2000) 'Young people's perceptions of mental health', *Children and Society*, vol 14, pp 60-72.

Backett-Milburn, K., Cunningham-Burley, S. and Davis, J. (2003) 'Contrasting lives, contrasting views? Understanding of health inequalities from children in differing social circumstances', *Social Science and Medicine*, vol 57, pp 613-23.

Baumer, J.H., Hunt, L.P. and Shield, J.P.H. (1998) 'Social disadvantage, family composition, and diabetes mellitus: prevalence and outcome', *Archives of Disease in Childhood*, vol 79, pp 427-30.

Beautrais, A.L. (2000a) 'Methods of youth suicide in New Zealand: trends and implications for prevention', *Australian and New Zealand Journal of Psychiatry*, vol 34, pp 413-19.

Beautrais, A.L. (2000b) 'Risk factors for suicide and attempted suicide among young people', *Australian and New Zealand Journal of Psychiatry*, vol 34, pp 420-36.

Bhugra, D., Desai, M. and Baldwin, D.S. (1999) 'Attempted suicide in West London I: rates across ethnic communities', *Psychological Medicine*, vol 29, pp 1125-30.

Biederman, J. and Faraone, S.V. (2002) 'Current concepts on the neurobiology of Attention-Deficit/Hyperactivity Disorder', *Journal of Attention Disorders*, vol 6, suppl 1, pp S7-16.

Boreham, R. and Prior, G. (1998) 'Self-reported health', in P. Prescott-Clarke and P. Primatesta (eds) *Health Survey for England: The health of young people 1995-1997. Volume 1: Findings*, London: The Stationery Office, pp 33-66.

Botting, B. (1997) 'Mortality in childhood', in F. Drever and M. Whitehead (eds) *Health inequalities: Decennial Supplement*, London: ONS, pp 83-94.

Bourne, J., Bridges, J. and Searle, L. (1994) *Outcast England: How schools exclude black children*, London: Institute of Race Relations.

Bramble, D. (2003) 'Annotation: the use of psychotropic medications in children: a British view', *Journal of Child Psychology and Psychiatry*, vol 44, pp 169-79.

Britton, A. and McPherson, K. (2001) 'Mortality in England and Wales attributable to current alcohol consumption', *Journal of Epidemiology and Community Health*, vol 55, pp 383-8.

Budd, T. (2003) *Alcohol-related assault: Findings from the British Crime Survey*, London: Home Office.

Byrne, M., Agerbo, E., Eaton, W.W. and Mortensen, P.B. (2004) 'Parental socio-economic status and risk of first admission with schizophrenia – a Danish national register based study', *Social Psychiatry and Psychiatric Epidemiology*, vol 39, pp 87-96.

Caldwell, C.H., Kohn-Wood, L.P., Schmeelk-Cone, K.H., Chavous, T.M. and Zimmerman, M.A. (2004) 'Racial discrimination and racial identity as risk or protective factors for violent behaviors in African American young adults', *American Journal of Community Psychology*, vol 33, pp 91-105.

Caprara, G.V. and Rutter, M. (1995) 'Individual development and social change', in M. Rutter and D.J. Smith (eds) *Psychosocial disorders in young people: Time trends and their causes*, Chichester: John Wiley & Sons Ltd, pp 35-66.

CAPT (Child Accident Prevention Trust) (2002a) *Child accident facts: Factsheet*, London: CAPT.

CAPT (2002b) *Home accidents: Factsheet*, London: CAPT.

Caspi, A., Taylor, A., Moffitt, T.E. and Plomin, R. (2000) 'Neighbourhood deprivation affects children's mental health: environmental risks identified in a genetic design', *Psychological Science*, vol 11, pp 338-42.

Casswell, S., Pledger, M. and Hooper, R. (2003) 'Socioeconomic status and drinking patterns in young adults', *Addiction*, vol 98, pp 601-10.

Christensen, P. and Prout, A. (2002) 'Anthropological and sociological perspectives on the study of children', in S. Greene and D. Hogan (eds) *Researching children*, London: Sage Publications.

Christoffersen, M.N., Poulsen, H.S. and Nielsen, A. (2003) 'Attempted suicide among young people: risk factors in a prospective register based study of Danish children born in 1966', *Acta Psychiatrica Scandivica*, vol 108, pp 350-8.

Coles, B. (1995) *Youth and social policy:Youth citizenship and young careers*, London: UCL Press.

Connolly, V., Unwin, N., Sherriff, P., Bilous, R. and Kelly, W. (2000) 'Diabetes prevalence and socioeconomic status: a population based study showing increased prevalence of type 2 diabetes mellitus in deprived areas', *Journal of Epidemiology and Community Health*, vol 54, pp 173-7.

Cooper, J., Appleby, L. and Amos, T. (2002) 'Life events preceding suicide by young people', *Social Psychiatry and Psychiatric Epidemiology*, vol 37, pp 271-5.

Coppock, V. (1997) '"Mad", "bad" or misunderstood?', in P. Scraton (ed) *Childhood in crisis*, London: UCL Press, pp 146-62.

Coupland, C., Hippisley-Cox, J., Kendrick, D., Groom, L., Cross, E. and Savelyich, B. (2003) 'Severe traffic injuries to children, Trent, 1992-7: time-trend analysis', *British Medical Journal*, vol 327, pp 593-4.

Crawford, M.J. and Prince, M. (1999) 'Increasing rates of suicide in young men in England during the 1980s: the importance of social context', *Social Science and Medicine*, vol 49, pp 1419-23.

Crawford, T.N., Cohen, P., Midlarsky, E. and Brook, J.S. (2001) 'Internalizing symptoms in adolescents: gender differences in vulnerability to parental distress and discord', *Journal of Research on Adolescence*, vol 11, pp 95-118.

Dennehy, A., Smith, L. and Harker, P. (1997) *Not to be ignored:Young people, poverty and health*, London: CPAG.

DfT (Department for Transport) (2002) *General review of progress towards the 2010 casualty reduction targets*, London: DfT.

DfT (2003) *Road casualties in Great Britain: Main results 2002. Statistics Bulletin (03)25*, London: DfT.

Diekstra, R. F.W., Kienhorst, C.W.M. and de Wilde, E.J. (1995) 'Suicide and suicidal behaviour among adolescents', in M. Rutter and D.J. Smith (eds) *Psychosocial disorders in young people: Time trends and their causes*, Chichester: John Wiley & Sons Ltd, pp 686-761.

DiGuiseppi, C., Roberts, I. and Speirs, N. (1999) 'Smoke alarm installation and function in Inner London council housing', *Archives of Disease in Childhood*, vol 81, pp 400-3.

Doggett, A.M. (2004) 'ADHS and drug therapy: is it still a valid treatment?', *Journal of Child Health Care*, vol 8, pp 69-81.

Dougherty, G., Pless, I. and Wilkins, R. (1990) 'Social class and the occurrence of traffic injuries and deaths in urban children', *Canadian Journal of Public Health*, vol 81, pp 204-9.

Dowswell, T. and Towner, E. (2002) 'Social deprivation and the prevention of unintentional injury in childhood: a systematic review', *Health Education Research*, vol 17, pp 221-37.

Drukker, M., Kaplan, C., Feron, F. and van Os, J. (2003) 'Children's health-related quality of life, neighbourhood socio-economic deprivation and social capital: a contextual analysis', *Social Science and Medicine*, vol 57, pp 825-41.

Engström, K., Diderichsen, F. and Laflamme, L. (2002) 'Socio-economic differences in injury risks in childhood and adolescence: a nation-wide study of intentional and unintentional injuries in Sweden', *Injury Prevention*, vol 8, pp 137-42.

Falaschetti, E. and Hirani, V. (2003) 'Blood pressure', in K. Sproston and P. Primatesta (eds) *Health Survey for England 2002: The health of children and young people*, London: The Stationery Office.

Farrington, D.P. (1995) 'Teenage antisocial behaviour', in M. Rutter (ed) *Psychological disturbances in young people: Challenges for prevention*, Cambridge: Cambridge University Press, pp 83-130.

Feltbower, R.G., McKinney, P.A., Campbell, F.M., Stephenson, C.R. and Bodansky, H.J. (2003) 'Type 2 and other forms of diabetes in 0-30 year olds: a hospital based study in Leeds, UK', *Archives of Disease in Childhood*, vol 88, pp 676-9.

Fergusson, D.M. and Lynsky, M.T. (1998) 'Conduct problems in childhood and psychosocial outcomes in young adulthood: a prospective study', *Journal of Emotional and Behavioural Disorders*, vol 6, pp 2-18.

Fombonne, E. (1995a) 'Depressive disorders', in M. Rutter and D.J. Smith (eds) *Psychosocial disorders in young people: Time trends and their causes*, Chichester: John Wiley & Sons Ltd, pp 544-615.

Fombonne, E. (1995b) 'Eating disorders', in M. Rutter and D.J. Smith (eds) *Psychosocial disorders in young people: Time trends and their causes*, Chichester: John Wiley & Sons Ltd, pp 616-85.

Freeman, H.L. and Stansfeld, S.A. (1998) 'Psychosocial effects of urban environments, noise and crowding', in A. Lundberg (ed) *The environment and mental health: A guide for clinicians*, Mahwah, NJ: Lawrence Erlbaum Associates, pp 147-73.

Furlong, A. and Cartmel, F. (1997) *Young people and social change: Individualisation and risk in late modernity*, Buckingham: Open University Press.

Furnham, A. and Adam-Saib, S. (2001) 'Abnormal eating attitudes and behaviours and perceived parental control: a study of white British and British–Asian school girls', *Social Psychiatry and Psychiatric Epidemiology*, vol 36, pp 462-70.

Graham, H. and Power, C. (2004) *Childhood disadvantage and adult health: A lifecourse framework*, London: Health Development Agency.

Gunnell, D., Lopatazidis, A., Dorling, D., Wehner, H., Southall, H. and Frankel, S. (1999) 'Suicide and unemployment in young people – analysis of trends in England and Wales, 1921-95', *British Journal of Psychiatry*, vol 175, pp 263-70.

Haarasilta, L., Marttunen, M., Kaprio, J. and Aro, H. (2001) 'The 12-month prevalence and characteristics of major depressive episode in a representative nationwide sample of adolescents and young adults', *Psychological Medicine*, 31, pp 1169-79.

Harrison, L. and Gardiner, E. (1999) 'Do the rich really die young? Alcohol-related mortality and social class in Great Britain, 1988-94', *Addiction*, vol 94, pp 1871-80.

Harrison, G., Gunnell, D., Glazebrook, C., Page, K. and Kwiecinski, R. (2001) 'Association between schizophrenia and social inequality at birth: case–control study', *British Journal of Psychiatry*, vol 179, pp 346-50.

Hawker, J.I., Olowokure, B., Sufi, F., Weinberg, J., Gill, N. and Wilson, R.C. (2003) 'Social deprivation and hospital admission for respiratory infection: an ecological study', *Respiratory Medicine*, vol 97, pp 1219-24.

Hawton, K., Houston, K. and Shepperd, R. (1999) 'Suicide in young people: study of 174 cases aged under 25 years based on coroners' and medical records', *British Journal of Psychiatry*, vol 175, pp 271-6.

Hawton, K., Fagg, J., Simkin, S., Bale, E. and Bond, A. (2000) 'Deliberate self-harm in adolescents in Oxford, 1985-95', *Journal of Adolescence*, vol 23, pp 47-55.

Hawton, K., Harriss, L., Simkin, S., Bale, E. and Bond, A. (2001) 'Social class and suicidal behaviour: the associations between social class and the characteristics of deliberate self-harm patients and the treatment they are offered', *Social Psychiatry and Psychiatric Epidemiology*, vol 36, pp 437-43.

Healey, A., Knapp, M. and Farrington, D.P. (2004) 'Adult labour market implications of antisocial behaviour in childhood and adolescence: findings from a UK longitudinal study', *Applied Economics*, vol 36, pp 93-105.

Helms, P.J. and Christie, G. (1999) 'Prospects for preventing asthma', *Archives of Disease in Childhood*, vol 80, pp 401-5.

Hertzman, C., Power, C., Matthews, S. and Manor, O. (2001) 'Using an interactive framework of society and lifecourse to explain self-related health in early adulthood', *Social Science and Medicine*, vol 53, no 12, pp 1575-85.

Hill, J. (2002) 'Biological, psychological and social processes in the conduct disorders', *Journal of Child Psychology and Psychiatry*, vol 43, pp 133-64.

Hippisley-Cox, J., Groom, L., Kendrick, D., Coupland, C., Webber, E. and Savelyich, B. (2002) 'Cross sectional survey of socioeconomic variation in severity and mechanism of childhood injuries in Trent, 1992-7', *British Medical Journal*, vol 324, pp 1132-4.

Hjern, A. and Bremberg, S. (2002) 'Social aetiology of violent deaths in Swedish children and youth', *Journal of Epidemiology and Community Health*, vol 56, pp 688-92.

Hollis, C. (2000) 'Adult outcomes of child- and adolescent-onset schizophrenia: diagnostic stability and predictive validity', *American Journal of Psychiatry*, vol 157, pp 1652-9.

Ireland, L. and Holloway, I. (1996) 'Qualitative health research with children', *Children and Society*, vol 10, pp 155-64.

Jensen, P.S., Kettle, L., Roper, M.T., Sloan, M.T., Dulcan, M.K., Hoven, C., Bird, H.R., Bauermeister, J.J. and Payne, J.D. (1999) 'Are stimulants overprescribed? Treatment of ADHD in four US communities', *Journal of American Academy of Child and Adolescent Psychiatry*, vol 38, pp 797-804.

Jones, J.M., Bennett, S., Olmsted, M.P., Lawson, M.L. and Rodin, G. (2001) 'Disordered eating attitudes and behaviours in teenaged girls: a school-based study', *Canadian Medical Association Journal*, vol 165, pp 547-52.

Judge, K. and Benzeval, M. (1993) 'Health inequalities: new concerns about the children of single mothers', *British Medical Journal*, vol 306, pp 677-80.

Karvonen, S., West, P., Sweeting, H., Rahkonen, O. and Young, R. (2001) 'Lifestyle, social class and health-related behaviour: a cross-cultural comparison of 15 year olds in Glasgow and Helsinki', *Journal of Youth Studies*, vol 4, pp 393-413.

Kessler, R.C. and Walters, E.E. (1998) 'Epidemiology of DSM-III-R major depression and minor depression among adolescents and young adults in the National Comorbidity Survey', *Depression and Anxiety*, vol 7, pp 3-14.

Koppel, S. and McGuffin, P. (1999) 'Socio-economic factors that predict psychiatric admissions at a local level', *Psychological Medicine*, vol 29, pp 1235-41.

Kutchins, H. and Kirk, S.A (1997) *Making us crazy: DSM – The psychiatric bible and the creation of mental disorders*, London: Constable.

Lader, D., Singleton, N. and Meltzer, H. (2000) *Psychiatric morbidity among young offenders in England and Wales*, London: ONS.

Laflamme, L. and Engström, K. (2002) 'Socioeconomic differences in Swedish children and adolescents injured in road traffic accidents: cross-sectional study', *British Medical Journal*, vol 324, pp 396-7.

Laing, G. and Logan, S. (1999) 'Patterns of unintentional injury in childhood and their relation to socio-economic factors', *Public Health*, vol 113, pp 291-4.

Lalloo, R., Sheiham, A. and Nazroo, J.Y. (2003) 'Behavioural characteristics and accidents: findings from the Health Survey for England, 1997', *Accident Analysis and Prevention*, vol 35, pp 661-7.

Leventhal, T. and Brooks-Gunn, J. (2000) 'The neighborhoods they live in: the effects of neighborhood residence on child and adolescent outcomes', *Psychological Bulletin*, vol 126, pp 309-37.

Linnet, K.M., Dalsgaard, S., Obel, C., Wisborg, K., Henriksen, T.B., Rodriguez, A., Kotimaa, A., Moilanen, I., Thomsen, P.H., Olsen, J. and Jarvelin, M.R. (2003) 'Maternal lifestyle factors in pregnancy risk of attention deficit hyperactivity disorder and associated behaviors: review of the current evidence', *American Journal of Psychiatry*, vol 160, pp 1028-40.

London Development Agency (2004) *Rampton revisited: The educational experiences and achievements of black boys in London schools*, London: London Development Agency Education Commission.

Lynsky, M., Degenhardt, L. and Hall, W. (2000) 'Cohort trends in youth suicide in Australia, 1964-1997', *Australian and New Zealand Journal of Psychiatry*, vol 34, pp 408-12.

Lyons, R.A., Jones, S.J., Deacon, T. and Heaven, M. (2003) 'Socioeconomic variation in injury in children and older people: a population study', *Injury Prevention*, vol 9, pp 33-7.

Lyons, R.A., Delahunty, A.M., Heaven, M., McCabe, M., Allen, H. and Nash, P. (2000) 'Incidence of childhood fractures in affluent and deprived areas', *British Medical Journal*, vol 320, p 149.

McCarron, P., Gunnell, D., Harrison, G.L., Okasha, M. and Davey Smith, G. (2003) 'Temperament in young adulthood and later mortality: prospective observational study', *Journal of Epidemiology and Community Health*, vol 57, pp 888-92.

MacGibbon, B. (1999) 'Inequalities in health related to transport', in D. Gordon, M. Shaw, D. Dorling and G. Davey Smith (eds) *Inequalities in health: The evidence presented to the Independent Inquiry into Inequalities in Health, chaired by Sir Donald Acheson*, Bristol: The Policy Press, pp 185-96.

Macmillan, R., McMorris, B.J. and Kruttschnitt, C. (2004) 'Linked lives: stability and change in maternal circumstances and trajectories of antisocial behaviour in children', *Child Development*, vol 75, pp 205-20.

McMunn, A., Primatesta, P. and Bost, L. (1998) 'Blood pressure', in P. Prescott-Clarke and P. Primatesta (1998) *Health Survey for England: The health of young people 1995-1997. Volume 1: Findings*, London: The Stationery Office, pp 109-50.

Madge, N. and Harvey, J.G. (1999) 'Suicide among the young – the size of the problem', *Journal of Adolescence*, vol 22, pp 145-55.

Mash, E.J. and Wolfe, D.A. (2002) *Abnormal child psychology* (2nd edn), Belmont, CA: Wadsworth.

Maughan, B., Brock, A. and Ladva, G. (2004a) 'Mental health', in ONS, *The health of children and young people*, London: ONS.

Maughan, B., Rowe, R., Messer, J., Goodman, R. and Meltzer, H. (2004b) 'Conduct disorder and oppositional defiant disorder in a national sample: developmental epidemiology', *Journal of Child Psychology and Psychiatry*, vol 45, pp 609-21.

Maynard, M., Gunnell, D., Emmett, P., Frankel, S. and Davey Smith, G. (2003) 'Fruit, vegetables, and antioxidants in childhood and risk of adult cancer: the Boyd Orr cohort', *Journal of Epidemiology and Community Health*, vol 57, no 3, pp 218-25.

Meltzer, H., Gatward, R., Goodman, R. and Ford, T. (2000) *The mental health of children and adolescents in Great Britain*, London: The Stationery Office.

Micklewright, J. (2002) *Social exclusion and children: A European view for a US debate*, CASE Paper 51, London: Centre for Analysis of Social Exclusion, London School of Economics and Political Science.

Miles, S. (2000) *Youth lifestyles in a changing world*, Buckingham: Open University Press.

Montgomery, S.M., Cook, D.G., Bartley, M.J. and Wadsworth, M.E.J. (1998) 'Unemployment, cigarette smoking, alcohol consumption and body weight in young British men', *European Journal of Public Health*, vol 8, pp 21-7.

Morrison, A., Stone, D.H., Redpath, A., Campbell, H. and Norrie, J. (1999) 'Trend analysis of socioeconomic differentials in deaths from injury in childhood in Scotland, 1981-95', *British Medical Journal*, vol 318, pp 567-8.

Morrow, V. (2001) 'Using qualitative methods to elicit young people's perspectives on their environments: some ideas for community health initiatives', *Health Education Research*, vol 16, pp 255-68.

Mulvany, F., O'Callaghan, E., Takei, N., Byrne, M., Fearon, P. and Larkin, C. (2001) 'Effect of social class at birth on risk and presentation of schizophrenia: case-control study', *British Medical Journal*, vol 323, pp 1398-401.

Nasman, E. (1994) 'Individualisation and institutionalisation of children', in J. Qvortup, M. Bardy, G. Sgritta and H. Wintersberger (eds) *Childhood matters: Social theory, practice and politics*, Aldershot: Avebury.

Nazroo, J. (1999) *Ethnicity and mental health: Findings from a national community survey*, London: Policy Studies Institute.

Nigg, J.T. and Hinshaw, S.P. (1998) 'Parent personality traits and psychopathology associated with antisocial behaviours in childhood Attention-Deficit Hyperactivity Disorder', *Journal of Child Psychology and Psychiatry and Allied Disciplines*, vol 39, pp 145-59.

Norris, C. and Lloyd, G. (2000) 'Parents, professionals and ADHD: what the papers say', *European Journal of Special Needs Education*, vol 15, pp 123-37.

PACTS (Parliamentary Advisory Council for Transport Safety) (2003) *PACTS Briefing Paper: Drinking and driving*, London: PACTS.

Patel, N. and Fatimilehin, I.A. (1999) 'Racism and mental health', in C. Newnes, G. Holmes and C. Dunn (eds) *This is madness: A critical look at psychiatry and the future of mental health services*, Ross-on-Wye: PCCS Books, pp 51-73.

Pickett, W., Garner, M.J., Boyce, W.F. and King, M.A. (2002) 'Gradients in risk for youth injury associated with multiple-risk behaviours: a study of 11,329 Canadian adolescents', *Social Science and Medicine*, vol 55, pp 1055-68.

Power, C. and Matthews, S. (1997) 'Origin of health inequalities in a national population sample', *Lancet*, vol 350, pp 1584-9.

Prescott-Clarke, P. and Primatesta, P. (eds) (1998) *Health Survey for England: The health of young people 1995-1997. Volume 2: Methodology and documentation*, London: The Stationery Office.

Primatesta, P. (2003) 'Respiratory health', in K. Sproston and P. Primatesta (eds) *Health Survey for England 2002: The health of children and young people*, London: The Stationery Office.

Primatesta, P., Bost, L. and McMunn, A. (1998) 'Respiratory symptoms and lung function', in P. Prescott-Clarke and P. Primatesta (eds) *Health Survey for England: The health of young people 1995-1997. Volume 1: Findings*, London: The Stationery Office, pp 151-90.

Prout, A. and Hallett, C. (2003) 'Introduction', in C. Hallett and A. Prout (eds) *Hearing the voices of children: Social policy for a new century*, London: RoutledgeFalmer.

Raat, H., Bonsel, G.J., Essink Bot, M.L., Landgraf, J.M. and Gemke, R.J. (2002) 'Reliability and validity of comprehensive health status measures in children: the Child Health Questionnaire in relation to the Health Utilities Index', *Journal of Clinical Epidemiology*, vol 55, pp 67-76.

Richardson, A. and Budd, T. (2003) 'Young adults, alcohol, crime and disorder', *Criminal Behaviour and Mental Health*, vol 13, pp 5-16.

Roberts, H., Smith, S. and Bryce, C. (1993) 'Prevention is better ...', *Sociology of Health and Illness*, vol 15, pp 447-63.

Roberts, I. and Pless, B. (1996) 'Social policy as a cause of childhood accidents: the children of lone mothers', *British Medical Journal*, vol 306, pp 1737-9.

Roberts, I. and Power, C. (1996) 'Does the decline in child injury mortality vary by social class? A comparison of class specific mortality in 1981 and 1991', *British Medical Journal*, vol 313, pp 784-6.

Rutter, M. (1995) 'Causal concepts and their testing', in M. Rutter and D.J. Smith (eds) *Psychosocial disorders in young people: Time trends and their causes*, Chichester: John Wiley & Sons Ltd, pp 7-34.

Rutter, M. (1999) 'Resilience concepts and findings: implications for family therapy', *Journal of Family Therapy*, vol 21, pp 119-44.

Rutter, M. and Smith, D.J. (1995) 'Time trends in psychosocial disorders in youth', in M. Rutter and D.J. Smith (eds) *Psychosocial disorders in young people: Time trends and their causes*, Chichester: John Wiley & Sons Ltd, pp 763-81.

Sauvola, A., Rasanen, P.K., Joukamaa, M.I., Jokelainen, J., Jarvelin, M.R. and Isohanni, M.K. (2001) 'Mortality of young adults in relation to single-parent family background – a prospective study of the Northern Finland 1966 birth cohort', *European Journal of Public Health*, vol 11, no 3, pp 284-6.

Sava, F. (2000) 'Is Attention Deficit/Hyperactivity Disorder an exonerating construct? Strategies for school inclusion', *European Journal of Special Needs Education*, vol 15, pp 149-57.

Schneiders, J., Drukker, M., van der Ende, J., Verhulst, F.C., van Os, J. and Nicolson, N.A. (2003) 'Neighbourhood socioeconomic disadvantage and behavioural problems from late childhood into early adolescence', *Journal of Epidemiology and Community Health*, vol 57, pp 699-703.

Simonoff, E., McGuffin, P. and Gottesman, I.I. (1994) 'Genetic influences on normal and abnormal development', in M. Rutter, E. Taylor and L. Hersov (eds) *Child and adolescent psychiatry* (3rd edn), Oxford: Blackwell Science, pp 129-51.

Simonoff, E., Elander, J., Holmshaw, J., Pickles, A., Murray, R. and Rutter, M. (2004) 'Predictors of antisocial personality – continuities from childhood to adult life', *British Journal of Psychiatry*, vol 184, pp 118-27.

Smith, A.S. and Farrington, D.P. (2004) 'Continuities in antisocial behavior and parenting across three generations', *Journal of Child Psychology and Psychiatry*, vol 45, pp 230-47.

Smith, D.J. (1995) 'Youth crime and conduct disorders', in M. Rutter and D.J. Smith (eds) *Psychosocial disorders in young people: Time trends and their causes*, Chichester: John Wiley & Sons Ltd, pp 389-489.

Smith, E.P., Walker, K., Fields, L., Brookins, C.C. and Seay, R.C. (1999) 'Ethnic identity and its relationship to self-esteem, perceived efficacy and prosocial attitudes in early adolescence', *Journal of Adolescence*, vol 22, pp 867-80.

Sproston, K. and Primatesta, P. (eds) (2003) *Health Survey for England 2002: The health of children and young people*, London: The Stationery Office.

Stanistreet, D. and Jeffrey, V. (2003) 'Injury and poisoning mortality among young men: are there any common factors amenable to prevention?', *Crisis*, vol 24, pp 122-7.

Starfield, B., Riley, A.W., Witt, W.P. and Robertson, J. (2002) 'Social class gradients in health during adolescence', *Journal of Epidemiology and Community Health*, vol 56, pp 354-61.

Stevenson, M., Jamrozik, K. and Spittle, J. (1995) 'A case-control study of traffic risk factors and child pedestrian injury', *International Journal of Epidemiology*, vol 24, pp 959-64.

Stiller, C., Quinn, M. and Rowan, S. (2004) 'Childhood cancer', in ONS, *The health of children and young people*, London: ONS.

Sweeting, H. and West, P. (1998) 'Health and age 11: reports from schoolchildren and their parents', *Archives of Disease in Childhood*, vol 78, pp 427-34.

Sweeting, H. and West, P. (2003) 'Fifteen, female and stressed: changing patterns of psychological distress over time', *Journal of Child Psychology and Psychiatry*, vol 44, pp 399-411.

Thapar, A., Fowler, T., Rice, F., Scourfield, J., van den Bree, M., Thomas, H., Harold, G. and Hay, D. (2003) 'Maternal smoking during pregnancy and Attention Deficit Hyperactivity Disorder symptoms in offspring', *American Journal of Psychiatry*, vol 160, pp 1985-9.

Timms, D. (1998) 'Gender, social mobility and psychiatric diagnoses', *Social Science and Medicine*, vol 46, pp 1235-47.

Tomlinson, S. (2005) 'Race, ethnicity and education under New Labour', *Oxford Review of Education*, vol 31, pp 153-71.

Towner, E., Jarvis, S., Walsh, S. and Aynsley-Green, A. (1994) 'Measuring exposure to injury risk in schoolchildren aged 11-14', *British Medical Journal*, vol 308, pp 449-52.

Wallace, S.A., Crown, J.M., Cox, A.D. and Berger, M. (1997) *Child and adolescent mental health*, Oxford: Radcliffe Medical Press.

Webb, L. (2002) 'Deliberate self harm in adolescence: a systematic review of psychological and psychosocial factors', *Journal of Advanced Nursing*, vol 38, pp 235-44.

West, P. (1988) 'Inequalities? Social class differentials in health in British youth', *Social Science and Medicine*, vol 27, pp 391-6.

West, P. (1997) 'Health inequalities in the early years: is there equalisation in youth?', *Social Science and Medicine*, vol 44, pp 833-58.

West, P. (1999) 'Youth', in D. Gordon, M. Shaw, D. Dorling and G. Davey Smith (eds) *Inequalities in health: The evidence presented to the Independent Inquiry into Inequalities in Health, chaired by Sir Donald Acheson*, Bristol: The Policy Press, pp 12-22.

West, P. and Sweeting, H. (2004) 'Evidence of equalisation in health in youth from the West of Scotland', *Social Science and Medicine*, vol 59, pp 13-27.

West, P., Sweeting, H. and Speed, E. (2001) 'We really do know what you do: a comparison of reports from 11 year olds and their parents in respect of parental economic activity and occupation', *Sociology*, vol 35, pp 539-59.

Williams, J.M., Currie, C.E., Wright, P., Elton, R.A. and Beattie, T.F. (1997) 'Socio-economic status and adolescent injuries', *Social Science and Medicine*, vol 44, pp 1881-91.

Willoughby, M. (2003) 'Developmental course of ADHD symptomatology during the transition from childhood to adolescence: a review with recommendations', *Journal of Child Psychology and Psychiatry*, vol 44, pp 88-106.

Wittchen, H.U., Nelson, C.B. and Lachner, G. (1998) 'Prevalence of mental disorders and psychosocial impairments in adolescents and young adults', *Psychological Medicine*, vol 28, pp 109-26.

Zito, J.M., Safer, D.J., dosReis, S., Gardner, J.F., Boles, M. and Lynch, F. (2000) 'Trends in the prescribing of psychotropic medications to preschoolers', *Journal of the American Medical Association*, vol 283, pp 1025-30.

SEVEN

Health inequalities during childhood and youth: policy and practice

Introduction

There is a paradox, as Chapter Six has shown, between the relative clinical invisibility of young people and high levels of social concern. Youth, allied with drugs, crime and antisocial behaviour, has arguably dominated domestic home affairs in the UK in the 1990s (Parker et al, 1998), with much of the response and the advocacy coming from the margins of health and welfare rather than mainstream medicine. This chapter, although focusing on the two main sources of inequalities in mortality and morbidity for children and young people, that is accidents and mental health, is also located firmly in the arena of health behaviour for it is delinquency, rather than the problems of conduct disorder that often lie at its heart, that has attracted the political profile and hence research attention. Given that delinquency itself is then but part of a larger spectrum of antisocial behaviour, including substance misuse and sexual promiscuity, the links to Chapters Eight and Nine are manifold.

The organisational difficulties consequent on interventions in early life were outlined in Chapter Five. Here, the challenge of assessing what works, for whom and in what circumstances is made yet harder by the age range encompassed. Traditional notions of bounded youth have, as Chapter Six has stressed, been challenged by the increasing delay before the vast majority of adolescents achieve financial and domestic independence. There is thus an extended period post-adolescence where one can no longer assume the existence of adult responsibilities. Arguably this may have some advantages in that the window for tackling childhood disadvantage may widen but chronological age becomes a less reliable guide to policy (Graham and Power, 2004) and, as we noted in Chapter Six, even this extension of childhood is differentiated by class.

Typically, intervention and policy do not accord equal emphasis across the 20 years of childhood and youth. Those focusing on accidents and injuries, together with nutrition, tend to place more emphasis on childhood, while those that focus on mental health, substance misuse and sexual health tend to place more stress on early youth. Few initiatives take late youth as their focus. Indeed, the lack of appropriate services for children in areas such as mental health has long been a cause for concern without the added complication that young people in late adolescence and beyond might also require a differentiated approach. It is to this uneven typology of evidence, policy and practice that we now turn.

Accidents

As Chapter Six has shown, injury is not only the most important cause of child death in the UK, but also has a steeper social class gradient than any other cause of death for this cohort. A child from the lowest social class is, for example, nine times more likely to die in a house fire than a child from a well-off home (Roberts, 2002). Safety inside the home is of paramount importance in early life with a large proportion of these injuries being potentially preventable. The wider horizons of older children, however, place the environment, play and being safe from traffic close to the top of their agendas (Roberts, 2002). Indeed, as Chapter Six has noted, the road environment is a key locus of risk in different guises across the age spectrum, accounting for two fifths of deaths among young people aged 15-24 in the category injuries and poisoning. The contribution of substance misuse to such deaths and injuries means one part of the preventative jigsaw for young people lies under that heading and is considered further in Chapter Nine, while the increasing significance of suicide and purposeful injury with age means another important literature is included under the review of mental health.

What works? Evidence and practice

Much of the literature focuses on accident prevention for the early years. Nearly half (48%) of the health promotion interventions included in Towner et al's (2001) systematic review, for example, were aimed at those aged four and under, with half targeting the youngest group of children covered by this chapter, those aged five to nine. Only just over one third included interventions aimed at the 10- to 14-year-old age group and most of these focused on the pre-teenage years. The majority of the studies, reflecting the significance of transport accidents, also focus on the road environment, only 5%, for example, encompassing the field of leisure or sport.

Unusually, within the compass of this book, there is evidence that single issue campaigns can be effective, particularly those focusing on safety equipment such as child-resistant packaging and smoke detectors. There is also a stronger emphasis than in most of the areas reviewed on the potential for environmental modification, ranging from alterations to the road system to physical barriers to injury such as window bars, cycle helmets and mouth guards. It is also notable, however, that, as in other policy fields, multimodal interventions, incorporating, for example, legislation, education, safety equipment and environmental modification, are the most likely to yield positive results. It follows that there is a movement, albeit tentative, away from reliance on individual/behavioural approaches to one that admits the need to change the culture of organisations or communities.

Road accidents involving children are more scattered than those involving adults, with an obvious relationship to the roads near home. There is now good evidence that area-wide engineering schemes and traffic calming measures, that is, schemes which reduce traffic and traffic speeds in residential areas, reduce accidents for this age group, decreasing traffic injuries on average by between 11% and 15% (Bunn et al, 2003; Liabo and Curtis, 2003). Much of this dates back to research begun in the 1980s by the Transport and Road Research Laboratory, which piloted a series of urban safety measures in five areas of high risk from road traffic accidents. This included an increase in the number of roundabouts, the banning of right turns and the provision of central refuges (Towner et al, 1993). Two key advantages are relatively low costs and interventions that, while focusing particularly on the most vulnerable, are effective for all ages. The introduction of 20mph speed limits was found, for example, to reduce injuries to child pedestrians by 70%, with those to cyclists reducing by nearly one half (Towner and Ward, 1998).

Significantly, such schemes also have the (often unmeasured) potential to increase cycling and walking at the neighbourhood level, together with the potential for children to play outdoors, with concomitant benefits for both health and the environment (Liabo and Curtis, 2003; Morrison et al, 2004). Research in Hertfordshire, for example, suggested not only that school children aged 10-13 burned up more calories walking to and from school than during weekly Physical Education (PE) lessons but also that letting children go out to play is "one of the best things that parents can do for their children's health", whereas structured leisure activities tend to be car borne (Mackett, 2004). Neighbourhood interventions also have greater capacity for addressing inequalities than traffic education, which tends to be disproportionately taken up by the middle classes (Liabo et al, 2003).

For cyclists there is some evidence that cycle training can improve safe riding behaviour and good evidence that cycle helmets offer protection from head and brain injuries, particularly at lower speeds (Towner and Ward, 1998). Educational campaigns to encourage the wearing of cycle helmets (primarily school-based) can then increase their use, most particularly among younger children and girls (Towner et al, 2001), while family encouragement and peer behaviour may also be important (Kendrick and Royal, 2003). Studies that followed the introduction of cycle helmet legislation for both adults and children in the Australian state of Victoria in 1990 stressed the significance of context, with the intervention building on 10 years of educational campaigns, together with helmet discounts and the support of the mass media. This had a positive influence on both the use of helmets and the incidence of injuries. However, it was also noted that there was a 10% reduction in child cyclists following the legislation and a 46% reduction in teenage cyclists, not only reducing the improvement attributable to helmets but also having the negative side-effect of apparently discouraging cycling among older children. A further inequalities dimension may be introduced by lower levels of helmet ownership in deprived areas (Kendrick and Royal, 2003). Further research is also required around motorcycle training schemes, the visibility of motorcyclists and motorcycles and the influence of engine size (Coleman et al, 1996).

The leisure environment, like roads, is similarly in the public domain and hence a legitimate target for legislation and intervention. Indeed, one review suggested that the costs of exercise to the health system might outweigh the benefits when the cost of injuries was taken into account (Nicholl et al, 1994, cited in NHS CRD, 1996). It has, however, been the subject of only limited evaluation (the effectiveness, for example, of beach guards, swimming lessons and protective equipment or rule changes) combined with limited surveillance of the distribution of injuries. For young children there is evidence that improvements to playground design, including the height of play equipment and the provision of specialised surface treatments can reduce both the frequency and severity of injuries (Towner and Ward, 1998). For adolescents there is similar support for environmental engineering changes to the sports environment and prophylactic injury prevention programmes. Legislation also appears effective for 15- to 24-year-olds whether in sports, road or workplace settings (Coleman et al, 1996), where, for example, the agricultural environment continues to be a source of considerable risk.

The home is less amenable than these environments to regulation. Fires, for example, are the second most important cause of injury to children under 15 after pedestrian injuries on the road, with smokers' houses posing a particular risk. Smokers' materials have been estimated to contribute to 35% of deaths and 20% of non-fatal injuries. The use of smoke detectors (as opposed to smoking cessation programmes) is well supported by research, particularly if high-risk households are targeted by means of home visits, education and the free distribution of safety devices (NHS CRD, 1996). Uptake is also amenable to counselling as part of primary care child health surveillance. Issues of installation, positioning and maintenance, however, often remain problematic and a recent systematic review points to the lack of evaluation looking beyond ownership and functioning to reduction in injury (DiGuiseppi and Higgins, 2001). The use of child-resistant containers is also well evidenced, as to a lesser degree are window bars and the design of domestic products (such as short kettle leads), but other interventions in the home environment often have limited proven impact on the requirement for medical attention, not least because of the inability of many studies to demonstrate small effects (Lyons et al, 2004).

One contributory factor, as Chapter Six signalled, is likely to be the significance of deprivation. Lucas (2003) draws on two systematic reviews (Roberts et al, 1996; Elkan et al, 2000) to suggest that home visiting (targeted in most instances at the wider welfare of those aged under two) can substantially reduce rates of accidental injury, particularly in families at high risk, such as those living in areas of deprivation, poor housing or from large families. As with similar reviews of parenting programmes, the large body of evidence is, however, based on North American experience and reduction in rates of injury tends to be one of many possible outcomes of a larger home visiting programme. Moreover, none of the reviews were able to establish what components of the home visiting programme were effective in reducing childhood injury in the home. Nevertheless, results such as those achieved by the Newcastle Play it Safe campaign and the suggestion that home visiting can be effective against both accidental and non-accidental injury point to the need for further research into the role of social support in preventing childhood injury (Towner and Ward, 1998).

Educational programmes alone appear to have little effect, irrespective of the form they take (including skills training, mass media exposure and targeted education courses) or the focus (such as a road safety programme for children, or parental awareness of the risks from drowning in the home). Box 7.1, however, provides an example of a controlled study that did demonstrate positive outcomes for both road safety and community empowerment. Research linking problem behaviour and accidents suggests measures targeted at high-risk children need to move beyond knowledge and skills to challenge the attitudes and habits that underlie many risky behaviours (West et al, 1998).

Box 7.1: Road safety training – the example of Drumchapel

In 1993 the Drumchapel area of Glasgow, then an area of high unemployment with low-rise rented housing, limited garden space, narrow roads and parking on the pavements, recorded a pedestrian casualty rate for five- to nine-year-olds six times the national average. Children aged 10-14 fared little better. A series of practical road safety training sessions for young children was therefore introduced at the request of the local community. This involved over 100 local parent volunteers receiving training in order that they in turn could train small groups of five- to seven-year-olds at the roadside.

Over 750 children from 10 local schools were specifically taught how to cross safely at parked vehicles and intersections and how to identify dangerous roadside locations, constructing safe routes to avoid them. This information was delivered in four to six weekly training sessions near the children's schools, each lasting 25-30 minutes. Before and after tests and comparison with a matched sample of control children found the judgement and behaviour of intervention children to have improved in all three skills areas, with the improvement maintained at two months. They also found intervention children to have a better conceptual understanding that they could apply to novel traffic situations. The skills levels of the control group were assessed to be several years behind. The study also stressed the improved contact between schools and the community that followed from parental involvement and the positive effect on community morale associated with local action (Thomson and Whelan, 1997).

Community programmes that involve local participation and use a broad range of interventions including education have the potential to reduce childhood injuries from a wide variety of causes and to develop a culture of safety. Conclusive proof of a positive and sustained impact on injury rates is, however, difficult to demonstrate conclusively (Towner and Dowswell, 2002). Many are based on the World Health Organization (WHO) safer community model, which was developed in Sweden in the 1980s and was founded on a mix of environmental and behavioural solutions, the involvement of a range of organisations, local ownership from the community, the availability of child safety products and the development of a long-term strategy based on accurate local surveillance systems (Towner et al, 2001). This reportedly resulted in a reduction in home-based accidents by 27% and a reduction in occupation accidents by 28%, suggesting that the promotion of safety measures in many settings simultaneously could be effective across the age spectrum, with multifactorial approaches offering more scope to modify behaviour (NHS CRD, 1996).

A similar study in New Zealand (see Box 7.2) suggests there is, however, a danger of interventions becoming too diffuse. Indeed, two further applications

Box 7.2: Community injury prevention – the Waitakere project

Waitakere is the sixth largest city in New Zealand with a multicultural population of 155,000. Between 1995 and 1997 it was the site of a community-based injury prevention pilot based on the WHO model. This established seven priority areas for intervention including the Maori and Pacific population, children, young people, alcohol and road accidents. It also established three intervention strategies: promotion; education and training; and advocacy and action for hazard reduction and environmental change. Project coordinators were appointed because of their community development experience and knowledge of appropriate cultural processes rather than their knowledge of injury prevention.

Evaluation established that, irrespective of the range of intervention areas, the primary focus throughout the implementation phases was child safety. This proved effective. Comparisons between Waitakere and a matched population of 147,000 revealed statistically significant reductions in child injury hospitalisations. It also revealed significantly higher levels of awareness of injury prevention safety messages and the acquisition of child safety items such as stair gates, fireguards, car restraints and protective sports equipment. Wider benefits were ascribed to embedding the project in local government. This resulted in better links with the local community and a corresponding increase in trust. It also raised the profile of injury prevention within an organisation that held a key role in influencing community safety structures and issues. The evaluation did, however, suggest that the whole range of injury prevention issues could not necessarily be effectively covered and the positive results in the child priority area indicated the merits of targeting the intervention (Coggan et al, 2000).

of the WHO model focusing on unintentional childhood injury in small communities suggest success, if measured only by a meaningful reduction in injury levels, will be elusive. This reflects the difficulties of developing appropriate injury surveillance systems (given the comparative rarity of death and serious injury) and the cost and difficulty of establishing local monitoring systems (Simpson et al, 2003). Instead, they highlight the importance of the model in developing community capacity and raising awareness, which, in turn, can prompt the political and environmental changes needed to reduce the risk of injury.

It is also important to note that legal and environmental change are often based on change in the climate of opinion resulting from educational campaigns, shaping culture and creating the imperative for government to act (Towner et al, 1993), changes to the drink driving laws, and the introduction of motorcycle helmets, for example. Education for professionals and policy makers also needs to be considered alongside that aimed at children and their parents.

Limitations to the evidence base

The evidence base for injuries and accidents is again dominated by North American literature. Only 17% of the interventions included in Towner et al's 2001 review, for example, were based in the UK. The authors also found that too few details were often given on either intervention or evaluation to establish exactly what works for whom, in what context. They also identified a need for good-quality measures of non-fatal injury (rather than a continued reliance on measures such as hospital admissions as a proxy) and gaps in the research findings including a paucity of information on older children and adolescents and interventions in the leisure/sports environment.

Perhaps the most significant deficit, given the pronounced socio-economic gradient outlined in Chapter Six, is the lack of information and focus on deprived areas and deprived groups (Towner et al, 2005). There is a lack of consideration of the differential impact of car restraints or the effect of introducing cycle paths in deprived areas, for example (Millward et al, 2003). Dowswell and Towner (2002) reviewed the world literature on childhood injuries for references to social deprivation and found only 32 papers. Moreover, these did not reflect the distribution of risk, placing the emphasis on the economic barriers to the ownership of safety devices such as cycle helmets and smoke detectors, rather than focusing on child pedestrian injuries. They also continued to target individuals' knowledge and behaviour rather than environmental changes. The significance of the urban/rural dimension has also been neglected with, for example, children in cars subject to higher fatality rates on rural roads due to the higher speeds. Significantly, the study of small communities in New Zealand noted earlier, also found that the most disadvantaged community focused on tangible outputs, particularly those relating to the physical environment, and sought practical support from similarly disadvantaged communities while the more affluent area sought to influence the local authority planning and policy process and networked internationally (Simpson et al, 2003).

Policy

The health of the nation (DH, 1992) aimed to reduce the death rate from unintentional injury in children aged 14 and under by one third by the year 2005 (from 6.7 per 100,000 to no more than 4.5 per 100,000). This was replaced in 1999 by targets established by *Saving lives: Our healthier nation* (DH, 1999), which aimed to reduce the death rate from accidents by at least one fifth and the rate of serious injury (across all age groups) by one tenth by 2010. Subsequently, the Road Safety Strategy (DETR, 2000) introduced the more stringent (and age-specific) aim of reducing the number of children killed and seriously injured by 50% over the same period. *Our healthier nation* also established a task force on accidental injuries, establishing the priority areas for children aged 0-15 as pedestrian injuries, fires and thermal injury, and play and recreation (Towner et al, 2005).

The key focus for policy, reflecting both the incidence of risk and the legitimacy of intervention, has been transport. Again there is a strong economic as well as health inequalities rationale, with road accidents costing over £16,000 million per annum and traffic calming schemes across England and Wales having the potential to save £357 million in reduced accidents (Liabo and Curtis, 2003). While interventions at the policy level may have the potential to reduce injuries in the road environment there is, however, very little evidence of efficacy in this area (Towner et al, 2001). There has, for example, been a reduction since the 1980s in the number of children injured and killed as pedestrians but a key contributory factor has been the reduction in child pedestrians, most notably because of the rise of the car-borne school run (Liabo and Curtis, 2003). Here, the proportion of children travelling to school by car has almost doubled since the 1980s (DfES, 2003), increasing the risks posed by road traffic at and near the school gate. Therefore, there needs to be a reliance on more than transport policy to reverse the situation first described in 1990 where children's issues in transport planning are marginalised by policies that seek to accommodate the growth in the demand for motor transport (Hillman et al, 1990, cited in Towner and Ward, 1998). Land-use policies, housing, social and fiscal policies all have, for example, a potential role to play in reducing accidents, often bringing debates around individual and social rights and responsibilities to the foreground.

The government's 1998 White Paper *A new deal for transport* introduced a number of new initiatives aimed at encouraging children to be less reliant on the car for school travel (DETR, 1998). Safe Routes to School encouraged local authorities to implement physical measures to improve safety for those walking and cycling, such as junction improvements and traffic calming, alongside travel awareness measures. This was furthered by the introduction of Local Transport

Plans (LTPs) in 1999, which required local authorities to look more widely and produce an integrated transport strategy (operative for five years) for reducing car use, while continuing to improve children's safety on the journey to school, including working with individual schools to develop School Travel Plans (STPs). There was also support from the Department for Education and Employment (DfEE) and the Department of Health (DH) in the shape of the Healthy Schools Programme (see Chapter Nine).

A survey in 1999 found this had resulted in relatively little activity (DETR, 1999). Only a quarter of local authorities had introduced STPs for at least one school and a further 44% had more limited school transport initiatives (typically focusing on single measures such as cycle training or traffic management near schools). Coverage was also very limited geographically, with STPs relating to only 2% of all schools, mostly within the primary sector. The research also suggested that little impact would have been made on the issue of inequalities, for although distribution was not analysed relative to social deprivation, most schemes were based in medium-sized towns with a population of 25,000-250,000. The plans did reflect the evidence base, however, with engineering measures being the most common ingredient and most having a multimodal emphasis, including walking and cycling initiatives alongside education. The research also revealed national policy to be challenged both by parents' reluctance to reduce car dependence (fuelled by issues of road and personal safety) and by the limited availability of resources. Most non-district authorities either had no budget at all for STPs or a budget of less than £50,000.

Some of these issues have been countered by the action plan *Travelling to school* (DfES, 2003), which aims to increase the number of completed plans to 3,000 by 2004, rising to 10,000 by 2006 and to increase coverage to nearly two fifths of all schools. The resource issue has also been addressed to a degree, with a £7.5 million per annum budget for school travel advisors available from 2004, initially for two years but now extended to 2008. These advisors will support local authorities and schools in producing travel plans and will focus in the first instance on secondary schools. From 2004 additional capital grants (typically £5,000 per primary school and £10,000 per secondary school) are also available for schools that complete a travel plan that will help fund measures such as cycle parking and lockers. Additionally, travel plans give access, via the LTP process, to capital investment for infrastructure change such as cycle routes, footpaths and traffic management (DfES, 2003). Good practice examples suggest schools can reduce car journeys by between one quarter and one third by a combination of interventions such as walking buses, cycle routes and drop-and-go sites at a distance from the school. Significantly, the planning process also stresses the improvements in school–community links, reductions in congestion and pollution and improvements in independent mobility – potentially countering the current concern with lack of physical activity and obesity. Kerbcraft schemes based on the Drumchapel Project (see Box 7.1) have, for example, been rolled out across

England, Wales and Scotland, with the initiative in England attracting £9 million to establish transferability across 64 local authorities (DfT, 2004).

Policies that concern other land uses, such as the location of shopping centres or health centres, can also generate traffic that, in turn, influences injury rates. Those that relate to schools again have particular relevance to children's travel patterns. In the 1970s in England, for example, an increase in school size was accompanied by increased school journey time with accompanying casualty rates (Preston, 1972), while parental choice has the potential to increase catchment areas still further. Policies affecting the private/public mix of traffic can also affect injury rates, with public transport associated with reduced road casualties and schemes such as the yellow school bus pilots and walking buses providing a potential alternative to using the car for school (Steer Davies Gleave, 2003).

The nature of the physical environment, as Chapter Six noted, is also important. Early studies found higher casualty rates in Victorian areas of terraced housing, where small gardens, a preponderance of on-street parking and few play areas increased risk. In such areas the frequent juxtaposition of high traffic volumes and speeds, poor housing design, more children than average walking to school and more children walking unaccompanied, alongside higher levels of family stress and differences in parental behaviour and knowledge has led, as in transport, to policies that aim to strengthen and involve communities. The creation of a safer environment is an integral part of Neighbourhood Renewal (see Chapter Eleven). Nine pilot Home Zones have also been established across England and Wales and a further four will be implemented by the Scottish Parliament. These aim to move beyond traffic calming to promote the social use of residential streets by improving street design and community involvement. They also prioritise pedestrians and cyclists so that the safety and quality of life of residents takes priority over traffic movements. One expected benefit is hoped to be a reduction in child casualties but additional benefits, such as a reduction in social isolation and casual crime, are also expected (www.homezoneschallenge.com).

Mental health

One in five children and young people is estimated to suffer from mental health problems with some 10% of 5- to 15-year-olds having a diagnosable mental health disorder. This suggests that around 1.1 million children and young people under the age of 18 would benefit from specialist services, with 45,000 of these having a severe mental health disorder (DH, 2004a). Within this spectrum the late teens and early twenties represent possibly the highest risk of mental health problems of any age group (Maughan et al, 2004) and, with respect to adolescents, probably one of the most neglected (Baruch, 2001). The overlap between the risk factors for psychiatric disorder and youth offending is particularly pronounced, with other key vulnerable groups including looked-after children, those with learning difficulties and the homeless.

Many of these young people will have multiple vulnerabilities, with the widest spectrum of risk and consequent cost to society (including poor educational attainment, limited employment prospects, insecure relationships, early parenting, involvement in crime and risk to health) contingent on conduct disorders and hyperactivity (Scott et al, 2001). Indeed, antisocial behaviour tends not only to be stable over time within individuals but also within families (Kazdin, 1995). There is thus a key role for interventions that reduce a range of negative impacts and negative chain reactions, open up new opportunities and neutralise harmful experiences (Rutter, 1999). Empirical evidence suggests, for example, that while resort to drugs or alcohol to cope with stress, dropping out of education, or early pregnancy and marriage, all increase the likelihood of a negative chain reaction, positive events such as success at school (not necessarily academic) can increase self-efficacy and self-esteem and hence increase control over key life events.

The 1999 ONS Survey on the Mental Health of Children and Adolescents in Britain (Meltzer et al, 2000) reports high rates of service use among those with mental health problems, including health, education, social services and the police. Only a small (but unknown) proportion, however, receive treatment from the Child and Adolescent Mental Health Service (CAMHS), and it has been suggested that, in common with other countries, most children who need mental health services are not receiving specialised care (Maughan et al, 2004). Around 40% of children with a mental health disorder are not currently receiving any specialist service (DH, 2004a). The majority of young people with mental health problems thus present to primary health, education or social services (where, one study found, the majority of looked-after adolescents had identifiable psychopathology, most commonly conduct disorders, overanxious disorders and depression [McCann et al, 1996]). The question as to what works has, therefore, a pronounced community component running alongside the need for specialist healthcare.

What works? Evidence and practice

The aetiology of emotional and behavioural disorders is, as Chapter Six has outlined, still poorly understood. Interventions have sought to address the range of contributory biological, psychological and social mechanisms. Arguably the key focus of social concern and hence research has, however, been the reduction of delinquency (a multicausal outcome measured by variables as diverse as stealing, fighting, lying and truancy), rather than the improvement of mental health per se. Delinquency itself is then but part of a larger spectrum of antisocial behaviour, spanning substance misuse, sexual promiscuity and dangerous driving (Farrington, 1996). Interventions in any of these areas that address risk or protective factors rather than symptoms have the potential, therefore, for widespread benefits. Many of these risks, however, militate against young people and their families either engaging with treatment programmes or remaining in treatment.

Protective factors are well established from longitudinal studies. The Newcastle

1000 Family Study, following children born in 1947, found that although delinquency was strongly correlated with multiple deprivation, those children from socially deprived backgrounds who stayed out of trouble tended to benefit from a positive temperament, good maternal and domestic care and educational achievements. The same factors proved protective in adolescence, with the addition of family contact with the school and the presence (for girls) of the natural father at home (Kolvin et al, 1990). The Cambridge Study in Delinquent Development, drawing on boys born in the early 1950s, similarly found economic deprivation, family criminality, parental mishandling and school failure to be key predictors of offending behaviour (Farrington, 1996).

The role of poverty mediated by parenting and education has thus long been established as key. There has been a similar long-standing interest in the cultivation of resilience – the ability to overcome such stress or adversity. This has been shown to relate to the development of a repertoire of coping strategies rather than a single protective factor (Rutter, 1999). It is now recognised, therefore, that greater cumulative impact is possible from interventions that address a combination of variables rather than single issues. It is also accepted that brief treatments are likely to have but limited effect given the range of contributory variables and that disorders such as early-onset conduct disorder may require continuing care or at least regular review. Little research has, however, been conducted on the wider structural barriers and enablers to mental well-being (see, for example, Crowley et al, 2004).

Parent training

A range of early intervention parenting programmes with a preventative emphasis has been shown to be effective in the early years. This continues to hold for childhood, with many of the interventions reviewed in Chapter Five actually directed at children up to the age of 10. Research suggests that the most effective parent training programmes for children of primary school age combine universal and selective elements, operate over the long term using a multicomponent, multisite model, and specifically increase the social competence of the children and the management skills of the parents, increasing the effectiveness of discipline and rewarding pro-social behaviour (Bor, 2004). On average, two thirds of children under the age of 10 whose parents take part in such a programme improve (Fonagy et al, 2002).

The evidence suggests that such interventions do not, however, work so well with adolescents with conduct disorder who require more in-depth approaches, such as functional family therapy (FFT) and multi-systemic treatment (MST) (Fonagy et al, 2002), both of which are designed to increase parental ability as well as address the specific problems of the child. The influence of the family also diminishes as children grow older to be replaced by the increased importance of peers. Given this apparent schism, and the earlier coverage of pre-adolescent issues, the remainder of this section focuses primarily on youth. Nevertheless, it should be remembered that many of the comprehensive interventions in infancy and preschool have positive effects (in terms, for example, of reduced offending and substance misuse and increased educational engagement), which extend across this whole period (see, for example, Schweinhart et al, 1993; Olds et al, 1998). This, combined with the more limited efficacy of later interventions, emphasises the importance attached to early intervention as well as the need to equip parents of adolescents with special skills.

Functional family therapy/multi-systemic treatment and multimodal interventions

FFT works from the premise that poor behaviour has a role within the family and that the family has to understand how they are actively maintaining the problem. Family relations are then addressed via both cognitive and behavioural therapy including, for example, aspects such as communication training and contingency management alongside the way family members are labelled. Research has supported its role in reducing delinquent behaviour over 25 years, particularly its ability to reduce repeat offending (Fonagy et al, 2002), but this may not necessarily apply in the case of conduct disorders as opposed to delinquency (Bor, 2004). It also suggests that rates of sibling delinquency can be reduced by inclusion in such programmes and that gains can be long lasting (Kazdin, 1995).

In contrast, it is suggested that MST is effective for children and adolescents with severe emotional and behavioural problems, with research having encompassed a variety of target groups and locations and having found a variety of positive outcomes. These range from decreased adolescent psychiatric symptoms, better school attendance and improved family outcomes to reduced arrest rates and time spent in institutions (Woolfenden et al, 2001; Bor, 2004). Littell et al (2004), in their proposed review of the effectiveness of MST, emphasise that its distinguishing feature is the multifaceted nature of the intervention, rather than the innovatory nature of any of its component parts. A second key is the model of clinical supervision, which requires daily contact with therapists and targets specific, well-defined problems and their underlying causes. It is also typically short term, embracing work with family, school and peer groups, and designed to avoid residential placement by working in the home and community. A notable advantage is the tendency to record relatively low attrition rates despite working with often quite troubled and disorganised families (Fonagy et al, 2002). However, positive outcomes tend to be restricted to the originators of the approach, emphasising the importance of training.

Cognitive behavioural therapies

Cognitive behavioural therapies (CBTs) address the way young people think as well as behave, typically including training in problem solving and social skills. Their use is supported in the treatment of aggression, anxiety disorders and phobias and depression, although their efficacy has not been convincingly demonstrated with respect to obsessive-compulsive disorder (Joughin, 2003). There is evidence, for example, that cognitive behavioural interventions and educational programmes may reduce suicide risk behaviours and stress by increasing personal control and coping skills including family involvement (Fonagy et al, 2002). CBT is also key to the treatment of conduct disorders in older children and adolescents where effectiveness has been demonstrated in combination again with parent training. In the specific case of young offenders, for instance, average reductions in recidivism of between 10% and 16% have been reported (Utting et al, 2002). However, as Fonagy et al (2002) also point out, there is no such thing as generic CBT – rather "particular packages that have been at least partly validated for children with specific problems and at particular developmental stages" (Fonagy et al, 2002, p 388).

School-based interventions

School-based interventions also receive renewed support, particularly if they are multimodal, sustained and involve both work in school and with parents (What Works for Children?, 2002). A systematic review of youth suicide prevention, for example, found a general lack of controlled studies but it did find some evidence that school, family and community-based studies could modify suicide-related risks if not suicidal behaviour (Crowley et al, 2004). The essence of such an evidence base supports interventions such as the Healthy Schools Initiative, advocating approaches that introduce teams to reduce crime and delinquency; highlight behavioural norms; develop social competencies; and focus on CBT for high-risk youth. However, while whole school policies to address bullying, for example, have been found to reduce levels of aggression within schools and address the mental health problems of both the bullied and bully, it is not known whether they can reduce aggressive behaviour of clinical severity (Fonagy et al, 2002). Schools can also provide an accessible route into psychotherapy, particularly for hard-to-reach groups in special schools or exclusion units, potentially normalising counselling, allowing benefits to be generalised beyond the clinical setting and allowing a wider preventative dimension to be incorporated (Baruch, 2001; Clarke et al, 2003).

In a precursor to the On Track Programme, the Home Office Programme Development Unit (PDU) provided funds between 1992 and 2000 for innovative local projects designed to address crime and criminal justice by providing early interventions in support of children at risk of offending. Mentoring was one area subjected to study, with the potential to address issues that lead to absenteeism, school exclusion, school failure and criminal activity at an early stage. Evaluation identified improvements in confidence, self-control, social awareness and relationships. However, it also found serious problems remained, such as behaviour, school attendance, exclusion and performance (St James-Roberts and Samlal Singh, 2001), attributed in part to the focused nature of the intervention and its limited duration. These limitations are, however, also borne out by a substantive literature review that concludes that mentoring alone is not effective in changing behaviour among those who are already truanting or involved in criminal activities, substance misuse or aggressive behaviour and may, indeed, exacerbate antisocial behaviour. Nevertheless, it can assist in the formation of stable relationships and, for young people who are failing to engage at school or within their community, this relationship might in itself be viewed as a positive outcome (Lucas and Liabo, 2003). Indeed, the literature continues to stress the importance of creating a sense of belonging as a protection against a range of disturbed behaviour (Hendry and Reid, 2000). The Dorset Healthy Alliance Project, outlined in Box 7.3 and

Box 7.3: The Dorset Healthy Alliance Project

The Dorset Healthy Alliance Project was initially a three-year school-based pilot designed to provide a targeted but non-stigmatising preventative service for children aged 9-16 and their families. A partnership project between education, health, probation and social services, it was based in a local secondary school and one of its primary feeders (with a further two schools acting as controls), and involved a project teacher in each school (full time in the case of the primary school), together with a social worker supporting both schools.

The aim was to reduce truancy, delinquency, disruptive behaviour in school, school exclusions and associated social, neighbourhood and family problems by intervening before the problems became unmanageable and helping families experiencing difficulties. Key components of the intervention included counselling, establishing networks of family support and interagency collaboration and providing a crisis team to support the teachers.

Reported outcomes included a resolution of child and family problems (including fewer child protection referrals), increased accessibility to support for families, improved educational achievements and a reduction in truancy and exclusion rates. Levels of theft from school, vandalism and substance misuse also decreased. Significantly, reduced delinquency was found to be most strongly associated with teenagers who enjoyed school. The intervention was also found to be cost-effective. There was an estimated 111% return on the preventative investment based on savings in special education and reduced thefts in school, rising to 250% if wider criminality was considered and potentially larger returns if factors such as child protection and health were also taken into account. The initiative was mainstreamed by the county in 1996 (Pritchard, 2001).

commissioned as part of this same PDU programme, provides evidence about the protective role that can be afforded by a positive school ethos.

Pharmacological treatments

Evidence from a number of randomised controlled trials (RCTs) (see Fonagy et al, 2002, for a comprehensive review) suggests the areas where psychopharmacological treatments (that is, medication) are the most effective. They are, for example, the first choice for Attention Deficit/Hyperactivity Disorder (ADHD), although diet may also be supportive and psychosocial treatments, such as parent training or behavioural therapy, can be useful adjuncts. Psychopharmacological treatments are also supported in the treatment of obsessive-compulsive disorder and depression and may be appropriate in the treatment of conduct problems and delinquency (oppositional disorder) in conjunction with psychosocial treatments such as parent training. In contrast, a significant rate of discontinuation of medication and relapse is found when it comes to eating disorders, where cognitive techniques tend to be more effective. FFT, for example, has been shown to be effective against anorexia nervosa in adolescents where the illness was not yet chronic.

Implications for practice

Recent reviews of the treatment of child and adolescent mental health problems in primary care set this emergent research in perspective, arguing that CAMHS are still unable to draw on a reliable base of evidence. A variety of interventions such as training for primary care professionals, educational interventions by nurses and management by specialists have all, for example, produced at best equivocal child outcomes (Bower et al, 2001). One contributory factor is that a large proportion of the available evidence does not reflect the comorbidity issues found in day-to-day clinical practice where many children and young people present with a range of problems.

Second, there has also been only limited evaluation of the different therapeutic approaches used specifically to treat psychological problems in children and adolescents (Derisley, 2004). Indeed, of over 200 different therapy techniques in clinical practice, it has been claimed most "have no evidence on their behalf" (Kazdin, 1995, p 77). A synthesis of psychosocial interventions for schizophrenia (NHS CRD, 2000), for example, was unable to find any reviews focused specifically on the care of adolescents and, among treatments and service provision for the wider population, often found it difficult to isolate the effective components of an intervention or replicate the results achieved by the pioneers of the treatment. A systematic review of treatments for deliberate self-harm similarly found only one study focused on adolescents despite its significance for this group (Hawton et al, 1998). Efficacy, as noted earlier, also varies considerably according to the focus of treatment.

Third, despite the political priority accorded to youth crime, relatively few community-based programmes for young offenders, such as educational re-integration, remand fostering or mentoring, have been convincingly evaluated in the UK (Shiner, 2000). Utting et al (2002), synthesising a number of meta-analyses of community-based programmes for young offenders, suggest three types of programme are capable of producing an above-average reduction in recidivism: those designed to improve personal and social skills; those focused on changing behaviour; and multiple service programmes combining several different approaches. Community-based programmes were also found to be more effective than those in custodial settings as were those that address the full range of offending-related problems. However, it has been suggested that some, such as the juvenile awareness schemes falling under the 'Scared Straight' banner, may even increase delinquency (Petrosino et al, 2002), while attrition rates may be higher among the more persistent offenders (Lobley and Smith, 1999).

The Youth Justice Board is funding the Youth Offending Teams (YOTs) in England and Wales to develop mentoring, re-integration into education, training and employment and remand fostering, alongside those areas that are clearly indicated by the evidence base discussed earlier, such as parenting support and cognitive behavioural programmes. Nevertheless, a review of reducing offending in children and young people (What Works for Children?, 2002) noted how frequently the UK still used punitive measures (such as electronic tagging and final warnings) without supporting rehabilitation, and how integrated packages such as referral orders often faced practical difficulties in, for example, finding people to supervise reparation activities. Not surprisingly, therefore, many of the measures had only a limited effect on re-offending and few addressed the problems that gave rise to involvement in crime.

One clear emergent trend is the move away from treating symptoms in isolation and towards offering treatment that acknowledges the importance of the family and social context. In parallel, therefore, the focus of treatment has shifted from the clinical setting to the community, and the success of the treatment is increasingly measured in a wide range of outcomes orientated towards normal development within the family and peer group. At the same time there has been an acceptance that many disorders are at least partially irreversible and that psychosocial interventions should be assessed not in terms of an ability to cure but by an improvement in functioning (Fonagy et al, 2002).

Limitations to the evidence base

A major challenge in the complex area of mental health surrounds the ability to generalise outcome data and the need to ensure findings are relevant to the delivery of services. This includes the establishment of boundaries within which any treatment should be applied and the necessary staff mix required to deliver the programme. Fonagy et al (2002) suggest that the ability to link intervention and improvement is easier to achieve with some treatments (particularly psychopharmacological therapies and CBT) and clinical populations than with others, leaving vacuums in the literature surrounding the less accessible populations and more complex treatments.

A number of outcome domains critical to successful treatment are also often neglected, such as peer relations, social competence, academic functioning and participation in activities. So, too, are individual and contextual variables. Treatments such as parent training, for example, are culturally sensitive, potentially limiting extrapolation from a primarily North American research base. They may also be sensitive to gender, with child–rearing and socio–economic factors appearing to be potentially more important risk factors for young females, while parental characteristics such as education and teenage parenthood pose more important risks for males (Farrington and Painter, 2004). There are also considerable variations within treatments. For example, it has been suggested that CBT is offered in so many different sequences and permutations that it should preclude the use of meta–analytic techniques (Ronen, 1997, cited in Derisley, 2004). Such shortfalls provide an obvious challenge to the assessment of the efficacy of any intervention, a challenge that is compounded by variations in individual response to all but the most severe psychosocial sensors, environmental disadvantages which overlap and genetic mediators.

Policy

The limited access to specialist mental health services for children and young people and the large number of young people being treated within tier one (by non–specialist health and social care workers, for example) was acknowledged by the Health Advisory Service in the 1990s when they identified a need to strengthen the interface between the CAMHS and primary–level services, including the establishment of Primary Mental Health Workers (PMHWs). It remains an issue today with the Child Poverty Review highlighting the importance of improving access to mental health services and the Children's National Service Framework (NSF) suggesting, as already noted, that around 40% of children with a mental health disorder are still not currently receiving any specialist service. Expenditure, for a client group that potentially embraces one tenth of all children and young people, is also limited. The CAMHS grant for 2005–06 stands at only £90.5 million and this represents a 35% increase on 2004-05.

Progress towards a better-funded, more holistic and more accessible service is slow. The Audit Commission, reporting in 1999, found spending on children's mental health to vary by a factor of seven between different authorities with very little relation to need. It also found limited access to specialist services from other than clinicians. Only 14% of referrals, for example, were from education or social services, with the majority of youth justice managers reporting problems of access and less than 1% of CAMHS time spent supporting tier one provision. A survey in 2000 similarly found that while most CAMHS offered joint education and training with agencies active at tier one, this was limited in extent and less than a third offered a wider range of work such as structured consultation, outpatient clinics and joint casework or had established PMHW posts (Bradley et al, 2003). Not surprisingly, such activity was concentrated in the larger and more developed CAMHS, compounding geographical inequalities.

CAMHS services have also traditionally catered only for young people up to the age of 16, taking the school leaving age as the marker of passage into adulthood. This sits uneasily with the increasing incidence of severe mental illness in late adolescence and suggests the need for a refocusing of services and policy. However, provision for the mental health needs of 16- and 17-year-olds still tends to fall into a gap between services for children and those for adults (HM Government and DH, 2004). In 1999, for example, services were available only to those aged under 16 in over one quarter of authorities (Audit Commission, 1999), while by 2004 only half were offering services up to a child's 18th birthday (DH, 2004a). Meanwhile, concern continues to be expressed as to the lack of awareness, training, resources and research available to support young people with mental health problems in primary care (Jacobson et al, 2002).

This was compounded by the fact that the NSF for Mental Health, introduced in 1999, focused only on adults. The corresponding framework for children was not introduced until 2004 as part of the NSF for Children, Young People and Maternity Services (DH, 2004b). It has been argued, however, that the CAMHS development strategies have raised the profile of mental health on an interagency basis while the new NSF has confirmed the expectation that a comprehensive CAMHS will be available in all areas by 2006. This should include early intervention and mental health promotion, be accessible to those aged 0-18 and incorporate an annual increase in services of at least 10%. However, the Department of Health (DH) also acknowledges that there is still a real need to establish the extent of existing deficits and assess the needs of those who currently receive a poor service. This includes those with a learning disability, autistic spectrum disorders or behavioural problems, minority ethnic groups and those who require inpatient services or are in the criminal justice system (DH, 2003).

Attempts to improve practice have also been commissioned. The CAMHS innovation grant, for example, was introduced in 1998 to develop innovative projects for young people with mental health problems. This attracted a budget of £4 million per annum across three years from the DH, and was matched by funding from local authorities and health authorities in the 24 English localities chosen for support. The aim was to improve child mental health and the quality of service provision (including access), support parents and carers in order to prevent family breakdown, increase the skills and confidence of the client group and increase their engagement with schools, thereby reducing school exclusions.

The national evaluation was, however, confounded by the variety of the projects and the diversity of their client groups (three key foci being early intervention, looked-after children and children with severe and complex needs, such as young offenders, those suffering from abuse and those at risk of suicide). Nevertheless, many projects were able to report a reduction in clinically significant problems, alongside a reduction in disruptive behaviour. Projects focusing on looked-after children also reported increased self-awareness, while the early intervention projects were able to increase parental confidence and educational engagement. Most projects also aimed to increase agency understanding of their client group and increase interagency working, with the majority able to increase the involvement of CAMHS with the most vulnerable children and increase the appropriateness of referrals into the service. All but one of the services continued to operate once innovation funding had ceased (Kurtz and James, 2002).

Policy has arguably been more dynamic and investment more responsive in the area of antisocial behaviour. In line with many other countries there is a separate justice system for juveniles, custody is seen as a last resort and the emphasis is placed instead on a combination of prevention, rehabilitation and sanction (Australian Institute of Criminology, 2002). Historically intervention has tended to oscillate between rehabilitative and punitive approaches. The emphasis in the 1970s, for example, was on non-secure community-based programmes but with the increase in violent youth crime in the late 1980s and early 1990s there was renewed interest in punishing delinquent youths and, following the 1991 Criminal Justice Act, a desire to hold parents responsible for their children's criminal actions. In contrast, the 1998 Crime and Disorder Act, reflecting the "evidence that those who begin offending at an early age are disproportionately likely to become serious and persistent offenders" (Utting et al, 2002, p 167) signalled a statutory aim of prevention across a range of services (Home Office, 1998). The subsequent introduction of Intensive Supervision and Surveillance Programmes also aims to provide community-based alternatives to custody, enabling offenders to remain in their homes, schools or employment (Audit Commission, 2004).

The idea that there should be collective responsibility to prevent youth offending, shared by a range of public and voluntary sector agencies, as well as the wider community, is now established policy. Multiagency YOTs were introduced in 2000, consequent on the 1998 Crime and Disorder Act, and are responsible for preventing offending and re-offending by young people. They are often the lead partners in prevention initiatives such as the Youth Inclusion Programme and mentoring schemes. Multiagency Crime and Disorder Reduction Partnerships (CDRPs), meanwhile, are responsible for cutting overall crime levels, a significant proportion of which also involves young people either as victims or offenders (Crime Concern, 2002).

Increased funding has also been directed towards youth crime, including the Youth Action Approach Programmes and On Track. On Track (see Box 7.4) was established by the Home Office in 1999 as part of its Crime Reduction

Box 7.4: Evidence-based practice – the On Track Programme

On Track operates via five main categories of community-based intervention clearly related to the evidence base outlined earlier and in Chapter Five: home visiting; preschool education; home–school partnerships; parenting support and training; and family therapy. An additional category for specialist interventions was also included to allow locally specific issues to be addressed.

Early results suggest that only one fifth of users are referred onto the projects as a result of targeting. However, universal provision does have the advantage of reducing stigma and allowing identification of other children and families in need of support while also potentially increasing exposure to non-delinquent peers. Preliminary output, based on a small number of individuals, tentatively suggests positive changes are being made to a number of risk and protective factors. Specifically, approximately one third of those identified as having risk factors with respect to parental discipline, family conflict, offending or antisocial behaviour and violent or aggressive behaviour were reported as showing improvements after intervention, as were one fifth of those at risk because of poor parental supervision. However, this related to only between 18 and 31 children.

Similar findings were made in terms of attainment, attendance and levels of exclusion with, for example, over one half of children identified as at risk because of frequently unauthorised absences judged to have changed and one third of those with previous education welfare contacts having no further contact. However, this similarly related to only 27 children at most (France et al, 2004a).

Programme. An early intervention programme, in terms both of age group and stage of problem, it targets children aged 4-12 in areas of high crime and deprivation who are at risk of becoming offenders. Its aim is to prevent antisocial behaviour and crime and to reduce the risk factors that predict future offending by adopting an evaluated partnership approach, involving local communities and focusing on small geographical areas. A budget of £30 million for the three-year period from September 2000 was used to establish 24 programmes.

The Youth Inclusion Programme similarly aims to reduce crime, together with arrest and truancy rates and exclusions, but for an older client group, those aged 13-16. Introduced in 1999 in the 70 most deprived neighbourhoods it has an overall budget of £20 million and was meant to focus on up to 50 young people who were recognised to be the most disaffected and at greatest risk of offending. However, participation is voluntary and while there appears to have been a reduction in arrest rates and the number of offences for which young people are arrested, there has been a parallel rise in truancy. Questions have also been raised over the relationship between the activities offered (such as environmental work, sport and arts) and the problems that give rise to involvement in crime (What Works for Children?, 2002).

Parenting Orders were also introduced in June 2000 as a means of sanction where a child has committed a criminal offence, persistently truanted or displayed seriously antisocial behaviour. These powers were extended by the 2003 Anti-social Behaviour Act (Home Office, 2003) to cover those who consistently behave badly in school. Attendance on a parenting programme is compulsory on issue of a Parenting Order and the YOTs have had to identify suitable services, resulting in the introduction of over 40 new parenting projects. Parenting programmes have, as noted earlier, not always worked well in reducing conduct disorders in adolescents. However, a number of YOTs are piloting a programme based on FFT, which will then have the advantage of application and evaluation in a specifically UK context. Not surprisingly, managing a difficult child has already been revealed as often only one component among high parental need, including debt, housing, personal relationships and health (Ghate and Ramella, 2002).

Traditional divisions have proved hard to break down in practice. The work of the YOTs still tends to be dominated by court and pre-court work, while their community safety partners focus on prevention, situational measures and civil orders such as Anti-Social Behaviour Orders (ASBOs). Yet, if the goal of reducing young people's involvement in crime is to be achieved, it has been argued, CDRPs need to influence work with the most prolific offenders and YOTs need to be involved in a range of preventive measures. These should range "from targeted provision, such as intensive mentoring, to impacting on universal services such as education, housing and employment, which make a critical difference to offending patterns in the long-term" (Crime Concern, 2002, p 4). The Audit Commission propounds a similar message. There is a need to convince health and mental health services of the crucial roles they have to play in meeting the wider needs of young offenders and a need to involve schools directly (Audit Commission, 2004). *Every child matters* (DfES, 2004) similarly argues for the colocation of front-line staff in Children's Centres, extended schools and health settings in order to increase the opportunities both for the early identification of risk and for the integrated planning and delivery of services.

New initiatives have also encountered considerable problems moving from policy to implementation. On Track, for example, in common with many other complex multiagency pilots, faced difficulties with the recruitment and retention of staff (it was a year after designation, for example, that all the pilots had a project coordinator in place [Hine and Harrington, 2004]), interagency relations and procedures, tensions between initiatives and the mainstream and tensions between potentially competing initiatives. It was particularly affected, for example, by the creation of the Children and Young People's Unit (CYPU), and the subsequent establishment of the Children's Fund to bridge the preventative gap between Sure Start (aimed at 0- to 4-year-olds) and Connexions (aimed at 13- to 19-year-olds), and the disbursal of its budget of £380 million (France et al,

2004b). This introduced a new set of priorities (which often subsumed On Track) and a new set of target areas (with funds being available for all local authorities in England and programmes tending to operate at, for example, city rather than neighbourhood level). On Track itself was also moved to the CYPU in 2001.

As well as increased collective responsibility, there has also, therefore, been a shift in emphasis towards preventative work (mirroring that undertaken with families in the early years in, for example, Sure Start areas), most particularly as delinquency has come to occupy a central position on the social exclusion agenda. The Children's Fund, On Track, and more generally the Neighbourhood Renewal Fund (NRF), for instance, have all introduced targeted neighbourhood services for older children and adolescents together with their families (see, for example, NSNR, 2000). In part, this reflects the fact that it is too difficult for preventative interventions to pinpoint individuals and families at risk, but it also reflects an acknowledgement of the wider physical and social environment, such as inadequate housing. This can be tackled within the context, for example, of general neighbourhood renewal programmes or specific community crime prevention programmes, potentially improving the ability to supervise children and offer improved recreational facilities, and to stimulate community confidence through factors such as estate design, neighbourhood management, tenant involvement and community wardens. There remains, however, a shortage of convincing evidence for the effectiveness of these programmes (Farrington, 1996). The TOGETHER campaign, launched by the Anti-Social Behaviour Unit in 2003 with the aim of improving the interagency response to antisocial behaviour, is also now targeting services at families with the most challenging problems in its 60 local authority action areas (Shelter, 2005).

Conclusion

This chapter, while charting uneven territory, sometimes even uncharted territory, has also found itself revisiting familiar places. The shift to prevention and the stress on partnership, factors already highlighted with respect to early life, have been apparent throughout. To strategies such as parent education, home visiting and preschool education we now join family therapy, home–school partnerships and community regeneration. The holistic nature of early intervention has again been underlined as improvements in one area, such as road safety, are increasingly seen to be linked to the wider social exclusion agenda and, via connections, for example, to physical activity and community cohesion, to a more inclusive definition of health and well-being. Similarly, renewed support has been found for the multifaceted intervention that acknowledges the significance of social context and the importance of responding to the spectrum of contributory factors. The enactment in 2004 of the Children Bill has given statutory impetus to this trend, widening the legal responsibility for safeguarding children and promoting their welfare to embrace all key agencies rather than social services alone. This includes an emergent role for the facilitator, whether this takes the form of the project officer in a community-based injury prevention project, the school traffic advisor, facilitating school transport plans, or the PMHWs bridging the gap between primary care and CAMHS.

These themes are not immediately obvious in Table 7.1, which draws on the review-level evidence to summarise the interventions that appear effective with respect to health inequalities at this stage of the lifecourse, and those where such evidence remains lacking. Indeed, the evidence base relating to childhood and youth largely focuses, as with early life and adulthood, on health behaviours – diet, physical activity, smoking and alcohol, subjects which form the focus of Chapter Nine. Even for the topics assessed in this chapter it can be seen to focus on what Towner et al (2005) describe as the proximate or intermediate factors (exposure to hazard and behaviour) rather than the wider social, political, cultural or economic factors that lead to the differential distribution of resources. However, Table 7.1 does serve to reinforce the picture of uneven and ad hoc progress presented in this chapter. This applies irrespective of whether we are talking about research, policy or service provision. The relative neglect of children and young people as a distinct client group evident in Table 7.1 is also beset by historical inequities. This difference between places has then been compounded by the tendency to target interventions via neighbourhood services and to pilot new initiatives in discrete geographical areas. The socio-economic manifestation of health inequalities is thus overlain by a complex and highly differentiated system of opportunity, measured by varying densities of initiatives and partnership players (Murdoch and Abram, 1998; Jones and Little, 2000).

The net of joined-up working is similarly not without its holes. Mainstream agencies are struggling to come to terms with a fast-moving policy agenda and to find the resources required to move beyond crisis, while simultaneously accommodating a series of short-term initiatives, many of which are in direct competition for staff and resources. Meanwhile, the area-based initiatives (ABIs) themselves face significant challenges in moving from policy to implementation, in offering evidence of effective practice and in shaping the mainstream. Reliance either on individual/behavioural approaches or on ABIs is constantly tempered by the need to change the culture of organisations or communities and the need to influence the larger policy-making process including education, legislation and the distribution of resources. We continue to expand the web of connections and tensions as we move now from the consideration of health inequalities per se to address inequalities in health behaviours and life trajectories.

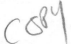
Table 7.1: Interventions during childhood and adolescence: summary of the evidence base relating to health inequalities

	Source
ACCIDENTS	
Roads	
There is good evidence that:	
Area-wide engineering schemes and traffic calming measures decrease traffic injuries	Systematic review
Child restraint loan schemes and legislation produce behavioural change	Systematic review
Cycle helmets offer protection from head and brain injuries, particularly at lower speeds	Overview
Educational campaigns and legislation can increase their use	Systematic review
There is reasonable evidence that cycle training can improve safe riding behaviour	Systematic review
Leisure	
There is some evidence that:	
Improvements to playground design can reduce both the frequency and severity of injuries	Overview
Environmental engineering changes to the sports environment and prophylactic injury prevention programmes reduce injuries to adolescents	Overview
Legislation is effective for 15- to 24-year-olds whether in sports, road or workplace settings	Overview
Home	
There is good evidence that smoke detectors and child-resistant containers reduce injury particularly if high-risk households are targeted	Systematic review/ overview
Less evidence attaches to window bars and the design of domestic products	Systematic review
Home visiting can substantially reduce rates of accidental injury	Overview
The role of education only reaches reasonable levels with respect to child/parent education to reduce pedestrian injuries and the use of car restraints	Overview
Multimodal interventions are the most likely to yield positive results	Systematic review
Lack of review-level evidence	
Leisure environment	
Older children	

(continued)

Table 7.1: Interventions during childhood and adolescence: summary of the evidence base relating to health inequalities (continued)

	Source
MENTAL HEALTH	
Parenting programmes with a preventative emphasis increase the social competence of children under 10 years and the management skills of their parents	Overview
Family and parenting interventions can reduce the time juvenile delinquents (aged 10-17) spend in institutions	Cochrane Review
CBT can be effective in the treatment of anxiety disorders, phobias and depression and (in combination with parent training) conduct disorders	Cochrane Review/ overview
FFT can reduce both delinquent behaviour and sibling delinquency	Overview
MST can prove effective with severe emotional and behavioural problems	Other review
Pharmacological treatments are effective for ADHD, particularly if supported by diet and psychosocial treatments (for example, parent training or behavioural therapy). Psychopharmacological treatments are also supported in the treatment of obsessive-compulsive disorder and depression and may be appropriate in the treatment of conduct problems and delinquency	Overview

Lack of review-level evidence

A specific focus on adolescents

Evaluation of community-based programmes for young offenders in the UK

References

Audit Commission (1999) *Children in mind: Child and adolescent mental health services (CAMHS) briefing paper*, London: Audit Commission.

Audit Commission (2004) *Youth justice 2004: A review of the reformed youth justice system*, London: Audit Commission.

Australian Institute of Criminology (2002) *What works in reducing young people's involvement in crime?*, Canberra: Australian Institute of Criminology.

Baruch, G. (2001) 'Mental health services in schools: the challenge of locating a psychotherapy service for troubled adolescent pupils in mainstream and special schools', *Journal of Adolescence*, vol 24, no 4, pp 549-70.

Bor, W. (2004) 'Prevention and treatment of childhood and adolescent aggression and antisocial behaviour: a selective review', *Australian and New Zealand Journal of Psychiatry*, vol 38, no 5, pp 373-80.

Bower, P., Garralda, E., Kramer, T., Harrington, R. and Sibbald, B. (2001) 'The treatment of child and adolescent mental health problems in primary care: a systematic review', *Family Practice*, vol 18, no 4, pp 373–82.

Bradley, S., Kramer, T., Garralda, M.E., Bower, P., Macdonald, W., Sibbald, B. and Harrington, R. (2003) 'Child and adolescent mental health interface work with primary services: a survey of NHS provider trusts', *Child and Adolescent Mental Health*, vol 8, no 4, pp 170–6.

Bunn, F., Collier, T., Frost, C., Ker, K., Roberts, I. and Wentz, R. (2003) 'Traffic calming for the prevention of road traffic injuries: systematic review and meta-analysis', *Injury Prevention*, vol 9, no 3, pp 200–4.

Clarke, M., Coombs, C. and Walton, L. (2003) 'School based early identification and intervention service for adolescents: a psychology and school nurse partnership model', *Child and Adolescent Mental Health*, vol 8, no 1, pp 34–9.

Coggan, C., Patterson, P., Brewin, M., Hooper, R. and Robinson, E. (2000) 'Evaluation of the Waitakere community injury prevention project', *Injury Prevention*, vol 6, no 2, pp 130–4.

Coleman, P., Munro, J., Nicholl, J., Harper, R., Kent, G. and Wild, D. (1996) *The effectiveness of interventions to prevent accidental injury to young persons aged 15-24 years: A review of evidence*, Sheffield: Medical Care Research Unit, University of Sheffield.

Crime Concern (2002) 'Keeping young people safe and out of trouble: joining up the community safety and youth offending agendas' (www.crimeconcern.org.uk), accessed 14 April 2005.

Crowley, P., Kilroe, J. and Burke, S. (2004) *Youth suicide prevention: Evidence briefing summary*, London: Health Development Agency.

Derisley, J. (2004) 'Cognitive therapy for children, young people and families: considering service provision', *Child and Adolescent Mental Health*, vol 9, no 1, pp 15–20.

DETR (Department of the Environment, Transport and the Regions) (1998) *A new deal for transport: Better for everyone*, London: The Stationery Office.

DETR (1999) *Research into levels of activity relating to school travel initiatives*, London: DETR.

DETR (2000) *Tomorrow's roads: Safer for everyone*, London: DETR.

DfES (Department for Education and Skills) (2003) *Travelling to school: An action plan*, Nottingham: DfES.

DfES (2004) *Every child matters: Change for children in the criminal justice system*, London: DfES.

DfT (Department for Transport) (2004) *Tomorrow's roads – safer for everyone: The first three year review. The government's road safety and casualty reduction targets for 2010*, London: DfT.

DH (Department of Health) (1992) *The health of the nation: A strategy for health in England and Wales*, London: HMSO.

DH (1999) *Saving lives: Our healthier nation*, London: The Stationery Office.

DH (2003) 'Getting the right start: the National Service Framework for Children. Emerging findings' (www.doh.gov.uk/nsf/children/gettingtherightstart), accessed 1 July 2004.

DH (2004a) *3779/CAMHS standard, National Service Framework for Children, Young People and Maternity Services*, London: DH.

DH (2004b) *National Service Framework for Children, Young People and Maternity Services*, London: DH.

DiGuiseppi, C. and Higgins, J. (2001) 'Interventions for promoting smoke alarm ownership and function (Cochrane Review)', *The Cochrane Library, issue 2, 2004*, Chichester: John Wiley & Sons Ltd.

Dowswell, T. and Towner, E. (2002) 'Social deprivation and the prevention of unintentional injury in childhood: a systematic review', *Health Education Research*, vol 17, no 2, pp 221-37.

Elkan, R., Kendrick, D., Hewitt, M., Robinson, J.J.A., Tolley, K., Blair, M., Dewey, M., Williams, D. and Brummell, K. (2000) 'The effectiveness of domiciliary health visiting: a systematic review of international studies and a selective review of the British literature', *Health Technology Assessment*, vol 4, no 13, pp iii-234.

Farrington, D. (1996) *Understanding and preventing youth crime*, York: Joseph Rowntree Foundation.

Farrington, D. and Painter, K. (2004) *Gender differences in offending: Implications for risk-focused prevention*, Online Report 09/04, London: Home Office.

Fonagy, P., Target, M., Cottrell, D., Phillips, J. and Kurtz, Z. (2002) *What works for whom? A critical review of treatments for children and adolescents*, London: The Guilford Press.

France, A., Hine, J. and Armstrong, D. (2004b) 'Implementing the On Track crime reduction programme: lessons for the future', in V. Harrington, S. Trikha and A. France (eds) *Process and early implementation issues: Emerging findings from the On Track evaluation*, London: Home Office, pp 44-53.

France, A., Hine, J., Armstrong, D. and Camina, M. (2004a) *The On Track early intervention and prevention programme: From theory to action*, London: Home Office.

Ghate, D. and Ramella, M. (2002) *Positive parenting: The national evaluation of the Youth Justice Board's parenting programme*, London: Youth Justice Board.

Graham, H. and Power, C. (2004) *Childhood disadvantage and adult health: A lifecourse framework*, London: Health Development Agency.

Hawton, K., Arensman, E., Townsend, E., Bremner, S., Feldman, E., Goldney, R., Gunnell, D., Hazell, P., van Heeringen, K., House, A., Owens, D., Sakinofsky, I. and TräskmanBendz, L. (1998) 'Deliberate self harm: systematic review of efficacy of psychosocial and pharmacological treatments in preventing repetition', *British Medical Journal*, vol 317, no 7156, pp 441-7.

Hendry, L. and Reid, M. (2000) 'Social relationships and health: the meaning of social "connectedness" and how it relates to health concerns for rural Scottish adolescents', *Journal of Adolescence*, vol 23, no 6, pp 705-19.

Hillman, M., Adams, J. and Whitelegg, J. (1990) *One false move...A study of children's independent mobility*, London: Policy Studies Institute.

Hine, J. and Harrington, V. (2004) *Delivering On Track*, London: Home Office.

HM Government and DH (Department of Health) (2004) *Choosing health: Making healthy choices easier*, London: HM Government and DH.

Home Office (1998) *Crime and Disorder Act (Chapter 37)*, London: The Stationery Office.

Home Office (2003) *Anti-social Behaviour Act (Chapter 38)*, London: The Stationery Office.

Jacobson, L., Churchill, R., Donovan, C., Garralda, E., Fay, J. and Members of the Adolescent Working Party, Royal College of General Physicians (2002) 'Tackling teenage turmoil: primary care recognition and management of mental ill health during adolescence', *Family Practice*, vol 19, no 4, pp 401-9.

Jones, O. and Little, J. (2000) 'Rural challenge(s): partnership and new rural governance', *Journal of Rural Studies*, vol 16, no 3, pp 171-83.

Joughin, C. (2003) 'Cognitive behaviour therapy can be effective in managing behavioural problems and conduct disorder in pre-adolescence' (www.whatworksforchildren.org.uk), What Works for Children Group, Evidence Nugget, September.

Kazdin, A. (1995) *Conduct disorders in childhood and adolescence*, Thousand Oaks, CA: Sage Publications.

Kendrick, D. and Royal, S. (2003) 'Inequalities in cycle helmet use: cross sectional survey in schools in deprived areas of Nottingham', *Archives of Disease in Childhood*, vol 88, no 10, pp 876-80.

Kolvin, I., Miller, F.J.W., Scott, D.M., Gatzanis, S.R.M. and Fleeting, M. (1990) *Continuities of deprivation?*, ESRC/DHSS Studies in Deprivation and Disadvantage No 15, Aldershot: Avebury.

Kurtz, Z. and James, C. (2002) *What's new: Learning from the CAMHS innovation projects. Executive summary*, London: DH.

Liabo, K. and Curtis, K. (2003) 'Traffic calming schemes to reduce childhood injuries from road accidents and respond to children's own views of what is important' (www.whatworksforchildren.org.uk), What Works for Children Group, Evidence Nugget, April.

Liabo, K., Lucas, P. and Roberts, H. (2003) 'Can traffic calming measures achieve the children's fund objective of reducing inequalities in child health?', *Archives of Disease in Childhood*, vol 88, no 3, pp 235-6.

Littell, J., Popa, M. and Forsythe, B. (2004) 'Multisystemic treatment for severe social, emotional, and behavioral problems in children and adolescents aged 10-17 (Protocol for a Cochrane Review)', *The Cochrane Library*, Chichester: John Wiley & Sons Ltd.

Lobley, D. and Smith, D. (1999) *Working with persistent juvenile offenders: An evaluation of the Apex Cue Ten project*, Edinburgh: The Scottish Office Central Research Unit.

Lucas, P. (2003) 'Home visiting can substantially reduce childhood injury' (www.whatworksforchildren.org.uk), What Works for Children Group, Evidence Nugget, April.

Lucas, P. and Liabo, K. (2003) 'One-to-one, non-directive mentoring programmes have not been shown to improve behaviour in young people involved in offending or anti-social activities' (www.whatworksforchildren.org.uk), What Works for Children Group, Evidence Nugget, April.

Lyons, R., Sander, L., Weightman, A., Patterson, J., Jones, S., Lannon, S., Rolfe, B., Kemp, A. and Johansen, A. (2004) 'Modification of the home environment for the reduction of injuries (Cochrane Review)', *The Cochrane Library*, Chichester: John Wiley & Sons Ltd.

McCann, J. B., James, A., Wilson, S. and Dunn, G. (1996) 'Prevalence of psychiatric disorders in young people in the care system', *British Medical Journal*, vol 313, no 7071, pp 1529-30.

Mackett, R. (2004) 'Making children's lives more active' (www.cts.ucl.ac.uk/research/chcaruse), accessed 14 April 2005.

Maughan, B., Brock, A. and Ladva, G. (2004) 'Mental health', in ONS (ed) *The health of children and young people*, London: ONS (www.statistics.gov.uk/children).

Meltzer, H., Gatward, R., with Goodman, R. and Ford, T. (2000) *Mental health of children and adolescents in Great Britain*, London: The Stationery Office.

Millward, L.M., Morgan, A. and Kelly, M.P. (2003) *Prevention and reduction of accidental injury in children and older people: Evidence briefing summary*, London: Health Development Agency.

Morrison, D., Thomson, H. and Petticrew, M. (2004) 'Evaluation of the health effects of a neighbourhood traffic calming scheme', *Journal of Epidemiology and Community Health*, vol 58, no 10, pp 837-40.

Murdoch, J. and Abram, S. (1998) 'Defining the limits of community governance', *Journal of Rural Studies*, vol 14, no 1, pp 41-50.

NHS CRD (National Health Service Centre for Reviews and Dissemination) (1996) 'Preventing unintentional injuries in children and young adolescents', *Effective Health Care*, vol 2, no 5, pp 1-16.

NHS CRD (2000) 'Psychosocial interventions for schizophrenia', *Effective Health Care*, vol 6, no 3, pp 1-8.

Nicholl, J., Coleman, P. and Brazier, J. (1994) 'Health and healthcare costs and benefits of exercise', *PharmacoEconomics*, vol 5, no pp 109-22.

NSNR (National Strategy for Neighbourhood Renewal) (2000) *Report of Policy Action Team 8: Anti-social behaviour*, London: The Stationery Office.

Olds, D., Henderson, C., Cole, R., Eckenrode, J., Kitzman, H., Luckey, D., Pettitt, L., Sidora, K., Morris, P. and Powers, J. (1998) 'Long term effects of nurse home visitation on children's criminal and anti-social behavior', *Journal of American Medical Association*, vol 280, no 14, pp 1238-44.

Parker, H., Aldridge, J. and Measham, F. (1998) *Illegal leisure: The normalization of adolescent recreational drug use*, London: Routledge.

Petrosino, A., Turpin-Petrosino, C. and Buehler, J. (2002) '"Scared Straight" and other juvenile awareness programs for preventing juvenile delinquency (Cochrane Review)', *The Cochrane Library, issue 3, 2004*, Chichester: John Wiley & Sons Ltd.

Preston, B. (1972) 'Statistical analysis of child pedestrian accidents in Manchester and Salford', *Accident Analysis and Prevention*, vol 4, no 4, pp 323-32.

Pritchard, C. (2001) *A family–teacher–social work alliance to reduce truancy and delinquency – The Dorset Healthy Alliance project*, RDS Occasional Paper No 78, London: Home Office.

Roberts, H. (2002) *What works in reducing inequalities in child health?*, Barkingside: Barnardo's.

Roberts, I., Kramer, M.S. and Suissa, S. (1996) 'Does home visiting prevent childhood injury? A systematic review of randomised controlled trials', *British Medical Journal*, vol 312, no 7022, pp 29-35.

Ronen, T. (1997) *Cognitive developmental therapy with children*, Chichester: John Wiley & Sons Ltd.

Rutter, M. (1999) 'Resilience concepts and findings: implications for family therapy', *Journal of Family Therapy*, vol 21, pp 119-44.

Schweinhart, L.J., Barnes, H.V. and Weikart, D.P. (1993) *Significant benefits: The High/Scope Perry preschool study through age 27*, Ypsilanti, MI: High/Scope Press.

Scott, S., Knapp, M., Henderson, J. and Maughan, B. (2001) 'Financial cost of social exclusion: follow up study of antisocial children into adulthood', *British Medical Journal*, vol 323, no 7306, pp 191-4.

Shelter (2005) *Shelter inclusion project: Two years on*, London: Shelter.

Shiner, M. (2000) *Doing it for themselves: An evaluation of peer approaches to drug prevention*, Briefing Paper 6, London: Drugs Prevention Advisory Service, Home Office.

Simpson, J., Morrison, L., Langley, J. and Memon, P. (2003) 'The process and impact of implementing injury prevention projects in smaller communities in New Zealand', *Health Promotion International*, vol 18, no 3, pp 237-45.

St James-Roberts, I. and Samlal Singh, C. (2001) *Can mentors help primary school children with behaviour problems?*, Home Office Research Study 233, London: Home Office Research, Development and Statistics Directorate.

Steer Davies Gleave (2003) *Evaluation of first yellow bus pilot schemes*, London: Report to the DfT.

Thomson, J. and Whelan, K. (1997) *A community approach to road safety education using practical training methods: The Drumchapel project*, Road Safety Research Report No 3, London: DfT.

Towner, E. and Dowswell, T. (2002) 'Community-based childhood injury prevention interventions: what works?', *Health Promotion International*, vol 17, no 3, pp 273-84.

Towner, E. and Ward, H. (1998) 'Prevention of injuries to children and young people: the way ahead for the UK', *Injury Prevention*, vol 4, suppl 1, pp S17–S25.

Towner, E., Dowswell, T. and Jarvis, S. (1993) *Reducing childhood accidents: The effectiveness of health promotion interventions: A literature review*, London: Health Education Authority.

Towner, E., Dowswell, T., Mackereth, C. and Jarvis, S. (2001) *What works in preventing unintentional injuries in children and young adolescents? An updated systematic review*, London: Health Development Agency.

Towner, E., Dowswell, T., Errington, G., Burkes, M. and Towner, J. (2005) *Injuries in children aged 0-14 years and inequalities*, London: Health Development Agency.

Utting, D., Vennard, J. and Scott, S. (2002) 'Young offenders in the community', in D. McNeish, T. Newman and H. Roberts (eds) *What works for children?*, Buckingham: Open University Press, pp 164-85.

West, R., Train, H., Junger, M., Pickering, A., Taylor, E. and West, A. (1998) *Childhood accidents and their relationship with problem behaviour*, Road Safety Research Report No 7, London: Road Safety Division, DETR.

What Works for Children? (2002) 'Research briefing. Reducing offending in children and young people: What works?' (www.whatworksforchildren.org.uk/docs.briefings), accessed 14 April 2005.

Woolfenden, S., Williams, K. and Peat, J. (2001) 'Family and parenting interventions in children and adolescents with conduct disorder and delinquency aged 10-17 (Cochrane Review)', *The Cochrane Library, issue 3, 2004*, Chichester: John Wiley & Sons Ltd.

EIGHT

Inequalities in health behaviours and the life trajectories of children and youth: research evidence

Introduction

In the previous two chapters, we focused on pathways and policies relating to health inequalities during childhood and youth. Clear social gradients were highlighted with regard to accidents, injuries and mental health. In other respects, however, evidence of social inequality in current health status is more equivocal. Mortality due to causes other than accidents and injuries shows much less class variation. Similarly, variation in many physical health indicators is neither substantial nor consistent. As noted in Chapter Six, the suggestion that childhood and youth is a period during which a process of equalisation takes place, social variations in health status disappearing, has been linked to a postmodern account of the potentially homogenising effects of globalisation on young people, factors such as peer groups and youth culture taking on greater significance than socio-economic background. This thesis would suggest that, due to globalisation, health inequalities based on 'modern' class divisions may begin to recede.

Against this, we have argued that health-damaging behaviours that are known to produce adverse health outcomes in later life *are* strongly subject to social gradients. Although attempts to explain socio-economic differences in unhealthy behaviours have mainly focused on adults, 'lifestyle patterns' tend to be established during childhood and youth. For example, early dietary habits shape later food preferences. The majority of smokers first experiment with smoking, are initiated into a smoking subculture and become addicted to tobacco during this period of the lifecourse. Similarly, major risk factors for the development of alcoholism in later life are the early onset of drinking and the heavy use of alcohol during late adolescence. The tendency to focus more attention on the health behaviours of adults than of young people has given rise to a relative dearth of information about how best to target interventions to tackle the development of problematic behaviours at this early stage (Droomers et al, 2003). Against this background, the first part of this chapter explores patterns of and risk factors associated with unhealthy behaviours during childhood and youth, with reference to diet and nutrition, physical exercise, substance use and sexual behaviour.

Continuities in health-damaging behaviours provide one important pathway linking early disadvantage to later outcomes. Continuities in socio-economic circumstances are another important reason why childhood disadvantage predicts poor health in adulthood. Educational outcomes can still be largely predicted on the basis of social classification. Similarly, the likelihood of entering the social care system (one of the strongest predictors of social exclusion in later life) significantly increases with social disadvantage. These critical determinants of young people's life trajectories are considered in the second part of this chapter.

Inequalities in health behaviours

Diet and nutrition

Due to the widely reported 'rising tide of obesity', the diet of British children and adolescents has been the focus of increasing attention by researchers, policy makers and the media. In addition to linking changes in the composition of children's diets to an increasing prevalence of overweight and obesity in childhood and adolescence, questions have been raised about the extent to which current dietary patterns provide children with the right balance of vitamins and minerals to support healthy growth and development. The longer-term implications of nutrition in childhood have also emerged as a concern. Dietary patterns in adulthood that are strongly associated with risk of cardiovascular disease, diabetes and many cancers may in part be established in childhood. It has also been proposed that childhood diet exerts an independent effect on health outcomes in later life.

Diet, nutrition and socio-economic status

Against this background, evidence that British schoolchildren eat relatively high amounts of processed foods and few fruits and vegetables has caused alarm. According to the 1997 National Diet and Nutrition Survey (NDNS) of 4- to 18-year-olds (Gregory et al, 2000, cited by Nessa and Gallagher, 2004), the most common foods eaten by children and adolescents in a typical week are chips, white bread, savoury snacks, biscuits, buns, cakes and pastries and chocolate confectionery, all of which had been eaten by at least three quarters of the children surveyed. A similar proportion had drunk carbonated soft drinks. Less than half of the young people had consumed any leafy green vegetables or bananas, and around a quarter had eaten citrus fruits. Just over half of the boys and girls had eaten cooked carrots and apples or pears and 59% of girls had eaten raw or salad vegetables. For boys, however, the most popular source of 'fruit and vegetables' were baked beans. Similar findings emerged in the 1995-97 and 2002 Health Surveys for England (HSE). The 1995-97 HSE found that less than a fifth of children aged 2-15 reported eating fruit and vegetables more than once every day. By contrast, a quarter of children ate sweet food such as biscuits, sweets and chocolate more than once every day (Bost et al, 1998). In the 2002 HSE, only 12% and 17% of 5- to 15-year-olds and 16- to 24-year-olds respectively ate five or more portions of fruits or vegetables a day (Deverill, 2003).

Despite concerns that many children are consuming more energy than they require (Chan, 1999), the NDNS found that average daily energy intakes fell below the recommended requirements for both boys and girls at all age groups, although protein intakes substantially exceeded recommended levels. Micronutrient deficiencies were identified in the survey. A total of 50% of 15- to 18-year-old girls and 45% of 11- to 14-year-old girls had iron intakes lower than the Lower Reference Nutrient Intake (LRNI). Teenage girls were also more likely to have lower than recommended intakes of magnesium, zinc, potassium and calcium, one quarter of 11- to 14-year-olds and one in five 15- to 18-year-olds having calcium intakes lower than the LRNI. Micronutrient deficiencies may stem in part from a tendency to miss meals, particularly breakfast. In a survey undertaken by the Schools Health Education Unit, 21% of girls aged 15-16 reported eating no breakfast, a further 19% just a drink and 15% no lunch the day before (Balding, 2001, cited by Lucas, 2003).

Both the 1997 NDNS and the 2002 HSE suggest that the dietary patterns of children and young people vary according to socio-economic status. In the latter, fruit and vegetable consumption increased with household income (Deverill, 2003). One in ten children in the lowest three income quintiles ate five or more portions a day compared with one in six in the highest income quintile. A similar pattern was observed in young adults, where 22% of young women in the highest income quintile ate five or more portions a day, compared with 16% in the lowest quintile. The difference was more marked among young men (22% in the highest income quintile compared with 12% in the lowest).

In the NDNS, young people from lower socio-economic households (manual working background, in receipt of benefits or in the bottom income quintile) were less likely to have consumed raw and salad vegetables, apples, pears and bananas and more likely to have eaten chips, sugar confectionery and burgers and kebabs. Despite this, total energy intakes of boys in households in the lowest income quintile were significantly lower than those of boys in the highest income bracket (no relationship was observed between energy intake and household wealth for girls). Children and adolescents from more advantaged socio-economic households had higher average daily intakes of protein, sugar and fat. The proportion of total energy they derived from starch was lower than for children living in more disadvantaged households.

The reasons why dietary patterns vary according to socio-economic status remain subject to debate. The concept of food poverty (a combination of price, availability and accessibility) is influential. Dowler (1999) suggests that low-income families rely on convenience-processed foods because they are relatively cheap, acceptable and predictable, with no waste and regular portion sizes. In comparison, fruit, leaner cuts of meat and wholemeal bread are viewed by the poor as luxury items. As noted in Chapter Four, a number of authors propose that food in the corner shops, convenience stores and the small independent supermarkets frequented by poorer people tends to be more expensive than in larger supermarkets. However, empirical evidence of higher food prices in deprived areas is contradictory. Social and cultural norms, knowledge and health motivation play a role in dietary patterns. For example, differences between ethnic groups can be greater than differences in income groups with respect to the consumption of vegetables and pulses. There is also growing interest in the way in which psychosocial factors associated with poverty shape health behaviours such as diet (see Chapter Ten).

Diet, nutrition and health outcomes

Diet in childhood and adolescence influences both proximate and long-term health and well-being. Short-term fasting (for example, by missing breakfast) is reported to affect cognition, memory, concentration and behaviour at school (Lucas, 2003). As well as the general fatigue brought about by anaemia, iron deficiency has been associated with impaired school performance (Chan, 1999). The consumption of sugar (particularly of non-milk extrinsic sugars) increases risk of tooth decay. In the oral health survey of the NDNS, evidence of dental caries (including active tooth decay and fillings) was found in 53% of 4- to 18-year-olds and evidence of unhealthy gums in 35%. Dental plaque was highest in 11- to 15-year-olds, where 51% were reported to have dental plaque, and was more prevalent in boys than in girls. Children in households of manual working background and where parents were in receipt of benefits were more likely to have experienced dental caries, particularly up to the age of 14. Regional differences in dental caries were observed, children and young people in Scotland experiencing the highest rates and those in London and the South East the lowest rates. The survey suggests that dental decay is associated with frequency of sugar consumption rather than total intake of sugar or sugar-containing foods (Walker et al, 2000).

In the long term, micronutrient deficiencies can have important consequences on health. Calcium, for example, influences bone formation and peak bone mass in early adulthood, which relate to the risks of rapid bone loss and osteoporosis in later life. As antioxidants in fruits and vegetables appear to protect against free radical mediated damage to DNA, the relatively low consumption of fruits and vegetables among young people in Britain should also cause concern. In the Boyd Orr Study, which involved a cohort with a 60-year follow-up, increased childhood fruit intake was inversely associated with cancer incidence in adulthood. A protective effect of vegetable consumption on cancer risk was not apparent in the study. However, as vegetables are, like fruit, a rich source of potentially anticarcinogenic compounds, the lack of association may have reflected the·

convention for prolonged cooking of vegetables at the time (pre-war) of the original survey (Maynard et al, 2003).

Another consequence of poor diet and nutrition is an increase in obesity. Childhood obesity is associated with a number of negative consequences in the short term and the longer term. Psychological/psychiatric problems and several cardiovascular risk factors (hyperlipidemia, hypertension and abnormal glucose tolerance) occur with increased frequency in obese children and adolescents. Reported increases in type II diabetes occurring in adolescence are probably related to the increase in obesity prevalence in this age group. A number of respiratory symptoms have also been associated with childhood obesity, including asthma, reduced lung capacity and sleep-related disordered breathing. In the longer term, obesity in childhood is a risk factor for adult obesity. There is also some evidence to suggest that overweight in adolescence increases adult cardiovascular morbidity and mortality independently of adult body mass index (BMI) (Reilly et al, 2003; Campbell et al, 2004).

Controversies in childhood diet and nutrition

Evidence of variations in diet according to socio-economic status, together with growing knowledge about the implications of poor diet in childhood for both proximate and long-term health, makes this an important area for health inequalities research and policy. However, this field of work is not without its controversies. Difficulties have arisen in quantifying the prevalence of overweight and obesity, in understanding the causes of this 'modern epidemic' and in linking risks for dietary problems with certain socio-economic and ethnic groups. While a BMI of 30 kg/m^2 is recognised internationally as a definition of adult obesity, BMI in childhood changes substantially with age. Previous studies have thus based estimates of overweight and obesity on the proportion of children exceeding BMI centiles in representative surveys. Typically, the 85th centile has been used to represent overweight and the 95th centile to represent obesity. In addition to leading (when standards are regularly updated) to "the self fulfilling prophecy that there will always be 15% overweight and 5% obesity" (Jebb and Prentice, 2001), these arbitrarily set cut-off points do not indicate thresholds at which overweight in children confers a risk to health. The use of different reference populations and different BMI centile cut-offs has also prevented international comparison of obesity trends and the monitoring of trends over time (Cole et al, 2000). To address these difficulties, a number of alternative measurements have been developed. A new internationally agreed reference standard for childhood obesity developed by Cole et al (2000) provides age- and sex-specific BMI cut-off points from 2-18 years of age that correspond to values of 25 kg/m^2 (overweight) and 30 kg/m^2 (obese) at age 18. Addressing concerns that BMI gives no indication of the distribution of body fat (in children, as in adults, centralised or abdominal fat carries an increased risk for health complications), reference data have also been provided on the waist circumferences of British children and adolescents, although these are expressed in centiles (McCarthy et al, 2001).

Using the new internationally agreed cut-off points, the NDNS found that 15.4% of 4- to 18-year-olds were overweight and 4% were obese (Jebb et al, 2004). These figures are slightly lower than those yielded by the 2002 HSE which, using the new international classification, found that 16.3% and 5.5% of boys aged 2-15 were respectively overweight and obese, while rates of overweight and obesity among girls were 20.3% and 7.2% respectively. The prevalence of overweight and obesity increases with age. In the 2002 HSE, 23% and 9.2% of young men aged 16-24 were respectively overweight and obese, while rates among young women were 21.2% and 11.5% (Stamatakis, 2003a). Most studies thus agree that British children and young people are getting fatter (Chinn and Rona, 2001; Rudolf et al, 2004).

Worryingly, some evidence suggests that the use of BMI may systematically underestimate the prevalence of obesity in young people (McCarthy et al, 2003). The waist circumferences of young people aged 11-16 have increased sharply (by an average of 6.9 cm between 1977-97 in boys and an average of 6.2 cm between 1987-97 in girls). These increases are greater than increases in BMI over the same period. Moreover, higher percentages of boys and girls exceed the 91st and 98th centiles for waist circumference than the equivalent centiles for BMI, suggesting that body composition may be changing over time, an increase in fat mass being obscured by a reduction in muscle mass. In 1997, 28% of boys and 38% of girls exceeded the 91st centile for waist circumference (used to represent overweight). A total of 14% and 17% of boys and girls respectively exceeded the 98th centile (the cut-off for obesity). As an accumulation of excess central fat affects levels of insulin and cholesterol, this has been identified as an important risk factor for both diabetes and heart disease. Thus, these trends in British children could have important implications for current and future morbidity.

Given evidence of an association between obesity and social disadvantage, these trends will also have important implications for health inequalities. In the 1997 NDNS, the risk of obesity was significantly higher in Social Classes IV and V than Social Classes I-III. Rates of obesity were also higher among Asian groups and children living in Wales and Scotland (Jebb et al, 2004). Secondary analysis of the 1999 HSE found little evidence of socio-economic gradients in overweight and obesity, although significant ethnic group differences were observed, African-Caribbean and Pakistani girls having an increased risk of being obese and Indian and Pakistani boys an increased risk of being overweight than the general population (Saxena et al, 2004). In the 2002 HSE, however, obesity was strongly associated with social disadvantage (as measured by household income quintile, occupational status and area deprivation), although the relationship between overweight and socio-economic status was less consistent.

Teasing out the factors that link lower socio-economic status with higher rates of overweight and obesity in childhood and youth is not straightforward as the statistical links between socio-economic status and obesity tend to be stronger than the association between obesity and behavioural risk factors. As noted earlier, for example, total energy intakes of boys in households in the lowest income quintile in the NDNS were significantly lower than those of boys in the highest income bracket. This corresponds with the 1995-97 HSE finding that *underweight* in boys aged 2-15 is skewed towards the poorest households. However, it does not explain the fact that the lower social classes are also at higher risk of being overweight. Some evidence suggests that dietary composition may be more significant than total energy intake to obesity. Although data from long-term studies are lacking, the consumption of starchy foods with a high glycemic index (such as white bread, refined cereals and potato products) has been linked to weight gain (Ludwig, 2000; Roberts, 2000; Brand-Miller et al, 2002). This hypothesis does accord with the fact that, in the NDNS, the proportion of total energy derived from starch was higher for children living in socially disadvantaged households.

The fact that the links between socio-economic status, health behaviours and obesity are not straightforward suggests that some care should be taken in assuming that the 'modern epidemic of fatness' stems from the "sedentary, sofa-lounging, fat-guzzling conditions of contemporary society" (Evans, 2003, p 88). Over-consumption of energy-rich diets and a lack of physical activity do contribute to the development of obesity in childhood and adolescence. However, there may be gender differences in the relative effects of diet and physical activity on weight gain (Steinbeck, 2001). A range of other factors also contribute to the development of obesity. As noted in Chapter Four, intrauterine growth retardation and rapid postnatal catch-up growth are believed to influence predisposition to obesity in later life. Susceptibility to obesity is also influenced by genetic factors, twin studies suggesting that at least 50% of the tendency towards obesity is inherited (Kiess et al, 2001). Thus, as in mental health, obesity is now understood to stem from a complex interaction between genes and environment.

The interpretation of socio-economic variations in the prevalence of obesity should be sensitive to its multifactorial causation or lower socio-economic and ethnic groups are in danger of being stigmatised "as pathologically unable to look after their bodies" (Evans, 2003, p 92). There are dangers that the portrayal of obesity and, increasingly, overweight, as a 'disease' may in itself contribute to psychological problems such as lowered self-esteem and depression in otherwise healthy adolescents. This 'obesity discourse' also ignores the fact that the relationship between obesity and adverse health outcomes appears to be mediated by other factors such as level of physical activity. For example, obese men who are moderately fit have a lower death rate than men who have a healthy weight but who are unfit (Brodney et al, 2000, cited by Evans, 2003). According to Evans (2003), the current focus on body shape, size and weight is simplistic, alarmist and stigmatising. He proposes that a more balanced approach is required that recognises that it is possible to be healthy and overweight at the same time.

It is important to recognise the danger of simplifying the relationship between socio-economic status and obesity and of stigmatising particular groups. Against this, there is plentiful evidence to suggest that diet in childhood should be taken very seriously. Thus, Evans' concerns about the extent to which children's diets and lifestyles are being increasingly subject to medical surveillance and control (Evans et al, 2003) must face equally legitimate concerns that many children are not enjoying the healthy diets that they need and deserve.

Physical activity

Although there is an extensive literature documenting the health benefits of regular physical activity in adults, activity–health relationships in children are not clear-cut (Livingstone et al, 2003). Low physical activity levels and sedentary behaviours are associated with an increased risk of weight gain and obesity in children and young people. More active children also tend to develop higher peak bone masses than their less active counterparts. Thus, regular weight-bearing exercise in pubertal girls may provide longer-term protection against osteoporosis (MacKelvie et al, 2003). There is some evidence that the cardiovascular profiles of active children are generally healthier (Boreham and Riddoch, 2001). In contrast to adults, however, where physical activity has been shown to affect cardiovascular risk factors positively, the correlation with physical activity and body fatness in children tends to be stronger than physical activity effects on cardiovascular risk factors (Steinbeck, 2001). This in part reflects the low prevalence of cardiovascular abnormality at this age. Finally, although some studies suggest that there is a behavioural carry forward of physical activity, active children being more likely to become active adults, data supporting the notion of physical activity tracking are weak (Livingstone et al, 2003). Much of the focus on physical activity in children has thus centred on its role in protecting against overweight and obesity.

Physical activity comprises a wider range of activities than those that are traditionally associated with 'exercise', 'sport' or 'PE'. Thus, while vigorous exercise may be the most effective way of improving cardiovascular fitness and strength, and weight-bearing activities are beneficial to muscular strength and bone health, evidence does suggest that cumulative moderate activity (such as walking, active play, dancing and helping with household chores) contributes to the prevention or reduction of obesity. Current recommendations state that all young people should participate in physical activity of at least moderate intensity for one hour per day (Rees et al, 2001). In the NDNS, only 61% of boys and 42% of girls aged 4–18 achieved this level (Rees et al, 2001). In the 2002 HSE, 70% of boys and 61% of girls aged 2–15 participated in physical activity for one hour or more. Among girls (but not among boys), overall participation rates in physical activity were found to decline with age after about age 10 (Stamatakis, 2003b). Both surveys suggest that participation in physical activity declines with age. In the 2002 HSE, 51% of young men and 28% of young women aged 16-24 participated in activity of at least moderate intensity for at least 30 minutes on five or more days a week.

It is not clear whether physical activity levels among British children are declining over time or not. Children are spending less time on physical activity in school. According to the Young People and Sport Survey commissioned by Sport England, 46% of young people surveyed in 1994 participated in two hours or more of PE lessons per week, compared to 32% in 1999. The proportion of school children spending less than one hour a week in PE rose from 5% to 18% over the same period. The decline in physical activity in school was in part compensated for by an increase in time spent undertaking physical activity out of school. During term times, however, only 24% of children spent more than 10 hours a week in physical activity outside school. During the summer holidays, 45% of children achieved at least this amount of exercise. However, more time was spent watching television or videos than participating in physical activity (Nessa and Gallagher, 2004).

Despite concerns that sedentary pastimes such as television watching have contributed to the rise in childhood obesity, Biddle et al (2004) found little association between television viewing and videogame playing and physical activity, suggesting that children and young people have time for both active and sedentary pursuits. Levels of accumulative moderate activity have been affected by the decline in the numbers of children who walk to school. The proportion of primary school children walking to school fell from 63% in 1992/94 to 54% in 1999/2001 (Nessa and Gallagher, 2004). There is also general agreement that parental physical activity has an influence on their children's activity, the likelihood of an active lifestyle significantly increasing if both parents are also active (Steinbeck, 2001). However, in contrast to studies of adults, socio-economic status has not been strongly associated with physical activity in children (Batty and Leon, 2002). Indeed, some evidence suggests that children from lower social classes are more likely to engage in sports and active play (Macintyre and Mutrie, 2004).

Substance misuse

While most young people in Britain do not expose themselves to major health risks, adolescence does appear to be a time of heightened risk taking. Some young people participate in sporting activities that have an element of risk, such as climbing and extreme sports, while others turn to more deviant activities such as joy-riding, illicit drug use and drinking. Although a distinction is generally drawn between positive and problematic risk behaviours, some researchers suggest that different forms of risk taking are underpinned by similar psychological factors (Plant and Plant, 1992; France, 2000). One explanation for heightened risk taking in adolescence is that experimentation is a normal and indeed healthy part of growing up. Insofar as trying out new activities helps young people to expand their horizons, gain mastery over new challenges, gain autonomy and form their own identities, risk taking serves to fulfil developmental needs. A second approach associates risk taking with the inherent need that young people have for sensation. Third, it has been proposed that risk taking reflects the fact that young people often view themselves as invulnerable and thus believe that the negative outcomes of risk taking cannot happen to them.

All of these approaches suggest that risk taking by young people is "natural, commonplace and, in some form or another, inevitable" (Plant and Plant, 1992, p 120). It is important nevertheless to acknowledge that, even if risk taking is a normal part of adolescence, the form that risk behaviour takes varies according to social and cultural context. Participation in 'positive' risk behaviours such as outdoor sports and international travel benefits from the provision of material resources and family/peer expectations that are more commonly associated with social advantage. By contrast, 'problematic' risk behaviours such as alcohol/drug misuse and dependence are more strongly associated with social deprivation. Young people with mental health disorders are at particularly high risk of substance misuse, which in turn exacerbates existing disorders. Thus, there are strong correlations between substance misuse and suicide, depression, conduct disorder, school drop-out and poor scholastic achievement. Substance misuse also contributes to other causes of mortality and morbidity such as accidents and injuries (Gilvarry, 2000).

Smoking

Although the use of tobacco is not associated with the array of social and behavioural problems that are linked to the use of alcohol and illicit drugs, cigarette smoking causes more health damage than any other psychoactive drug (Plant and Plant, 1992, p 33). Most smokers start smoking in their teenage years and the majority of young regular smokers smoke into their middle age (Jefferis et al, 2003). Persistent smoking contributes to adult disease and death from cancers, cardiovascular disease and respiratory disorders (see Chapter Ten), although smokers who quit by their thirties avoid most of the mortality risk attributable to smoking (Doll et al, 2004). Cigarette smoking during adolescence (particularly among those who start smoking young) has also been shown to be associated with increased risk for alcohol, cannabis, hard drug and multiple drug disorders, although a causal connection between adolescent smoking and subsequent substance misuse has not been established (Lewinsohn et al, 1999).

Few teenagers in the UK are unaware of the health consequences of cigarette smoking. Yet, according to the English Survey on Smoking, Drinking and Drug Use among Young People in 2002, 16% of English school children in 2002 had tried smoking by 11 years of age and by the age of 15, 63% had smoked cigarettes

(Natarajan and McManus, 2003). A proportion of children and adolescents who experiment with cigarettes go on to become regular smokers. A total of 20% of boys and 26% of girls aged 15 in the 2002 survey were regular smokers who smoked at least one cigarette a week. The prevalence of smoking increases further after the age of 16. In the 2002 HSE, 33% of young men and 35% of young women aged 16-24 reported that they were current cigarette smokers. Comparisons of the 1997 HSE with the 2003 HSE suggest that there has been a decrease in smoking by young men (from 37%). However, there has been little change in children's smoking levels, nor in the smoking of young women between the two periods (Wardle and Hedges, 2003).

A range of factors influences the uptake of regular smoking among children and young people (see Tyas and Pederson, 1998). Children whose parents, siblings and friends smoke are more likely to take up the habit (Green et al, 1991; Withers et al, 2000). Conversely, when young people's primary contacts are with non-smokers, they are less likely to engage in this behaviour. The impact of family influences on the uptake of regular smoking appears to be greater at younger ages. Thereafter the effect of friends' smoking far outweighs that of family members' (West et al, 1999). Younger teenagers, then, are less likely to smoke when their parents and siblings do not smoke, when their parents voice strong opposition to smoking, monitor their children's behaviour, use positive/authoritative parenting, are supportive and participate in activities with their children (Kobus, 2003). There is also a strong association between adolescent smoking and family structure, children being significantly less likely to smoke when they are living with both of their biological parents (Bjarnason et al, 2003; Griesbach et al, 2003).

The association between parental smoking and smoking initiation among young teenagers suggests that the strong socio-economic gradient that exists in adult smoking should be preceded in youth. However, research evidence of a relationship between social class and smoking in young people has been inconsistent (West et al, 1999). This may be a reflection of the definition of smoking adopted (Sweeting and West, 2001). The category 'current smoker' does not distinguish between those who smoke one or two cigarettes a week and those who smoke more than 10 cigarettes a day. When level of smoking is considered, a strong class gradient exists between teenagers in the lowest social classes who are the heaviest smokers and those from professional backgrounds who are the lightest smokers (Sweeting and West, 2001). In the 2002 HSE, for example, mean levels of saliva cotinine were over four times higher in boys aged 4-15 from the lowest household income quintile than in boys from the highest quintile. In both boys and girls, cotinine levels increased in a stepwise fashion with declining household income.

While the impact of family smoking on smoking uptake appears to decline at mid-youth, friends' smoking is of continued significance. There is a range of perspectives on the relationship between the uptake of smoking and friendship groups (Kobus, 2003). On the one hand, young people may simply select their friends on the basis of their smoking characteristics (peer selection). On the other hand, peers may somehow influence smoking initiation. For example, being surrounded by others who smoke may convey the message that smoking is an enjoyable and socially acceptable activity. Peer groups may also create an internal self-pressure to smoke, young people believing that by trying cigarettes they will avoid potential exclusion by peers and gain social approval. Concerns have been expressed that teenage girls in particular perceive that cigarette smoking contributes to the portrayal of a popular, cool and sexy image. It is important to note, however, that peer group membership often deters smoking, even current smokers discouraging their friends from using tobacco. Individual factors such as anxiety, self-esteem, psychopathology and relationships with parents and teachers may also affect the way in which young people select and respond to influences around them.

Some research suggests that the relative roles of peer selection and peer influence may vary according to gender. Reviewing a number of North American studies that have examined the relationship between the social reputation of groups and tobacco use, Kobus (2003) notes a distinction between trouble-making boys and 'top girls', groups that are both likely to smoke. The former engage in a range of risk-taking behaviours including drinking, drug misuse and fighting. Their smoking does not appear to be related to difficulties in resisting peer pressure, but instead to reflect their personal motivations to smoke. Thus, these youth select each other as friends, smoking behaviour preceding group formation (although the fact that peer influence reinforces smoking behaviour cannot be ruled out). By contrast, smoking initiation among 'top girls' is subject to peer influence. 'Top girls' choose to smoke (as well as drink, use drugs, wear the 'right' clothes and date boys) in order to maintain their status at the top of the social hierarchy (Kobus, 2003, p 48). The likelihood that they will continue to smoke is also influenced by peer friendships (Fergusson et al, 1995a). For example, smoking may be seen as a way of breaking the ice in new situations, asking someone for a cigarette providing an 'opening line' (Seguire and Chalmers, 2000). This has important implications for smoking cessation as adolescents who smoke regularly and whose friends all smoke are less likely to quit (Paavola et al, 2001).

As noted earlier, the growing impact of influences outside the family (for example, the peer group and youth culture) in adolescence and the diminishing role of family characteristics has been linked with an 'equalisation of health' in youth. In later youth, smoking levels continue to be characterised by a social gradient, although this is not as strong as in early youth. In the 2002 HSE, for example, mean levels of saliva cotinine among men and women aged 16-24 in the bottom income quintile were respectively 1.7 and 2.6 times higher than in men and women from the top quintile.

Evidence that stereotypes or images held about social identities affect decisions about tobacco use in youth throws some light on the role that cigarette advertising may play in influencing smoking among young people. Theoretical and empirical evidence exists for a causal relationship between tobacco promotional activities and both the onset of smoking and progression to established smoking (Choi et al, 2002; Pierce et al, 2002; Lovato et al, 2003). Thus, smoking by young people in Britain has also been influenced by wider contextual factors. During the period September 2001 to August 2002, tobacco advertising expenditure in the UK amounted to £25 million, excluding sponsorship and indirect advertising (ASH, 2004). In addition, tobacco companies have traditionally invested heavily (an estimated £78 million a year) in the sponsorship of sport to promote their brands. Through this medium, millions of viewers watching motor racing, snooker and rugby were exposed to images of smoking. Following the implementation of the 2003 Tobacco Advertising and Promotion Act, however, most forms of tobacco advertising and promotion (on billboards, in newspapers and websites and, from 2005/06, through international sports sponsorship) are now banned in the UK. There is considerable international evidence to suggest that the introduction of a tobacco advertising ban results in a reduction in tobacco consumption. However, concerns have been expressed about the ability of tobacco companies to find other ways of advertising their products through, for example, the marketing of clothing and accessories with a shared brand name. In addition, Action on Smoking and Health (ASH) suggests that some tobacco companies have set up covert websites to attract young people. These typically contain information about nightclubs or other events where cigarettes are promoted (ASH, 2004). Thus, the impact of this advertising ban on the prevalence and levels of cigarette smoking among British youth has yet to be seen.

Alcohol consumption

In certain respects, alcohol is different to illicit drugs and cigarettes. Drinking is legal and, for most sections of the community, socially acceptable. Thus, most young people in Britain have parents who drink and come into contact with other adults who drink. In contrast to tobacco, even moderate amounts of which cause health damage, light to moderate alcohol intake has been associated with reduced risk of cardiovascular disease (Brenner et al, 2001; Trevisan et al, 2004). However, the protective effect of alcohol is subject to debate (Marmot, 2001), some researchers arguing that observed associations are a reflection of certain lifestyle factors in light to moderate drinkers (lower levels of smoking and obesity), and the fact that people who abstain from drinking (and who appear to be at greater risk of cardiovascular disease) may do so *because* they feel unwell (Wannamethee and Shaper, 1999; Wouters et al, 2000).

If evidence of the protective effect of alcohol is equivocal, most studies agree that high intakes of alcohol are associated with increased morbidity and mortality (Hart et al, 1999). Most alcohol-related diseases take years to develop and are comparatively rare in young people. However, the early onset of drinking and the heavy use of alcohol during late adolescence are risk factors for the development of alcoholism in later life (Chou and Pickering, 1992; Hemmingsson and Lundberg, 2001). Alcohol is also an important contributory factor to deaths in young people by injury and poisoning (Stanistreet and Jeffrey, 2003). There is a strong association between binge drinking, crime and disorder among young men, 39% of binge drinkers in the 1998/99 Youth Lifestyles Survey admitting to having committed an offence and 60% admitting criminal and/or disorderly behaviour during or after drinking alcohol (Richardson and Budd, 2003). As noted in Chapter Six, between a third and a quarter of all violent crimes are alcohol-related, high levels of alcohol consumption characterising both offenders and the victims of assault (Budd, 2003). Alcohol consumption also affects the sexual behaviour of heterosexual young people, increasing the likelihood of early-onset sexual intercourse and unprotected sex (Fergusson and Lynskey, 1996). This may have implications for unwanted pregnancies and sexually transmitted diseases, including HIV (Murgraff et al, 1999).

Unfortunately, UK teenagers, together with those in a number of other Northern European countries, have among the highest levels of alcohol consumption in Europe (Plant and Miller, 2001). According to the European School Survey Project on Alcohol and Other Drugs, which included more than 90,000 students aged 15-16 in 1999, 28% of British teenagers reported being drunk on 10 or more occasions over the past 12 months. Heavy drinking sessions typically occur during weekend evenings and were reported to be associated with a number of adverse effects relating to sexual behaviour and delinquency (Plant and Miller, 2001).

High rates of alcohol intoxication are a reflection of a general increase in alcohol consumption among young people. According to the English Survey on Smoking, Drinking and Drug Use among Young People in 2002, the proportion of 11- to 15-year-olds who drink at least once a week increased from 13% in 1992 to 20% in 2002 (Blenkinsop, 2003a). Average weekly consumption of alcohol over the same period increased from 6.0 to 10.6 units. By 2002, boys and girls aged 15 had average weekly alcohol intakes of 14.3 and 11.4 units respectively. They were, moreover, familiar with a wide range of alcoholic drinks. Of the 47% of 15-year-olds who had drunk in the past week, 72% had consumed beer, lager or cider, 68% alcopops, 65% spirits and 41% wine. Beer, lager and cider accounted for the largest proportion of total alcohol consumption in boys, while girls drank proportionately higher amounts of spirits and alcopops (Blenkinsop, 2003b). Although provisions to prevent the sale of alcohol to underage drinkers are being more rigorously enforced, evidence suggests that they are not effectively restricting access to alcohol. This partly reflects the fact that teenagers are less likely to buy alcohol from off-licences and more likely to obtain it from their friends and relatives.

Among young men and women, alcohol consumption increases with age, peaking at around age 20-21 for young men with respect to mean weekly units consumed and around age 18-20 for young women. Thereafter weekly alcohol consumption declines (Erens, 2003). In the 2002 HSE, 42% of young men aged

SCINDLER + BICRA

16–24 exceeded the recommended limit of 21 units a week (up from 33% in the 1997 HSE) and 32% of young women drank more than 14 units (up from 22%). Mean consumption on the heaviest drinking day in the past week was estimated as 11.2 units for young male drinkers and 6.7 units for young female drinkers. The prevalence of binge drinking (consuming twice the recommended daily limit) was 61% among men and 52% among women. Binge drinking among young women (but not young men) has increased significantly since 1998 (the year when questions on the heaviest drinking day were introduced to the HSE), when 38% of young females were estimated to consume six or more units on their heaviest drinking day (Erens, 2003).

Young people drink alcohol for a range of reasons. Psychological factors common to all risk-taking behaviour are likely to play a role, children using alcohol to experience the adult world, satisfy their curiosity, test out their own limits and to have fun (Robson, 2001). Family socialisation processes such as modelling, supervision, norms and relationships are also at work. Adolescents whose parents drink alcohol are more inclined to drink themselves. Droomers et al (2003) suggest that inadequate parenting, poor parental monitoring and control, poor parental support, poor family cohesion or bonding, positive parental norms or tolerance of alcohol and family alcohol problems are linked to increased adolescent alcohol consumption. Links between parental alcohol misuse and the presence of alcohol problems in offspring may suggest a genetic contribution (Gilvarry, 2000). Peer influences are also significant, particularly among older children. For example, in a longitudinal study, Fergusson et al (1995b) found that association/affiliation with substance-using peers at the age of 15 independently predicted abusive or hazardous alcohol consumption at the age of 16.

Research evidence of a relationship between socio-economic status and heavy drinking in youth is very mixed. Studies in New Zealand suggest that socio-economic background affects adolescent alcohol consumption substantially, young people from more disadvantaged backgrounds being more likely to drink larger amounts of alcohol (Droomers et al, 2003) and to binge drink (Casswell et al, 2003), while young people from more advantaged backgrounds drank more frequently, but in smaller amounts. In England, by contrast, there is little evidence to suggest that young people's alcohol use is linked to social disadvantage. In the 2002 HSE, young men and women from the highest income quintile had the highest mean consumption of alcohol units and were most likely to have drunk over 50 units in the previous week. Binge drinking did not vary consistently by household income, although young women in the highest income quartile were more likely to have consumed six or more units on their heaviest drinking day than young women from the bottom income quintile.

It is possible that the lack of a link between social disadvantage and alcohol abuse in the 2002 HSE reflects the failure to distinguish severity criteria for alcohol 'problems'. Regular excessive drinking is not synonymous with alcohol misuse and alcohol dependence and may be subject to different risk factors

(Holly and Wittchen, 1998). Thus, the HSE may have failed to capture the subgroup of 'problem drinkers' who are reaching criteria for alcohol dependence. Although Swedish research suggests that risk of alcoholism is not strongly associated with social class of origin, young adults with high levels of alcohol dependency are at risk of downward social mobility that in turn produces social class inequalities (Hemmingsson et al, 1999). A second subgroup worthy of further analysis comprises young people who have both alcohol dependency and a comorbid mental health problem such as conduct disorder. In such cases, similar sets of individual, family and environmental factors appear to be at work that are strongly associated with social disadvantage.

Illicit drug use

As well as having among the highest levels of alcohol consumption, young Britons have been identified as the most drug-involved in Europe. According to the European School Survey Project carried out in 1995, over 40% of 15- to 16-year-olds surveyed in the UK had tried at least one drug. Scottish adolescents were particularly likely to have experienced an illicit drug (50.1% of those surveyed, compared to 39.6% in England). Only Ireland (37%) came anywhere near these levels, with the European norm being around 10% (Parker, 2001, p 2). Similar proportions of 15-year-olds in the English Survey on Smoking, Drinking and Drug Use among Young People admitted to having tried drugs. By 2002, 43% of boys and 38% of girls had tried drugs (excluding volatile substances), 25% and 18% respectively in the last month (McManus and Natarajan, 2003). The Northern Regions Longitudinal Study (which included volatile substances) identified slightly higher levels of regular drug use. A total of 52.5% of younger cohort 15-year-olds sampled in the North of England had tried drugs and 32.2% had taken at least one drug in the past month (Egginton et al, 2001).

The Northern Regions Longitudinal Study suggests that drug-trying rates rise with age, but perhaps begin to plateau at around 17 years. Significant differences were observed between sixth formers and those who left secondary school after taking their GCSEs. Almost 65% of 17-year-old school leavers had tried a drug. 17.9% were regular users and 27.6% intended to try drugs again (that is, were 'potential users'). By contrast, 53.1% of sixth formers had tried a drug, 23.5% were potential users and 14.5% regular users. The drugs involved in trying episodes also varied between the two groups. School leavers reported substantially higher rates of use for all drugs, except legal herbal 'highs'. Drugs where relative use by school leavers was most significantly higher than that of sixth formers included tranquillisers, heroin (tried by a very small minority), amphetamines and LSD. In absolute terms, cannabis and nitrates were the most popular drugs tried by both groups (Egginton et al, 2001).

Adolescent drug use is often associated with deviancy and personal, social and educational deficits, particularly in the North American literature. Researchers involved in the Northern Regions Longitudinal Study have consistently challenged this picture, arguing that during the 1990s, drug use by youth became normalised (Parker et al, 1998). This was particularly the case for cannabis, but also nitrates, amphetamines and, equivocally, LSD and ecstasy, which were associated with the dance club scene. Features of normalisation included the widespread availability and use of recreational drugs; cultural acceptance of social drug use, which is no longer seen to belong to an unknown subcultural world; and the broad socio-economic profile of young people using recreational drugs (Parker et al, 1998). For example, dance club users come disproportionately from higher social groups and are usually in higher education or employment (Measham et al, 2001).

The Northern Regions Longitudinal Study certainly suggests that English adolescents who try, occasionally use, or regularly use, illicit drugs are not personally, educationally or socially atypical. In this study, neither 'race', parental occupation, school attainment nor, in the younger cohort, gender predicted drug involvement. Regular drug users were more likely to live in single-parent families, to have poorer personal relationships with their parents and to go out in the evenings unsupervised. Early smoking and early regular drinking were also significant predictors of drug use. In general, however, at least in terms of their own age cohort, drug-using youth could not be described as atypical, unconventional or deviant. Indeed, like the significant minority of college/ university students who are heavy drinkers and drug users, many will eventually become overtly successful and productive citizens (Egginton et al, 2001).

The largely conventional identity of many young drug users lies at the heart of the normalisation thesis with respect to recreational drug use. However, it is important to point out that heroin and cocaine are not included in this thesis (Parker et al, 1998). This reflects the fact that fewer young people experiment with these drugs; they are more physically addictive and, rather than being accommodated into leisure time, heroin tends to pull people into lifestyles that centre on obtaining funds to continue their habit. In contrast to the wide range of social backgrounds of recreational drug users, heroin use is found primarily in deprived communities, among marginalised young men with poor educational and occupational prospects. A qualitative survey of 86 young heroin users in four English towns found significant levels of relative poverty, childhood disruption, family difficulties (including alcohol or drug problems), school truancy and early onset of smoking and drinking (Measham et al, 2001). Heroin dependency often reinforces delinquent and criminal behaviour, leads to a breakdown of relationships with parents and relatives, is associated with a range of personal health problems and raises major childcare and child protection issues (Parker, 2001). It is thus strongly linked with and further exacerbates social exclusion.

Although the normalisation thesis is quite controversial, it can be seen as a pragmatic response to the fact that there are now too many young people experimenting with drugs to pathologise. The distinction between 'normal' recreational drug use and 'problematic' use of more addictive drugs is not, however, without its problems. Dance clubbers, for example, are at the serious end of recreational drug use, taking large amounts of different drugs, including Class A ecstasy and cocaine (Measham et al, 2001). Because of their social profiles and self-regulated drug use very few are likely to be caught up in the criminal justice system. This raises the question of whether their Class A drug use is less 'problematic' than that of poor, unemployed drug users simply by virtue of the fact that they are middle class and can afford their habit. Further, it should not be assumed that recreational drug use has no adverse effects. A high proportion of drug users on the club scene report physical and psychological health problems and have been admitted to an Accident and Emergency Department as a result of both drug use and injury (Measham et al, 2001). The rise in heroin use can also be seen as an unwanted consequence of the normalisation of recreational drug use (Parker et al, 2001), general tolerance of drugs among young people and the wider availability of harder drugs breaking down previous barriers to experimenting with this drug. Thus, there is a blurring of the boundaries between 'recreational' and 'problematic' drug use. It nevertheless remains the case that drug users with the greatest problems with regard to health, well-being and future social and economic trajectories are those using heroin and crack cocaine in Britain's poorest communities.

Sexual health

Concern about the sexual behaviour of adolescents and young adults has grown in recent years, in part because of the recognition that rates of teenage pregnancy are particularly high in the UK, but also due to the fact that sexually transmitted infections (STIs) are increasingly prevalent in this age group. Teenage pregnancy (but not occurrence of STIs) is significantly associated with early age of first intercourse and evidence suggests that the age at which young people first have sex has steadily declined (Wellings et al, 2001). Over the last 10 years, age at first sexual intercourse has dropped from 17 to 16 years in the UK. In 2000, 26% of women and 30% of men aged 16-19 were under 16 years of age at first sexual intercourse (Munro et al, 2004). Rising rates of sexual activity among young teenagers have become a particular cause of concern, although surveys vary in their estimates of sexual activity by age. In a 1997 survey of 13- to 14-year-old school pupils in central and southern England, 6.7% of boys and girls reported already having sexual intercourse (Bonell et al, 2003), while 18.0% of 13- to 14-year-old boys and 15.4% of girls in east Scotland reported having sexual intercourse. For nearly three quarters of these, their first such experience had occurred before their 13th birthday (Wight et al, 2000). Other studies support these higher estimates of the numbers of teenagers aged 12 and 13 who are becoming sexually active. In eastern England, for example, 20% of 13-year-olds in a school-based survey of 13- to 18-year-olds reported that they had already had either full or oral sexual intercourse with a partner (Burack, 1999). A good proportion of young teenagers regret their first experience of sexual intercourse, 32% of girls and 27% of boys in the east Scotland study feeling that this had happened too early (Wight et al, 2000).

Early age of first intercourse and teenage pregnancy are associated with lower socio-economic status (Bonell et al, 2003; McLeod, 2001). This relationship is in part mediated by family influences such as living with a single parent, having older sexually active siblings, parental values concerning teenage sexual activity, quality of communication about sex and poor parental supervision (Wellings et al, 1999; Miller, 2002). In particular, father absence is associated with elevated risk for early sexual activity (Woodward et al, 2001; Ellis et al, 2003). Early adolescent conduct problems, which are themselves associated with social, family and personal disadvantage, predict early-onset sexual activity (Fergusson and Woodward, 2000). Low educational aspirations and problems with school also appear to be associated with attitudes and practices regarding sex. For example, in the central and south England survey, dislike of school was significantly associated with early sex, as well as expectations of having sex before the age of 16, a belief that most peers were already sexually active and expecting to be a parent by the age of 20 (Bonell et al, 2003). Finally, there may be an additional neighbourhood effect, attitudes and behaviour of peers shaping the sexual behaviour of children growing up in deprived communities (McCulloch, 2001).

Teenage pregnancy and motherhood

During the 1990s, teenage pregnancy was identified as a major public health 'problem' in the UK. As we discuss below, this conceptualisation is not without its critics. It was based, however, on the recognition that national rates of teenage pregnancy were higher than those in most other developed countries. The teenage birth rate in the UK was similar to that in other Northern European countries in the 1970s. Continental birth rates fell in the following two decades, but this was not the case in the UK. Countries such as Norway, Sweden, Denmark, Germany and the Netherlands, which have teenage pregnancy rates that are considerably lower than those of the UK, also have an earlier and more open approach to sexual issues in schools and in families. This is associated, in the Netherlands at least, with later ages at first sexual intercourse, better communication and forward planning between partners, more effective contraceptive use and lower levels of subsequent regret (Ingham, 2000). There are some signs that, since the late 1990s, conception rates in under 18-year-olds in England and Wales have started to decline. Nevertheless, large numbers of teenage girls are affected. In 2001, 41,000 women under the age of 18 conceived, over 22,000 of whom continued with their pregnancies (data derived from the Office for National Statistics [ONS]). Thus, a significant number of children are living with a teenage mother.

While teenage pregnancy is strongly associated with socio-economic disadvantage, the relationship is even more pronounced for early motherhood. This is because a significant proportion of conceptions by girls under the age of 18 results in abortion and young women in areas that are socially deprived are less likely to use abortion to resolve unplanned pregnancy than their counterparts in wealthier areas (Lee et al, 2004). In 2001, 45.7% of the 41,000 pregnancies that occurred in women under 18 years of age in England and Wales resulted in a termination (data derived from the ONS). In under 16-year-olds, the abortion rate rose to 55.8%. Young women's pregnancy decisions reflect their social and economic circumstances. Pregnancy can be a calamity for those who expect to become better educated, better skilled and to pursue a career. By contrast, motherhood can represent a rational and meaningful life option for women with low expectations of education and the job market (Geronimus, 1997, cited by Arai, 2003). Thus, a young woman's decision whether to continue with a pregnancy or not is strongly shaped by her social and economic prospects.

The fact that, for some women, early child-bearing can be seen as a positive and rational behaviour does not sit easily with the tendency to depict early pregnancy and motherhood as problematic and even pathological (Arai, 2003). This reflects an understanding that teenage pregnancy is associated with poor health and socio-economic consequences. It is often assumed, for example, that premature parenthood *causes* future poverty by affecting educational attainment and employment opportunities, thus creating long-term benefit dependency and poverty. However, the adverse socio-economic outcomes faced by young mothers are at least in part accounted for by individual and family background (Jaffee, 2002; Chevalier and Viitanen, 2003). Indeed, some researchers go so far as to suggest that the life trajectories of socially disadvantaged women are little altered by teenage pregnancy and that, rather than wait for cumulative exposure to poverty to increase risks of poor pregnancy outcomes, it makes more sense for such women to have their children in their teens (Geronimus, 1992, cited by Rich-Edwards, 2002).

Questions have also been raised as to whether poor health outcomes associated with teenage pregnancy (for example, anaemia, pregnancy-related hypertension, low birth weight, prematurity, intrauterine growth retardation and neonatal mortality) are attributable to age of mother or other factors. A large review of research suggested that, other than a modest increase in prematurity, low birth weight and neonatal death when maternal age is less than 16, age has little effect. Instead, the relationship between adverse outcomes and teenage pregnancy is confounded by social, economic and behavioural factors such as smoking (Cunnington, 2001). It is also debatable whether poor psychosocial adjustment, poor parenting skills and associated developmental and behavioural problems in the children of teenage parents reflects the impact of maternal age (on maternal role satisfaction, mother–infant interaction, attitudes to child discipline and realistic expectations of infant behaviour and development) or restricted access to information and education, which can occur at any age (Lawlor and Shaw, 2002).

Thus, the idea that teenage pregnancy should be conceptualised as a public health 'problem' is not without its critics. It is nevertheless the case that women who become pregnant in their teens are more likely to experience problems during pregnancy, to engage in health-damaging behaviours, and to experience adverse birth outcomes than their older counterparts. As noted in Chapter Four, evidence suggests that teenage mothers are the most likely of all age groups to lack support from partners and the wider community, and to experience depression and anxiety. According to the 2002 HSE, mothers aged 16-24 were significantly less likely to have planned their pregnancies (43%) than older women (over 70%), and were more likely to report relationship problems, a lack of social support, and unhappiness about their pregnancy. The 2002 HSE also found lower rates of protective behaviour among young mothers. Those aged 16-24 were more likely to smoke during pregnancy (34% compared to 12% aged 35 and over) and less likely to take folate supplementation before and during pregnancy. As to be expected, all of these factors also varied according to income status (Blake, 2003; Herrick and Kelly, 2003). However, the fact that these risk factors may have more to do with socio-economic position than age should not detract from the fact that teenage mothers and their children are a highly vulnerable group.

Sexually transmitted infections

Young people generally have a higher number of sexual partners, a greater number of concurrent partnerships and change partners more often than older age groups (HPA et al, 2003). As a result they are more vulnerable to acquiring an STI. Unfortunately, sexual health has deteriorated in recent years – surveillance data indicated a rise in the prevalence of acute STIs since 1999, with a particularly steep increase being noted for those aged 24 years and under. Between 1997 and 2002, diagnoses of chlamydia, gonorrhoea and new HIV infections have doubled and new diagnoses of syphilis have increased ninefold (data derived from the Health Protection Agency [HPA]). Rates of chlamydia, gonorrhoea and genital warts were highest among females aged 16-19 and males aged 20-24 (HPA et al, 2003, p 44). In 2002, women aged 16-24 accounted for 72% of all female chlamydia diagnoses, 66% of gonorrhoea (40% of females cases were under the age of 20), 62% of syphilis (although rates of syphilis in young people remain low) and 61% of genital warts reported by genitourinary medicine (GUM) clinics in England, Wales and Northern Ireland. Rates of genital herpes simplex are also highest among males and females aged 16-24. Risk exposure to HIV is more evenly distributed, people aged 16-24 accounting for just over 10% of all reports of new HIV diagnoses in 2002 (Brown, et al, 2004). However, high rates of other STIs and evidence of increasing unsafe sexual behaviour in this age group means that they may be increasingly vulnerable to HIV infection (Munro et al, 2004, p 7).

If left untreated, many STIs are associated with serious health consequences such as cervical cancer, pelvic inflammatory disease (PID), ectopic pregnancy, infertility and congenital complications. It is estimated that nearly 40% of cases of PID in women might be attributable to prior infection with chlamydia (Munro et al, 2004). Because most chlamydia infections in women are asymptomatic, this STI is particularly subject to under-diagnosis and treatment. Thus, while surveillance data from GUM clinics suggests a prevalence rate of 1.2% in women aged 16-19 (HPA et al, 2003), 3% of women aged 18-24 in the 2002 National Survey of Sexual Attitudes and Lifestyle who provided a urine sample were infected with chlamydia (Munro et al, 2004, p 5). High rates of gonorrhoea in young people are also of concern as, like chlamydia, this can lead to PID, ectopic pregnancy and infertility. In contrast to genital chlamydia, gonorrhoea tends to be a highly concentrated disease, with high rates being found in urban deprived populations and among black minority ethnic populations (HPA et al, 2003, p 31). Gonococcal rates in London represent over 40% of all diagnoses in the UK and rates are over 10 times higher in black minority ethnic populations compared with other ethnic groups living in London (Munro et al, 2004, p 5). Almost half of heterosexual diagnoses of syphilis in London between 2001-03 occurred in black ethnic groups. HIV infection rates are also significantly higher among black minority ethnic populations, the majority of whom are black Africans, although rates in black Caribbeans have increased rapidly in recent years (HPA et al, 2003, p 47).

Sexual abuse

One group of women that appears to be particularly susceptible to acquiring sexually transmitted infections is those who report a history of childhood sexual abuse (CSA), perhaps because CSA increases the likelihood of certain risk behaviours such as sexual compulsivity and substance misuse (Petrak et al, 2000). CSA has also been linked to a range of other social, medical and psychological consequences, including educational and occupational difficulties, depression, antisocial behaviour and teenage pregnancy (Frothingham et al, 2000; Roberts et al, 2004). Survivors of CSA are more likely to experience parenting difficulties, for example in establishing clear generational boundaries with their children. They may be more permissive as parents, and may be more likely to use harsh physical discipline (DiLillo and Damashek, 2003). Evidence shows that the abused are also more prone to become the abusers of the next generation.

Establishing the prevalence of CSA is complicated by definitional and other methodological considerations. Sexual abuse involves forcing or enticing a child or young person to take part in sexual activities which may involve physical contact (penetrative and non-penetrative) or non-contact activities such as involving children in looking at, or in the production of, pornographic material or watching sexual activities, or encouraging children to behave in sexually inappropriate ways (Creighton, 2003, p 7). Prevalence figures will thus vary according to the definition used. For example, a 1991 survey found that, using the most rigorous definition, 4% of women and 2% of men aged 16-21 reported a history of CSA that involved "some form of penetration or coerced/forced masturbation where the abuser was at least five years older". The broadest definition, "any event/interaction that the young person reported as unwanted/ abusive before they were 18", gave prevalence figures of 59% for women and 27% for men (Kelly et al, 1991, cited by Creighton, 2004). In a more recent UK survey of young adults aged 18-24, prevalence rates similarly varied according to whether contact was involved or not, 16% of women and 7% of men reporting CSA that involved sexual contact, while 21% of women and 11% of men reported any CSA (Cawson et al, 2000).

Evidence of the prevalence of abuse also varies according to the source of information used. Creighton (2004) uses the analogy of an iceberg of abuse, where only a tiny portion is recorded (in criminal statistics or on Child Protection Registers). Many other children have not been recognised as being victims of abuse or, if they have been recognised, have not been reported or registered. Between April 2002 and March 2003, for example, there were 1,880 reported offences of 'gross indecency with a child under the age of 14' in England and Wales and by the end of March 2003 around 3,000 children and young people had been placed on Child Protection Registers due to sexual abuse (data derived from the National Society for the Prevention of Cruelty to Children [NSPCC]). Yet, as noted earlier, survey data indicates far higher prevalence levels. Officially recorded rates of CSA in England are also significantly lower than registered rates in Australia, Canada and the US (Creighton, 2004).

Because a very small proportion of CSA is likely to be formally recorded, evidence of socio-economic differences in risk of sexual abuse has to be treated very carefully. A study of convicted and cautioned abusers in the West Midlands found high rates of unemployment among perpetrators (Morris et al, 1997). Children who are placed on Child Protection Registers are also drawn disproportionately from socially disadvantaged families (Sidebotham et al, 2002). However, although such families may possess more of the internal and external factors that have been shown to be associated with child abuse in general, they are also subject to more social surveillance (Creighton, 2004, p 15). Thus, in the absence of socially referenced national statistics, it is impossible to confirm whether risk of CSA varies according to social class.

Inequalities in life trajectories: the role of education and social care

Evidence presented to date demonstrates how powerfully circumstances in childhood shape health inequalities in later life. So far, however, we have only focused on *direct* links between health and health risk factors in childhood and adult health. Examples include the association between slow intrauterine growth and health outcomes in later life; the significantly higher risk that children with mental health problems face for adult psychiatric disorders; the links between poor diet and nutrition in childhood and risk of adult cancer and obesity; and continuities in health-damaging behaviours such as smoking.

Continuity in health and health risk factors is thus one mechanism by which childhood circumstances are linked to health inequalities in later life. A second mechanism is the continuity experienced by many children in their socio-economic circumstances, social disadvantage in childhood predicting social position in adult life, which in turn influences adult health (Graham and Power, 2004). This relationship may be mediated and indeed amplified by child health itself. For example, chronic illness in childhood or delayed growth due to factors such as poor nutrition and disrupted sleep may impact on educational performance and subsequent labour market position (Blane, 1999). Similarly, early health-related behaviours may influence later life chances, data from the US National Longitudinal Survey of Youth suggesting that frequent hard drug use in youth has a negative impact on future labour market participation and earnings (Burgess and Propper, 1998). It is important to note, however, that the impact of early health and health-related behaviours is likely to vary according to socio-economic status, the education and employment prospects of those from socially advantaged backgrounds being less affected than those in less advantaged socio-economic groups.

In the final section of this chapter, we consider the impact of two factors of the socio-economic trajectories of children and young people: education and the experience of being in care. While the education system provides an example of the way in which differential opportunities are spread throughout society, looked-after children are an unusually vulnerable group who are known to be at particular risk of poor mental, physical and psychological well-being, during childhood and youth as well as later life. As such, they should be a key target group for health inequalities policies.

Inequalities in education

Education plays a critical role in the link between childhood disadvantage and adult disadvantage, as parental background is a significant determinant of educational performance and educational performance determines access to key opportunities in adult life. The well-educated are at lower risk of unemployment and are more likely to obtain better-paid jobs than those with poor qualifications, data from consecutive Labour Force Surveys suggesting that the earnings premium associated with each additional year of education may be as high as 10% (Walker and Zhu, 2003). A higher income reduces the incentive to engage in criminal activity as well as the frustration that might otherwise lead to crime (Feinstein, 2002a). It also allows individuals to live in better conditions, consume more nutritious food, buy better healthcare and so on (Feinstein, 2002b). For example, analysis of National Child Development Study data found that, by the age of 37, one third of those with very low skills levels did not own their own home, compared with under 10% of men and women with good skills (Bynner and Parsons, 1997, cited by Sparkes, 1999). Those with higher educational qualifications tend to enjoy more control over their working lives, more variety and challenge in their work and greater job satisfaction, factors that may be associated with improved psychosocial health, immunological status and healthier behaviours (see Chapter Ten). Finally, education appears to exert an independent effect on health-related behaviours, those with better qualifications being more likely to exercise and control their diet and less likely to smoke than their less educated counterparts, even after controlling for factors such as income (Feinstein, 2002b; Lawlor et al, 2005).

Given the associations between adult life chances and school outcomes, current levels of educational attainment suggest that many children are facing serious future disadvantage. In 2003/04, 4.2% of English pupils aged 16 obtained no GCSE passes and 24.3% gained no passes at grades A–C (DfES, 2004a). Both of these groups are at high risk of exclusion from further education, training or employment (Sparkes, 1999). They are also more likely to come from a background of socio-economic disadvantage. Using the government's indicator for low income, pupils eligible for free school meals (FSM) are significantly less likely to achieve the national benchmark of five GCSE passes at grades A–C (26.3% compared to 56.2% of pupils not eligible for free school meals in 2004 [DfES, 2005]). This social gap is reflected in access to university places, which is increasingly important for success in the workplace. Here, evidence suggests that the education gap is widening over time. Between the early 1980s and late 1990s, the proportion of children from the richest quarter of families who had completed a degree by the age of 23 increased from 20% to almost a half. Over the same period, the number of graduates among the poorest quarter of families increased from 6% to just 9% (*The Observer*, 2005).

There are also significant ethnic differences in school performance, with children of Chinese, Indian, Irish, and Mixed White and Asian heritage achieving above the national average at GCSE level, while Black, Mixed White and Black Caribbean, Pakistani and Bangladeshi children score below the national average (DfES, 2005). Socio-economic status and ethnicity are also strongly associated with school exclusion and children who are excluded from school are at significantly higher risk of experiencing longer-term problems. African-Caribbean boys, children in care and children with special educational needs are over-represented in exclusion statistics and the outcomes for these groups tend to be worse than for other excluded children. There is a strong association between exclusion, crime and delinquency, children with a record of poor attendance and exclusion being more likely to have a record of offending and vice versa.

The educational attainment of excluded children is also considerably lower on average than that of non-excluded children (Parsons et al, 2001).

The substantive effects of social origin on educational outcomes have long been recognised and variously attributed to genetic factors; parental education and involvement; family structure (for example, family size, lone-parent status and institutional care); neighbourhood effects such as community cohesion; and school factors, such as intake mix, peer influences, leadership, resources, school ethos and quality of teaching (Sparkes, 1999; Rutter and Maughan, 2002). Evidence suggests that non-school factors are a more important source of variation in educational attainment than differences in the quality of education that students receive (Thomas and Mortimore, 1996; Gibson and Asthana, 1998). This does not mean, however, that children from socially disadvantaged backgrounds are condemned to educational failure. Schools can and should make a difference. Notwithstanding the government's targeted interventions at schools in disadvantaged areas, however (see Chapter Three), there are strong grounds for arguing that the British education system is not fulfilling its potential to tackle social inequality.

First, social class differences in educational attainment are larger when children leave the English school system than when they enter it. Data from the 1970 Birth Cohort Survey, which recorded the results of development tests given to a subsample of 1,292 children at four different ages, found that although children's attainment was already structured by social class at 22 months of age, social class differences became even more extreme by the age of 10. Children of low socio-economic status who had low attainment at 22 months were still likely to have low attainment eight years on. By contrast, children with high socio-economic status were more likely to show high attainment at the age of 10, even if their attainment was low at 22 months (Feinstein, 2003). Socio-economic differences in national curriculum assessment and GCSE performance similarly become more pronounced as children become older. In 2002-03, 69% and 80% of seven-year-old children eligible for FSM attain the expected level for reading and mathematics respectively. This compared to 88% and 93% of non-FSM eligible children. By age 11, 54% and 53% of FSM children reached the expected level in English and mathematics compared to 79% and 76% of non-FSM children. By the age of 14, only 44% and 46% of FSM children attained the expected levels, compared to 74% and 75% of non-FSM eligible children (DfES, 2004b). By later adolescence, social divisions widen further, as reflected by differences in GCSE performance and entrance to university.

Second, data from the Programme for International Student Assessment (PISA) show that the UK currently falls within the least egalitarian half of OECD (Organisation for Economic Co-operation and Development) countries with regard to both equality of opportunity and equality of outcomes (Green, 2003). A total of 61% of differences in outcomes between schools in the UK can be explained by school social intake characteristics (measured by parental occupational level, wealth and 'cultural capital'), compared to the OECD average of 34%. As measured by the slope of the socio-economic gradient (reflecting the effect of student background on performance), the UK is one of the most unequal countries. By contrast, most of the Nordic countries and East Asian states have well above average equity levels. The distribution of performance is also relatively wide in the UK, suggesting that the weakest students are allowed to fall further behind than in countries with more equal outcomes such as Finland, Korea and Japan. Significantly, these countries also show that it is possible to combine high average standards with high levels of equity (Green, 2003).

The example of countries where educational outcomes are more equal suggests that Britain could do more to address the strong class divide that exists in education. In Chapter Three, however, we noted that countries that have actively promoted the marketisation of their comprehensive systems tend to be characterised by relatively high levels of educational inequality, while those that are more genuinely comprehensive have higher levels of equity. Thus, notwithstanding the introduction of a number of policies targeting schools in highly deprived areas, the government's current strategy of improving schools through choice and competition is unlikely to close the educational gap between the disadvantaged and their peers.

Inequalities in vulnerability: the case of looked-after children

While education plays a key role in the transmission of advantage and disadvantage across the generations, one of the most powerful predictors of social exclusion in adult life is the experience of being in care. At any one time, around 60,000 children are being looked after by local authorities, 40% of whom are aged 10 or under. Most (80%) enter care because of abuse or neglect or for family reasons. Two thirds live in foster care and one in 10 in children's homes (SEU, 2003). There is a well-established link between deprivation and children coming into care, factors such as unemployment, low income, inadequate accommodation and lone-parent status threatening the stability of family life.

The poor educational participation and performance of looked-after children has become a focus of policy concern, not least because educational disadvantage leads to disadvantage in other areas. As noted in Chapter Four, neglect and abuse in the first few years of life has long-term consequences for learning and behaviour and many looked-after children have experienced significant adversity in early life. Frequent movement within the care system, school exclusion and non-attendance have also been linked to educational under-achievement. Some estimates suggest that children in care are 10 times more likely to be excluded than those outside the care system (Brodie, 2000; Goddard, 2000). All of these factors are reflected in the relatively poor educational performance of looked-after children. In 2003, 53% achieved the expected level in national curriculum assessments at age seven, 42% at age 11 and 23% at age 14. The comparable percentages for all children in England were 85%, 78% and 69% respectively.

Only 9% of looked-after children obtained at least five GCSEs at grades A–C, compared with 53% of all children (DfES, 2004c). Thus, as with educational inequality in general, differences between the educational performance of looked-after children and other school children become increasingly pronounced with age.

There is a high incidence of mental health problems and psychiatric disorders among looked-after children, although measurement differences (such as the age range of subjects) give rise to a wide range of prevalence estimates. According to the ONS, 45% of children in care aged 5–17 have mental disorders, over four times higher than for all children (SEU, 2003). Levels of mental disorders are higher among boys, older children and those living in residential homes. A study of adolescents (aged 13–17) looked after by an Oxfordshire local authority found that 96% in residential units and 57% in foster care had a psychiatric disorder (McCann et al, 1996). The most common diagnosis was conduct disorder (28%), followed by overanxious disorder (26%); 23% suffered from major depressive disorder, a worryingly high prevalence compared to rates within the community. A more recent study of children aged 8–19 living in residential homes in Leeds found similar rates of emotional and behavioural difficulties (93%), including post-abuse issues; 14% had had an episode of self-harm (Nicholas et al, 2003). High rates of conduct disorder among looked-after children are associated with high rates of criminal behaviour. In 2003, 10% of looked-after children aged 10 or over were cautioned or convicted for an offence during the year, three times the rate for all children of this age (DfES, 2004c).

The poor mental health of children living in residential homes in part reflects selection. Children with severe behavioural difficulties or emotional problems are often considered unsuitable for placement in foster homes, are more likely to experience breakdowns in their placements and thus more likely to be looked after in residential homes. However, the childcare system can itself present risks for mental health problems. US research suggests that children in residential facilities are more vulnerable to abuse than those who live in families. Several high-profile cases have involved the sexual abuse of children by staff, although evidence suggests that physical abuse and inappropriate restraint are more common forms of institutional maltreatment. Children in residential care also appear to be at greater risk of physical and sexual assault from their peers than staff members, a questionnaire survey of children from 48 different care homes finding that 13% of children had been sexually taken advantage of by a peer while in care and four in ten had been bullied (Barter, 2003).

While the physical health of looked-after children does not appear to be significantly worse than that of children living in their own homes, unmet needs have been identified with respect to health promotion. A case control study in South West Wales found that, compared to children living at home, looked-after children were less likely to be fully immunised, to visit a dentist regularly and to have received advice on health behaviours despite the fact that they were more likely to smoke and use illegal drugs (Williams et al, 2001). The low uptake of immunisation and other preventive activities could in part reflect the difficulty of keeping track with health needs when there are frequent placements. A study of the health information available on teenagers in residential care found significant gaps and inconsistencies in record keeping, making it very difficult to monitor the implications of past health, development and family history for current health concerns (Bundle, 2001).

Higher than average rates of poor mental health, drug use and antisocial behaviour combined with low educational attainment significantly increase the likelihood that looked-after children will experience social exclusion in later life. In 2003, 22% of 16-year-old looked-after children were unemployed the September after leaving school compared to 7% of all school leavers (DfES, 2004c). Unemployment, insufficient support during the transition from care to adult life and the lack of safety nets that other young people can fall back on place care leavers at additional risk of homelessness. A total of 20% of care leavers experience some form of homelessness within two years of leaving care and 30% of young single homeless people have been in care (Stephens, 2002). While economic exclusion, mental health problems and drug or alcohol misuse are themselves triggers for homelessness, being homeless exacerbates such problems. Risk of sexual exploitation and violence from others is also very high among the homeless population. Other adverse outcomes for young people who have been in care include teenage pregnancy, parenting problems and high rates of criminal activity. Over a quarter of prisoners were in care as children. Young people who have been in care are two-and-a-half times more likely to become teenage parents and the children of women who have spent time in care are themselves two-and-a-half times more likely to go into care than their peers (SEU, 2003).

The poorer educational, economic, social and health outcomes of looked-after children in part reflect the significant adversity that many such children have experienced in their early lives. However, some of their problems have also been attributed to the childcare system itself (Jackson and Thomas, 1999). A number of policy initiatives have sought to improve outcomes for children in care. For example, the Department of Health (DH) Quality Protects Programme sets targets which include a reduction in the number of placement changes for children and improvements to the care-leaving packages that local authorities provide. The 2000 Children (Leaving Care) Act (England and Wales) entitles looked-after children to support from their local authority until they are 21 years old. This includes advice from a Personal Advisor and a pathway plan, a key element of which is accommodation. Local Connexions services have been established to provide information, advice and guidance to young people. National minimum standards have been published for children's homes and fostering services and joint guidance issued by the DH and the Department for Education and Skills (DfES) on the education of children and young people in public care.

All of these reforms are aimed at improving the life chances of children in care. However, the complexity of problems faced by looked-after children, together with continued resource and capacity problems, are important barriers to change (SEU, 2003). The way in which British childcare and particularly residential care is structured may also contribute to its poor outcomes. Since the 1990s, there has been a steady reduction in residential care provision and a shift in the use of foster placements. Residential care is thus treated as a short-term option for children who have not been successfully placed with families. However, evidence from other countries such as Israel suggests that residential care can lead to more satisfactory outcomes if it creates a stable, living experience for children who grow up with both the same peer group and the same carers and who have considerable help and support with their education (Jackson and Thomas, 1999). Examples such as these suggest that, while residential care in Britain continues to be seen as a last resort, young people living in residential homes will remain one of the most vulnerable groups with respect to both social exclusion and health inequalities.

The policy implications

As noted in Chapter Six, rather less attention has been paid to the significance of health inequalities in childhood and youth than in other stages of the lifecourse. In addition to reflecting the assumption that this is a 'healthy age', the relative neglect of children and young people in health inequalities research may be an outcome of the belief that this is a period during which a process of equalisation of health takes place, influences outside the family such as the school, the peer group and youth culture weakening the effects of family background. In fact, as this chapter has indicated, there are strong continuities between social origin and social status of destination and parental socio-economic circumstances remain a major determinant of young people's life chances. Factors such as parental occupation, education and income explain a far higher proportion of the variation in school performance in the UK than in Western countries on average, suggesting that, rather than equalising life chances, a strong class divide persists in British education. This plays a critical role in linking social disadvantage in childhood with social and health disadvantage in adult life. Level of education is not only strongly associated with income level, quality of employment, housing, food, access to leisure and so on, all of which are factors that impinge on adult health (see Chapter Ten). It also independently shapes propensity to adopt and maintain healthy lifestyles, those with higher qualifications being less likely to smoke and more likely to control their diet and exercise than their less educated counterparts, even after controlling for factors such as income.

The strong association between parental socio-economic status and educational performance suggests that the equalisation thesis has been somewhat overplayed. The persistence of social inequalities in terms of health risks and behaviours also suggests that social origin remains a critical determinant of health outcomes. Dietary patterns during childhood and youth vary significantly according to socio-economic status, young people from lower socio-economic backgrounds consuming lower amounts of fruit and vegetables and higher proportions of refined and particularly starchy foods. As a result, children and young people in the poorest households are at higher risk of being overweight and obese. Problems of underweight have also been noted in boys from lower-income households, suggesting that weight distribution among socially disadvantaged children may be becoming increasingly U-shaped. This has serious implications for health inequalities in both the short and longer terms.

Problematic risk behaviours such as smoking and hard drug misuse during youth are also more strongly associated with social deprivation. Yet, although it is during this stage of the lifecourse that most people are first initiated into substance use, there has been a relative dearth of information on the health behaviours of young people. Evidence presented earlier suggests that the significance of variations in health behaviours during childhood and youth to health inequalities in adulthood should not be underestimated. Most smokers, for example, start smoking in their teenage years. Those who are in social networks where cigarette smoking is the norm are significantly more likely to take up the habit, leading to both social and neighbourhood concentration in the prevalence of smoking. A strong class gradient exists between teenagers in the lowest income groups who are the heaviest smokers and those from professional backgrounds who are the lightest smokers. While the social gradient in smoking is not as pronounced in later youth, young men and women from poorer backgrounds are more likely to smoke and to maintain their habit during later adulthood (see Chapter Ten).

Evidence of socio-economic variations in alcohol and drug use varies according to the definition of substance use that is adopted. Most UK surveys suggest a positive relationship between alcohol consumption and social status, young men and women from higher income groups drinking more frequently and in larger amounts. Similarly, use of cannabis, nitrates and amphetamines does not appear to be strongly associated with social deprivation, although young people who leave school at 16 appear to be more likely to have tried drugs than those who stay on to achieve higher qualifications. Against this, highly 'problematic' drug and alcohol use does appear to be strongly associated with social disadvantage. There are strong correlations between alcohol dependence and mental health disorders, both of which are associated with relative poverty, family difficulties, school drop-out and poor educational achievement. Heroin addiction and, increasingly, addiction to crack cocaine are also strongly associated with social deprivation, delinquent and criminal behaviour, poor educational performance and unemployment.

Although sexual behaviour has consequences for current morbidity, as reflected in the increasing prevalence of sexually transmitted diseases in young people, early sexual activity can also be conceived as part of a pathway leading to later adult circumstances. Children who start having sexual intercourse at an early age are significantly more likely to become pregnant as teenagers, to leave school early, to have poor employment prospects and to be lone mothers. There is some debate as to whether teenage pregnancy itself changes the life trajectories of these young women, whose adverse socio-economic outcomes are at least in part accounted for by individual and family background. However, few disagree that teenage mothers are a vulnerable group whose economic prospects are significantly worse than those of women who defer motherhood.

As with other areas of health inequality, a wide range of risk factors has been implicated in the likelihood of engaging in health-damaging behaviours, suggesting a need for multidimensional policy approaches that are addressed at a number of levels (individual, family, school and wider community). Chapter Nine evaluates evidence, policy and practice relating to a range of interventions targeting nutritional status, substance use and sexual health. As in previous chapters exploring policy and practice (and reflecting the current body of effort), the focus is primarily on so-called downstream initiatives. Again, however, the point is made that individual risk factors are shaped by the wider context, signalling the need for focused policy initiatives to be complemented by structural solutions. Of these, we consider efforts to promote greater educational equity to be of considerable importance. A case for greater universalism and less targeting can also be made on the grounds that, for most modifiable health-risk factors in childhood and youth, there is an incremental gradient across the social spectrum. This suggests that rather than purely focusing on 'poor' and 'socially excluded' young people, policies targeting this age group should have a broader reach (Batty and Leon, 2002).

References

Arai, L. (2003) 'Low expectations, sexual attitudes and knowledge: explaining teenage pregnancy and fertility in English communities: insights from qualitative research', *The Sociological Review*, vol 51, no 2, pp 199-217.

ASH (Action on Smoking and Health) (2004) *Tobacco advertising and promotion*, Fact Sheet No 19, London: ASH.

Balding, J. (2001) 'Food choices and weight control', in J. Balding, *Young people in 2000*, Exeter: SHEU.

Barter, C. (2003) *Abuse of children in residential care*, London: NSPCC.

Batty, G. and Leon, D. (2002) 'Socioeconomic position and coronary heart disease risk factors in children and young people: evidence from UK epidemiological studies', *European Journal of Public Health*, vol 12, pp 263-72.

Biddle, S.J., Gorely, T., Marshall, S.J., Murdey, I. and Cameron, N. (2004) 'Physical activity and sedentary behaviours in youth: issues and controversies', *Journal of the Royal Society for the Promotion of Health*, vol 124, pp 29-33.

Bjarnason, T., Davidaviciene, A.G., Miller, P., Nociar, A., Pavlakis, A. and Stergar, E. (2003) 'Family structure and adolescent cigarette smoking in eleven European countries', *Addiction*, vol 98, pp 815-24.

Blake, M. (2003) 'Infant health', in K. Sproston, and P. Primatesta (eds) *Health Survey for England 2002: Maternal and infant health*, London: The Stationery Office.

Blane, D. (1999) 'The life course, the social gradient and health', in M. Marmot and R.G. Wilkinson (eds) *Social determinants of health*, Oxford: Oxford University Press, pp 64-80.

Blenkinsop, S. (2003a) 'Drinking, frequency and purchase', in R. Boreham and S. McManus (eds) *Smoking, drinking and drug use among young people in England in 2002*, London: The Stationery Office, pp 91-8.

Blenkinsop, S. (2003b) 'Prevalence of drinking', in R. Boreham and S. McManus (eds) *Smoking, drinking and drug use among young people in England in 2002*, London: The Stationery Office, pp 71-90.

Bonell, C.P., Strange, V.J., Stephenson, J.M., Oakley, A.R., Copas, A.J., Forrest, S.P., Johnson, A.M. and Black, S. (2003) 'Effect of social exclusion on the risk of teenage pregnancy: development of hypotheses using baseline data from a randomised trial of sex education', *Journal of Epidemiology and Community Health*, vol 57, pp 871-6.

Boreham, C. and Riddoch, C. (2001) 'The physical activity, fitness and health of children', *Journal of Sports Science*, vol 19, pp 915-29.

Bost, L., Primatesta, P. and McMunn, A. (1998) 'Anthropometric measures and eating habits', in P. Prescott-Clarke and P. Primatesta (eds) *Health Survey for England: The health of young people 1995-1997. Volume 1: Findings*, London: The Stationery Office, pp 67-108.

Brand-Miller, J.C., Holt, S.H., Pawlak, D.B. and McMillan, J. (2002) 'Glycemic index and obesity', *American Journal of Clinical Nutrition*, vol 76, pp 281S-5S.

Brenner, H., Rothenbacher, D., Bode, G., Marz, W., Hoffmeister, A. and Koenig, W. (2001) 'Coronary heart disease risk reduction in a predominantly beer-drinking population', *Epidemiology*, vol 12, pp 380-2.

Brodie, I. (2000) 'Children's homes and school exclusion; redefining the problem', *Support for Learning*, vol 15, pp 25-9.

Brodney, S., Blair, S. and Lee, C. (2000) 'Is it possible to be overweight and fit and healthy?', in C. Bouchard (ed) *Physical activity and health*, Champaign, IL: Human Kinetics, pp 355-71.

Brown, A.E., Sadler, K.E., Tomkins, S.E., McGarrigle, C.A., LaMontagne, D.S., Goldberg, D., Tookey, P.A., Smyth, B., Thomas, D., Murphy, G., Parry, J.V., Evans, B.G., Gill, O.N., Ncube, F. and Fenton, K.A. (2004) 'Recent trends in HIV and other STIs in the United Kingdom: data to the end of 2002', *Sexually Transmitted Infections*, vol 80, pp 159-66.

Budd, T. (2003) *Alcohol-related assault: Findings from the British Crime Survey*, London: Home Office.

Bundle, A. (2001) 'Health of teenagers in residential care: comparison of data held by care staff with date in community child health records', *Archives of Disease in Childhood*, vol 84, pp 10-14.

Burack, R. (1999) 'Teenage sexual behaviour: attitudes towards and declared sexual activity', *British Journal of Family Planning*, vol 24, pp 145-8.

Burgess, S. and Propper, C. (1998) *Early health related behaviours and their impact on later life chances: Evidence from the US*, CASE Paper 6, London: Centre for Analysis of Social Exclusion, London School of Economics and Political Science.

Bynner, J. and Parsons, S. (1997) *It doesn't get any better: The impact of poor basic skill attainment on the lives of 37 year olds*, London: Basic Skills Agency.

Campbell, K., Waters, E., O'Meara, S., Kelly, S. and Summerbell, C. (2004) 'Interventions for preventing obesity in children (Cochrane Review)', *The Cochrane Library, issue 1, 2004*, Chichester: John Wiley & Sons Ltd.

Casswell, S., Pledger, M. and Hooper, R. (2003) 'Socioeconomic status and drinking patterns in young adults', *Addiction*, vol 98, pp 601-10.

Cawson, P., Wattam, C., Brooker, S. and Kelly, G. (2000) *Child maltreatment in the United Kingdom: A study of the prevalence of child abuse and neglect*, London: NSPCC.

Chan, W. (1999) 'Nutritional needs of school children', in N. Donovan and C. Street (eds) *Fit for school: How breakfast clubs meet health, education and childcare needs*, London: New Policy Institute, pp 8-10.

Chevalier, A. and Viitanen, T.K. (2003) 'The long-run labour market consequences of teenage motherhood in Britain', *Journal of Population Economics*, vol 16, pp 323-43.

Chinn, S. and Rona, R.J. (2001) 'Prevalence and trends in overweight and obesity in three cross sectional studies of British children, 1974-94', *British Medical Journal*, vol 322, pp 24-6.

Choi, W.S., Ahluwalia, J.S., Harris, K.J. and Okuyemi, K. (2002) 'Progression to established smoking: the influence of tobacco marketing', *American Journal of Preventive Medicine*, vol 22, pp 228-33.

Chou, S.P. and Pickering, R.P. (1992) 'Early onset of drinking as a risk factor for lifetime alcohol-related problems', *British Journal of Addiction*, vol 87, pp 1199-204.

Cole, T., Bellizzi, C., Flegal, K. and Dietz, W. (2000) 'Establishing a standard definition for child overweight and obesity worldwide: international survey', *British Medical Journal*, vol 320, pp 1240-53.

Creighton, S. (2003) *Child protection statistics: Child protection in the family*, London: NSPCC.

Creighton, S. (2004) *Prevalence and incidence of child abuse: International comparisons*, London: NSPCC.

Cunnington, A. (2001) 'What's so bad about teenage pregnancy?', *Journal of Family Planning and Reproductive Health Care*, vol 27, pp 36-41.

Deverill, C. (2003) 'Fruit and vegetable consumption', in K. Sproston and P. Primatesta (eds) *Health Survey for England 2002: The health of children and young people*, London: The Stationery Office.

DfES (Department for Education and Skills) (2004a) *GCSE and equivalent results for young people in England, 2003/04 (Provisional)*, London: DfES.

DfES (2004b) *National curriculum assessment and GCSE/GNVQ attainment by pupil characteristics in England, 2002 (final) and 2003 (provisional)*, London: DfES.

DfES (2004c) *Outcome indicators for looked after children: Twelve months to 30 September 2003, England*, SFR 13/2004, London: DfES.

DfES (2005) *National curriculum assessment GCSE and equivalent attainment and post-16 attainment by pupil characteristics, in England 2004*, London: DfES.

DiLillo, D. and Damashek, A. (2003) 'Parenting characteristics of women reporting a history of childhood sexual abuse', *Child Maltreatment*, vol 8, pp 319-33.

Doll, R., Peto, R., Boreham, J. and Sutherland, I. (2004) 'Mortality in relation to smoking: 50 years' observations on male British doctors', *British Medical Journal*, vol 328, pp 1519-33.

Dowler, E. (1999) 'Families and food poverty', in N. Donovan and C. Street (eds) *Fit for school: How breakfast clubs meet health, education and childcare needs*, London: New Policy Institute, pp 23-7.

Droomers, M., Schrijvers, C.T.M., Casswell, S. and Mackenbach, J.P. (2003) 'Occupational level of the father and alcohol consumption during adolescence: patterns and predictors', *Journal of Epidemiology and Community Health*, vol 57, pp 704-10.

Egginton, R., Aldridge, J. and Parker, H. (2001) 'Unconventional? Adolescent drug triers and users in England', in H. Parker, J. Aldridge and R. Egginton (eds) *UK drugs unlimited: New research and policy lessons on illicit drug use*, Basingstoke: Palgrave, pp 31-50.

Ellis, B.J., Bates, J.E., Dodge, K.A., Fergusson, D.M., Horwood, L.J., Pettit, G.S. and Woodward, L. (2003) 'Does father absence place daughters at special risk for early sexual activity and teenage pregnancy?', *Child Development*, vol 74, pp 801-21.

Erens, B. (2003) 'Alcohol consumption', in K. Sproston and P. Primatesta (eds) *Health Survey for England 2002: The health of children and young people*, London: The Stationery Office.

Evans, J. (2003) 'Physical education and health: a polemic or "let them eat cake"!', *European Physical Education Review*, vol 9, pp 87-101.

Evans, J., Evans, B. and Rich, R. (2003) '"The only problem is, will children like their chips": education and the discursive production of ill-health', *Pedagogy, Culture and Society*, vol 11, pp 215-40.

Feinstein, L. (2002a) *Quantitative estimates of the social benefits of learning 1: Crime*, Research Report No 5, London: Centre of Research on the Wider Benefits of Learning.

Feinstein, L. (2002b) *Quantitative estimates of the social benefits of learning 2: Health (depression and obesity)*, Research Report No 6, London: Centre of Research on the Wider Benefits of Learning.

Feinstein, L. (2003) 'Do schools counteract early performance differences between children from different social backgrounds?', *Economica*, vol 70, pp 73-97.

Fergusson, D.M. and Lynskey, M.T. (1996) 'Alcohol misuse and adolescent sexual behaviors and risk taking', *Pediatrics*, vol 98, pp 91-6.

Fergusson, D.M. and Woodward, L.J. (2000) 'Educational, psychosocial, and sexual outcomes of girls with conduct problems in early adolescence', *Journal of Child Psychology and Psychiatry and Allied Disciplines*, vol 41, pp 779-92.

Fergusson, D.M., Lynskey, M.T. and Horwood, L.J. (1995a) 'The role of peer affiliations, social, family and individual factors in continuities in cigarette smoking between childhood and adolescence', *Addiction*, vol 90, pp 647-59.

Fergusson, D.M., Horwood, L.J. and Lynskey, M.T. (1995b) 'The prevalence and risk factors associated with abusive or hazardous alcohol consumption in 16 year olds', *Addiction*, vol 90, pp 935-46.

France, A. (2000) 'Towards a sociological understanding of youth and their risk-taking', *Journal of Youth Studies*, vol 3, pp 317-31.

Frothingham, T.E., Hobbs, C.J., Wynne, J.M., Yee, L., Goyal, A. and Wadsworth, D.J. (2000) 'Follow-up study eight years after diagnosis of sexual abuse', *Archives of Disease in Childhood*, vol 83, pp 132-4.

Geronimus, A. (1992) 'The weathering hypothesis and the health of African American women and infants: evidence and speculation', *Ethnicity and Disease*, vol 2, pp 207-21.

Geronimus, A. (1997) 'Teenage childbearing and personal responsibility: an alternative view', *Political Science Quarterly*, vol 112, pp 405-30.

Gibson, A. and Asthana, S. (1998) 'Schools, pupils and exam results: contextualising school performance', *British Educational Research Journal*, vol 24, pp 269-82.

Gilvarry, E. (2000) 'Substance abuse in young people', *Journal of Child Psychology and Psychiatry*, vol 41, pp 55-80.

Goddard, J. (2000) 'The education of looked after children', *Child and Family Social Work*, vol 5, pp 79-86.

Graham, H. and Power, C. (2004) *Childhood disadvantage and adult health: A lifecourse framework*, London: Health Development Agency.

Green, A. (2003) 'Is UK education exceptionally unequal? Evidence from the IALS and PISA surveys', *Forum*, vol 45, pp 67-70.

Green, G., Macintyre, S., West, P. and Ecob, R. (1991) 'Like parent like child? Associations between drinking and smoking behaviour of parents and their children', *British Journal of Addiction*, vol 86, pp 745-58.

Gregory, J., Lowe, S., Bates, C., Prentice, A., Jackson, L., Smithers, G., Wenlock, R. and Farron, M. (2000) *National diet and nutrition survey: Young people aged 4 to 18 years*, London: The Stationery Office.

Griesbach, D., Amos, A. and Currie, C. (2003) 'Adolescent smoking and family structure in Europe', *Social Science and Medicine*, vol 56, pp 41-52.

Hart, C.L., Smith, G.D., Hole, D.J. and Hawthorne, V.M. (1999) 'Alcohol consumption and mortality from all causes, coronary heart disease, and stroke: results from a prospective cohort study of Scottish men with 21 years of follow up', *British Medical Journal*, vol 318, pp 1725-9.

Hemmingsson, T. and Lundberg, I. (2001) 'Development of alcoholism: interaction between heavy adolescent drinking and later low sense of control over work', *Alcohol and Alcoholism*, vol 36, pp 207-12.

Hemmingsson, T., Lundberg, I. and Diderichsen, F. (1999) 'The roles of social class of origin, achieved social class and intergenerational social mobility in explaining social-class inequalities in alcoholism among young men', *Social Science and Medicine*, vol 49, pp 1051-9.

Herrick, J. and Kelly, Y. (2003) 'Maternal health', in K. Sproston, and P. Primatesta (eds) *Health Survey for England 2002: Maternal and infant health*, London: The Stationery Office.

Holly, A. and Wittchen, H.U. (1998) 'Patterns of use and their relationship to DSM-IV abuse and dependence of alcohol among adolescents and young adults', *European Addiction Research*, vol 4, pp 50-7.

HPA (Health Protection Agency), SCIED (Scottish Centre for Infection and Environmental Health, ISD (Information and Statistics Division, Scotland), National Public Health Service for Wales, CDSC (Communicable Disease Surveillance Centre) Northern Ireland and UASSG (Unlinked Anonymous Surveys Steering Group) (2003) *Renewing the focus: HIV and other sexually transmitted infections in the United Kingdom in 2002*, London: HPA.

Ingham, R. (2000) 'Doctors should advise adolescents to abstain from sex: the case against', *British Medical Journal*, vol 321, pp 1521-2.

Jackson, S. and Thomas, N. (1999) *On the move again? What works in creating stability for looked after children*, Ilford: Barnado's.

Jaffee, S.R. (2002) 'Pathways to adversity in young adulthood among early childbearers', *Journal of Family Psychology*, vol 16, pp 38-49.

Jebb, S.A. and Prentice, A. (2001) 'Single definition of overweight and obesity should be used', *British Medical Journal*, vol 323, p 999.

Jebb, S.A., Rennie, K.L. and Cole, T.J. (2004) 'Prevalence of overweight and obesity among young people in Great Britain', *Public Health Nutrition*, vol 7, pp 461-5.

Jefferis, B., Graham, H., Manor, O. and Power, C. (2003) 'Cigarette consumption and socio-economic circumstances in adolescence as predictors of adult smoking', *Addiction*, vol 98, pp 1765-72.

Kelly, L., Regan, L. and Burton, S. (1991) *An exploratory study of the prevalence of sexual abuse in a sample of 16-21 year olds*, London: PNL Child Abuse Studies Unit.

Kiess, W., Galler, A., Reich, A., Müller, G., Kapellen, T., Deutscher, J., Raile, K. and Kratzsch, J. (2001) 'Clinical aspects of obesity in childhood and adolescence', *Obesity Reviews*, vol 2, pp 29-36.

Kobus, K. (2003) 'Peers and adolescent smoking', *Addiction*, vol 98, suppl 1, pp 37-55.

Lawlor, D.A. and Shaw, M. (2002) 'Too much too young? Teenage pregnancy is not a public health problem', *International Journal of Epidemiology*, vol 31, pp 552-4.

Lawlor, D.A., Batty, G., Morton, S., Clark, H., Macintyre, S. and Leon, D. (2005) 'Childhood socioeconomic position, educational attainment, and adult cardiovascular risk factors: the Aberdeen children of the 1950s cohort study', *American Journal of Public Health*, vol 95, pp 1245-51.

Lee, E., Clements, S., Ingham, R. and Stone, N. (2004) *A matter of choice? Explaining national variations in teenage abortion and motherhood*, London: Joseph Rowntree Foundation.

Lewinsohn, P.M., Rohde, P. and Brown, R.A. (1999) 'Level of current and past adolescent cigarette smoking as predictors of future substance use disorders in young adulthood', *Addiction*, vol 94, pp 913-21.

Livingstone, M.B., Robson, P.J., Wallace, J.M. and McKinley, M.C. (2003) 'How active are we? Levels of routine physical activity in children and adults', *Proceedings of the Nutritional Society*, vol 62, pp 681-701.

Lovato, C., Linn, G., Stead, L.F. and Best, A. (2003) 'Impact of tobacco advertising and promotion on increasing adolescent smoking behaviours', *Cochrane Database of Systematic Reviews 2003, issue 3*, Art. No. CD003439.

Lucas, P. (2003) 'Breakfast clubs and school fruit schemes: promising practice' (www.whatworksforchildren.org.uk), What Works for Children Group, Evidence Nugget, April.

Ludwig, D.S. (2000) 'Dietary glycemic index and obesity', *Journal of Nutrition*, vol 130, 2S suppl, pp 280S-283S.

McCann, J.B., James, A., Wilson, S. and Dunn, G. (1996) 'Prevalence of psychiatric disorders in young people in the care system', *British Medical Journal*, vol 313, pp 1529-30.

McCarthy, H.D., Ellis, S.M. and Cole, T.J. (2003) 'Central overweight and obesity in British youth aged 11-16 years: cross sectional surveys of waist circumference', *British Medical Journal*, vol 326, p 624.

McCarthy, H.D., Jarrett, K.V. and Crawley, H.F. (2001) 'Development of waist circumference percentiles in British children aged 5.0-16.9', *European Journal of Clinical Nutrition*, vol 55, pp 902-7.

McCulloch, A. (2001) 'Teenage childbearing in Great Britain and the spatial concentration of poverty households', *Journal of Epidemiology and Community Health*, vol 55, pp 16-23.

Macintyre, S. and Mutrie, N. (2004) 'Socio-economic differences in cardiovascular disease and physical activity: stereotypes and reality', *Journal of the Royal Society for the Promotion of Health*, vol 124, pp 66-9.

MacKelvie, K.J., Khan, K.M., Petit, M.A., Janssen, P.A. and McKay, H.A. (2003) 'A school-based exercise intervention elicits substantial bone health benefits: a 2-year randomized controlled trial in girls', *Pediatrics*, vol 112, pp e447-e452.

McLeod, A. (2001) 'Changing patterns of teenage pregnancy: population based study of small areas', *British Medical Journal*, vol 323, pp 199-203.

McManus, S. and Natarajan, L. (2003) 'Drug use', in R. Boreham and S. McManus (eds) *Smoking, drinking and drug use among young people in England in 2002*, London: The Stationery Office, pp 99-121.

Marmot, M.G. (2001) 'Alcohol and coronary heart disease', *International Journal of Epidemiology*, vol 30, pp 724-9.

Maynard, M., Gunnell, D., Emmett, P., Frankel, S. and Davey Smith, G. (2003) 'Fruit, vegetables, and antioxidants in childhood and risk of adult cancer: the Boyd Orr cohort', *Journal of Epidemiology and Community Health*, vol 57, no 3, pp 218-25.

Measham, F., Aldridge, J. and Parker, H. (2001) 'Unstoppable? Dance drug use in the UK club scene', in H. Parker, J. Aldridge and R. Egginton (eds) *UK drugs unlimited: New research and policy lessons on illicit drug use*, Basingstoke: Palgrave, pp 80-97.

Miller, B.C. (2002) 'Family influences on adolescent sexual and contraceptive behaviour', *Journal of Sex Research*, vol 39, pp 22-6.

Morris, I., Scott, I., Mortimer, M. and Barker, D. (1997) 'Physical and sexual abuse of children in the West Midlands', *Child Abuse and Neglect*, vol 21, pp 285-93.

Munro, H., Davies, M. and Hughes, G. (2004) 'Adolescent sexual health', in ONS, *The health of children and young people*, London: ONS.

Murgraff, V., Parrott, A. and Bennett, P. (1999) 'Risky single occasion drinking amongst young people – definition, correlates, policy and intervention: a broad overview of research findings', *Alcohol and Alcoholism*, vol 34, pp 3-14.

Natarajan, L. and McManus, S. (2003) 'Smoking prevalence and cigarette consumption', in R. Boreham and S. McManus (eds) *Smoking, drinking and drug use among young people in England in 2002*, London: The Stationery Office, pp 23-38.

Nessa, N. and Gallagher, J. (2004) 'Diet, nutrition, dental health and exercise', in ONS, *The health of children and young people*, London: ONS.

Nicholas, B., Roberts, S. and Wurr, C. (2003) 'Looked after children in residential homes', *Child and Adolescent Mental Health*, vol 8, pp 78-83.

Observer, The (2005) 'Class divisions bar students from university', 16 January.

Paavola, M., Vartiainen, E. and Puska, P. (2001) 'Smoking cessation between teenage years and beyond', *Health Education Research*, vol 16, pp 49-57.

Parker, H. (2001) 'Unbelievable? The UK's drugs present', in H. Parker, J. Aldridge and R. Egginton (eds) *UK drugs unlimited: New research and policy lessons on illicit drug use*, Basingstoke: Palgrave, pp 1-13.

Parker, H., Aldridge J. and Egginton, R. (eds) (2001) *UK drugs unlimited: New research and policy lessons on illicit drug use*, Basingstoke: Palgrave, pp 31-50.

Parker, H., Aldridge, J. and Measham, F. (1998) *Illegal leisure: The normalisation of adolescent recreational drug use*, London: Routledge.

Parsons, C., Godfrey, R., Howlett, K., Hayden, C. and Martin, T. (2001) 'Excluding primary school children: the outcomes six years on', *Pastoral Care*, December, pp 4-15.

Petrak, J., Byrne, A. and Baker, M. (2000) 'The association between abuse in childhood and STD/HIV risk behaviours in female genitourinary (GU) clinic attendees', *Sexually Transmitted Infections*, vol 76, pp 457-61.

Pierce, J.P., Distefan, J.M., Jackson, C., White, M.M. and Gilpin, E.A. (2002) 'Does tobacco marketing undermine the influence of recommended parenting in discouraging adolescents from smoking?', *American Journal of Preventive Medicine*, vol 23, pp 73-81.

Plant, M. and Miller, P. (2001) 'Young people and alcohol: an international insight', *Alcohol and Alcoholism*, vol 36, pp 513-15.

Plant, M. and Plant, M. (1992) *Risk takers: Alcohol, drugs, sex and youth*, London: Routledge.

Rees, R., Harden, A., Shepherd, J., Brunton, G., Oliver, S. and Oakley, A. (2001) *Young people and physical activity: A systematic review of barriers and facilitators*, London: EPPI-Centre, Institute of Education.

Reilly, J.J., Methven, E., McDowell, Z.C., Hacking, B., Alexander, D., Stewart, L. and Kelnar, C.J.H. (2003) 'Health consequences of obesity', *Archives of Disease in Childhood*, vol 88, pp 748-52.

Rich-Edwards, J. (2002) 'Teen pregnancy is not a public health crisis in the United States: it is time we made it one', *International Journal of Epidemiology*, vol 31, pp 555-6.

Richardson, A. and Budd, T. (2003) 'Young adults, alcohol, crime and disorder', *Criminal Behaviour and Mental Health*, vol 13, pp 5-16.

Roberts, R., O'Connor, T., Dunn, J., Golding, J. and the ALSPAC Study Team (2004) 'The effects of child sexual abuse in later family life: mental health, parenting and adjustment of offspring', *Child Abuse and Neglect*, vol 28, pp 525-45.

Roberts, S.B. (2000) 'High-glycemic index foods, hunger, and obesity: is there a connection?', *Nutrition Reviews*, vol 58, pp 163-9.

Robson, W.J. (2001) 'Alcohol misuse', *Archives of Disease in Childhood*, vol 84, pp 95-7.

Rudolf, M.C.J., Greenwood, D.C., Cole, T.J., Levine, R., Sahota, P., Walker, J., Holland, P., Cade, J. and Truscott, J. (2004) 'Rising obesity and expanding waistlines in schoolchildren: a cohort study', *Archives of Disease in Childhood*, vol 89, pp 235-7.

Rutter, M. and Maughan, B. (2002) 'School effectiveness findings 1979-2002', *Journal of School Psychology*, vol 40, pp 451-75.

Saxena, S., Ambler, G., Cole, T.J. and Majeed, A. (2004) 'Ethnic group differences in overweight and obese children and young people in England: cross sectional survey', *Archives of Disease in Childhood*, vol 89, pp 30-6.

Seguire, M. and Chalmers, K.I. (2000) 'Late adolescent female smoking', *Journal of Advanced Nursing*, vol 31, pp 1422-9.

SEU (Social Exclusion Unit) (2003) *A better education for children in care*, London: ODPM.

Sidebotham, P., Heron, J., Golding, J. and the ALSPAC Study Team (2002) 'Child maltreatment in the "Children of the Nineties": deprivation, class, and social networks in a UK sample', *Child Abuse and Neglect*, vol 26, pp 1243-59.

Sparkes, J. (1999) *Schools, education and social exclusion*, CASE Paper 29, Centre for Analysis of Social Exclusion, London School of Economics and Political Science.

Stamatakis, E. (2003a) 'Anthropometric measurements, overweight and obesity', in K. Sproston and P. Primatesta (eds) *Health Survey for England 2002: The health of children and young people*, London: The Stationery Office.

Stamatakis, E. (2003b) 'Physical activity', in K. Sproston and P. Primatesta (eds) *Health Survey for England 2002: The health of children and young people*, London: The Stationery Office.

Stanistreet, D. and Jeffrey, V. (2003) 'Injury and poisoning mortality among young men – are there any common factors amenable to prevention?', *Crisis*, vol 24, pp 122-7.

Steinbeck, K.S. (2001) 'The importance of physical activity in the prevention of overweight and obesity in childhood: a review and an opinion', *Obesity Reviews*, vol 2, pp 117-30.

Stephens, J. (2002) *The mental health needs of homeless young people: Bright futures: Working with vulnerable young people*, London: The Mental Health Foundation and Barnado's.

Sweeting, H. and West, P. (2001) 'Social class and smoking at age 15: the effect of different definitions of smoking', *Addiction*, vol 96, pp 1357-9.

Thomas, S. and Mortimore, P. (1996) 'Comparison of value-added models for secondary school effectiveness', *Research Papers in Education*, vol 11, pp 279-95.

Trevisan, M., Dorn, J., Falkner, K., Russell, M., Ram, M., Muti, P., Freudenheim, J.L., Nochajaski, T. and Hovey, K. (2004) 'Drinking pattern and risk of non-fatal myocardial infarction: a population-based case-control study', *Addiction*, vol 99, pp 313-22.

Tyas, S.L. and Pederson, L.L. (1998) 'Psychosocial factors related to adolescent smoking: a critical review of the literature', *Tobacco Control*, vol 7, pp 409-20.

Walker, A., Gregory, J., Bradnock, G., Nunn, J. and White, D. (2000) *National diet and nutrition survey: Young people aged 4 to 18 Years. Volume 2: Report of the oral health survey*, London: The Stationery Office.

Walker, I. and Zhu, Y. (2003) 'Education, earnings and productivity: recent UK evidence', *Labour Market Trends*, March, pp 145-52.

Wannamethee, S.G. and Shaper, A.G. (1999) 'Type of alcoholic drink and risk of major coronary heart disease events and all-cause mortality', *American Journal of Public Health*, vol 89, pp 685-90.

Wardle, H. and Hedges, B. (2003) 'Cigarette smoking', in K. Sproston and P. Primatesta (eds) *Health Survey for England 2002: The health of children and young people*, London: The Stationery Office.

Wellings, K., Wadsworth, J., Johnson, A., Field, J. and Macdowall, W. (1999) 'Teenage fertility and life chances', *Reviews of Reproduction*, vol 4, pp 184-90.

Wellings, K., Nanchahal, K., Macdowall, W., McManus, S., Erens, B., Mercer, C.H., Johnson, A.M., Copas, A.J., Korovessis, C., Fenton, K.A. and Field, J. (2001) 'Sexual behaviour in Britain: early heterosexual experience', *Lancet*, vol 358, pp 1843-50.

West, P., Sweeting, H. and Ecob, R. (1999) 'Family and friends' influences on the uptake of regular smoking from mid-adolescence to early adulthood', *Addiction*, vol 94, pp 1397-412.

Wight, D., Henderson, M., Raab, G., Abraham, C., Buston, K., Scott, S. and Hart, G. (2000) 'Extent of regretted sexual intercourse among young teenagers in Scotland: a cross sectional survey', *British Medical Journal*, vol 320, pp 1243-4.

Williams, J., Jackson, S., Maddocks, A., Cheung, W.-Y., Love A. and Hutchings, H. (2001) 'Case-control study of the health of those looked after by local authorities', *Archives of Disease in Childhood*, vol 85, pp 280-5.

Withers, N.J., Low, J.L., Holgate, S.T. and Clough, J.B. (2000) 'Smoking habits in a cohort of U.K. adolescents', *Respiratory Medicine*, vol 94, pp 391-6.

Woodward, L.J., Horwood, L.J. and Fergusson, D.M. (2001) 'Teenage pregnancy: cause for concern', *New Zealand Medical Journal*, vol 114, pp 301-3.

Wouters, S., Marshall, R., Yee, R.L. and Jackson, R. (2000) 'Is the apparent cardioprotective effect of recent alcohol consumption due to confounding by prodromal symptoms?', *American Journal of Epidemiology*, vol 151, pp 1189-93.

NINE

Inequalities in the health behaviour of children and youth: policy and practice

Introduction

Normal childhood and adolescent development is arguably characterised first by immature and then by inconsistent behaviour, compounded by a sense of invulnerability, experimentation, and a limited concern for future health. This scenario is complicated by two quite different imperatives. On the one hand, young people now face earlier and more intensive exposure to high-risk behaviour, with social and media attitudes encouraging them to look and act older than their years (NSNR, 2000). On the other hand, as Chapter Six has established, there is an increasing delay before the vast majority of adolescents achieve financial and domestic independence. There is thus an extended period post-adolescence where one can no longer assume a requirement to conform and where conspicuous consumption may be an important motivation (Parker et al, 1998).

Social variations are manifest in these risk behaviours and, as Chapter Eight demonstrated, childhood and adolescence, long-held as a period of relative equality in health, is now increasingly perceived as a period of extreme inequality in terms of health behaviour and attendant risk with both immediate and long-term implications. The risk-taking behaviours that can be described as problematic in childhood and youth, such as smoking, drinking, other drug use, early sexual activity and poor eating habits, are all associated with one another (Tyas and Pederson, 1998). The recent attention given to the so-called obesity epidemic has helped extend the profile of social concern to still younger children, albeit with a more explicit focus on health.

The complex relational web between risk factors and detrimental outcomes militates against compartmentalisation. It demands that the connections are made, challenging the preoccupation with symptoms rather than causes and pointing to the need to address the whole person, not just one or two risk factors (Millward et al, 2004). This chapter focuses on three significant areas where health behaviour is markedly unequal, that is: diet and nutrition; substance abuse; and sexual health; together with education and employment.

Diet and nutrition

Poor diet in childhood, as Chapter Eight has shown, is associated with both poor child and later adult health. Interventions fall under two related heads. First, there have been long-standing efforts to improve nutritional status, by both food supplementation (ranging from the school-based provision of milk and school meals to the current focus on fruit and vegetables) and efforts to address food poverty. Second, there has been a more recent emphasis on weight-related disorders, primarily obesity. The incidence of dental caries is a further corollary of poor nutritional status, with less than half of all children disease-free on starting school (Walker et al, 2000), a reflection of the frequency and amount of sugar being consumed.

Food supplementation: food poverty and modern malnutrition

It has been suggested that the government's National Diet and Nutrition Survey (NDNS) exposes a pattern of modern malnutrition, especially in low-income families (Gregory et al, 2000). Chapter Eight has shown how such dietary deficiencies show a social class and income gradient, with households in the lowest income brackets consuming less fresh fruit and vegetables, skimmed milk, fish, fruit juices and breakfast cereals than average, despite spending a greater proportion of their income on food than those in better-off households.

One contributory factor is believed to be food poverty, with those living in the poorest areas having reduced access (although the reasons for this are debated) to good-quality affordable food. Despite suggestions that adults in poverty protect their children's diets at the expense of their own (Dowler and Calvert, 1995), it has been suggested that one in 50 children do not get three meals a day (Dowler et al, 2001). Social and cultural norms, knowledge and health motivation are important in this equation. Skipping breakfast, for example, is particularly common among adolescent girls, while one in ten girls aged 15-18 report being either a vegan or vegetarian, and those under 25 typically eat half as many fruit and vegetables as those in the 55-64 age group (Gregory et al, 2000). Interventions that address food poverty have the potential to reduce inequalities in diet and expenditure among the poorest families and have formed an important component of the government's Neighbourhood Renewal Strategy (see Chapter Eleven), while interventions that aim to improve nutritional status have the potential to reduce health inequalities if they are targeted at those in greatest need.

Weight-related disorders

Since the 1980s the prevalence of obesity has increased so dramatically that by 1998 the World Health Organization (WHO) declared it a global epidemic. In the UK it has similarly become a public health priority, with incidence of obesity trebling between 1980 and 2001. As Chapter Eight demonstrated, the prevalence of overweight and obesity among children of all ages is increasing as part of this trend, with national statistics suggesting upwards of one fifth of all children are now either overweight or obese, and local studies producing much higher proportions (Bundred et al, 2001; Rudolf et al, 2001). Pertinently, although the risk factors for a range of health disorders increase with weight, many of the problems for overweight/obese children are deferred to later life, leading some to suggest that "the most important long-term consequence of childhood obesity is persistence into adulthood" (Mulvihill and Quigley, 2003, p 14). This too is a risk that increases with the age of the child and the severity of the obesity. The yearly cost has been estimated as £0.5 billion in terms of treatment costs to the National Health Service (NHS) and more than £2 billion in terms of the impact on the wider economy (NAO, 2001). As with adults, it is an area where socio-economic, ethnic and national inequalities exist. The causes, as we have already noted, include not just an increasingly sedentary lifestyle, reliance on the car and changing eating habits (reflecting, for example, longer working hours and less food preparation at home) (NAO, 2001), but also genetic factors. Many are areas that health professionals are unable to change in isolation.

The increased prevalence of obesity has largely overshadowed other weight-related disorders such as anorexia nervosa and bulimia nervosa which, as Chapter Six has shown, are both comparatively rare and higher among higher social classes. The literature is equivocal about the relationship between the prevalence of such eating disorders and the prevention of obesity but emphatic about the high incidence of dieting and shape/weight-related concerns among older children and teenagers, factors that are not captured by such statistics. The difficulty is determining when these constitute abnormal eating attitudes and behaviour carrying a high degree of risk and when they are part of the natural course of adolescence (Pratt and Woolfenden, 2004). There is a strong argument, therefore, for considering the range of weight-related disorders under one public health umbrella.

What works? Evidence and practice

In considering the efficacy of key interventions attention is focused on three salient areas: breakfast clubs (which aim to improve nutritional status within a specific context), healthy eating initiatives (which take a more broad-based approach to nutritional status) and efforts to prevent and treat obesity.

Breakfast clubs

Children who have no breakfast may be at risk from adverse health effects in the long term, and adverse educational and social effects in the short term as a consequence of poor concentration and behaviour in school, together with poor socialisation, bullying and erratic attendance (Street, 1998). An overview of breakfast clubs (Ani and Grantham-McGregor, 1998) suggests they may confer corresponding short-term benefits on classroom behaviour (including active class participation and peer interaction), cognition, academic outcomes and school attendance, with such effects more noticeable in poorly nourished children. They can also provide a safe place for children to meet their friends before school (Lucas, 2003). However, the findings reviewed were largely from outside either Europe or North America. Beneficiaries were thus not only more likely to be undernourished than children in the UK but also less likely to attend school regularly. Those studied also tended to fall into the 9- to 12-year-old age group, whereas in countries such as the UK it may be adolescents who are most at risk of skipping meals and least likely to take part in breakfast schemes (Lucas, 2003).

The Department of Health (DH) established a pilot in 1999/2000 to develop school-based breakfast clubs, with the aim of developing preferences for healthy eating and establishing a positive start to the school day by providing breakfast for those who would otherwise start the school day hungry. Funds were allocated to 253 clubs, with approximately two thirds of these based in primary schools, and were focused on the more deprived areas targeted already by, for example, Health Action Zones (HAZs), Education Action Zones (EAZs) or Sure Start. A national evaluation of this pilot found only modest benefits with respect to social, nutritional, educational and psychological well-being. However, children and parents alike regarded "school breakfast clubs as capable of precipitating *at least* a degree of positive change across a broad spectrum of outcomes", including dietary behaviour, social relations and reductions in family stress at the start of the day (Shemilt et al, 2003, p 110). Meanwhile, three quarters of the surveyed clubs felt they had improved attendance (see also Shemilt et al, 2004) and punctuality, with four fifths claiming improvements in concentration and half an improvement in academic performance during morning lessons.

Similar positive outcomes were revealed by a previous sample of 35 clubs in the UK, with organisers reporting a calmer start to the day, better parent/teacher dialogue, improved social cohesion among pupils and less disruptive behaviour (Street and Kenway, 1999). However, there was still concern over early arrivals, children not taking breakfast (including those who spent breakfast club money on snacks before arriving at school) and an inability to reach those with the greatest problems of punctuality, attendance or need (Lucas, 2003). Nevertheless, a recent survey of award-winning clubs by the New Policy Institute suggested that most of these clubs were attracting a disproportionate number of children claiming free school meals (FSM), a group that is less likely to eat breakfast at home (Harrop and Palmer, 2002). The evaluation of the national DH pilot (set up in areas with some degree of multidimensional adversity) similarly suggested they were capable of "reaching families likely to be most in need of support including some families at risk of or experiencing social exclusion" (University of East Anglia, 2002, p 8). Use here was greatest among families where a parent was experiencing marked levels of emotional stress or where children had high levels of overall difficulties. A randomised controlled trial (RCT) also found a higher proportion of breakfast club attendees had borderline or abnormal conduct and a higher total difficulties score (Shemilt et al, 2004).

Healthy eating initiatives

A systematic review of interventions designed to promote healthy eating (Roe et al, 1997) suggests the key is similarly behavioural change, with the intervention matched to the population characteristics, as opposed to the more traditional provision of information. Effective interventions include a supportive family, social and structural environment, a personal approach with contact sustained over time, multiple strategies that address barriers to change and influence the local environment, and training for those involved in the delivery and support of such programmes. Interestingly, such interventions appear to be more successful in reducing fat intake and blood cholesterol than in supplementing intake of starchy foods or fruit and vegetables (Roe et al, 1997). However, even such targeted interventions are only producing reductions in total fat intake as a proportion of dietary energy in line with the UK population target set by *The health of the nation* (DH, 1992) (–3%), while the parallel aim was to increase the consumption of fruit and vegetables and starchy foods by at least 50%.

This problem is well illustrated by a cluster randomised trial of 43 primary schools in South Wales and the South West of England, where the introduction of fruit tuck shops was found to have only limited impact on pupils' fruit consumption and to produce no significant difference between intervention and control schools in pupils' intake of fruit or other snacks. Indeed, only 70,000 fruits were sold in the 23 intervention schools over the year, equating to just 0.046 fruits per pupil per day, and four schools had closed their fruit tuck shops by the end of the intervention year (Moore et al, 2000; Moore, 2001). A whole school intervention that increased the provision of fruits and vegetables in school (via tuck shops and school lunches), as well as providing information for parents, children and teachers, together with tasting opportunities and practical food preparation, found little more success. Evaluation found that children in the intervention schools increased their fruit intake more than those in the control school, and their knowledge about fruits and vegetables was also greater, but the changes were only modest (Anderson, 2001).

Food Dudes (see Box 9.1) represents a further step towards adopting a comprehensive approach to altering eating behaviour, introducing peer group example and a reward system. The programme has been conducted with incremental changes to context, age group, socio-economic profile of the children, and administration (moving from programme staff to school staff). It has now been rolled out in parts of Scotland, Wales, England and Ireland and is the subject of ongoing evaluation.

Box 9.1: A behavioural approach to increasing fruit and vegetable consumption

The Food Dudes are a group of slightly older peers introduced to primary school-aged children by video. In the course of their adventures, they are seen to enjoy eating a variety of fruit and vegetables and invite the viewers to eat these foods and join their struggle to save the health of the children of the world. Prizes such as stickers and pencils are awarded to children who consume sufficient quantities of targeted foods. As well as everyday vegetables and fruit these include a number of new foods presented in the form of snack packs of raw fruit and vegetables at break time and as cooked additions to the lunch menu.

Typical results showed snack time consumption of fruit and vegetables doubling from baseline to intervention, with canteen consumption of vegetables trebling in one school. These results were maintained at a six-month follow-up. Importantly, the largest gains in terms of additional fruit and vegetable consumption were shown for those children who ate the least at the outset with, for example, those who ate only 4% of their fruit and vegetables at baseline increasing to 68% and 38% respectively during the intervention.

Evaluation established that both the video and the rewards scheme were required to produce significant results, while merely making the fruit and vegetables available, particularly at lunchtime, had no effect. Success was attributed to the way the programme encouraged children repeatedly to try the fruit and vegetables so that they acquired a taste for these and came to see themselves as fruit and vegetable eaters. The study also found good generalisation of effect both in terms of foods consumed (extending to non-target fruit and vegetables) and context (with increased consumption at school also recorded at home and increased consumption at snack time also noticeable at lunchtime) (Lowe et al, nd).

Obesity: prevention and treatment

A recent systematic review of interventions for the prevention of obesity in children found "the mismatch between the prevalence and significance of the condition and the knowledge base from which to inform preventative activity" to be "remarkable and an outstanding feature of this review" (Campbell et al, 2002, p 12). Others stress the limitations of review-level evidence itself for decision making about policy and practice in such a complex and relational field, an area that is impossible to capture in quantitative outcomes alone (Mulvihill and Quigley, 2003).

As far as prevention goes, the strongest evidence of effectiveness focuses on multifaceted school-based programmes, that is, programmes that promote physical activity, the modification of dietary intake and the targeting of sedentary behaviours (Mulvihill and Quigley, 2003). Such interventions have been found to be particularly effective for girls. Planet Health, for example, was a multifaceted behavioural intervention that targeted 11- to 13-year-olds in the three areas just described, but with a strong emphasis on reducing television viewing (Gortmaker et al, 1999). Two years later it found reduced prevalence of obesity among girls in the intervention schools and fewer obese girls in the intervention group but no significant differences for boys. Two possible reasons were the more pronounced reduction in television viewing among the girls and a greater increase in their fruit and vegetable consumption, resulting in a smaller daily increment in total energy intake.

The one UK study included within the systematic reviews (see Box 9.2) found, however, that positive changes in attitudes and environment were accompanied by few significant changes in behaviour, and suggested that the prevailing social and environmental forces require much larger public health control measures (Sahota et al, 2001a). A more recent UK school-based preventative programme similarly found no clear intervention effect and stressed the need for reinforcement beyond the school setting (Warren et al, 2003). Such community-based interventions, by definition, do not focus just on children and adolescents and

Box 9.2: A multifaceted school-based programme for obesity

The APPLES study focused on 10 primary schools in Leeds, randomly allocated to either the intervention or control group. The intervention was designed to influence diet and physical activity as well as knowledge, and was underpinned by the Health Promoting Schools philosophy, involving the whole school community (including parents, teachers and catering staff) (Sahota et al, 2001b). It also took sustainability into account by using existing staff to deliver the programme (Campbell et al, 2002). Components included teacher training, modification of school meals, the development of school action plans targeting the curriculum, physical education, tuck shops and playground activities.

Process evaluation showed that the APPLES intervention was successful in producing changes at the school level, in terms of changing the ethos of the schools and the attitudes of the children, but had little effect on children's behaviour other than a modest increase in the consumption of vegetables (Sahota et al, 2001a). Data were collected on 634 children aged 7-11 years but after one year in the programme there was no difference in change in Body Mass Index (BMI) between the children in the two groups, nor any difference in dieting behaviour. Indeed, fruit consumption was lower in obese children in the intervention group and sedentary behaviour was higher in overweight children in the intervention group. Global self-worth was, however, higher in obese children in the intervention group although not reflected in other psychological measures (dietary restraint, body shape preference and self-perception).

are considered more generally in Chapter Eleven. With respect specifically to young people the limited data available make it difficult to conclude that one strategy or combination of strategies is more important than others in the prevention of childhood obesity (Campbell et al, 2002).

There is even less evidence for the preventative effectiveness of school-based health promotion interventions (focusing on the classroom curriculum to reduce sedentary behaviours such as television and video games), and a lack of evidence as to the effectiveness of school-based physical activity on a standalone basis (NHS CRD, 2002). However, Campbell et al (2002) suggest that the most promising interventions focus on simple reductions in sedentary behaviours with lifestyle activities sustainable across the lifecycle (such as walking and cycling) likely to be the most effective. There is also evidence that there are different issues affecting primary and secondary schools, with a sharp drop off in sports uptake in the upward transition and an increase in canteen, tuck shop and vending machine access to food.

Family-based behavioural modification programmes that involve parents via family therapy and target these same three areas (dietary education, physical activity and a reduction in sedentary behaviours), together with regular visits to a paediatrician, also lack the same weight of evidence as multifaceted school-based interventions, but do show limited evidence of effectiveness. In contrast, there is a lack of evidence to support family-based health promotion programmes as a preventative measure (despite the fact that these too include a strong focus on dietary and health education, increased activity and sustained contact with children and parents) (Mulvihill and Quigley, 2003). This suggests the potential importance of the behavioural modification/family therapy element.

With respect to the treatment of obesity, Summerbell et al (2004) synthesised the results of 18 RCTs that focused on lifestyle interventions (all having some form of dietary input, physical activity and behavioural therapy), and that observed participants for a minimum of six months. Most were, however, based in hospital settings and focused on small, homogenous, motivated groups. As a result their review, as with the issue of prevention, found little generalisable evidence of what works. Indeed, none of the studies were conducted in the UK although all were undertaken in societies where there is a similar "unrelenting progression towards weight gain", militating against the maintenance of weight loss (Summerbell et al, 2004, p 7).

It is the family as opposed to the school that tends to be the locus for successful interventions at the treatment stage, most specifically family-based interventions involving at least one parent alongside the child, and combining physical activity and health promotion with the targeting of sedentary behaviour (Mulvihill and Quigley, 2003). For primary school children evidence supports multifaceted family behaviour modification programmes, where the parent acts as the agent of change (and components include parenting, communications skills training and child management alongside diet, exercise and reductions in sedentary

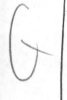

behaviour). The value of the parental influence may, however, vary with the age of the child, providing more benefits to younger (more compliant) children. Evaluation of effectiveness is also compromised by the disparate nature of the interventions (and an inability to isolate the effective components of any such programme), so that overall there remains insufficient evidence to recommend family-based behaviour modification programmes as an effective treatment (NHS CRD, 2002). There is, nevertheless, limited evidence for behaviour modification programmes that lack parental involvement, suggesting the support of parents is important to the process and that treatments need to be individualised.

Story (1999) draws on a non-systematic literature review of 12 school-based interventions targeted at overweight children (the large majority with a no-treatment control and based on physical activity and nutritional education). Eleven out of twelve found a reduction in the percentage of children classified as overweight in the intervention group, with an average decline in individual body weight of 10%. Interventions again tended to be more effective where children were younger and weight problems the most intense. However, Story (1999) also highlights the stigma potentially attaching to school-based treatments, with the possibility of psychosocial damage; few studies of school-based treatments have thus been conducted since 1985 with the school acting instead as a potentially powerful preventative arena.

LeMura and Maziekas (2002), drawing on a meta-analysis of laboratory-based exercise programmes, also demonstrate the effectiveness of exercise treatment programmes, the three most favoured interventions being low-intensity, long-duration exercise; aerobic exercise with high repetition resistance training; and exercise programmes in conjunction with behaviour modification. The translation of effective laboratory-based strategies to a non-clinical setting is often, however, problematic. The results from a series of small trials in the US (Epstein et al, 1985, reviewed in Summerbell et al, 2004) suggest again that while lifestyle exercise (such as walking or running), aerobics and callisthenics may all produce significant reductions in weight, it is the former that is the most likely to produce sustained change. Finally, while the National Institute for Clinical Excellence (NICE) has approved the use of two drugs in the management of adult obesity, orlistat and sibutramine, neither are currently recommended for use with younger age groups (NICE, 2001).

The evidence for sustained effective weight loss treatments is thus small, partly because to have any effect interventions need to be complex and partly because such interventions do not alter the context of the obese child's environment external to the family. Additionally, as Summerbell et al (2004) point out, a problem of epidemic proportions requires commensurate resources in prevention and treatment in order to achieve change. Successful strategies require action to create environments that support prevention and maintenance (that is, upstream rather than individual interventions), and need to address the range of obesogenic factors (sports and leisure, family, high-energy foods, education and information)

(Blair et al, 2003). Encouragingly, however, it has been suggested that lifestyle behaviours that contribute to and sustain obesity in adults are less well-established in children and may be more amenable to change (Edmunds et al, 2001).

Other weight-related disorders

Pratt and Woolfenden (2004), considering interventions for preventing eating disorders in children and adolescents, were similarly unable to draw any firm conclusion about the effectiveness of eating disorder programmes in childhood and adolescents. Again, a variety of approaches (encompassing the acquisition of knowledge, the modification of eating and risk behaviours and efforts to increase social well-being), a diversity of target groups and a paucity of admissible RCTs, limited the evidence base. However, the correlation between such eating disorders and overweight status, low self-esteem, depression, suicidal ideation and substance misuse, indicates the need again to take a holistic approach to the identification and amelioration of risk factors, together with the identification of protective factors.

Limitations to the evidence base

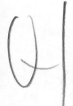

The limitations to the available evidence base are emerging as a dominant subtext within this book. Here the diversity of the studies (with numerous intervention components), their methodological quality (including recruitment base), size, and duration, limits the generalisability and reproducibility of the findings concerning obesity, as does the US focus and the concentration on children aged 7-12. This is compounded by difficulties in the measurement of childhood obesity, measures of diet and physical activity (which are often weak estimates of actual behaviour) and a limited understanding of the interface between an individual's behaviour and their environment. Several studies that effected change in the short term found these changes were not maintained at subsequent follow-ups, suggesting (as indicated by the behavioural change literature) the need for sustained rather than time-limited interventions.

Roe et al (1997), considering healthy eating interventions, found a similar reliance on findings from the US and a neglect of the adolescent population. They suggest there are too few well-evaluated studies to identify the most effective outcomes for any given target group. There is also a marked neglect of patient-related variables, including gender, ethnicity, socio-economic status and psychological status, reflecting the general dearth of evidence in relation to public health interventions that address health inequality issues (Mulvihill and Quigley, 2003), together with a neglect of the characteristics of those lost from follow-up.

Policy

The issues of diet and obesity have been on the political agenda since the 1990s, albeit with a primary emphasis on the adult population. *The health of the nation* (DH, 1992) introduced targets in these areas and this was reinforced by both the *Independent Inquiry into Inequalities in Health* (Acheson, 1998), which recommended increasing the availability and accessibility of foodstuffs to reduce health inequalities throughout life, and *Saving lives: Our healthier nation* (DH, 1999). This emphasis has been maintained by the Public Health White Paper, *Choosing health* (HM Government and DH, 2004), which took reducing obesity and improving diet and nutrition as one of its six overarching priorities. It is also supported by the 2004 Spending Review Objectives, where one of the joint targets for the DH, Department for Education and Skills (DfES) and the Department for Culture, Media and Sport (DCMS) is to halt the year-on-year rise in obesity among children under the age of 11 by 2010 in the context of a broader strategy to tackle obesity in the population as a whole (DfES, 2004a).

A first theme, and one that reflects the evidence base, has been the increased emphasis on a 'settings' approach to health promotion, in which schools and communities are identified as the locus for multiple and reinforcing health-promoting actions. The concept of the healthy school was developed by the WHO in the early 1980s in order to encourage a whole school approach to personal and community health (see, for example, Lister-Sharp et al, 1999). It recognises, for example, that classroom education on nutrition is undermined if healthy food choices are not available in school meals and in school tuck shops. This produced a raft of health-promoting school programmes across the UK, which were consolidated and extended by the Healthy Schools Programme, a joint DH and Department for Education and Employment (DfEE) initiative launched in England in 1998. This aims to improve standards of health and education and to tackle health inequalities by making children, teachers, parents and local communities more aware of the opportunities that exist in schools for improving health. The focus on the school may be of particular importance in rural areas where young people do not have easy access to health and other services.

An important part of the Programme is the National Healthy School Standard (NHSS), a national guidance and accreditation process to support the development of healthy schools, which includes the requirement to promote healthier food within schools and to provide education about healthy eating. The standard is now increasingly focused on achievements at school level and concerned to target the most disadvantaged. Schools themselves are expected, for example, to demonstrate how they are contributing to targets around health inequalities, social inclusion and raising achievements, while those schools where FSM eligibility is 20% or more are expected to implement the standard most closely, achieving NHSS Level Three by March 2006 (DH and DfES, 2003a). A review of the NHSS suggested it has been instrumental in providing a structure for health promotion work and curriculum development and increasing motivation to act. Related improvements in pilot schools included improvements in attendance, bullying, self-esteem and the school environment, that is, areas beyond academic achievement, with the standard felt to mirror the broad view that young people take of health (Rivers et al, 2000). Success is, however, highly dependent on the standard being accorded a high profile at senior level in local health and education authorities, having a similarly high level of support at school level and being backed by adequate human and financial resources, including the ability to renegotiate external catering contracts. There have also been problems involving young people systematically, and little evidence to date of any real difference between schools according to level reached (Warwick et al, 2004).

Within this holistic context many would argue that the role of school meals has long been neglected. School lunches were once considered a means of enabling needy and undernourished children to benefit from school education. Their contribution to the health of children had been tentatively recognised by the re-introduction after 20 years of national minimum nutritional standards for schools in 2001. This was, however, set against the growth of commercial sponsorship in school meals and catering contracts awarded to firms who had but a weak commitment to providing nutritious meals. It was also set against the low FSM uptake, thought to be caused in part by the stigma and bullying associated with targeting (Riley, 2005). Both act to constrain the potential of school meals to confer nutritional advantage.

There has also been a lack of any serious challenge to advertising or attention to the power of marketing to make healthier choices more attractive, alongside a lack of research into the negative effects of junk food. Meanwhile, the food industry continues to offer a range of incentives to schools to allow the sale of their produce on school sites, or indeed commands a contractual presence by virtue of the Private Finance Initiative (where they operate in tandem with the construction companies to secure a range of catering and vending contracts). Given the time it took to ban tobacco, despite conclusive evidence as to its adverse impact on health, the task of redefining where, when and how unhealthy foods may be marketed in the interest of public health, is likely to be major challenge. *Choosing health* has signalled the intention to start to address the issue, albeit in the future, with a strategy to restrict the advertising and promotion to children (including sponsorship, vending machines and packaging) of foods and drinks that are high in fat, salt or sugar (HM Government and DH, 2004).

Similar plans to consider the introduction of nutrient-based standards for school meals were given a much needed impetus by a television series presented by celebrity chef Jamie Oliver. This raised the profile of school lunches dramatically, stressing not only the limited per capita spend and the wide-ranging consequences of poor diet but also the endemic resistance to healthy eating among many school children and their parents. The government consequently pledged £280 million (over three years from September 2005) to improve school meals, with per capita spend rising from 37p to (the still very low figure of) 50p per child in primary schools and 60p in secondary schools. This will be reinforced by accredited training qualifications for school caterers, new statutory requirements (from 2006) for nutrient-based primary and secondary standards and revised school meal standards to cover the whole school day (thus including, for example, vending machine sales). Significantly, this reinforces moves already made by the Scottish Executive and Welsh Assembly to introduce and resource higher standards, suggesting, as with a number of other aspects of the health inequalities agenda, a more progressive approach outside England. However, criticism continues to focus on the available resources (given, for instance, the dismantling of the kitchen infrastructure) and the lack of a curriculum in schools to teach children to purchase, prepare and cook healthy food. More pervasively, the Child Poverty Action Group (CPAG) suggests universal provision of school meals is fundamental to ensuring increased uptake from low-income homes (Riley, 2005).

Other components of the Healthy Schools Programme include the National Healthy Schools Network, Wired for Health, Cooking for Kids and Safer Travel to School (which focuses on strategies to reduce car journeys to school where safer, healthier alternatives exist). A series of related initiatives build on this school focus and the integrated approach between education and health. The proportion of young people spending two hours or more in physical education lessons at school fell, for example, from 46% in 1994 to 33% in 1999 (CYPU, 2001), with nearly one fifth of school children spending less than one hour per week on physical education (Nessa and Gallagher, 2004), half the NHSS standard. The government's plan for sport (DCMS, 2000) therefore included a focus both on young people and the educational infrastructure. This incorporated a health inequalities dimension with lottery-funded school sports coordinators to be established initially in the 600 communities in the greatest need and lottery resources channelled, via Sport England, to disadvantaged areas: areas with Sports Action Zone, EAZ or Excellence in Cities funding. It also established specialist sports colleges. This was reinforced in 2002 by the Physical Education, School Sports and Club Links Strategy, which aims to build on the emerging network of specialist sports colleges to develop 400 school sport partnerships by 2006, supported by teachers released to act as secondary school sports coordinators and primary/special school link teachers (DfES and DCMS, 2003). Funding of £459 million was dedicated to the strategy in 2002 with a further £519 million identified in 2004 for the period 2006-08. Further support has been given by a Public Service Agreement (PSA) target that aims to increase the percentage of 5- to 16-year-olds who spend a minimum of two hours each week on high-quality Physical Education (PE) and school sport within *and beyond* the curriculum from 25% in 2002 to 75% by 2006 (DfES, 2004a). By 2003-04 62% of pupils in school within a school sport partnership were reported to have met this target, although as yet only 6,500 of England's 12,000 schools fall into this category.

Breakfast clubs can similarly be seen as a response to a number of key public policy drivers: childcare, education, nutrition and social inclusion, although their status remains ambiguous and insecure, in part probably because of this breadth of remit (Harrop and Palmer, 2002). Adequate coverage is also a real problem for so many of these targeted initiatives. The New Policy Institute (Street and Kenway, 1999) estimated that there were some 400-600 breakfast clubs in 1999, catering for perhaps 0.5% of primary school-aged children, a figure that contrasts markedly with the suggestion that one third of all children may start the day without breakfast. Breakfast clubs in more deprived areas are also highly dependent on external funding since it is unlikely that they will ever be able to charge enough to cover their costs. As with childcare, the political emphasis on new starts and the provision of start-up funding has also left many clubs in financial difficulty (while the task of securing ongoing funding is a disincentive to establishment, particularly in primary schools, which have higher staffing ratios and lower rates of attendance). Staffing is a further critical barrier because of the early start and the restricted hours. However, the holistic emphasis is gradually encouraging more schools to view such clubs as part of their mainstream activities rather than an additional service, with concurrent opportunities to provide staffing, for example, from school budgets (Harrop and Palmer, 2002).

Given the increasing evidence of a link between nutrition and school performance and behaviour many would argue that this is a wise investment of educational resources but, paradoxically, these clubs do not always offer a nutritious and well-balanced meal. A survey of award-winning breakfast clubs by the New Policy Institute found most had adopted a 'give them what they want philosophy' in order to ensure good take-up of breakfast or sometimes to restrict costs (Harrop and Palmer, 2002, p 25). Fresh foods are thus cut back with the club focusing (as in resource-constrained households) on popular foods that they know the children will eat. As a consequence health and nutrition and access for families on a low income are both frequent casualties – suggesting the need for increased emphasis on the importance of breakfast, the involvement of health professionals and increased subsidies for those who cannot afford to participate (Street and Kenway, 1999).

Another relatively high-profile response has been the Five-a-Day Programme in England. Established by *The NHS Plan*, where it was linked to *The NHS Cancer Plan* (DH, 2000) and the National Service Framework for Coronary Heart Disease (NSF for CHD), it aims to increase people's awareness of the importance of having access to, and eating, at least five portions of vegetables and fruit a day. Key elements are the National School Fruit Scheme, which entitles children aged between four and six to a free piece of fruit each day at school, and community initiatives developed by primary care organisations and their partners for people living in disadvantaged areas, together with work with the food industry, including growers and caterers, to improve the general public's access to fruit and vegetables. The National Audit Office (NAO) has also suggested that the

DH and DfES should consider a performance target for fruit and vegetables in schools, while the Children's NSF also directs attention to the broader issues of healthy diet and physical activity.

Effective political strategies against weight-related disorders are similarly recognised as those that (drawing on the albeit tentative evidence base) work at a number of levels (individual, group and community), and address both circumstantial barriers to change (such as affordability and access) and attitudinal barriers (such as dietary perceptions, health-related knowledge, cooking skills and peer pressure) (HDA, 2002). Within the NHS, primary and community health professionals such as general practitioners (GPs), health visitors and school nurses, offer the greatest contact with overweight/obese children. Research conducted by the NAO in 1999 found, however, that while 83% of health authorities had identified obesity as a public health issue in their Health Improvement Programme, only 28% had actually taken action to address this and plans tended to address the issue via cancer and CHD strategies, rather than a dedicated obesity strategy, suggesting a corresponding neglect of childhood and adolescence (NAO, 2001). Key staff have long been subject to a number of competing priorities. School nurses, for instance, are significantly bound up in child protection as well as immunisation work, which limits their ability to work on prevention or increase their public health role, despite the rhetoric of both *Choosing health* (HM Government and DH, 2004) and the NSF for Children and Young People.

Substance abuse

Cigarette smoking is the major preventable cause of premature mortality in industrialised countries. Reducing its prevalence among adults is thus central to policies to improve health and to reduce socio-economic inequalities. Given that most smokers start smoking in their teenage years, and that heavy smoking in adolescence is associated with a higher risk of smoking long term, childhood and early youth would be expected to be key periods for primary prevention. Indeed, with 16% of 11-year-olds in England having already experimented with smoking, it has been suggested that programmes may have to target children as young as four to eight years of age if they are to intervene before behavioural patterns become established (NHS CRD, 1999). The proportion of young people smoking on a regular, weekly basis has remained relatively stable across the 1990s with, as Chapter Eight has shown, 20% of boys and 26% of girls aged 15 smoking at least one cigarette a week.

The pattern of alcohol consumption, the first and most widely consumed recreational drug used by young people, has similarly shown no obvious trend when measured by frequency over the 1990s, with approximately one fifth of 11- to 15-year-olds drinking in the past week. However, the average weekly consumption of alcohol among young people has increased substantially (Rowan,

2004), and the UK heads the European league table in terms of the prevalence of binge drinking and youthful intoxication. Contributory factors include increasingly sophisticated subsector marketing and increases in the alcoholic content of the drinks sold.

Alcohol dependence is surprisingly common even at this early stage in the lifecourse, with misuse carrying a range of immediate risks of harm both to the young person and to others. In Europe one in four deaths of young men aged 15-29 is attributable to alcohol, while in the UK 18,000 young people are estimated to be scarred for life each year as a result of drunken assaults (Foxcroft et al, 2003). The age of initiation is linked to the lifetime alcohol dependency rate (although use does not track as strongly into adulthood as cigarette smoking) (Graham and Power, 2004). As Chapter Eight has shown, research also suggests that alcohol may act as a gatekeeper to other drug use, with exclusive use of either cigarettes or illegal drugs being negligible. Changes to its normative status might thus influence a range of substance use, as well risky and premature sexual behaviour. It is estimated that the cost of alcohol misuse approaches £20 billion a year, including crime and antisocial behaviour and lost productivity as well as damage to health (Cabinet Office, 2004).

The situation with respect to other drugs is more complex, reflecting both the range of available substances and the patterns of consumption. Not only does the UK have the highest rates of drug use in Europe, comparable to those found in the US, but research also suggests that official statistics underestimate both experimentation and usage. As Chapter Eight has shown, two fifths of young people aged 15 have tried one or more street drugs, most commonly cannabis. Until recently, however, it was suggested that there had been a de facto bifurcation of recreational and hard drug use, with 99% of the cost of drug misuse in England and Wales attributed to the 250,000 Class A drug users of all ages, 100,000 of whom are possibly young people (Drugs Strategy Directorate, 2002). The related socio-economic costs are nevertheless immense (estimated at between £10 and £17 billion a year) for Class A drug use alone (not least because of the existence of strong links with crime), with recreational use by young people estimated to cost a further £28 million a year (Canning et al, 2004). This is reflected in the annual drugs-related expenditure which, at £1.5 billion for 2005/06, dwarfs that seen for any other intervention discussed in this book. Meanwhile, the increasing use of heroin and cocaine by adolescents and young adults within recreational settings, poly-drug use and the mixing of drugs and alcohol provide a further challenge for policy and practice. Perceptions of substance use as recreational can also act as a barrier to accessing help (Wincup et al, 2003). Each year it is estimated that 20,000 young people become adult problem drug users (DfES, 2005), and problems cluster among the most vulnerable.

What works? Evidence and practice

While interventions often target a range of drugs, they appear to be more common with respect to tobacco and other drug use than with respect to alcohol. This is probably a response to social attitudes, with a general acceptance of sensible alcohol use as opposed to a concern for abstinence. Most, reflecting the stage of lifecourse, also focus on primary prevention, with some secondary prevention to address substance misuse and limited interventions around the issue of dependence. The acceptance of links to social exclusion also means substance misuse is increasingly seen as an integral part of the larger youth agenda, particularly in neighbourhood renewal areas and in conjunction with vulnerable groups such as the homeless, care leavers and youth offenders (Home Office, nd).

Both adolescent nicotine dependence and social circumstances influence adult smoking (Jefferis et al, 2003). Interventions seeking to reduce nicotine dependence in isolation are, therefore, unlikely to be effective in reducing the socio-economic gradients in smoking. Rather, they need to address both the pharmacological and social pathways into adult smoking. This has meant both an increasing emphasis on social influences within educational programmes and the introduction of community interventions that address the decision to smoke within a broad social context.

Thomas (2002), while acknowledging the key influence of culture on smoking, presents a typically US-centric view of behavioural interventions in schools designed to prevent children from starting smoking. As in many other areas, he finds little evidence to support the provision of information alone, and only equivocal evidence to support interventions based on social learning theory/ social influence, including, for example, discussions around the incidence of smoking, its social consequences, peer, family and media influences on smoking and tobacco refusal skills. One reason is likely to be (as in Box 9.3) the focus on the school environment alone without recourse to the wider social and cultural context. The same class of programmes was also found to be the most effective by earlier meta-analyses. Rooney and Murray (1996), for example, suggested social influence programmes could reduce smoking by between 5% and 30%.

Outcomes, it has been suggested, might also be improved by supplementation with interventions designed to increase generic social competence (improving social skills, reducing stress and increasing self-esteem in the classroom, for example, without a specific anti-smoking emphasis). However, a key limiting factor for any school-based educational programmes for early youth is the degree to which different groups participate in school life and identify with the institution. Kobus (2003), in reviewing peer group influences, found that by their early teens disenfranchised groups related to activities outside school and to age-heterogeneous groups in the larger community. This potentially limits the impact of school-based educational programmes to their more pro-social peers, while other vulnerable groups such as truants and the excluded are, by definition, unable to participate and require a more targeted approach. Regular smokers, for

Box 9.3: Educational interventions in isolation

The Hutchinson Smoking Prevention Project (Peterson et al, 2000) ran for 15 years, from 1984 to 1999, and was sustained across eight subsequent school years, following participants for two years after leaving school. However, no effect of intervention on prevalence of smoking was found either at school leaving or at later follow-up. This may have been because the intervention lacked key features present in more successful programmes, because it was based predominantly in low-risk areas (mainly white, rural schools), or because it ignored key differences between the schools, such as smoking incidence, when delivering the curriculum (Thomas, 2002).

The European Smoking Prevention Framework Approach, focusing initially on 20,000 non-smoking 13-year-olds in six European countries, is designed eventually to encompass adolescents, schools, parents and out-of-school activities. The first phase of the intervention focused on a teacher-led school-based programme that included social influence processes and training in refusal skills with variable parental or community components across at least five lessons.

Few significant short-term effects were attributable to the framework. However, in Spain, the experimental group reported positive psychological effects, with higher scores relating to attitudes towards smoking, intention to smoke and self-efficacy. Significant (although modest) preventative behavioural effects were also observed in Spain and Finland, with the experimental group recording fewer students starting to smoke. In contrast, counterproductive cognitive effects were found in the UK. Here there was no significant difference between the number of lessons delivered in experimental and control regions, lessons were also shorter than in many of the European comparators, they did not include refusal skills training or social pressure/influence and there were no supporting parental or community activities (de Vries et al, 2003).

example, are twice as likely to be absent from school as non–smokers (Charlton and Blair, 1989). Breeze et al (2001), focusing on drugs prevention discourses, also suggest that the emphasis on resistance and risk sits uneasily with what they describe as a cost-benefit consumerist hedonistic perspective, wherein young people are comfortable with their drug use and lack significant guilt but still have inadequacies in their knowledge base.

Another limitation is the intensity and duration of the intervention. Most schools teach health education as part of personal health and social education (PHSE). However, it has been suggested that 20–30 lessons during adolescence may be required to influence smoking behaviour (Prochaska, 2000; Tobler et al, 2000). This is a major demand on the curriculum alongside potentially similar claims from other PHSE targets, and contrasts markedly with the limited time allocated within many of the reviewed interventions. MacKintosh et al (2000), describing a multicomponent drugs intervention programme that still amounted to only 11–25 hours for the majority of students, emphasised the need not only to consider the time available but also the degree to which social influence is capable of forming the basis of harm reduction as opposed to primary prevention interventions, and the degree to which it can be effective with older adolescents.

An alternative is to ally school-based interventions with actions in the community, such as parent education, work with youth organisations, and campaigns ranging from those aiming to reduce cigarette sales to minors to those aiming to reduce cardiovascular diseases across the age range (see Box 9.4). Like those designed to improve generic social competence, such programmes have not been rigorously evaluated (Thomas, 2002), and little support has been found for their effectiveness. Where positive results have been found, the interventions have again been informed by social learning theory, emphasising the importance of creating negative attitudes towards smoking and reducing the intention to smoke (Sowden et al, 2004). An authoritative positive parenting

Box 9.4: School-based interventions within the context of wider community activity

The North Karelia Project started as a community-wide cardiovascular disease prevention programme in this Finnish province in 1972. It ran for eight years with a focus on mass communication and community organisation (Vartiainen et al, 1998), then, between 1978 and 1980, two school-based educational components were added in order to prevent smoking among young people (aged 12-13 at the time of intervention). These programmes ran for two years and involved two pairs of matched schools (one urban, one rural) based in the intervention community (one pair receiving a teacher-led programme of smoking prevention sessions, the other a health educator-led programme). Both teachers and peer leaders were trained to deliver anti-smoking messages. A third pair of schools (selected from a province outside the intervention area) acted as a control. Participants were followed up 15 years later at the age of 28, and mean lifetime cigarette consumption was found to be 22% lower among those in the intervention community than those in the control area (Vartiainen et al, 1998).

Two studies in the UK (Action Heart, based in Rotherham and Stopping them Starting, based in Cardiff) compared school/community-based interventions (including the involvement of key workers, health promotion and peer-led health education) with school-based interventions alone. These studies found no significant differences (Baxter et al, 1997; Gordon et al, 1997). One possible explanation is that the Finnish study introduced the school component into a long-established community intervention that included adult smoking cessation programmes, while in the two UK studies, the community intervention was the 'optional extra', running parallel to the school-based component.

style has also been found to be protective, in contrast to a permissive, distracted family environment (Tyas and Pederson, 1998), findings that reinforce the emphasis placed on parenting in early life. Indeed, a comprehensive review of child and adolescent mental health treatments found that family therapy was "superior to other treatment modalities" in reducing substance misuse (Fonagy et al, 2002, p 324).

The literature suggests that mass media campaigns can have a significant and cost-effective impact in this area, reducing cigarette consumption and de-normalising smoking, particularly if their focus is on the industry's manipulation of youth and the negative effects of second-hand smoke (Lantz et al, 2000). However, only a limited number of studies have employed a controlled design to this end and these do not provide strong evidence of effectiveness. Sowden and Arblaster (1999) found only two. Both were intensive programmes, repeated across three or four years and based on social learning theory (including, for example, refusal skills and resistance to advertising pressures). Both had an effect on intermediate outcomes such as attitudes towards smoking and intentions to smoke in the future as well as smoking rates. In both cases, too, the successful interventions utilised a mass media programme in conjunction with school-based education (as opposed to no intervention or school-based intervention only), suggesting the increased potency of broad-based interventions.

In contrast, the enforcement of the law relating to cigarette sales to underage youth appears to have a limited impact on smoking behaviour. In a synthesis of interventions aimed at preventing the sale of tobacco to minors, few communities achieved sustained levels of high compliance, and there was little consequent effect on youth perceptions of access to tobacco or on the prevalence of smoking. However, it has been suggested that there is a threshold level of compliance, above which access can be reduced, and that if such compliance can reduce consumption by 5% it would be as cost-effective as any other prevention activities (Stead and Lancaster, 2004).

A recent meta review confirmed that the main focus for the primary prevention of drug use is adolescents in schools. It also reported that primary prevention programmes are unlikely to have a major impact on drug use or drug problems, that the impact of drug prevention programmes tends to be confined to the gateway drugs of alcohol, tobacco and cannabis rather than illicit drugs, and that most British interventions are not properly evaluated (Canning et al, 2004). The challenge of tackling health inequalities in this manner was further highlighted by the fact that school-based initiatives were found to be more effective with non-users (where they may delay start) and lower-risk adolescents (where they may raise awareness and challenge normative beliefs) rather than with those at a high risk. High-risk families are also less likely to be involved with parent-orientated programmes. There was, however, some support for interactive programmes, with those led by peers that addressed the social influences of substance use being the most effective (Tobler et al, 2000). Additional features of effective programmes were intensity (more than 10 sessions) and reinforcement via booster sessions (Canning et al, 2004). A distinction may also be made between peer delivery (which appears to have limited ability to make users stop but may reinforce abstinence and limit drug-using repertoires) and peer development programmes. The latter provide a basis for working with more vulnerable young people and appear able to foster the educators' self-esteem and maturity and change their existing patterns of drug use (Shiner, 2000). The young person who is delivering the programme thus tends to benefit the most. Interestingly, a consideration of peer-led sexual health programmes suggests, however, that it may be not the inclusion of a peer per se but rather the ability of the provider to facilitate learning and their comfort with the subject matter, that may be important (Ellis and Grey, 2004).

Parker et al (2001) note that young adolescents in the late 1990s, despite having more access to drugs, had slightly lower rates of drug trying and recent drug taking and were less likely to be current smokers and drinkers. However, they suggest this was largely independent of official interventions. They advocate abandoning the search for abstinence solutions in favour of management strategies: a national secondary prevention programme to target adolescent recreational drug triers and users in order to prevent their progression to harder drugs, and initiatives to minimise harm from problematic drug use. Clubbers in their early twenties, for instance, are often poly-drug users who confound the image of the socially excluded criminal who resorts to Class A drugs, yet can face problems with their physical and psychological health and are unlikely to be seen by treatment programmes (Measham et al, 2001). Targeted public health messages for young heroin users have similarly been suggested to harness their contemplation to change, avoid overdosing and prevent the switch from smoking to injecting. In general, however, while the effectiveness of prevention programmes has been demonstrated with respect to the acquisition of knowledge, this does not extend to drug-using behaviour for the most vulnerable groups, as measured by prevention or delay in onset (Millward et al, 2004). A review of the grey literature similarly found evidence of projects that had engaged with young people and produced better services but little evidence that this prevented, delayed or modified risky behaviour. This was attributed in part to the absence of effective evaluation. It did, however, add further support to one of the underlying themes of this book – the movement away from single-issue interventions towards combined interventions that address a cluster of risks (Coomber et al, 2004).

A systematic review of over 50 psychosocial and educational interventions aimed at the primary prevention of alcohol misuse for those aged 25 and under was similarly unable to come to any firm conclusions concerning the nature of effective prevention in the short or medium term. Nearly half of the interventions reviewed proved ineffective, there was little to distinguish effective interventions from the ineffective and the former failed to convince with respect to either pattern or scale of outcomes (Foxcroft et al, 2003). Research based in Australia suggests one of the contributory factors may again be the emphasis on abstinence or delayed use. A school-based programme focusing instead on harm reduction goals was able to produce significant changes in consumption (including harmful and hazardous consumption) and the harm associated with consumption, alongside the more normal changes in knowledge and attitudes. These were all sustained to varying degrees across the programme, although diminishing by the final follow-up 17 months after programme delivery (McBride et al, 2004).

The American Strengthening Families Programme, initiated for families where one parent was involved in a methadone maintenance programme or attending a substance misuse outpatient centre, was highlighted as of potential interest. Here the aim was to enhance the quality of parenting and to reduce problem behaviour, with reduced substance use in older children and reduced adolescent drug use at follow-up incidental to a larger improvement in child behaviour and family relationships. Home visits by nurses in the prenatal period and early childhood to high-risk families were similarly found, 15 years later, to be reflected in reduced cigarette and alcohol consumption and behavioural problems related to alcohol and drugs in the by then adolescent children (Olds et al, 1998). This again demonstrates the importance of broad-based parenting programmes beyond their efficacy in early life (see Chapter Five). As with smoking, the more recent emphasis on community-based interventions was also considered to hold promise (Foxcroft et al, 2003). Minimum drinking age laws can also be effective in preventing alcohol-related accidents and injuries with review-level evidence also suggesting that lower blood alcohol concentration laws can similarly reduce accidents involving young and inexperienced drivers (Mulvihill et al, 2005). However, neither of these have been tested in a UK context.

In contrast to the equivocal evidence relating to prevention, there is robust research evidence from the National Treatment Outcome Research Study that treatment for drug dependence is effective, with consequent gains in health, crime reduction and risky behaviours such as injecting and sharing injecting (Edmunds et al, 1999; Gossop et al, 2001; Sondhi et al, 2002). Efficacy, as always, depends on the characteristics of the regimes and very little is known about treatment outcomes for young people (HAS, 2001). The National Treatment Outcome Research Study, for example, covers all those aged 16-58 without reporting separately on effectiveness for young people (although the majority of the clients studied were in their late twenties and early thirties) (Gossop et al, 1998). Across the study group as a whole, however, one third achieved abstinence from illicit opiates in community settings, rising to one half in residential settings after four to five years (Gossop et al, 2001).

A review of adolescent treatment outcomes (Williams et al, 2000) found similar levels of reduction with again an allied improvement in illegal behaviour, together with health and school functioning. Significant relapse rates are, however, also recorded not least because over 90% of adolescents in substance misuse treatment programmes have demonstrated psychiatric comorbidity, which reduces treatment compliance and predicts poor long-term outcomes (HAS, 2001). The reported improvements in other domains such as confidence, self-esteem and coping strategies suggest, however, a base for sustained intervention. This is supported by more descriptive studies (see, for example, Crome et al, 1998) that similarly find improvements across a broad range of functions and high levels of retention within the service despite multiple disadvantages.

Limitations to the evidence base

The studies reviewed varied in terms of the location, duration and type of intervention considered, the age range of the participants, base rates of substance use and outcomes measured. Behavioural approaches often seek to address tobacco, alcohol and drug use, and even antisocial behaviour, together. While commonalities suggest this is a sensible approach, it makes it difficult to compare outcomes and community interventions are similarly very difficult to evaluate. The European Smoking Prevention Framework Approach evaluation (see Box 9.3) illustrates well the difficulties of isolating the effective characteristics of such interventions, even within the dictates of a common framework, particularly when the intervention seeks to accommodate local needs and to account for different national baselines (de Vries et al, 2003). The US bias to the available literature also means that potentially important cultural differences are in danger of being ignored, while variations within the target population are often neglected or unreported. There is a lack of attention, for example, to ethnicity (Markham et al, 2001), while the emphasis on school-based primary prevention has tended to exclude those most at risk. The impact on long-term behaviour has also been neglected in favour of changes in attitude, knowledge and the development of resistance skills, with a parallel emphasis on self-reported behaviour at the expense of more objective measures of drug use such as saliva and blood tests (Canning et al, 2004).

Policy

The cultural context for reducing the initiation and incidence of smoking is probably now at its most supportive. In contrast with nutrition there is active market intervention with, for example, bans on tobacco advertisements including the withdrawal of tobacco sponsorship, enforcement of under-age sales, proof of age cards and rules on the location of cigarette vending machines. These, together with widespread restrictions on smoking in public spaces, combine to reduce opportunities for smoking and make it less socially acceptable, while taxation makes it costly. In the UK it is also illegal to sell tobacco to anyone under the age of 16 (although not for them to smoke it), although enforcement and compliance are often problematic.

Within this largely supportive environment, the White Paper *Smoking kills* (DH, 1998a) (see Chapter Five) identified young people as a priority for the smoking cessation strategies introduced from April 1999 and set targets to reduce smoking among children in England from 13% to 9% or less by 2010, with a fall to 11% by 2005. Subsequent surveys of English smoking cessation service coordinators found, however, that the programmes had made little progress either in attracting young people or in developing services for them, and that those suffering from smoking-related illnesses were given a higher priority (Coleman et al, 2002; Pound et al, 2005). Even where services were offered, these were seen to be peripheral to a primarily adult-focused strategy and did not cater for those below the age of 16. Not surprisingly, therefore, the Health Development Agency (HDA) found there was almost "no good evidence of effective smoking cessation interventions for young people, nor much experience in the UK of setting up and running such interventions" (HDA, 2004, p 1). Such findings reinforce the impression of a preoccupation with primary prevention for this age group, irrespective of substance concerned, and illustrate the difficulty in translating a change in policy into practical response. Similarly, there have been few reported trials of cessation programmes and few young people are counselled to quit as a part of a routine medical consultation. In contrast, descriptive studies suggest many teenage smokers are motivated to quit, and that the use of nicotine replacement therapy (NRT) for adolescents should be reconsidered (Lantz et al, 2000).

The UK drugs strategy was formalised in the early 1990s in response to the widespread emergence of problematic heroin use in many poor communities, followed by the unprecedented expansion in young people's recreational drug trying. *Tackling drugs together* (HMSO, 1994) has been criticised for being strong on the 'war on drugs' rhetoric and weak in all other respects (Parker et al, 2001). A key legacy, however, was the creation of Drug Action Teams (DATs), which brought key players such as the police, probation, health, education, social services, drugs services and voluntary and community organisations together at the local level. This includes a dedicated budget for the treatment of young people (80% of DATs now provide treatment services for young people), together with a sum of money to be spent on support for education in schools (including teacher training and the Healthy Schools Programme) that is directed to the local education authority (LEA).

Tackling drugs to build a better Britain (Cabinet Office, 1998), conceived by New Labour as a 10-year strategy to 2008, similarly employed an essentially UK approach, with almost every health, welfare, care and control and enforcement official expected to play a role in a local multiagency partnership approach to dealing with drugs. The strategy had four key goals (with accompanying targets), one of which was to help young people resist drug misuse, together with the protection of communities from drug-related antisocial and criminal behaviour, the identification of drug-driven or related offending in the criminal justice system and the reduction in the availability of drugs on the streets. Significantly, the latter is the least developed and, together with the changes in the criminal justice system and the emphasis on young people, marks a shift away from enforcement in this area towards prevention and treatment. With £250 million of new money in the first five years and an annual expenditure of £1.3 billion per annum, critics have, however, queried the lack of success (Parker et al, 2001).

The strategy was thus further updated in 2002, including a focus on Class A drugs that emphasises education, prevention and treatment, and a further increase in resources, with planned direct annual expenditure rising further to nearly £1.5 billion in 2005/06. Young people are again one of four priority areas for these new resources, including education campaigns focusing on Class A drugs, support for families and increased outreach and community treatment, while changes to the youth justice system include provision for testing and referral for treatment on arrest and as a condition of community sentences. The aim is to support 40,000-50,000 vulnerable young people per annum by 2006, with research suggesting that criminal justice intervention schemes are highly cost-effective in terms of savings to health and welfare as well as the criminal justice system itself (Millward et al, 2004).

One contributory element, expected to accommodate one tenth of this target group, is the Positive Futures Programme. This is a sports-based social inclusion project aimed at 10- to 19-year-olds in the 57 most disadvantaged communities, where sports and arts are being used as part of what is described as a 'relationship strategy' to reconnect marginalised young people with local services, to develop skills to resist drugs and reduce offending and, critically, to re-enter education (Positive Futures, 2004). Also key are the Youth Offending Teams (YOTs), juvenile custody (together expected to support 12,000) and the drug treatment agencies (a further 5,000). However, the main mechanism continues to be local health and education services and Connexions, which together are expected to provide nearly 60% of this target provision, a threefold increase on 2002. The Jobcentre Plus Progresss2work Initiative, introduced in 2002, also aims to help drug users find and sustain employment (Drugs Strategy Directorate, 2002).

A further key change has been the reclassification of cannabis as a Class C drug. Previous to January 2004 the processing of young people for cannabis possession dominated policing contact, increasing the friction with young people, potentially making reintegration into the education system or employment difficult and accounting for the equivalent of 500 full-time officers a year (May et al, 2002). These resources could have been more effectively directed towards prevention and treatment. There has also been a relaxation in targets, explicitly acknowledging the difficulty of reducing illicit drug use per se among all under 25-year-olds and the inability to reduce Class A drug use by 50% by 2008. The focus is now on achieving general reductions in Class A and frequent drug use, particularly among the most vulnerable.

The Updated National Drugs Strategy has in turn been revisited under the auspices of *Every child matters* (DfES, 2005) in an attempt to ensure an integrated service for vulnerable children with an enhanced preventative element. This also introduced a targeted geographical approach with High Focus Areas. These are areas with high levels of local need and inadequate levels of service provision where progress towards the new objectives of reformed delivery, strengthened accountability, increased service and workforce capacity and a focus on the needs of the most vulnerable young people is expected to be more rapid than average (DfES, 2005). This more integrated approach is emphasised by two developments already discussed. The first is the assumption of lead policy responsibility by the DfES (which shares responsibility with the Home Office for target delivery). The second is the assumption of local operational responsibility and target delivery by the Directors of Children's Services (with the DAT chairs) through the medium of the Children and Young People's Plans due to be produced in April 2006 (DfES, 2005).

The final part of the triad is represented by the Alcohol Harm Reduction Strategy for England (Cabinet Office, 2004). This focuses on reducing the harm caused by crime and antisocial behaviour (seen as primarily an urban problem) alongside the harm caused to health because of binge and chronic drinking. While youth is not an explicit target, the 5.9 million binge drinkers (technically those who consume above twice the recommended daily guidelines but more commonly considered those who drink to get drunk) are generally aged under 25. One of the key strategies also focuses on changing behaviour and culture via improved education and communication and young people are again the prime target. Ofcom has also reviewed the rules on broadcast advertising of alcohol to ensure that from January 2005 advertisements do not appeal particularly to the under-18s or link alcohol with sexual activity or behavioural attributes such as daring or aggression (HM Government and DH, 2004).

Unlike drugs policy, the relatively large population who have alcohol problems is less likely to have contact with the criminal justice system and this cannot, therefore, be used as a trigger for treatment. Instead, the first port of call is more likely to the health system, particularly Accident and Emergency Departments, together with schools and, for example, mental health assessments or YOTs. Here, both increased training and effective screening procedures are required if such contacts are to act as key entry points for secondary and tertiary interventions. At present, for example, there is little specific reference to drugs or alcohol even in the *Framework for the assessment of children in need and their families* (DH et al, 2000).

As noted already, school programmes have been seen as attractive vehicles for primary prevention because most schools already teach health education as part of PHSE. The results of school interventions have, however, often been disappointing, with competing priorities among (non-statutory) PHSE targets as well as pressure from the national curriculum. Drugs education (including alcohol and tobacco) is now a planned component of PHSE, with Citizenship a statutory part of the national secondary curriculum since September 2003, and the majority of schools having a drugs education policy. This aims to increase pupils' knowledge about the range of drugs (including the risks attached), examine their attitudes towards drugs and drug users and develop the personal and social skills to communicate, make effective choices and ask for help when needed (DH and DfES, 2003b). It is also one of the NHSS themes, moving away from the school's role in developing knowledge and skills towards influencing behaviour. The government, reflecting concerns over the requirement for secondary prevention, is also considering how substance misuse education can be provided in post-16 education settings.

The Connexions service, the DfES career and academic planning service for 13- to 19-year-olds, also holds a wider supportive role in secondary and further education. Personal Advisors are trained to address individual and social problems, including the use of drugs and alcohol. Priority is given to young people at risk of disaffection and underachievement and the evidence base would suggest that such an approach might be able to address the paradox that while knowledge about the harmful effects of a behaviour appears not to be protective, it seems to become more relevant when personalised (Tyas and Pederson, 1998).

Despite the political imperative to create coherent strategies with an explicit focus on young people, critical services for young people continue to be absent or under great pressure, particularly with respect to alcohol and drugs misuse. DATs, as the local delivery arm of the drugs policy, have ensured some local treatment is available for young people. However, the Health Advisory Service suggests there is still a lack of understanding that children's services are not just an extension of adult drug services (HAS, 2001). Meanwhile, the recent introduction of the alcohol harm reduction strategy means the response time in this area has been limited. It has been suggested that there is now an established need for a dedicated, specialist therapeutic social care and health service (covering drugs, alcohol, mental health and sexual health) to back up the operation of the Connexions service. The introduction of Children's Trusts by 2008 (see Chapter Five) should begin to address these issues.

Sexual health

The sexual health of young people in the UK is poor. As Chapter Eight has noted, there is a high incidence of risky sexual behaviour, allied with high rates of teenage pregnancy and an increase in sexually transmitted infections (STIs), with teenagers and young adults bearing a disproportionate part of the burden (Ellis and Grey, 2004). Together, this forms a considerable cluster of risk that carries significant implications for future health and fertility. It is also a risk that varies considerably with gender, socio-economic background, education, ethnicity and locality (NHS CRD, 1997; Aggleton et al, 1998). Teenage mothers, for example, tend to be disadvantaged at the outset and this is often compounded by the early transition to motherhood which can cause stress on adolescent relationships, compromise antenatal health and further affect educational attainment and longer-term opportunities, often resulting in long-term benefit dependency and poverty (Chevalier and Viitanen, 2003; Swann et al, 2003). Consequently, it is increasingly accepted that policy and practice must address not only sexual behaviour and the range of adverse health and social outcomes but also the determinants of risk.

What works? Evidence and practice

Despite arguments for joined-up action and a holistic approach to the needs of young people, evidence as to what works tends to focus on the prevention of teenage pregnancy and effective support for teenage parents and their children. A recent review of the prevention of STIs found, however, that nearly half the included studies focused on young people, with 14 out of 26 looking at sex education programmes in schools (Ellis and Grey, 2004). This found that school-based sex education programmes can be effective in reducing sexually risky behaviour among adolescents and that they are more effective if begun before the onset of sexual activity. By increasing condom use, delaying initiation and reducing the frequency of sex, STI programmes also potentially reduce unintended pregnancy (Kirby, 1999, cited in HDA, 2001). However, a key limitation (as with substance misuse) is that the adolescent population attending school is generally at a low risk and interventions need to be able to target high-risk youth. This is compounded by a lack of evidence as to the effectiveness of interventions designed to reduce inequalities in sexual health. However, a number of studies do emphasise the links between behaviour, education and wider social opportunities, and use the link to suggest attention be paid to socio-political intervention including the improvement of educational and employment opportunities (Ellis and Grey, 2004).

There have been two main approaches to unintended pregnancy: educational (primarily again school-based) interventions and the provision and delivery of contraceptive and counselling services (NHS CRD, 1997). In marked contrast to this focus, it has been argued persuasively that raising expectations of girls from a very young age has a direct effect on the chances of their becoming a teenage mother, and that policy should instead target educational opportunities and aspirations from the pre-primary phase onwards (Cheesbrough et al, 2002).

Education

DiCenso et al (2002), focusing on RCTs alone, suggest there is little if any evidence to support the effectiveness of primary prevention strategies, with the exception of multifaceted approaches to life skills and pregnancy. However, a broader synthesis of systematic reviews and meta-analyses (Swann et al, 2003) suggests there is good evidence to support school-based sex education linked to contraceptive services, alongside the community-based delivery of education, development and contraceptive services; youth development programmes; and family outreach (see also Dennison, 2004). These are strategies that focus on early intervention in the lifecourse and acknowledge the need to empower young people within personal relationships, as well as addressing continuing low levels of knowledge and constraints to contraceptive access and use (Wellings, 1998). They improve chances of eventual condom or other contraceptive use without increasing sexual activity (Cheesbrough et al, 2002).

The majority of evaluations of educational approaches are, typically, US-based. These suggest that successful interventions are characterised by a sound theoretical base, intervene before patterns of behaviour are established and take a participatory, personalised age-appropriate approach. They also include practical skills such as improvements in communication (negotiating protected sex and the use of contraception remains problematic) and focus clearly on reducing one or more sexual behaviours that lead to unintended pregnancy or STI infection (Meyrick and Swann, 1998). Additionally, the literature emphasises the need for integration and a broad-based approach, closing the gap between education and health and raising awareness of the range of issues impinging on sexual health (see Box 9.5). Such a collaborative, multiagency approach is considered particularly apposite where the young people concerned fall into the hard-to-reach or vulnerable category (HDA, 2001).

Box 9.5: Changes in rates of under-16 conceptions

Limited reductions in the rate of teenage pregnancy in England and Wales conceal markedly different trajectories at the health authority level. Changes in the under-16 conception rate at this scale ranged from an increase of 55% to a decrease of 28% in the period 1992-96. Research, focusing on the experience in the 20 best and 20 worst authorities, attempted to identify the factors that were associated with these differential changes. It found that authorities where the teenage pregnancy rate was decreasing were more likely than those at the other end of the spectrum to have introduced specialist services, better-trained staff in schools, consultation with young people, active health promotion, and the involvement of youth services, alongside greater cooperative working between agencies. It concluded that "those areas that addressed the issue more comprehensively were rewarded with reductions in rates" (Ingham et al, nd, p 11).

Communication within the family about sex has been found to be significantly associated with rates of teenage pregnancy (Wellings et al, 1998), although an authoritative review finds insufficient evidence to link communication and sexually risky behaviour (Ellis and Grey, 2004). Children whose parents adopt a more realist-humanist approach are likely to learn more from their parents about sexual matters than those who adopt a moralistic one. In the Netherlands, for example, where teenage pregnancy rates are six times lower than they are in

Britain, and sex is discussed more openly in the home, research suggests young people are both better informed about sexual health and contraception and more sexually competent (using contraception and able to define the role of sex within a relationship). Young people also engage in more mixed-sex out-of-school activities, discuss problems with friends of both sexes and subscribe to weaker gender stereotypes than in Britain, where cultural expectations continue to link successful masculinity to number of sexual encounters and performance (Aggleton et al, 1998). A total of 85% of young people in the Netherlands are estimated to use contraception at first intercourse compared to 66% of 16- to 19-year-olds in the UK and 50% of those aged under 16 (SEU, 1999). It may also be significant that there has been an increase in what has been termed the 'Double Dutch' method of combined condom and pill use in an effort to reduce both teenage pregnancy and protect against STIs, which would also increase contraceptive effectiveness among young people. In the US a recent drop in the very high rates of teenage pregnancy have similarly been ascribed to changed contraceptive methods, with increased use of contraceptive injections and implants.

Programmes that offer educational support or improve job prospects may also motivate young people to avoid pregnancy (NHS CRD, 1997). Box 9.6 emphasises the key roles of economy and education.

Box 9.6: Structural influences on sexual health

In Sweden, teenage birth rates have decreased by three quarters since 1970 and are currently almost five times smaller than those in the UK. Context is undoubtedly important. The majority (70%) of 13- to 17-year-olds still live with both their natural parents and there is a tradition of liberal attitudes to youthful sexual activity, combined with a long history of sex education in schools and contraceptive services that not only target young people but also provide routine chlamydia screening. Figures from the United Nations Children's Fund (UNICEF) also show the rates of 15- to 19-year-olds out of full-time education in Sweden is less than half that in the UK (Munro et al, 2004). Significantly, however, Sweden experienced a period of economic stagnation in the late 1990s. This has been accompanied by an increase in teenagers not enrolled in high school standard programmes, a cut-back in school budgets, including those for sex education, increased non-attendance and social segregation. At the same time there has been an increase in teenage abortions and chlamydia infections and an increase in other risk-taking behaviours such as smoking and drug use (Edgardh, 2002).

Few programmes have attempted to tackle the underlying socio-economic and environmental factors associated with an increased risk of pregnancy. Qualitative research suggests, for example, that the most vulnerable and socially disadvantaged (children in care, the homeless, those who have suffered sexual abuse or who have mental health problems) often have difficulties forming and maintaining relationships and feel they have little control over their lives, while sex tends to lack any significant meaning or value. They are thus likely to gamble with contraception as part of a broader pattern of risk taking (Hughes et al, 1999). As Chapter Five emphasised, some of the solutions are likely to lie in interventions initiated at a much earlier age. Day care for disadvantaged children, for example, has been shown to lower pregnancy rates among these children as adolescents (Zoritch et al, 2000).

Contraception and counselling

The next stage is to ensure contraceptive use and protection from STIs at first intercourse and at all subsequent events. Research shows an association between conception rates and the type of contraceptive services available locally, with clinics, particularly youth-orientated clinics, encouraging use and reducing pregnancy rates (Clements et al, 1998). Successful contraceptive services aimed at young people focus on access to a wide variety of settings and consider both physical accessibility (location, for example, on bus routes) and timing (such as availability after school or on a drop-in basis). They also provide trained and selected staff, services targeted specifically at boys and men, and services that are integrated so that contraception is available not only alongside other sexual health services but alongside services that move beyond health. It is also important to utilise key presenting opportunities such as emergency contraception and offer a long-term service that is sensitive to local needs and the characteristics of local high-risk groups, and to ensure that young people are aware of the various options available to them subsequent to unprotected sex or conception.

Less is known about the experiences and sexual health needs of young lesbians and gay men. Indeed, it has been suggested that one of the reasons for poor contraceptive use among young heterosexuals is the tension between health promotion/safe sex messages and cultural and gendered expectations. Girls, who as a group tend to have the most difficulty dealing with condoms, tend to remain the ones expected to negotiate their use (Hillier et al, 1998).

Secondary prevention

Initiatives to prevent adverse health and social outcomes have been divided into four key groups: antenatal care; social support and parenting; preschool education and support; and parental education support. These are all areas that, as Chapter Five demonstrated, are critical to life chances. This established that parenting programmes per se are effective in changing parenting practices and improving behaviour problems in young children (Barlow and Stewart-Brown, 2000) as well as improving aspects of maternal psychosocial health including anxiety, depression and self-esteem (Barlow and Coren, 2003), while early education programmes can improve longer-term outcomes for children with disadvantaged backgrounds. Coren and Barlow (2003) also conducted a Cochrane Review of the best evidence relating specifically to parenting programmes aimed at improving outcomes for teenage mothers and their children. The results, while limited by methodological problems, indicate that parenting programmes are similarly effective in improving a range of outcomes for both teenage parents and their infants, including maternal sensitivity, identity, self-confidence and the infants' responsiveness to their parents. They suggest that, as with the wider class of parenting programmes, group-based interventions may be a more supportive and helpful strategy than individual interventions, while fathers are typically neglected. There are also a number of approaches that allow teenage mothers to continue formal education while increased flexibility concerning educational re-entry is similarly attracting increased political attention.

The pilot Sure Start Plus Programme (see Box 9.7), introduced in 1999, provides a nationally evaluated example of an intervention designed to reduce the risk of

---

Box 9.7: Secondary prevention: the example of Sure Start Plus

Sure Start Plus has sought to influence mainstream services in order to make them more accessible to pregnant teenagers, provide new services and provide training for professionals. National evaluation suggests the intervention has been most successful in addressing the social isolation and low self-confidence of young women. Users are reported as finding the programme user-friendly and providing high-quality information and advice in areas such as housing, benefits, education, health and relationships. However, it has been less successful in encouraging young mothers to breastfeed for at least six weeks, in reaching young fathers and black and minority ethnic parents, or in developing appropriate group work (Wiggins et al, 2003). These are all areas where the evidence base (see Chapter Five) suggests resources should be focused.

Some of the local programmes were still not completely functional two years into the intervention. Constraints included staff recruitment, an appropriate partnership board, lack of resources, limited national/strategic guidance and lack of a clear identity. Doubts have also been expressed about the tensions between target-driven guidance and the desire for individual empowerment, mechanisms for learning from one another and sustainability once funding ends in 2006, with concomitant job insecurity. Indeed, even the move to the Children, Young People and Families Directorate has been seen by some Regional Teenage Pregnancy Coordinators as posing a threat for the programme, which now has to establish credibility and attract resources not only within the teenage pregnancy agenda but the larger child and family programme. This may weaken the health link and has prompted fears that specialist pregnancy advisors will be replaced by generic young people advisors (Rosato et al, 2004). The programme has received 4,000 referrals, close to its current carrying capacity.

long-term social exclusion and poverty resulting from teenage pregnancy and teenage parenthood by taking an individually tailored yet broad-based approach to supporting teenage parents.

Limitations to the evidence base

Teenage pregnancy rates remained relatively constant for the three decades from 1969 but fell between 1998-2000 by 6% (Botting et al, 1998), suggesting that policy may be beginning to have an impact. As in many areas reviewed, the evidence base is, however, often insufficient to support particular interventions. Reviews conducted for the Health Education Authority and its successor body the Health Development Agency comment on the poor methodological quality of many of the studies covered and the focus on different outcomes, which makes synthesis difficult. The diversity of approaches also militates against conclusions about the efficacy of universal programmes as opposed to initiatives targeting particularly vulnerable groups such as non-school attendees, looked-after children, the homeless, children of teenage parents and some black and minority ethnic groups. Nevertheless, there is evidence for interventions that increase knowledge and skills (via education and family-based approaches), reduce risk (by increasing service quality and uptake) and prevent adverse health and social outcomes (by increasing access to information, advice, counselling and social support) (Meyrick and Swann, 1998; Swann et al, 2003). Young people are not considered a priority group for HIV prevention initiatives so, in an area where there is very little review-level evidence relating even to the high-risk groups in the UK population and no review-level evidence about addressing inequalities, there is no consideration of interventions to prevent HIV transmission (Ellis et al, 2003).

Policy

As Chapter Eight noted, the teenage birth rate in the UK was similar to that in other Northern European countries in the 1970s but was not subject to the same subsequent decrease. Sexual health (including STIs and unplanned conceptions among young people) was, therefore, one of the five priority areas established by *The health of the nation* (DH, 1992). This introduced a target of reducing unplanned conceptions to those aged under 16 to 4.8 per 1,000 by 2000 (from a baseline of 9.6 per 1,000 in 1989/91). However, by 1996/98 the rate had only been reduced to 9.0 per 1,000.

It was the Green Paper, *Our healthier nation* (DH, 1998b) that saw teenage pregnancy for the first time as a social issue related to structural issues. Internationally, a marked correlation had been noted between countries with high rates of live births to teenagers and high levels of relative deprivation, poor educational achievement and family breakdown (SEU, 1999). The significance had also been noted of high levels of income inequality, high proportions of teenage parents, and a benefit system that did not require lone parents to work until their children had left school, alongside low levels of contraceptive use. The Teenage Pregnancy Strategy, with a budget of £60 million across the first three years, was thus a product of the Social Exclusion Unit's interdepartmental remit. It focused on better prevention, aiming to halve the rate of conceptions among those under the age of 18 (and reduce conception rates in those under the age of 16) across a decade. This is now encapsulated in a joint DH/DfES Public Service Agreement (PSA), and an 8.6% improvement has been recorded, the conception rate for 15- to 17-year-olds having fallen from 46.6 per 1,000 in 1998 to 42.6 per 1,000 in 2002.

It also focuses on increased support for teenage parents. The specific target here was to have 60% of teenage mothers learning or in employment by 2010. The strategy also acknowledged the range of related issues such as housing and social support, advocating, for example, that no lone parent under the age of 18 should be placed in a lone tenancy and that teenage pregnancy coordinators be appointed jointly by health and local authorities to pull together local services. Towards this end those aged under 16 are now required to finish their full-time education and receive help with childcare. For lone parents of employable age the New Deal for Lone Parents (NDLP) provides a package of support around preparation for work. Revisions to the scheme mean that it is now available to all, not just those claiming Income Support and with dependent children of school age.

Meanwhile, as noted earlier, the cross-departmental pilot programme, Sure Start Plus, was introduced to reduce the risk of long-term social exclusion and poverty resulting from teenage pregnancy and teenage parenthood. Funded initially for three years to March 2004 under the auspices of the Sure Start Unit it was extended to April 2006 and responsibility transferred to the Teenage Pregnancy Unit, where it too became part of the national Teenage Pregnancy Strategy. Shortly afterwards the Teenage Pregnancy Unit itself was moved from the DH to the new Children, Young People and Families Directorate, DfES. Sure Start provides coordinated support to pregnant teenagers and teenage parents under 18 years via a Personal Advisor who coordinates a tailored support package. It also addresses the health inequalities agenda by being based in 20 HAZs (or former HAZs) in England, selected additionally for having high rates of teenage pregnancy.

There is thus a growing acceptance that education and socio-economic status are two of the strongest factors predicting teenage pregnancy and adverse health outcomes. This is reflected in the growing number of structural solutions: the availability of day care, the concern for increasing numbers in education post-16, the tentative emergence of family policy and demands for the provision of appropriate housing. The body of effort remains, however, focused on primary and secondary prevention (interventions that increase knowledge, enhance social/relationship skills, improve access to services and other resources and facilitate their effective use) rather than offering any serious challenge to socio-economic disadvantage.

The children of teenage mothers also constitute a high-risk group alongside their mothers (Coren et al, 2003). They risk higher infant mortality rates, lower birth weights, developmental and behaviour problems and lower school attainment (Botting et al, 1998), together with an increased likelihood of childhood accidents and hospital admittance. Contributory factors have been examined in the preceding chapters on early life, and include a lack of preconception healthcare, higher than average rates of smoking during pregnancy and postnatal depression, limited breastfeeding, a lack of knowledge of child development and a lack of effective parenting skills. A reduction in teenage pregnancy was therefore also identified as one of the key interventions for the NHS if it was to achieve its health inequalities target in the area of infant mortality. However, there is also an analytical tendency to confuse young mothers with single mothers, unmarried mothers with unsupported mothers and unplanned pregnancies with unwanted pregnancies. Outcomes, as Chapter Eight has stressed, are not universally negative nor attributable necessarily to age (Aggleton et al, 1998).

The Sexual Health and HIV Strategy (DH, 2001) also highlights young people as a target group for specific health information and prevention. It seeks to reduce the transmission of STIs and HIV, as well as reducing the prevalence of undiagnosed infections and unintended pregnancy rates and the stigma associated with STIs and HIV. The initial roll-out of the chlamydia screening programme in England, for example, targets selected groups of women under the age of 25, such as those attending genitourinary medicine (GUM) clinics, women seeking terminations and those having their first cervical smear. However, it is restricted at the outset to just 10 sites. Sex education in schools also now has to include education about HIV/AIDS and other STIs. The system is, however, under disproportionate pressure. Between 1991 and 2001, the number of new episodes dealt with by GUM clinics rose by 143%, reaching 1.3 million in 2001. In some clinics, patients had to wait for up to 28 days for a routine appointment, and in 5% of clinics there was a delay of up to a week for urgent appointments (Munro et al, 2004). This increase in workload and waiting times has implications for the treatment of all populations using these clinics, but particularly for a subpopulation such as adolescents, where embarrassment and stigma along with poor communication skills and poor treatment-seeking behaviour may already be barriers to accessing advice. In Sweden, awareness of sexual health among 16- to 23-year-olds was found to be highest among those who had contact with the healthcare system.

Education and employment

Education has been a pervasive theme within this chapter. We have seen how knowledge about health behaviours remains a key weapon within the primary preventative agenda, albeit one that tends to be most effective in the hands of those at lowest risk. We have seen how the school has become a key locus for health promotion interventions, such as improved nutrition and physical activity. We have also noted how the complex relational web between risk factors and detrimental outcomes challenges the preoccupation with symptoms and demands that behavioural interventions make the link to education and wider social opportunities. Chapter Three looked at educational policies across the lifecourse while Chapter Eight looked at the direct role that education plays in determining health inequalities. Here we focus on educational interventions at the community level.

A number of initiatives have been introduced aimed specifically at schools or areas with high levels of social disadvantage and poor educational attainment. The first of these were EAZs. Introduced in two competitive rounds from 1999 EAZs were archetypal new labour partnership projects, predicated on support from business and innovation. They were designed to tackle a range of attainment-related issues, including the quality of teaching, social inclusion and support for pupils and their families, with each of the 73 zones focusing on two or three secondary schools together with their primary feeder schools. McKnight et al (2005), reviewing their contribution, concur with Ofsted in suggesting that they did more to tackle inclusion than standards, establishing homework and breakfast clubs and improving the motivation, attitudes and self-esteem of pupils. However, their impact on standards was largely confined to the youngest pupils.

In 1999 the programme was succeeded by the Excellence in Cities programme. This covered a far larger geographical area (encompassing one third of local education authorities [LEAs] and schools), involved more substantial funding and was a more prescriptive programme, including learning support units and learning support mentors. The programme also focused primarily on secondary schools, including the introduction of City Learning Centres. It appears to have had a more significant effect on attainment and attendance, with evaluation finding the greatest improvements among those with lower levels of attainment and attributing this to both the focused strategy and the fact that responsibility for implementation lies with the schools themselves. However, in both cases very considerable disadvantages remain and it has again been suggested this may require more radical reforms to mainstream funding rather than just a continuation of targeted initiatives (McKnight et al, 2005).

The role of schools in inclusion has also continued to receive recognition via the Extended Schools' Strategy. This expects all schools over time to provide a core offer of extended services, including study support, parental support, family learning and improved referral to multiagency support alongside a childcare component as established by the 10-year Childcare Strategy. There is also a new statutory duty on schools, established by the 2000 Education Act, to safeguard children and promote their welfare (DfES, 2004b).

Considerable political emphasis, as Chapter Three noted, has also been placed on participation in higher education. For children aged 16-plus who attend full-time courses at school or college, a means-tested Education Maintenance Allowance (EMA) was introduced on a pilot basis in 1999, with the aim of encouraging children from lower-income families to continue in education. It is now available nationally, with approximately half of all 16-year-olds in England estimated to be eligible and allowances ranging from £10 to £30 per week depending on family income. At the same time young people not in employment are entitled to lower rates of Income Support than those aged 25 or over, with the basic rate for a single person aged 16-17 standing at only £32.50 a week. Entry to employment is thus being deferred. A PSA target aiming to increase participation in higher education towards 50% of those aged 18-30 and to increase fair access (DfES, 2004a) has also been established.

Those aged 18-30 were also the focus of the government's first welfare-to-work programme – the New Deal for Young People (NDYP). Its aim is to increase employment and long-term employability by a tailored package of support (delivered by a Personal Advisor) that combines advice, training, support (including the identification and resolution of barriers to employment) and other assistance, including work experience. It was introduced into 12 pathfinder areas in January 1998 and then launched, almost immediately, across Britain in April 1998. At that time almost 120,000 young people were long-term unemployed, with a further 15,000-20,000 young people becoming eligible each month (NAO, 2002). Additionally, young rough sleepers were given immediate access to the New Deal gateway (SEU, 1998).

The initial target was to move 250,000 young people off benefits and into work by 2002. This target was actually met by September 2000, with 339,000 participants having ceased claiming Jobseeker's Allowance by October 2001 and experiencing at least one spell of sustained employment, 240,000 of whom were known to have moved to unsubsidised sustained jobs. However, this needs to be put into the context of the labour market, where youth unemployment was decreasing rapidly. The net effect of the programme has thus been estimated as a reduction in youth unemployment of 35,000 and an increase in youth employment of 15,000 across the first two years of its operation (many having entered education or training). This was achieved at a net cost of about £140 million per annum or between £5 and £8,000 per person of any age brought into employment as a result of the scheme (NAO, 2002). The most dramatic impact was on those registered as unemployed for over a year, where a fall of almost 95% was recorded between April 1997 and April 2002 (from 90,700 to 5,100).

Little is known about the quality of jobs taken by NDYP leavers, but a national survey has suggested high levels of job satisfaction and some evidence of wage progression, with evidence identifying the individualised help from the Personal Advisors as the key element of success (see Finn, 2003). Subsequent patterns of unemployment are also considered to resemble the newly rather than the long-term unemployed. Other assessments have, however, been less favourable, suggesting about one third of those who participated in NDYP returned to unemployment and about one in five of those who did obtain a job failed to retain it for 13 weeks (Finn, 2003). An increased emphasis on job entry targets is also thought to be undermining the original focus of the programme.

Subsequent changes to the programme, following the government's Green Paper, *Towards full employment in a modern society* (DWP, 2001), have aimed to increase flexibility, the involvement of employers and the focus on barriers to employment. Significantly, however, the unemployment rate for 16- to 17-year-olds who are outside this policy envelope has not fallen, and this younger age group (which is likely to include some of the most disadvantaged) appears neglected by policy makers unless in education or training (Hills and Stewart, 2005). Evaluations of NDLP suggest this is also making a net if modest impact (Finn, 2003). It has been estimated that employment rates among lone parents are approximately five percentage points higher than they would have been in the absence of New Labour's policies (McKnight, 2005).

Conclusion

In seeking to establish the links between the evidence base, policy and practice as it relates to health behaviours for young people, we have been confounded by the age range subsumed within this stage of the lifecourse. We have been challenged by the difficulties in separating normal behaviour from risky behaviour and the risky from the problematic, and confronted by the lack of evidence as to how to target problematic behaviour at an early stage. Unlike the health inequalities discussed in Chapter Seven, it is not necessarily a shift, in one sense, to prevention that is required in the behavioural realm – the research evidence suggests that preventative strategies are most effective among those at lowest risk. Rather it is a shift to the acceptance and effective management of risky health. However, it is also a shift to elemental prevention that is required – addressing the structural determinants of health inequalities such as education and employment. Table 9.1 summarises those interventions that the evidence base indicates as effective in improving health behaviours at this stage of the lifecourse, together with key areas where the review-level evidence is still lacking.

This chapter has drawn a familiar picture of connections within this realm of risky behaviour, such that problems tend not to occur singly but at least in tandem. The stress on social pathways and links to the social inclusion agenda recognise this interconnectivity, as does the use of adult advisors or mentors to provide social and emotional support and practical signposting across a range of initiatives such as Connexions and Sure Start Plus. Beneath these recent (and often geographically partial introductions), however, critical services for children and youth are often absent or partial, while mainstream services commonly still operate in parallel. There is a recognised need for one-stop services and multiagency provision that are geared towards the holistic needs of young people (Millward et al, 2004), yet organisational barriers continue to prevent effective service organisation. The fragmentation of responsibility means costs and benefits are unlikely to fall in the same place and agencies remain unaware that antisocial behaviour in childhood leads to high costs for them (Scott et al, 2001).

It has also become apparent that while interventions often succeed in changing knowledge and attitudes, the link to behavioural change is much more tenuous. Not surprisingly, given the age group under consideration, the school has emerged as a key locus for preventative intervention. The NHSS epitomises the search for multifactorial change that can impact simultaneously on the linked triad of health inequality, social inclusion and education, extend beyond the immediate school community and become embedded in mainstream policy, increasing the chances for sustained and durable intervention. Potentially universal interventions, irrespective of whether we are talking about breakfast clubs, substance abuse or sexual health, tend, however, not to reach those most in need. Area-based initiatives (ABIs), such as HAZs, EAZs and Sure Start, have been employed to target intervention, as have initiatives that target particular hard-to-reach groups, such as arrest referral schemes, community projects that seek the views of ethnic groups and initiatives such as Positive Futures that offer diversionary activities for marginalised young people (Millward et al, 2004).

The role of the family has also received renewed attention not just because of its potentially protective role but also as a necessary locus for treatment. There continues, however, to be less research on the role of statutory agencies, particularly the contribution of welfare agencies (Graham and Power, 2004). As we move to consider adulthood, family structure continues to be critical but the intersection with structural factors such as employment and housing also becomes central.

Table 9.1: Interventions during childhood and adolescence: summary of the evidence base relating to health behaviours

	Source
NUTRITIONAL STATUS	
Obesity	
Two key reviews (one on treatment and one on prevention) suggest no direct conclusions can be drawn with confidence	Cochrane Review
There is some evidence that multifaceted school-based programmes that promote physical activity, modify diet and target sedentary behaviour can reduce the prevalence of obesity among school children	Review of reviews
There is less evidence that preventative efficacy attaches to any of these elements alone or to a multifaceted focus on the family	Review of reviews
Multifaceted family behaviour modification programmes can be effective in the targeted treatment of obesity	Review of reviews
Healthy eating	
Healthy eating interventions can prompt behavioural change and reduce fat intake and blood cholesterol but such reductions tend to be minimal (approximately −3% total fat intake)	Other review
Breakfast clubs	
In developing countries breakfast clubs may improve classroom behaviour, cognition, academic outcomes and school attendance in the short term	Review
Lack of review-level evidence	
Information on adolescents	
Studies from the UK	
Sustainable weight-loss treatments	
Interventions for preventing eating disorders	
Upstream interventions	
DRUGS (INCLUDING ALCOHOL AND TOBACCO)	
Smoking	
There is a lack of high-quality evidence about the effectiveness of combinations of social influences and social competence approaches in school	Cochrane Review
Enforcement of the law relating to cigarette sales to under-age youth can have an effect on retailer behaviour, but the impact on smoking behaviour is likely to be small	Cochrane Review
There is some support for the effectiveness of community-wide interventions in helping to prevent the uptake of smoking in young people based again on social learning theory/the social influences approach	Cochrane Review
There is some evidence that the mass media can be effective in preventing the uptake of smoking in young people in conjunction with other interventions	Cochrane Review
There is review-level evidence that increasing the price of cigarettes reduces tobacco use among both adolescents and young adults	Review of reviews
Alcohol	
No firm conclusions about the effectiveness of psychosocial and educational interventions aimed at the primary prevention of alcohol misuse for those aged under 25 in the short and medium term are possible	Cochrane Review

(continued)

Table 9.1: Interventions during childhood and adolescence: summary of the evidence base relating to health behaviours (continued)

	Source
Alcohol (contd)	
There is some evidence for effectiveness of peer-led prevention programmes and interactive programmes that foster the development of interpersonal skills. This also applies to smoking	Review of reviews
Minimum legal drinking age laws prevent alcohol-related crashes, supported by lower blood alcohol concentration laws	Review of reviews
Drugs	
Very little is known about treatment outcomes for young people	Overview
Family therapy appears to be superior to other treatment modalities in reducing substance misuse	Overview
Lack of review-level evidence	
Effectiveness of community programmes	
Interventions that focus on youth	
Initiatives to prevent progression to harder drugs and minimise harm from problematic drug use	
SEXUAL HEALTH	
There is good evidence to support school-based sex education; education linked to contraceptive services alongside the community-based delivery of education, development and contraceptive services; youth development programmes; and family outreach (but this is not supported by RCTs)	Review of reviews
STI campaigns increase condom use and can delay initiation and reduce the frequency of sex, potentially reducing unintended pregnancy as well	Review of reviews
Programmes that offer educational support or improve job prospects may motivate young people to avoid pregnancy	Overview Cochrane Review
Parenting programmes and antenatal care programmes may be effective in improving outcomes for both teenage mothers and their infants	Cochrane Review
Lack of review-level evidence	
Early fatherhood	
Upstream interventions versus poverty and disadvantage	
Interventions relating to the UK	

References

Acheson, D. (1998) *Independent Inquiry into Inequalities in Health*, London: The Stationery Office.

Aggleton, P., Oliver, C. and K.R. (1998) *The implications of research into young people, sex, sexuality and relationships*, London: Health Education Authority.

Anderson, A. (2001) 'The development and evaluation of a novel school based intervention to increase fruits and vegetables intake in children', in Food Standards Agency (ed) *Encouraging consumption of fruit and vegetables by young people through school based interventions: Report from the Food Standards Agency seminar (22.11.01)*, London: Food Standards Agency, p 2.

Ani, C. and Grantham-McGregor, S. (1998) 'The effects of breakfast on educational performance, attendance and classroom behaviour', in N. Donovan and C. Street (eds) *Fit for school: How breakfast clubs meet health, education and childcare needs*, London: New Policy Institute, pp 11-17.

Barlow, J. and Coren, E. (2003) 'Parent-training programmes for improving maternal psychosocial health (Cochrane Methodology Review)', *The Cochrane Library*, Chichester: John Wiley & Sons Ltd.

Barlow, J. and Stewart-Brown, S. (2000) 'Behaviour problems and group based parenting education programmes', *Developmental and Behavioral Pediatrics*, vol 21, no 5, pp 356-70.

Baxter, A., Milner, P., Hawkins, S., Leaf, M., Simpson, C., Wilson, K., Owen, T., Higginbottom, G., Nicholl, J. and Cooper, N. (1997) 'The impact of heart health promotion on coronary heart disease lifestyle risk factors in schoolchildren: lessons learnt from a community-based project', *Public Health*, vol 111, pp 231-7.

Blair, M., Stewart-Brown, S., Waterston, T. and Crowther, R. (2003) *Child public health*, Oxford: Oxford University Press.

Botting, B., Rosato, M. and Wood, R. (1998) 'Teenage mothers and the health of their children', *Population Trends*, vol 93, pp 19-28.

Breeze, J., Aldridge, J. and Parker, H. (2001) 'Unpreventable? How young people make and remake drug taking decisions', in H. Parker, J. Aldridge and R. Egginton (eds) *UK drugs unlimited: New research and policy lessons on illicit drug use*, Basingstoke: Palgrave, pp 51-79.

Bundred, P., Kitchiner, D. and Buchan, I. (2001) 'Prevalence of overweight and obese children between 1989 and 1998: population-based series of cross-sectional studies', *British Medical Journal*, vol 322, no 7277, pp 1-4.

Cabinet Office (1998) *Tackling drugs to build a better Britain: The government's ten-year strategy for tacking drug misuse*, Cm 3945, London: The Stationery Office.

Cabinet Office (2004) *Alcohol harm reduction strategy for England*, London: The Stationery Office.

Campbell, K., Waters, E., O'Meara, S., Kelly, S. and Summerbell, C. (2002) 'Interventions for preventing obesity in children (Cochrane Review)', *The Cochrane Library*, Chichester: John Wiley & Sons Ltd.

Canning, U., Millward, L., Raj, T. and Warm, D. (2004) *Drug use prevention among young people: A review of reviews: Evidence briefing summary*, London: Health Development Agency.

Charlton, A. and Blair, V. (1989) 'Absence from school related to children's and parental smoking habits', *British Medical Journal*, vol 298, pp 90-2.

Cheesbrough, S., Ingham, R. and Massey, D. (2002) *Reducing the rate of teenage conceptions. A review of the international evidence on preventing and reducing teenage conceptions: The United States, Canada, Australia and New Zealand*, London: Health Development Agency.

Chevalier, A. and Viitanen, T.K. (2003) 'The long-run labour market consequences of teenage motherhood in Britain', *Journal of Population Economics*, vol 16, no 2, pp 323-43.

Clements, S., Stone, N., Diamond, I. and Ingham, R. (1998) 'The spatial distribution of teenage conceptions within Wessex', in K. Wellings (ed) *Promoting the health of teenage and lone mothers: Setting a research agenda*, London: Health Education Authority, pp 71-81.

Coleman, T., Pound, E. and Cheater, F. (2002) *National survey of the new smoking cessation services: Implementing the smoking kills White Paper*, Nottingham: University of Nottingham.

Coomber, R., Millward, L., Chambers, J. and Warm, D. (2004) *A rapid interim review of the 'grey' literature on risky behaviour in young people aged 11-18 with a special emphasis on vulnerable groups*, London: Health Development Agency.

Coren, E. and Barlow, J. (2003) 'Individual and group-based parenting programmes for improving psychosocial outcomes for teenage parents and their children (Cochrane Review)', *The Cochrane Library*, Chichester: John Wiley & Sons Ltd.

Coren, E., Barlow, J. and Stewart-Brown, S. (2003) 'The effectiveness of individual and group-based parenting programmes in improving outcomes for teenage mothers and their children: a systematic review', *Journal of Adolescence*, vol 26, no 1, pp 79-103.

Crome, I.B., Christian, J. and Green, C. (1998) 'Tip of an iceberg? Profile of adolescent patients prescribed methadone in an innovative community drug services', *Drugs: Education, Prevention and Policy*, vol 5, no 2, pp 195-7.

CYPU (Children and Young People's Unit) (2001) *Building a strategy for children and young people: Consultation document*, London: CYPU.

DCMS (Department for Culture, Media and Sport) (2000) *A sporting future for all: The government's plan for sport*, London: DCMS.

de Vries, H., Mudde, A., Kremers, S., Wetzels, J., Uiters, E., Ariza, C., Vitoria, P., Fielder, A., Holm, K., Janssen, K., Lehtuvuori, R. and Candel, M. (2003) 'The European Smoking Prevention Framework Approach (ESFA): short-term effects', *Health Education Research*, vol 18, no 6, pp 649-63.

Dennison, C. (2004) *Teenage pregnancy: An overview of the research evidence*, London: Health Development Agency.

DfES (Department for Education and Skills) (2004a) *Autumn performance report 2004: Achievement against Public Service Agreement targets, 2000-2004*, Cm 6399, London: DfES.

DfES (2004b) *Every child matters: Change for children in schools*, London: DfES.

DfES (2005) *Every child matters: Change for children, young people and drugs*, London: DfES.

DfES and DCMS (Department for Culture, Media and Sports) (2003) *Learning through PE and sport: A guide to the physical education, school sport and club links strategy*, London: DfES and DCMS.

DH (Department of Health) (1992) *The health of the nation: A strategy for health in England and Wales*, London: HMSO.

DH (1998a) *Smoking kills*, London: The Stationery Office.

DH (1998b) *Our healthier nation: A contract for health*, CM 3852, London: The Stationery Office.

DH (1999) *Saving lives: Our healthier nation*, London: The Stationery Office.

DH (2000) *The NHS Cancer Plan*, London: DH.

DH (2001) *The national strategy for sexual health and HIV*, London: DH.

DH and DfES (2003a) *National Healthy Schools Standard: Confirming healthy school achievement*, London: DH and DfES.

DH and DfES (2003b) *National Healthy Schools Standard: Drugs education (including alcohol and tobacco)*, London: DH and DfES.

DH, DfEE (Department for Education and Employment) and Home Office (2000) *Framework for the assessment of children in need and their families*, London: The Stationery Office.

DiCenso, A., Guyatt, G., Willan, A. and Griffith, L. (2002) 'Interventions to reduce unintended pregnancies among adolescents: systematic review of randomised controlled trials', *British Medical Journal*, vol 324, p 1426.

Dowler, E. and Calvert, C. (1995) *Nutrition and diet in lone-parent families in London*, London: Family Policy Studies Centre.

Dowler, E. and Turner, S. With Dobson, B. (2001) *Poverty bites: Food, health and poor families*, London: Child Poverty Action Group.

Drugs Strategy Directorate (2002) *Updated drug strategy*, London: Home Office.

DWP (Department for Work and Pensions) (2001) *Towards full employment in a modern society*, Cm 5984, London: DWP.

Edgardh, K. (2002) 'Adolescent sexual health in Sweden', *Sexually Transmitted Infections*, vol 78, pp 352-6.

Edmunds, L., Waters, E. and Elliott, E. (2001) 'Evidence based management of childhood obesity', *British Medical Journal*, vol 323, no 7318, pp 916-19.

Edmunds, M., Hough, M., Turnbull, P. and May, T. (1999) *Doing justice to treatment: Referring offenders to drug services*, Drugs Prevention Advisory Service Briefing Paper 2, London: Home Office.

Ellis, S. and Grey, A. (2004) *Prevention of sexually transmitted infections (STIs): A review of reviews into the effectiveness of non-clinical interventions*, London: Health Development Agency.

Ellis, S., Barnett-Page, E., Morgan, A. and Taylor, L. (2003) *HIV prevention: A review of reviews assessing the effectiveness of interventions to reduce the risk of sexual transmission*, London: Health Development Agency.

Epstein, L., Wing, R., Koeske, R. and Valoski, A. (1985) 'A comparison of lifestyle exercise, aerobic exercise, and calisthenics on weight loss in obese children', *Behaviour Therapy*, vol 16, pp 345-56.

Finn, D. (2003) 'Employment policy', in N. Ellison and C. Pierson (eds) *Developments in British social policy 2*, Basingstoke: Palgrave Macmillan, pp 111-28.

Fonagy, P., Target, M., Cottrell, D., Phillips, J. and Kurtz, Z. (2002) *What works for whom? A critical review of treatments for children and adolescents*, London: The Guilford Press.

Foxcroft, D., Ireland, D., Lister-Sharp, D., Lowe, G. and R.B. (2003) 'Primary prevention for alcohol misuse in young people (Cochrane Review)', *The Cochrane Library*, Chichester: John Wiley & Sons Ltd.

Gordon, I., Whitear, B. and Guthrie, D. (1997) 'Stopping them starting: evaluation of a community-based project to discourage teenage smoking in Cardiff', *Health Education Journal*, vol 46, pp 42–50.

Gortmaker, S., Peterson, K., Wiecha, J., Sobal, A., Dixit, S., Fox, M. and Laird, N. (1999) 'Reducing obesity via a school-based interdisciplinary intervention among youth', *Archives of Pediatrics and Adolescent Medicine*, vol 153, no 4, pp 409–18.

Gossop, M., Marsden, J. and Stewart, D. (1998) *NTORS at one year: The national treatment outcome research study: Changes in substance use, health and criminal behaviours one year after intake*, London: DH.

Gossop, M., Marsden, J. and Stewart, D. (2001) *NTORS after 5 years: Changes in substance use, health and criminal behaviour during the five years after intake*, London: National Addiction Centre.

Graham, H. and Power, C. (2004) *Childhood disadvantage and adult health: A lifecourse framework*, London: Health Development Agency.

Gregory, J., Lowe, S., Bates, C., Prentice, A., Jackson, L., Smithers, G., Wenlock, R. and Farron, M. (2000) *National diet and nutrition survey: Young people aged 4-18 years*, London: The Stationery Office.

Harrop, A. and Palmer, G. (2002) *Improving breakfast clubs: Lessons from the best*, London: New Policy Institute.

HAS (Health Advisory Service) (2001) *The substance of young needs: Review 2001*, London: HAS.

HDA (Health Development Agency) (2001) *Teenage pregnancy: An update on key characteristics of effective interventions*, London: HDA.

HDA (2002) *Cancer prevention: A resource to support local action in delivering the NHS Cancer Plan*, London: HDA.

HDA (2004) *Smoking interventions with children and young people*, Better Health for Children and Young People, HDA Briefing No 6, London: HDA.

Hillier, L., Harrison, L. and Warr, D. (1998) '"When you carry condoms all the boys think you want it": negotiating competing discourses about safe sex', *Journal of Adolescence*, vol 21, no 1, pp 15–29.

Hills, J. and Stewart, K. (2005) 'A tide turned but mountains yet to climb?', in J. Hills and K. Stewart (eds) *A more equal society?*, Bristol: The Policy Press, pp 325–46.

HM Government and DH (Department of Health) (2004) *Choosing health: Making healthy choices easier*, London: HM Government and DH.

HMSO (1994) *Tackling drugs together*, London: HMSO.

Home Office (nd) *Tackling drugs as part of neighbourhood renewal*, London: Home Office.

Hughes, K., Cragg, A. and Taylor, C. (1999) *Young people's experiences of relationships, sex and early parenthood: Qualitative research*, London: Health Education Authority.

Ingham, R., Clements, S. and Gillibrand, R. (nd) *Factors affecting changes in rates of teenage conceptions 1991 to 1997*, London: Teenage Pregnancy Unit.

Jefferis, B., Graham, H., Manor, O. and Power, C. (2003) 'Cigarette consumption and socio-economic circumstances in adolescence as predictors of adult smoking', *Addiction*, vol 98, no 12, pp 1765-72.

Kirby, D. (1999) 'Reflections on two decades of research on teen sexual behavior and pregnancy', *Journal of School Health and Place*, vol 69, no 3, pp 89-94.

Kobus, K. (2003) 'Peers and adolescent smoking', *Addiction*, vol 98, suppl 1, pp 37-55.

Lantz, P., Jacobson, P., Warner, K., Wasserman, J., Pollack, H., Berson, J. and Ahlstrom, A. (2000) 'Investing in youth tobacco control: a review of smoking prevention and control strategies', *Tobacco Control*, vol 9, no 1, pp 47-63.

LeMura, L. and Maziekas, M. (2002) 'Factors that alter body fat, body mass, and fat-free mass in pediatric obesity', *Medicine and Science in Sports and Exercise*, vol 34, no 3, pp 487-96.

Lister-Sharp, D., Chapman, S., Stewart-Brown, S. and Sowden, A. (1999) 'Health promoting schools and health promotion in schools: two systematic reviews', *Health Technology Assessment*, vol 3, no 22, pp 1-207.

Lowe, F., Horne, P., Tapper, K., Madden, P., Woolner, J., Le Noury, J. and Doody, M. (nd) *Changing the nation's diet: A programme to increase children's consumption of fruit and vegetables*, Working Paper 3, Bangor: University of Wales.

Lucas, P. (2003) 'Breakfast clubs and school fruit schemes: promising practice' (www.whatworksforchildren.org.uk), What Works for Children Group, Evidence Nugget, April.

McBride, N., Farringdon, F., Midford, R., Meuleners, L. and Phillips, M. (2004) 'Harm minimization in school drug education: final results of the school health and alcohol harm reduction project (SHAHRP)', *Addiction*, vol 99, no 3, pp 278-91.

MacKintosh, A., Stead, M., Eadie, D. and Hastings, G. (2000) *NE choices: Results of a multi-component drugs prevention programme for adolescents*, Drugs Prevention Advisory Service Briefing Paper 14, London: Home Office.

McKnight, A. (2005) 'Employment: tacking poverty through "work for those who can"', in J. Hills and K. Stewart (eds) *A more equal society?*, Bristol: The Policy Press, pp 23-46.

McKnight, A., Glennerster, H. and Lupton, R. (2005) 'Education, education, education ...: an assessment of Labour's success in tackling education inequalities', in J. Hills and K. Stewart (eds) *A more equal society?* Bristol: The Policy Press, pp 47-68.

Markham, W.A., Featherstone, K., Taket, A., Trenchard-Mabere, E. and Ross, M. (2001) 'Smoking amongst UK Bangladeshi adolescents aged 14-15', *Health Education Research*, vol 16, no 2, pp 143-56.

May, T., Warburton, H., Turnbull, P. and Hough, M. (2002) *Times they are a-changing: Policing of cannabis*, York: Joseph Rowntree Foundation.

Measham, F., Aldridge, J. and Parker, H. (2001) 'Unstoppable? Dance drug use in the UK club scene', in H. Parker, J. Aldridge and R. Egginton (eds) *UK drugs unlimited: New research and policy lessons on illicit drug use*, Basingstoke: Palgrave, pp 80–97.

Meyrick, J. and Swann, C. (1998) *An overview of the effectiveness of interventions and programmes aimed at reducing unintended conceptions in young people*, London: Health Education Authority.

Millward, L., Warm, D., Coomber, R., Chambers, J. and Kelly, M. (2004) *Evidence for effective drug prevention in young people: A summary of findings arising from research activity to date*, Wetherby: Health Development Agency.

Moore, L. (2001) 'Are fruit tuck shops in primary schools effective in increasing pupils' fruit consumption? A randomised controlled trial', in Food Standards Agency (ed) *Encouraging consumption of fruit and vegetables by young people through school based interventions: Report from the food standards agency seminar (22.11.01)*, London: Food Standards Agency, p 5.

Moore, L., Paisley, C. and Dennehy, A. (2000) 'Are fruit tuck shops in primary schools effective in increasing pupils' fruit consumption? A randomised controlled trial', *Nutrition and Food Science*, vol 30, no 1, pp 35–8.

Mulvihill, C. and Quigley, R. (2003) *The management of obesity and overweight: An analysis of reviews of diet, physical activity and behavioural approaches*, London: Health Development Agency.

Mulvihill, C., Taylor, L., Waller, S., with Naidoo, B. and Thom, B. (2005) *Prevention and reduction of alcohol misuse*, London: HDA.

Munro, H., Davis, M. and Hughes, G. (2004) 'Adolescent sexual health', in ONS (ed) *The health of children and young people*, London: ONS (www.statistics.gov.uk/children).

NAO (National Audit Office) (2001) *Tackling obesity in England: Report by the Comptroller and Auditor General*, London: The Stationery Office.

NAO (2002) *The New Deal for Young People*, London: The Stationery Office.

Nessa, N. and Gallagher, J. (2004) 'Diet, nutrition, dental health and exercise', in ONS (ed) *The health of children and young people*, London: ONS (www.statistics.gov.uk/children.

NHS CRD (National Health Service Centre for Reviews and Dissemination) (1997) 'Preventing and reducing the adverse effects of unintended teenage pregnancies', *Effective Health Care*, vol 3, no 1, pp 1–12.

NHS CRD (1999) 'Preventing the uptake of smoking in young people', *Effective Health Care*, vol 5, no 5, pp 1–12.

NHS CRD (2002) 'The prevention and treatment of childhood obesity', *Effective Health Care*, vol 7, no 6, pp 1–12.

NICE (National Institute for Clinical Excellence) (2001) *Guidance on the use of sibutramine for the treatment of obesity in adults*, London: NICE.

NSNR (National Strategy for Neighbourhood Renewal) (2000) *Report of Policy Action Team 12: Young people*, London: The Stationery Office.

Olds, D., Henderson, C., Cole, R., Eckenrode, J., Kitzman, H., Luckey, D., Pettitt, L., Sidora, K., Morris, P. and Powers, J. (1998) 'Long term effects of nurse home visitation on children's criminal and anti-social behavior', *Journal of American Medical Association*, vol 280, no 14, p 1238-44.

Parker, H., Aldridge, J. and Egginton, R. (2001) *UK drugs unlimited: New research and policy lessons on illicit drug use*, Basingstoke: Palgrave.

Parker, H., Aldridge, J. and Measham, F. (1998) *Illegal leisure: The normalization of adolescent recreational drug use*, London: Routledge.

Peterson, A.V., Kealey, K.A., Mann, S.L., Marek, P.M. and Sarason, I.G. (2000) 'Hutchinson smoking prevention project: long-term randomised trial in school-based tobacco use prevention: results on smoking', *Journal of the National Cancer Institute*, vol 92, no 24, pp 1979-91.

Positive Futures (2004) *Positive Futures impact report: Engaging with young people*, London: Home Office Drugs Strategy Directorate.

Pound, E., Coleman, T., Adams, C., Bauld, L. and Ferguson, J. (2005) 'Targeting smokers in priority groups: the influence of government targets and policy statements', *Addiction*, vol 100, suppl 2, pp 28-35.

Pratt, B. and Woolfenden, S. (2004) 'Interventions for preventing eating disorders in children and adolescents (Cochrane Review)', *The Cochrane Library*, Chichester: John Wiley & Sons Ltd.

Prochaska, J.O. (2000) 'Stages of change model for smoking prevention and cessation in schools', *British Medical Journal*, vol 320, no 7232, p 447.

Riley, A. (2005) *Fact sheet: School meals*, London: CPAG.

Rivers, K., Aggleton, P., Chase, E., Downie, A., Mulvihill, C., Sinkler, P., Tyrer, P. and Warwick, I. (2000) *Setting the standard: Research linked to the development of the national healthy school standard (NHSS)*, London: DH and DfEE.

Roe, L., Hunt, P., Bradshaw, H. and Rayner, M. (1997) *Health promotion interventions to promote healthy eating in the general population: A review*, London: Health Education Authority.

Rooney, B. and Murray, D. (1996) 'A meta-analysis of smoking prevention programs after adjustment for errors in the unit of analysis', *Health Education Quarterly*, vol 23, pp 48-64.

Rosato, M., Wiggins, M., Austerberry, H. and Oliver, S. (2004) *Summary of interim findings*, London: Sure Start Plus National Evaluation.

Rowan, S. (2004) 'Drug-use, smoking and drinking', in ONS (ed) *The health of children and young people*, London: ONS (www.statistics.gov.uk).

Rudolf, M., Sahota, P., Barth, J. and Walker, J. (2001) 'Increasing prevalence of obesity in primary school children', *British Medical Journal*, vol 322, no 7294, pp 1094-5.

Sahota, P., Rudolf, M., Dixey, R., Hill, A., Barth, J. and Cade, J. (2001a) 'Randomised controlled trial of primary school based intervention to reduce risk factors for obesity', *British Medical Journal*, vol 323, no 7320, pp 1029-32.

Sahota, P., Rudolf, M., Dixey, R., Hill, A., Barth, J. and Cade, J. (2001b) 'Evaluation of implementation and effect of primary school based intervention to reduce risk factors for obesity', *British Medical Journal*, vol 323, no 7320, pp 1027-9.

Scott, S., Knapp, M., Henderson, J. and Maughan, B. (2001) 'Financial cost of social exclusion: follow up study of antisocial children into adulthood', *British Medical Journal*, vol 323, no 7306, pp 191-4.

SEU (Social Exclusion Unit) (1998) *Rough sleeping: Report by the Social Exclusion Unit*, www.socialexclusionunit.gov.uk.

Shemilt, I., O'Brien, M., Thoburn, J., Harvey, I., Belderson, P., Robinson, J. and Camina, M. (2003) 'School breakfast clubs, children and family support', *Children and Society*, vol 17, no 2, pp 100-12.

Shemilt, I., Harvey, I., Shepstone, L., Swift, L., Reading, R., Mugford, M., Belderson, P., Norris, N., Thorburn, J. and Robinson, J. (2004) 'A national evaluation of school breakfast clubs: evidence from a cluster randomized controlled trial and an observational analysis', *Child: Care, Health and Development*, vol 30, no 5, pp 413-27.

Shiner, M. (2000) *Doing it for themselves: An evaluation of peer approaches to drug prevention*, Drugs Prevention Advisory Service Briefing Paper 6, London: Home Office.

Sondhi, A., O'Shea, J. and Williams, T. (2002) *Arrest referral: Emerging findings from the national monitoring and evaluation programme*, Drugs Prevention Advisory Service Briefing Paper 18, London: Home Office.

Sowden, A. and Arblaster, L. (1999) 'Mass media interventions for preventing smoking in young people (Cochrane Review)', *The Cochrane Library*, Chichester: John Wiley & Sons Ltd.

Sowden, A., Arblaster, L. and Stead, L. (2004) 'Community interventions for preventing smoking in young people (Cochrane Review)', *The Cochrane Library*, Chichester: John Wiley & Sons Ltd.

Stead, L. and Lancaster, T. (2004) 'Interventions for preventing tobacco sales to minors (Cochrane Review)', *The Cochrane Library*, Chichester: John Wiley & Sons Ltd.

Story, M. (1999) 'School-based approaches for preventing and treating obesity', *International Journal of Obesity*, vol 23, suppl 2, pp S43-S51.

Street, C. (1998) 'Introduction', in N. Donovan and C. Street (eds) *Fit for school: How breakfast clubs meet health, education and childcare needs*, London: New Policy Institute, pp 1-8.

Street, C. and Kenway, P. (1999) *Food for thought: Breakfast clubs and their challenges*, London: New Policy Institute.

Summerbell, C., Ashton, V., Campbell, K. J., Edmunds, L., Kelly, S. and Waters, E. (2004) 'Interventions for treating obesity in children (Cochrane Review)', *The Cochrane Library*, Chichester: John Wiley & Sons Ltd.

Swann, C., Bowe, K., McCormick, G. and Kosmin, M. (2003) *Teenage pregnancy and parenthood: A review of reviews*, London: Health Development Agency.

Thomas, R. (2002) 'School-based programmes for preventing smoking (Cochrane Review)', *The Cochrane Library*, Chichester: John Wiley & Sons Ltd.

Tobler, N., Roona, M., Ochshorn, P., Marshall, D., Streke, A. and Stackpole, K. (2000) 'School-based adolescent drug prevention programs: 1998 meta-analysis', *Journal of Primary Prevention*, vol 20, no 4, pp 275-336.

Tyas, S. and Pederson, L. (1998) 'Psychosocial factors related to adolescent smoking: a critical review of the literature', *Tobacco Control*, vol 7, winter, pp 409-20.

University of East Anglia (2002) *A national evaluation of school breakfast clubs: Evaluation summary, part 1*, Norwich: University of East Anglia.

Vartiainen, E., Paavola, M., McAlister, A. and Pekka, P. (1998) 'Fifteen-year follow-up of smoking prevention effects in the North Karelia Youth Project', *American Journal of Public Health*, vol 88, no 1, pp 81-5.

Walker, A., Gregory, J., Bradnock, G., Nunn, J. and White, D.M. (2000) *National diet and nutrition survey: Young people aged 4 to 18 years. Volume 2: Report of the oral health survey*, London: The Stationery Office.

Warren, J.M., Henry, C.J.K., Lightowler, H.J., Bradshaw, S.M. and Perwaiz, S. (2003) 'Evaluation of a pilot school programme aimed at the prevention of obesity in children', *Health Promotion International*, vol 18, no 4, pp 287-96.

Warwick, I., Blenkinsop, S., Aggleton, P., Eggers, M., Chase, E.I.S., Schagen, S., Zuurmond, M. and Scott, E. (2004) *Evaluation of the impact of the national healthy school standard*, London: Thomas Coram Research Unit and the National Foundation for Educational Research.

Wellings, K. (1998) 'Introduction', in K. Wellings (ed) *Promoting the health of teenage and lone mothers: Setting a research agenda*, London: Health Education Authority, pp 1-31.

Wellings, K., Wadsworth, J., Johnson, A. and Field, J. (1998) 'Correlates of teenage birth', in K. Wellings (ed) *Promoting the health of teenage and lone mothers: Setting a research agenda*, London: Health Education Authority, pp 32-42.

Wiggins, M., Austerberry, H., Rosato, M., Sawtell, M. and Oliver, S. (2003) *Service delivery study: Interim findings*, London: Sure Start Plus National Evaluation.

Williams, R., Chang, S. and Addiction Centre Adolescent Research Group (2000) 'A comprehensive and comparative review of adolescent substance abuse treatment outcome', *Clinical Psychology: Science and Practice Summary*, vol 7, no 2, pp 138-66.

Wincup, E., Buckland, G. and Bayliss, R. (2003) *Youth homelessness and substance use: Report to the drugs and alcohol research unit*, Home Office Research Study 258, London: Home Office Research, Development and Statistics Directorate.

Zoritch, B., Roberts, I. and Oakley, A. (2000) 'Day care for preschool children', *The Cochrane Library*, Chichester: John Wiley & Sons Ltd.

TEN

Health inequalities during adulthood: research evidence

Introduction

The development of lifecourse approaches to health inequalities has not only addressed the neglect of early life influences in a literature previously dominated by a concentration on adult risk factors for chronic adulthood disease (Davey Smith, 2003). It has also begun to challenge existing research on the relative contribution of such risk factors. For most of the postwar period, research focused on the role of so-called lifestyle factors in determining risk for chronic disease. The individualistic and potentially victim-blaming nature of such research attracted considerable criticism, which may go some way towards explaining why the psychosocial hypothesis (which explicitly considers the role of *social* inequality in producing ill health) was so warmly received. Indeed, psychosocial interpretations of the effects of social inequality on population health were accepted as common wisdom by the late 1990s.

More recent research has begun to question the relative significance of this pathway. For example, recent empirical data do not support the notion that current markers of social capital and the psychosocial environment account for health differences between countries. Early life circumstances 70 years before may be as, if not more, significant. This is certainly suggested by the type of evidence presented in Chapters Four and Six, which shows that socio-economic and psychosocial conditions during early childhood have a powerful impact on health, behaviour and achievement across the lifecycle.

While there is considerable current research interest in the relationship between childhood disadvantage and adult health, this should not result in the pendulum swinging away from a concern with adult risk factors to an excess concentration on early life influences. First, as we proposed in Chapter Two, the jury is still out on the psychosocial hypothesis and, at an individual level at least, there is strong evidence of a causal association between social support, mental health and physical health. Second, lifecourse research suggests that *both* childhood and adult circumstances influence health variations (Kuh et al, 2003). We examine such research in the first part of this chapter and describe the complex picture that emerges of the determinants of social inequalities in adult mortality. For example, evidence suggests that the relative importance of early and later life determinants of mortality varies according to cause of death. The differential effects of childhood and adult exposures may also change over time.

Although biological programming theories and, more recently, lifecourse research, has resulted in a re-evaluation of the relative significance of adult risk factors, it is nevertheless accepted that socio-economic circumstances during adulthood do have a role to play in the production of health inequalities. Lifestyle factors, psychosocial health, exposure to unsafe physical environments and access to key services are all of interest here. The chapter goes on to examine the significance of such influences, starting with lifestyle factors (smoking, diet and nutrition, physical exercise and substance misuse). The role of factors that impact on psychosocial well-being are then assessed, including poor social support and 'unhealthy' neighbourhoods. Finally, the ways in which material living conditions (income, employment, housing and the physical environment) and access to health services influence health are considered.

The relative role of early and later life influences on adult health

As noted in Chapter Two, by the late 1990s, three broad lifecourse models had been offered as explanations for socio-economic differences in risk of disease (Hertzman et al, 2001). The latency or critical period model drew attention to the way in which exposure to adversity in early life has long-term health effects. Pathway models focused on the ways in which poor childhood conditions influence social trajectories into and throughout adulthood that impact on health; while the accumulation model suggested that exposures gradually accumulate over time to increase the risk of chronic disease, poor circumstances throughout life conferring the greatest risk of poor health in adulthood through a type of dose–response relationship.

In practice, disadvantage during critical periods in early life directs many children onto negative life trajectories that reinforce cumulative disadvantage that in turn shapes future pathways. Thus, biological and social risk factors during different life stages not only influence health independently, but interactively and cumulatively. This poses some difficulties for separating out different effects (Hallqvist et al, 2004), and suggests a strong case for a less polarised and more integrative approach to lifecourse epidemiology that avoids treating these models as mutually exclusive paradigms. Thus, it is broadly agreed today that early life factors, chains of risk, material deprivation and the conventional risk factors identified by adult lifestyle models can *all* have a bearing on adult health, although the relative strengths of these effects may vary across different cohorts and health outcomes (Graham, 2002).

Against this background, there is a need to explore the relative importance of health risk factors during childhood and adulthood to *different* health outcomes. This, it is argued, may improve understanding of disease aetiology and inform the targeting of appropriate policies (Claussen et al, 2003). The task of isolating the effects of childhood and adult factors is complicated by the fact that, due to the continuity experienced by many children in their socio-economic circumstances, social disadvantage in early and later life tends to be linked (Davey Smith et al, 1998). Birth cohort studies that track their subjects from birth through life provide an important source from which the effects of early life, cumulative and contemporary circumstances can be modelled. However, the earliest birth cohort study members in Britain were born in 1946 and have not yet reached the age at which inequalities in key health indicators (including premature mortality) are fully manifest (Berney et al, 2000a, p 80). Thus, a number of alternative strategies have been used to model the effects of social disadvantage over the lifecourse (Wadsworth, 1997). These include studies in which subjects from earlier surveys or clinical populations are traced and followed up. One of the best known is the Boyd Orr cohort, in which follow-up data were collected from a sample of traced surviving members of a cohort of children surveyed between 1937 and 1939 (Gunnell et al, 1996, 1998; Blane et al, 1999; Berney et al, 2000b; Holland et al, 2000). Census data collected at different times have also been linked with death registration data in order to examine the impact of childhood and adulthood social circumstances on adult mortality (Claussen et al, 2003; Næss et al, 2004).

Such advances in study design and analytical strategies have allowed the analysis of independent associations between health outcomes and socio-economic circumstances in childhood and adulthood, that provide useful insights into the role played by exposures during different states of the lifecourse to disease aetiology. For example, adult mortality from stomach cancer, respiratory tuberculosis and stroke is more strongly related to historical levels of infant mortality (at the time at which these adults were born) than mortality from coronary heart disease (CHD) and lung cancer (Leon and Davey Smith, 2000). This finding is in agreement with the notion that people dying of respiratory tuberculosis in old age may have been initially infected in their early years and that early exposure to *Helicobacter pylori* is a key factor in the aetiology of stomach cancer. It also suggests that risk for stroke may be influenced by exposure (for example, to infection) in childhood. By contrast, factors in adult life are, as expected, more significant to the development of lung cancer.

Other studies confirm that the relative effect on disease and mortality of socio-economic conditions in childhood varies according to cause. For example, in the Scottish Collaborative Study, deaths from haemorrhagic (but not ischaemic) stroke and stomach cancer were most strongly associated with social class at birth and number of siblings (a factor related to risk of childhood infection), while deaths from lung cancer and accidents and violence were clearly influenced by exposures acting during adult life (Davey Smith et al, 1998; Hart and Davey Smith, 2003). Risk for psychiatric mortality also appears to be most strongly associated with adult social position (Claussen et al, 2003).

Other symptoms and conditions have been linked to factors across the lifecourse. For example, childhood circumstances appear to have an enduring effect on risk for obesity, although this can be modified in later years (Langenberg et al, 2003). Similarly, it is generally agreed that early childhood adversity establishes important biological risk factors for CHD while adult social position shapes key health behaviours that exacerbate risk in a cumulative fashion. When accumulation of risk is significant, the relative effects of childhood adversity and adult socio-economic circumstances tend to vary between cohorts. For example, in the British women's heart and health study, a range of cardiovascular disease risk factors were associated with both childhood and adult social position, but the association between insulin resistance and childhood social position was particularly strong (Lawlor et al, 2002). The Oslo Mortality Study similarly found that deaths from cardiovascular disease (the majority of which were due to CHD) were more strongly associated with childhood than adult social circumstances (Claussen et al, 2003). By contrast, in the Whitehall II Study, CHD morbidity was more strongly related to adult socio-economic status than to the father's social class (Marmot et al, 2001).

Differences between cohorts in the relative effects of early and later life exposures reflect the fact that socio-economic circumstances during childhood and adulthood and the exposures they produce vary with time and place. For instance, improving social conditions over the course of the 20th century appear to have contributed to declining rates of *Helicobacter pylori* and falling rates of death from stomach cancer in the UK (Davey Smith et al, 1998). In other countries such as Russia, Chile and Japan, however, high rates of infant mortality (and thus presumably of childhood diarrhoea and *Helicobacter pylori*) were maintained in the early decades of the 20th century and these are reflected in continuing high rates of stomach cancer mortality towards the end of the 20th century (Davey Smith, 2003).

Changes in the distribution of diseases mean that, over time, diseases with predominantly early life determination (for example tuberculosis, stomach cancer and haemorrhagic stroke) have declined in importance while those with adulthood determination (for example, lung cancer and accidental/violent death) or determination over the lifecourse (for example, CHD, ischaemic stroke and breast cancer) have become of relatively greater importance (Davey Smith, 2003 p xlvi). This shift in dominance from early life determination of mortality risk to a greater determination of adulthood influences took place after 1930, and would be expected to be reflected in a shift in the relative role of early and later life exposures in mortality at the end of the 20th and beginning of the 21st centuries.

Strong associations between mortality/disease risk factors and socio-economic conditions in childhood have certainly been noted in older cohorts such as the British women's heart and health study (born between 1920 and 1941), the Boyd Orr cohort (born around 1930) and children born between 1923 and 1939 in the ONS Longitudinal Study for England and Wales (Frankel et al,

1999; Lawlor et al, 2002; Curtis et al, 2004). These suggest that the widening gap in mortality rates that coincided with the growth in income inequality during the 1980s may have been less of a reflection of short-term government policies than the profound inequalities that existed between different socio-economic groups in the 1920s and 1930s. In 1931, the infant mortality rate in Manchester ranged from 44 per 1,000 in the best ward to 143 per 1,000 in the worst (Whitehead et al, 1997). Economic depression exacerbated existing divides. For example, during the 1930s, deprivation and high unemployment were particular problems in Scotland, Northern England and Wales, compared to the south of Britain, a pattern that was to be echoed in the geographical distribution of mortality in the 1980s and 1990s.

With improvements in postwar living conditions, including exposure to food rationing and broad welfare and educational reforms designed to promote a more equitable start in life, one would expect to see a reduction in the relationship between childhood socio-economic conditions and mortality in adulthood. However, analysis of the 1946 British birth cohort found no evidence of this (Kuh et al, 2002a). Early life factors were also found to be significantly associated with self-rated health at the age of 33 in the 1958 British birth cohort (Hertzman et al, 2001), and several studies of more recent cohorts suggest that childhood adversity continues to play a significant role in the development of psychological disorders (see Chapter Six). In contrast to the first decades of the 20th century, a significant proportion of pregnant women today smoke. Relative poverty has grown in the postwar period due to a widening in the distribution of income (Church and Whyman, 1997). Absolute improvements in living standards have not, moreover, eradicated problems of early life adversity. During the late 1980s and early 1990s, widespread concerns were expressed about the implications of low incomes for the health and nutrition of children and pregnant women (Davey Smith and Kuh, 1996; Wadsworth and Kuh, 1997), while today particular attention is being paid to the consequences of economic distress for quality of parenting. Thus, while the extent to which the widening mortality gap of the 1980s and 1990s can be attributed to government policies during this period is debatable, growing income polarisation and child poverty may well be reflected in growing health inequalities in the mid-21st century.

Although early life factors appear to remain significant to health inequalities, several studies of younger cohorts suggest that the effects of cumulative and current adult position have indeed become stronger (Hertzman et al, 2001; Pensola and Martikainen, 2004). As discussed in Chapter Eight, there is significant continuity in key health behaviours, many of which are established during childhood and youth. Pathway effects are also evident in the ways in which behavioural/emotional status during adolescence and educational qualifications play a critical role in shaping future adult position. Finally, socio-economic circumstances during adulthood have been directly implicated in the production of health inequalities. These are considered in the following section.

Adult socio-economic position and health risk factors

As already noted, for much of the postwar period, risk for chronic disease was largely associated with environmental factors in adult life. The focus within this paradigm was largely on so-called lifestyle factors (notably smoking, but also diet, physical activity and alcohol consumption), with relatively little attention being paid to other influences in later life. This was to change in the 1980s, which, in addition to seeing a revival of interest in the role of early life factors, saw the beginnings of a psychosocial theory of health inequalities. The publication of the Black Report in 1980, with its sympathy for materialist explanations for health inequalities, together with concerns that an individualistic focus on health-damaging behaviours amounted to victim blaming, also promoted interest in the role of relative material deprivation in health exclusion. Evidence of the contribution made by each of these groups of factors is considered next.

Health and lifestyle

After the Second World War, adult chronic diseases became a major public health concern as mortality rates from cancer and CHD took on increasing significance. In 1948, a major US prospective study on heart disease was set up in Framingham, Massachusetts. In addition to testing the pathological precursors of CHD (hypertension and elevated cholesterol), this considered the importance of other diseases, being overweight, physique and a number of personal habits (diet, alcohol consumption, smoking and physical activity) to heart disease. This study, together with Doll and Hill's (1954) prospective study of 40,000 doctors, which showed that smoking was a risk factor for lung cancer, CHD and chronic bronchitis, was to play an important role in the development of postwar epidemiology, with its strong focus on the role of adult lifestyle in risk for chronic disease (Kuh and Davey Smith, 1997).

Cigarette smoking

There is a general consensus that the lifestyle factors identified in the Framingham study do play an important role in chronic disease aetiology. Of these, cigarette smoking is responsible for the greatest burden of premature death. Some estimates suggest that about half of all persistent cigarette smokers are killed by their habit, a quarter while still in middle age (35-69 years) (Doll et al, 2004). In addition to increasing risk for lung and other cancers (particularly of the mouth, pharynx, larynx and oesophagus), smoking is associated with death from chronic obstructive pulmonary disease (COPD), including chronic bronchitis and emphysema. By increasing the hardening of the artery walls (atherosclerosis), making the blood clot more easily and increasing blood cholesterol, risk of CHD, peripheral vascular disease and stroke is increased among smokers. Smoking can also damage reproductive health in women and men. Women who smoke more than 20 cigarettes a day are three times less likely to become pregnant than non-smokers, while men who smoke produce on average fewer sperm and have a higher proportion of sperm with defects (Crofton and Simpson, 2002).

Lifelong smokers are at greatest risk of such health outcomes. Monitoring smoking-related mortality among British doctors over a 50-year period, Doll et al (2004) found that among men born around 1920, prolonged cigarette smoking from early adult life tripled age-specific mortality rates, but cessation at the age of 50 halved the hazard, while cessation at the age of 30 avoided almost all of it. The families of smokers are also vulnerable to the effects of passive smoking, rates of cot death, acute and respiratory disease being higher among children whose parents smoke, while the non-smoking partners of smokers and those exposed to high levels of smoke in other settings are at increased risk of lung cancer, CHD, chronic respiratory disease and asthma (Crofton and Simpson, 2002; Whincup et al, 2004). In the UK, an estimated £410 million a year is spent treating childhood illness related to passive smoking. In adults, passive smoking accounts for at least 1,000 deaths in non-smokers, at an estimated cost of about £12.3 million a year at 2002 prices (Parrott and Godfrey, 2004).

As noted in Chapter Eight, most smokers start in their teenage years, and rates of smoking among both men and women are highest among young people. In 2002/03, the proportion of adults who smoked was greatest among those aged 20-24 (37% of men and 38% of women). It then steadily declined with increasing age to 17% of men and 14% of women aged 60 and over (data derived from the Office for National Statistics [ONS]). In contrast to young people where, due to its higher prevalence, smoking is not so strongly associated with social disadvantage, there is a strong social gradient in rates of current smoking among adults. In 2001, 34% of those whose household reference person was in a routine occupation smoked, compared with only 15% of those in higher professional and higher managerial households (ONS and DH, 2003). The main reason for this growing social divide with age is that people from poorer, more disadvantaged social groups are less likely to quit than those from more advantaged groups.

A number of factors play a role in socio-economic differences in smoking cessation, including degree of dependence, social support, marital status and the proportion of smokers in the household (Chandola et al, 2004a). Level of nicotine dependence increases systematically with deprivation according to indicators such as time to first cigarette of the day, perceived difficulty of going the whole day without smoking, numbers of cigarettes smoked and intensity with which each cigarette is smoked (Jarvis and Wardle, 1999). Higher levels of dependence among people in the lowest social classes are already evident in youth. Young people who live in families where cigarette smoking is the norm and where cigarettes are readily available tend to be heavier smokers than those who live in families that voice opposition to smoking. With age, wider social networks relating to work and neighbourhood join family influences in shaping the extent to which smoking is socially sanctioned (Stead et al, 2001). Again, the social environments of the poor and disadvantaged are more likely to tolerate or encourage smoking than challenge the habit. This has important implications for smoking cessation. Notwithstanding knowledge levels about the harmful effects of cigarette smoking or indeed level of dependence, when one's partner, friends and working colleagues all smoke, it is very hard to quit.

As well as belonging to social networks in which smoking is a culturally ingrained behaviour, a perceived lack of social support can make it difficult for people to give up smoking. This may be as much a reflection of the personal and material circumstances of people's lives as an objective lack of social contact and support. For example, in Hilary Graham's study of smoking among working-class mothers (Graham, 1993), there was not a strong association between smoking status and access to family and friendship networks (although smokers did appear to be less well-integrated in the neighbourhoods in which their lived). However, smoking was strongly associated with additional caring responsibilities (caring alone, caring for more children and for children in poorer health) and disadvantaged material circumstances. Smokers were more likely to report periods of feeling alone and isolated and to describe their habit as a way of structuring time for themselves and keeping going under stress. Subsequent studies confirm that, for women living in disadvantaged circumstances who are experiencing anxiety and stress, smoking may be perceived as an important coping mechanism (Tod, 2003). Such research suggests that efforts to promote smoking cessation cannot target nicotine dependence alone, but should also address the wider social, cultural and psychological aspects of smoking (Copeland, 2003).

Diet and nutrition

After smoking, diet and nutrition are often identified as a key area for action in reducing adult chronic disease. In 1986-87, the prevalence of obesity among males and females aged 16-64 was 7% and 12% respectively. By 2002, 22% of men and women had a Body Mass Index (BMI) above 30 (www.heartstats.org). Obesity has been identified as an independent risk factor for premature death and is strongly associated with a range of other conditions which are themselves risk factors for chronic disease, notably hyperlipidaemia, hypertension and insulin resistance (Jebb, 2002). The rise in overweight and obesity has thus been of particular concern. Diets lacking in particular nutrients may also increase risk for disease. For example, evidence suggests an inverse association between intake of antioxidant nutrients, carotenoids, folates and other substances found in fruits and vegetables and risk of cancers (Johnson, 2002). Diets rich in fruit and vegetables have also been implicated in the promotion of skeletal health (in which calcium also plays a role) and, although evidence is mixed, there is research interest in the role played by dietary polyphenols (for example, found in wine, red onions and black tea) in reducing risk of cardiovascular disease (New, 2002; Williamson, 2002).

As noted in Chapter Eight, dietary patterns in childhood are subject to significant social gradients. These continue into adulthood where lower social status has been associated with low fruit and vegetable consumption (Billson et al, 1999; Pollard et al, 2001), high saturated fat intake (Boniface and Tefft, 2002) and low intake of wholegrain foods (Lang et al, 2003). Socio-economic trends in obesity are less clear-cut. Obesity in women has consistently been associated with lower social class. In the 1998 Health Survey for England (HSE), 31% of women aged 16+ in Social Class V were obese, compared with 15% of women in Social Class I. Among men, by contrast, obesity is not as strongly associated with social class, affecting 20% of men in Social Class V in 1998, compared with 12% in Social Class I.

According to the 2000/01 National Diet and Nutrition Survey (NDNS) of adults aged 19-64, BMI in men and women is significantly associated with a range of dietary factors, including percentage total energy intake from protein, carbohydrates and sugars and reported dieting (Rushton et al, 2004), suggesting that the current rise in obesity and its adverse health consequences reflect behavioural choices. Finding higher levels of weight concern and dieting among higher socio-economic groups, Wardle and Griffith (2001) propose that deliberate efforts at weight control do form part of the protection against weight gain. However, a growing body of work suggests that differences in BMI by social class cannot be attributed to lifestyle alone, but are formed at least partly during childhood. Predictors of adult obesity include a high maternal BMI before pregnancy, low growth in utero and during infancy and a high BMI during adolescence (Hardy et al, 2000; Laitinen et al, 2001; Erikkson et al, 2003). Rapid childhood growth has also been associated with an increased risk of adult obesity, although findings are mixed, some studies suggesting that low growth and/or thinness during childhood is a predictor of later obesity (Wright et al, 2001; Kuh et al, 2002b).

Evidence of the role played by early life factors to the pathogenesis of adult obesity casts doubt on the validity of a simple adult lifestyle account of obesity and its health risks. However, the fact that intergenerational mobility has the potential to reverse the effects of early disadvantage on obesity (Langenberg et al, 2003) is suggestive of an accumulation rather than a latency model. The mechanisms linking obesity to adverse health outcomes also appear to operate over the lifecourse rather than during adulthood alone. For example, evidence suggests that overweight in adolescence increases adult cardiovascular mortality and morbidity independently of adult BMI (Reilly et al, 2003; Campbell et al, 2004; Hardy et al, 2004). Such findings suggest the possibility of reducing adult obesity and its health risks by developing interventions that target women of child-bearing age, pregnant women, infants, children and adolescents. Many authors nevertheless agree that nutritional intervention in adulthood remains an effective means of reducing individual and population risk for chronic disease (see Chapter Eleven). In addition to supporting weight control, this can increase intake of nutrients that, as noted earlier, are protective against chronic disease.

Physical activity

As we discussed in Chapter Eight, the relationship between obesity and adverse health outcomes also appears to be mediated by other factors such as level of physical activity, obese men who are moderately fit having a lower death rate than men who have a healthy weight but who are unfit. Rates of physical activity among adults vary significantly according to socio-economic status (Bartley et al, 2000). According to the 2002 General Household Survey (GHS), only 30% of those aged 16+ whose household reference person was in a routine occupation had participated in at least one sport, game or physical activity (excluding walking) in the past four weeks, compared with 59% of those in higher professional and managerial households. Including walking, respective rates of participation in physical activity were 44% and 75%. The social gradient in physical activity was more pronounced for women than men, standardised ratios for female participation in at least one sport, game or physical activity ranging from 76 in the routine occupational group to 131 in the higher professional and managerial group. For men, the equivalent standardised ratios were 82 and 117 (data derived from the ONS). As physical activity in adults has been shown to positively affect cardiovascular risk factors, this is another aspect of adult lifestyle that provides an appropriate focus for intervention.

Substance misuse

Most research on the role of adult lifestyle in risk for chronic disease has focused on diet, smoking and physical activity. Other lifestyle factors that can present serious risks to health include alcohol and drug misuse, although this remains a relatively minor cause of mortality. In 2000, 5,543 deaths in England and Wales were classified as alcohol-related deaths (more than double the number in 1979). A marked rise in alcohol-related deaths in younger age groups has been noted. This is likely to reflect increased alcohol consumption and changing consumption patterns such as binge drinking. Hepatitis C infection, associated with intravenous drug use between the late 1960s and early 1980s, may also be contributing to increased numbers of deaths by cirrhosis in those now aged 40-60 (Baker and Rooney, 2003).

Despite evidence of the growing normalisation of illicit drug use (see Chapter Eight), total numbers of drug-related deaths also remain small. In 2001, 1,623 deaths were categorised as deaths caused by 'drug misuse' (deaths where the underlying cause was poisoning, drug abuse or drug dependence and where any of the substances controlled under the 1971 Misuse of Drugs Act were involved). Around 49% of male deaths related to drug misuse had an underlying cause of mental and behavioural disorders and 37% involved suicide. In women, by contrast, suicide formed the largest proportion of deaths related to drug misuse (65%) (Griffiths, 2003). Heroin, morphine and methodone are responsible for the majority of deaths related to drug misuse. The highest mortality rates from these substances occur in the North West, Yorkshire and the Humber, and in local authorities that are located in some of the largest urban areas and in a few coastal and regional centres. Common characteristics of such authorities include a high proportion of unemployed people, those living in either social or terraced housing and a high proportion of the population in partially skilled and unskilled manual occupations. This is consistent with other findings that deaths related to drug misuse are more common among unemployed and deprived people (Uren, 2001).

Explaining socio-economic variation in lifestyle factors

While there is general agreement that behavioural risk factors during adulthood play a significant role in the production of health inequalities, care should be taken to ensure that efforts to encourage more healthy lifestyles take full account of the factors that give rise to socio-economic differences in health behaviours. At present, these are poorly understood (Wardle and Steptoe, 2003). In the 1970s and 1980s, studies showed that social differences in health behaviours did not reflect differences in knowledge. Although the lack of correlation between knowledge and behaviour has since been questioned (Wardle et al, 2000), such findings reinforced the belief held by those to the right of the political spectrum that health-related behaviour was a matter of individual choice. The resulting policy focus on changing individual behaviour led many to propose that poorer people were effectively being blamed for their adverse health outcomes and that, rather than being viewed as the cause of health inequalities, socio-economic differences in health behaviours should themselves be seen as an outcome of differences in material circumstances.

One response to the critique of individualistic explanations of health inequalities has been to explore the role of direct material constraints on the choices of those living in poor environments. Several authors propose that economic constraints contribute to the unhealthy food choices observed among low socio-economic groups in industrialised countries, as diets based on refined grains, added sugars and added fats are more affordable than the recommended diets based on lean meats, fish, fresh vegetables and fruit (Darmon et al, 2003, 2004; French, 2003; Drewnowski, 2004). Current UK policy is influenced by the belief that low-income groups have difficulties regarding the access and affordability of fruits and vegetables. However, others caution against attributing unhealthy diets to a simple lack of money (Dibsdall et al, 2003; Robinson et al, 2004).

Recent research questions whether absolute poverty is the main barrier to promoting healthier lifestyles or whether psychosocial factors associated with poverty are more significant. Although many people are aware of the health-damaging effects of smoking, unhealthy diets and a lack of physical exercise, an orientation towards thinking about the present may make them unwilling to change their behaviours in order to prevent future disease (Dibsdall et al, 2003). Drawing on the Omnibus Survey of the ONS, future salience and frequently thinking about things to do to stay healthy were found to be independently related to the likelihood of carrying out healthy behaviours. Both factors were associated with socio-economic status, nearly half of respondents in semi-skilled and unskilled classes stating that they did not think about either the short-term or long-term future very often compared to only a third of those in Social Classes I and II. Those who expressed a strong belief in the role of chance on health were also more likely to smoke, have sedentary lifestyles and diets low in fruit and vegetables, regardless of their sense of personal control. Again, 'chance locus of control' was characterised by a social gradient, suggesting that one of the factors mediating socio-economic differences in healthy lifestyles may be a tendency to trust in luck (Wardle and Steptoe, 2003). This should not be interpreted as a reflection of fecklessness among the poor. It may be a rational response to the fact that, because the health of poorer people is overwhelmed by factors beyond their control, they have less to gain from healthy choices than people in good social circumstances who believe, quite correctly, that they can improve their health by healthy living (Blaxter, 1990). Against this background, it is important to understand the factors that constrain individual behaviour and produce health risks above and beyond those associated with personal lifestyle. Research suggests that these relate to both the psychosocial environment and material deprivation.

Health inequalities and the psychosocial environment

As noted in Chapter Two, the academic debate on the relationship between income inequality and population health has become "something of a minefield" (Whitehead and Diderichsen, 2001, p 165). However, certain aspects of the psychosocial hypothesis are widely accepted. At an individual level, there is good evidence to suggest that social participation, supportive social networks and a positive sense of well-being are protective of health. Psychosocial factors also offer a possible explanation for contextual or neighbourhood effects, evidence for which is consistent if modest. The significance of such factors to health inequalities lies in the suggestion that, at both individual and neighbourhood levels, poorer people are more likely to live in unhealthy social environments than affluent people.

Individual-level evidence

At the individual level, psychosocial processes may mediate the relationship between low socio-economic status and poor mental and physical health by influencing health-related behaviours (see earlier discussion on health and lifestyle), and producing acute or chronic patho-physiological changes. Here it is argued that people of low socio-economic status have lower levels of perceived mastery and control than individuals of higher socio-economic status, and are more likely to experience feelings of hopelessness, hostility and low self-esteem. These factors can in turn elicit a "cascade of cognitive, affective and biological responses" (Adler and Snibbe, 2003, p 121), psychosocial stress increasing risk for depression and anxiety which, as well as being well-defined psychiatric disorders in their own right, may mediate the relationship between socio-economic status and cardiovascular disease. As discussed in Chapter Two, neuroendocrine reactivity has been identified as an important mechanism here, raised levels of hormones such as cortisol, epinephrine and norepinephrine producing immediate effects such as increased heart rate and blood vessel constriction as well as long-term metabolic effects relating to cholesterol levels, central obesity and risk for CHD.

Systematic reviews suggest that evidence for an independent causal association between depression and CHD is strong and consistent, pertaining to both men and women and to various age groups (Hemingway and Marmot, 1999; Bunker et al, 2003). Risk for CHD appears to be directly related to the severity of depression, Bunker et al (2003) reporting that minor depression results in a one- to twofold increase in CHD and major depression a three- to fivefold increase, increased risks of a similar order to those produced by more conventional CHD risk factors such as smoking. Depression in patients after myocardial infarction also seems to be of prognostic importance. Evidence of a causal association between anxiety and CHD is more mixed, some studies suggesting that acute anxiety is predictive of sudden cardiac death while others produce null findings. And no clear association has been identified between hostility (including type A behaviour) and CHD. Indeed, some evidence suggests that hostility may offer a protective effect with respect to prognosis. Other psychosocial factors that have been examined in relation to risk for CHD include social network structure and quality of social support and work-related 'stressors'. The number of a person's social contacts and the support that they provide both appear to play an important role in both the onset of CHD and its prognosis, an association that exists for men and women and various age groups (Bunker et al, 2003). Evidence for a relationship between work characteristics (including job control, demands and strain) and CHD is more mixed, although this may reflect a need to further clarify the particular components of work-related stress that might be of aetiological importance. As unemployment and low-quality employment have been implicated in risk for a range of health outcomes (the relationship between work and health is discussed later in this chapter), this remains an area of intense research interest.

It is important to point out that much of the research that has taken place around the association between socio-economic status and psychosocial well-being has focused on white middle-aged men. Yet, this association is likely to vary according to ethnicity and gender due to factors such as discrimination and gender roles. For example, psychosocial domestic conditions (reflected by both the level of household and family demands and the resources available to help cope with these demands) may have a greater effect on the health of women compared with men (Chandola et al, 2004b). By contrast, data from the 1958 British birth cohort study suggests that work factors have a greater impact on socio-economic differences in psychological distress in men than women (Matthews et al, 2001). Work characteristics were also important for inequalities in depressive symptoms in men in the Whitehall II Study, while a combination of work and material disadvantage predicted depressive symptoms in women (Stansfeld et al, 2003). Analysis of the British Household Panel Survey (BHPS) showed that transitions from paid employment to either unemployment or long-term sick leave were associated with increased psychological distress for both men and women (Thomas et al, 2005). Gender differences in the role played by work-related factors thus appear to vary between cohorts. This is to be expected since gender roles, the significance accorded to work and potential conflicts between home and work vary according to socio-economic status and social norms and are highly context specific (Chandola et al, 2004c).

The impact of exposure to psychosocial stressors also varies across the lifecourse, although the extent to which childhood adversity contributes to adult psychological well-being by setting psychological tendencies (a latency model), chains of risk (a pathway model) or contributing as part of an accumulation of exposure is not fully understood. Power et al (2002) report that both childhood and adult life factors contribute to the development of inequalities in psychological distress and suggest an accumulation model. In this study, which used data from the 1958 British birth cohort, the principal childhood factors were ability at age seven (for both sexes) and adverse environment (institutional care for men and low class for women). Adult life factors varied, with stronger effects for work factors (job strain and insecurity) for men and qualifications on leaving school, early child-bearing and financial hardship for women. Lifecourse effects may also vary according to psychosocial outcome. For example, a study of Finnish men found that while adult socio-economic position was associated with all measures of psychosocial functioning under investigation, childhood socio-economic position was associated with cynical hostility and hopelessness in adulthood, but not depression (Harper et al, 2002).

While there remain some uncertainties about the role that psychosocial pathways play in the production and maintenance of health inequalities, there is no doubt that, when psychosocial well-being is treated as a health *outcome*, the scale of the problem is considerable. According to the 2000 British National Survey of Psychiatric Morbidity, one in six adults aged 16-74 years has a neurotic disorder such as anxiety, depression or phobias (ONS, 2001). Over a quarter of those interviewed reported hazardous drinking patterns (38% of men and 15% of women), with 7% showing symptoms of alcohol dependence. Prevalence of neurotic disorder is associated with socio-economic status, significantly higher levels being found among those living in rented accommodation and with no access to a car. However, risk for depression and anxiety does not appear to vary according to level of educational attainment (Lewis et al, 2003). Similarly, analysis of the BHPS found that education had no significant impact on self-reported mental health status (Andres, 2004). Because unemployment not only results in financial insecurity but also loss of status, identity, regular activity and social contacts, it emerges as a significant risk factor for low levels of psychological well-being (Montgomery et al, 1999; Andres, 2004). According to the Social Exclusion Unit of the Office of the Deputy Prime Minister, over 900,000 adults in Britain claiming Incapacity Benefit or Severe Disablement Allowance report mental health problems as their primary condition, with particularly high claimant rates in the North (ODPM, 2004). The proportion of those whose mental health problems preceded or succeeded unemployment is unknown. Lower socio-economic status and unemployment also predict prognosis for those with mental health problems.

Evidence suggests that merely having a job does not protect against negative psychological consequences. Quality of work is important. Key measures of the 'psychosocial work environment' include high psychological job demands, low job control, low reward, high strain, passive work and lack of social support (Marmot et al, 1999; Siegrist and Marmot, 2004). As noted already, research findings linking work characteristics and health outcomes are mixed, some studies yielding null or weak results (for example, Jonsson et al, 1999; Rosvall et al, 2002; Pelfrene et al, 2003; Lallukka et al, 2004), while others find that poor quality of work is positively associated with health-damaging behaviours, sickness absence, poor self-rated health, cardiovascular risk factors, depression and anxiety (North et al, 1996; Bosma et al, 1997; Niedhammer et al, 1998; Vahtera et al, 2000; d'Souza et al, 2003; Gimeno et al, 2004). According to the Social Exclusion Unit, in 2001-02 around half a million people in Britain thought that work-related stress was making them ill. However, the highest levels of stress were not reported by the lowest status workers but by teachers, nurses and managers (ODPM, 2004).

Area-level effects

As we discussed in Chapter Two, the idea that the social and physical environment in which people live has an effect on their health status over and above that produced by individual characteristics emerged as an important research theme in the 1990s. Psychosocial processes are believed to play some part in the creation of area-level effects on individual health because deprived areas are more likely than areas inhabited by socially advantaged people to have higher levels of noise, toxins and pathogens; more social conflict, crowding and crime; less access to recreational facilities, healthy foods and other means of restoring and maintaining health; and less social support – all factors that can contribute to increased levels of stress (Macintyre et al, 1993; Easterlow et al, 2000; Adler and Snibbe, 2003).

Evidence suggests that residents in deprived areas are significantly more likely to identify problems with their neighbourhood. According to the 2001 English Housing Condition Survey, 60% of households living in poor, predominantly council-built areas regarded litter and rubbish as a problem or a serious problem. Half similarly regarded fear of burglary, as did 44% concerning the general level of crime, vandalism and hooliganism and troublesome teenagers/children (ODPM, 2003). Perceptions of crime and fear of crime are not always related to absolute levels of criminal activity. However, Home Office data suggest that more serious antisocial behaviour problems are indeed more prevalent in the most deprived areas. A number of factors are at work. As discussed in Chapter Eight, children from socially disadvantaged families are at higher risk of developing conduct disorders and this risk may be exacerbated by neighbourhood factors (such as the built environment of high-rise housing estates). The prevalence of problem drinking also increases in the lowest socio-economic group and alcohol is a significant contributory factor in crimes that involve damage to property and violence to others.

There is little systematic evidence linking fear of crime and health (Green et al, 2002). However, it is plausible to suggest that fear results in stress and is thus part of a psychosocial pathway that links socio-economic circumstances to health outcomes. At a practical level, fear of crime also restricts mobility and reduces opportunities for health-promoting activities such as social and community involvement and use of services (Whitley and Prince, 2005). Several studies suggest that fear of crime is significantly associated with social and mental well-being. However, its impact may be more pronounced for certain subgroups such as low-income mothers and people with mental ill health (Whitley and Prince, 2005).

In some areas, psychosocial stressors associated with area-level factors are intensified by what becomes a self-reinforcing cycle of neighbourhood decline. The most run-down and neglected neighbourhoods with the highest levels of graffiti, litter, vandalism and crime are not surprisingly the most unpopular. Population turnover rates are higher (further undermining the development of social cohesion). However, choices to move are very limited for owner-occupiers who, due to falling house prices, may be trapped and for council tenants in London and the South where choices to move are limited (DETR, 1999). Due to low demand, such areas may be used disproportionately in allocation policies to rehouse deprived families, the concentration of which has been linked to localised pockets of antisocial behaviour (NSNR, 2000). All of these factors can contribute to a high sense of dissatisfaction in areas of high deprivation. According to a household survey carried out in 12 of the country's most unpopular (low demand) local areas, 34% were dissatisfied with their neighbourhood (rising to 55% in Salford and 80% in Burnley); 39% of respondents had been victims of crime and the same percentage felt unsafe walking out alone after dark; 41% said that there was not a strong sense of community; 38% wanted to move out of their present home. One of the general features of the resident populations of these unpopular areas was that they were relatively poor. Only a third of all adults were working and two thirds of renters received Housing Benefit (DETR, 1999).

Health inequalities and material deprivation

Despite widespread support among health inequalities researchers for the role played by material deprivation in health inequalities, epidemiological studies suggest that, individually, factors such as unemployment and poor housing make modest contributions to the total socio-economic gradient in health. However, care should be taken in assuming that material deprivation no longer plays a role in the production of health inequalities in British society. According to the accumulation model, the significance of this factor lies in the way in which different aspects of disadvantage cluster over time and place. Shaw et al (1999, p 102) suggest that the cumulative experience of advantage and disadvantage gives rise to a social structure that is finely graded with respect to socio-economic differentials. Thus, the material explanation of health inequalities lends itself as well to observations of the stepwise gradient in health outcomes as the psychosocial hypothesis.

Work and health

Work impinges on health status in a number of ways, from the direct effects of occupational exposures to more indirect effects via psychosocial pathways. Certain occupations (for example, coal mining and agricultural work) have traditionally been associated with an increased risk of injury and particular diseases. Due to changes in employment patterns such as the decline in manufacturing industries and the strengthening of policies relating to occupational health and safety, such health hazards are no longer viewed as the main causes of ill health related to work (Marmot and Feeney, 1996). However, occupational road accidents remain a major but largely unrecognised source of work-related deaths and injuries (Blane, 1999).

If occupational health hazards are no longer a main cause of ill health, the lack of any occupation is a clear health risk factor. As noted earlier, unemployment is significantly associated with ill health as defined by subjectively rated health, experienced symptoms, illness measures and mortality. For example, among an initially healthy group of working-aged men and women in Britain who were followed up over a 10-year period, the risk of experiencing a limiting illness among unemployed people was over twice that of employed people and for those who had not been economically active in the previous year, the risks were even greater (Bartley et al, 2004a). Unemployed people also suffer a substantially increased risk of premature death. According to the 1997 *Decennial Supplement* (Drever and Whitehead, 1997), men and women who were unemployed in 1981 had excess mortality of about 33% over the period 1981-92. Neither pre-existing ill health, nor social class, nor marital status (for women) could account for this raised mortality suggesting that, although selection may play a role in the link between unemployment and poor health (ill health increasing the likelihood of unemployment), unemployment is itself a cause of a worsening of health status (Bethune, 1997; Korpi, 2001).

There are important gender differences in the relation between employment status and ill health (Stronks et al, 1995). Among registered unemployed women and men, the risk factors linking unemployment to ill health appear to be similar (Leeflang et al, 1992). However, although the labour market position of women has undergone significant change since the 1970s, paid employment (particularly full-time employment) is still not universal for women in Britain. Married British women are often dependent on male breadwinners, and many lone women are dependent on poverty-level social benefits. This shapes the relative role played by one's own and one's partner's socio-economic status in the health of men and women.

The occupational status of female partners does not appear to strongly affect health and health risk factors among men. By contrast, a partner's occupational status is a significant determinant of women's health (Arber and Lahelma, 1993; Arber, 1996; Lahelma et al, 2000; Bartley et al, 2004b). This may in part reflect the relationship between a partner's employment status, material living conditions and financial insecurity, men's unemployment having particularly adverse consequences for the health of their wives. The power relations associated with different family roles may also be significant to the fact that behavioural risk factors among women are independently related to a partner's socio-economic position (Bartley et al, 2004b). Men are also affected by social roles at home, evidence from the Whitehall II Study suggesting that relatively high-grade male civil servants were at increased risk of anxiety and depression if they reported low control at home (Griffin et al, 2002).

Although much research has focused on the psychological consequences of unemployment, health effects have also been directly attributed to financial hardship. The 1980s and early 1990s saw a fall in the real value of both the lowest wages and benefits in the UK and an increasing gap between the incomes of the richest and poorest sections of society. This trend has been linked to the growth of health inequalities during the 1980s (assuming that factors during adulthood present significant risks to health). Since Labour came to power in 1997, several policies have been introduced that are directed at improving the incomes of the poor. Even so, in 2002-03, 17% of the population (and 21% of children) in Britain lived in low-income households before the deduction of housing costs.

After housing costs are deducted, rates of income poverty are around 7% and 11% higher (data derived from the ONS).

As discussed in Chapter Three, evidence suggests that a significant proportion of low-income families face real financial hardship as indicated by levels of indebtedness and reported difficulties affording food, clothing, consumer durables and leisure facilities. It is important to note that non-working families are not the only households to be affected (although they are particularly vulnerable). A significant proportion of British households comprise adults working for very low pay. According to the data drawn from the Labour Force Survey and Annual Survey of Hours and Earnings, in 2003 26% of men and 46% of women aged 22 and over earned less than £7 per hour, well below the Council of Europe's Decency Threshold of £7.57 (two thirds of average earnings). A total of 5% of adult men and 15% of adult women earned less than £5 per hour (data derived from the ONS). Such figures suggest that a key factor mediating the relationship between work and health could be poverty.

Housing and the environment

Even for adults in full-time employment, home is a key health locale and site of health-related behaviours. Interest in the public health consequences of substandard housing dates back to Victorian times, which saw the gradual introduction of state regulation concerning overcrowding, sanitation and basic housing standards. During the 20th century, substantial public resources were committed to directly providing a social housing sector. The quality of housing built under the first council housing programme 'homes fit for heroes' is generally acknowledged to have been high. In the 1950s and 1960s, the social housing sector became more focused on people displaced by slum clearance, in part through the development of high-rise blocks, and it is likely that the stigma of council housing stems from this period. Even so, a substantial proportion of the British population lived in social housing by the late 1970s.

With the privatisation of council housing (through the 'right to buy') in the 1980s, increasing rents in the council sector and a decline in the level of house building by local councils, the size of this sector shrunk from a peak of 32% of all housing in Britain in 1977 to 13% in 2001. As discussed in Chapter Three, council housing has acquired a residual role and council tenants have become more homogeneous, increasingly sharing characteristics associated with poverty. Against this background, it is hardly surprising that marked differences exist between the health status of social sector tenants and owner-occupiers. What is less clear is the extent to which these differences reflect other risk factors associated with low socio-economic status or can be directly attributed to differences in housing conditions between different sectors.

Accumulating evidence suggests that differences in housing quality play a role in the production of health inequalities according to tenure (Pollack et al, 2004).

The most deprived areas are characterised by greater concentrations of older, typically private sector rented housing and post-1945 social sector terraced and flatted accommodation. In 2001, for example, social rented dwellings comprised 40% of the stock in the most deprived 10% of English wards, compared to 5% in the least deprived 10% of wards. The social sector and, outside the South East, the private rented sector, are not only more likely to house poorer people, but the quality of their housing stock is poorer than that of the owner-occupied and registered social landlord (housing association) sectors. Setting a standard for 'decent homes' on the basis of state of repair, facilities and services, degree of thermal comfort and fitness for habitation, the 2001 English House Condition Survey found that 43% of local authority stock were 'non-decent', compared to 29% of owner-occupied dwellings and 28% of housing association homes. The highest proportion of non-decent dwellings was found in the private rented sector (49%), which had the highest failure rates on thermal comfort (40%), and was around twice as likely to fail on fitness (11%) and disrepair (17%) as any other sector. Some 42% of the poorest households were found to live in non-decent homes, groups identified as being particularly vulnerable by the 2001 English House Condition Survey, including people who live alone, minority ethnic groups and households with no one in full-time employment (ODPM, 2003).

Reviewing research on the relationship between housing and health, Dunn (2000) distinguishes between studies that propose that people who are already unhealthy are selected through public housing allocation policies into substandard housing conditions (for example, Smith, 1990; Robinson, 1998), and those that suggest that poor housing is a direct cause of poor physical and mental health. Regarding physical health, several studies examining evidence of a causal link between substandard housing and health inequalities have focused on the link between dampness and mould and ill health (Packer et al, 1994; Hopton and Hunt, 1996; Williamson et al, 1997). Exposure to moisture, a consequence of inadequate heating, insulation and ventilation, is in itself associated with increased risk of respiratory symptoms such as sore throat and nocturnal cough (Koskinen et al, 1999). In addition, condensation causes mould, fungi and other micro-organisms to grow. Many moulds in damp houses are allergenic and provide a food supply for house mites, which are also potential allergens (Wilkinson, 1999). Both have been linked to respiratory conditions, including asthma and common colds as well as allergic diseases such as allergic rhinitis and atopic dermatitis (Koskinen et al, 1999; Kilpelainen et al, 2001). However, some authors argue that home dampness and mould present only a small increased risk of respiratory symptoms (Peat et al, 1998).

In practice, it is difficult to distinguish the effects of dampness from those of cold housing on health as cold housing and damp housing tend to be closely related. Some evidence suggests that being unable to keep the home warm enough in winter is more strongly associated with health outcomes than damp housing

(Evans et al, 2000). This is supported to some extent by the results of a pilot intervention that, following the installation of central heating to damp houses occupied by children previously diagnosed with asthma, observed a significant reduction in respiratory symptoms (Somerville et al, 2000). Excess winter mortality among older people continues to be an important public health problem in Britain, risk of dying increasing with both a reduction in winter temperatures and a lack of central heating (Aylin et al, 2001; Healy, 2003). There is some evidence of an 'inverse housing law' in Britain, those areas where the climate is most severe tending to have the worst-quality housing (Blane et al, 2000). As those on low incomes are more likely to live in poorly constructed housing and are less able to afford to heat their homes adequately, risk of cold housing is particularly associated with poverty. Health effects also vary according to age, the very old and the very young being most vulnerable. Finally, it is not only cold temperatures that appear to affect health. Investigation of daily mortality counts in Greater London over a 21-year period found a linear relation between temperature and mortality above about 19°C. Again, older people are particularly vulnerable (Hajat et al, 2002).

Other aspects of the home environment that have been implicated in poor physical health include unsafe cooking and heating appliances, which can release harmful contaminants such as carbon monoxide, hydrocarbons and particulate matter; environmental radon, which has been linked to risk of lung cancer; inadequate ventilation, which is not only associated with the presence of mould, but with levels of air contaminants including environmental tobacco smoke; and potentially harmful building materials such as leaded paint, lead pipes, fibre board materials which can release formaldehyde, and textured ceilings which may contain asbestos. Stairways, stairwells and loose carpets have been associated with risk of accidents. Fires are also a major cause of mortality, particularly among poorer people who are more likely to smoke (Wilkinson, 1999; Howden-Chapman, 2004).

Wider neighbourhood conditions can also impact on physical health status. For example, living near to a major road has been associated with excess risk of stroke mortality due to exposure to road traffic pollution (Maheswaran and Elliott, 2003). Undertaking a systematic review of epidemiological papers examining the effects of ambient particulates, Mindell and Joffe (2004) suggest that there is moderate to strong evidence of a causal link between exposure and a range of health outcomes, including respiratory and circulatory disease at all ages, COPD and asthma in people aged 65+ and asthma in children and young adults. The authors conclude that at current UK levels, ambient particulates are causing adverse health effects in urban areas. A European study of 19 major cities similarly concluded that current levels of air pollution have a non-negligible effect on public health, although overall levels of particulates in Western Europe were found to be lower than in the Eastern European and Mediterranean cities in the study (Medina et al, 2004). It is important to note, however, that the validity of ambient monitoring data as a reflection of actual personal exposure varies according to the air pollutant in question. Such data are good surrogates for daily fine particle exposures but less so for gaseous traffic-related pollutants such as nitrogen dioxide and carbon monoxide that show small-area spatial variation. Thus, city-level data do not reflect the extent to which air pollution exposure is differentially distributed according to socio-economic status (O'Neill et al, 2003).

Many studies suggest that, due to housing market dynamics, poor and minority ethnic neighbourhoods are more likely to be located near to dense traffic and noxious industrial facilities than wealthy neighbourhoods. Lower socio-economic status may also affect susceptibility to air pollution through co-exposure to other pollutants in the home and at work (increasing the overall dose of pollutants) or through its association with predisposing health conditions and behaviours. Diabetes and smoking-related lung conditions appear to increase people's vulnerability to air pollution. For example, deposition of particles is relatively higher among people who have COPD. If both exposures and susceptibilities vary across socio-economic gradients, air pollution may play a more significant role in the production of health inequalities than has previously been acknowledged (O'Neill et al, 2003).

In addition to physical health outcomes, poor housing can impact on mental health in a number of ways. A range of housing conditions including noise, overcrowding and disrepair has been linked to increased levels of stress (Smith et al, 1993). High-rise housing can present problems for older people and women carrying shopping and small children, and make it more difficult for parents to supervise their children playing outside (Howden-Chapman, 2004). Dunn (2002) suggests that consideration be given to the notion of metaphorical homelessness in terms of rootlessness, proposing that control, autonomy and social support are as important in the home environment as the workplace. Insofar as the meaning of home is an accepted psychological and social construct, it is intuitive to suggest a relationship between housing, health and well-being, and this has been empirically supported by a number of studies (Weich et al, 2002; Macintyre et al, 2003; Pollack et al, 2004).

Although housing has been a relatively neglected area in health inequalities research, the strong relationship between homelessness and health is widely accepted. This relationship reflects health selection and the direct pathological effects of homelessness and affects both those living in temporary accommodation and rough sleepers. For example, the effects of health selection are reflected by the fact that those in poor health are more likely to be unemployed and less likely to be able to afford housing, increasing the risks of homelessness (Wilkinson, 1999). People with mental health problems are at particularly high risk of becoming homeless. The Social Exclusion Unit estimates that 30% to 50% of people sleeping rough suffer from mental health problems, which, for about 88%, existed before they went on the street (SEU, 1998).

Poor health can cause homelessness. However, homelessness tends in turn to exacerbate existing risks to poor health. Around 50% of people sleeping rough are heavy drinkers and 20% are drug addicts (SEU, 1998). Problems of substance misuse often precede homelessness but tend to become more pronounced with the stresses of sleeping rough. Substance misuse is associated with a range of physical problems including cirrhosis, overdoses and accidents. Injecting drug use also brings problems such as abscesses, infected injecting sites, risk of hepatitis and HIV infection through shared needles. Finally, homelessness can independently cause ill health through the difficulties of maintaining hygiene, obtaining an adequate diet and through promoting psychological distress and depression. Lack of security, together with the high level of stigma and discrimination experienced by this group, increases the risk of violent attack and rape. Physical health problems such as respiratory diseases (including tuberculosis), musculoskeletal problems (particularly relating to feet), dermatological disorders, including infestations, digestive problems and neurological disorders are also common among the homeless (RCP, 1994). As a result, rough sleepers aged between 45 and 64 have a death rate 25 times that of the general population (www.mungos.org).

Not all homeless people are, of course, living on the street. While numbers of rough sleepers have gradually declined since 1997, the number of homeless households living in temporary accommodation in England more than doubled, reaching 100,000 in 2004. Problems facing these families, many of which comprise children, include the psychological distress of insecurity; social isolation and lack of social support; stigmatisation; and educational disruption and disadvantage. People who are living in temporary accommodation are more likely to suffer from poor physical, mental and emotional health than the general population. For instance, they have a higher incidence of infection, illness and accidents and are more likely to attend hospital Accident and Emergency Departments (ODPM, 2005).

Access to health services

In contrast to the substantial body of research investigating the role of socio-economic position in producing variations in health *status*, relatively little work has been undertaken into inequalities in health *care*. Research highlighting the role of factors such as early life programming and events throughout the lifecourse in determining health variations has perhaps fostered the belief that direct medical intervention has had a limited part to play in what is essentially a public health issue. Societal factors remain the key determinant of disease incidence. However, the perception that access to healthcare makes only a minor contribution to health variations has been challenged by the burgeoning literature on evidence-based medicine that demonstrates significant improvements in disease incidence, quality of life and mortality following the use of particular treatments or procedures. In response, policy statements have again begun to emphasise the importance of ensuring equitable access to the National Health Service (NHS).

Despite growing support for the concept of healthcare equity, evidence of inequalities in the accessibility and use of NHS services has been and remains equivocal. While early studies suggested that there was a 'pro-rich' bias in healthcare provision (Tudor Hart, 1971; West and Lowe, 1976), Powell (1990) found little evidence to support claims that the NHS exhibits the inverse care law. Reports that poorer social groups had lower than predicted rates of utilisation (Townsend and Davidson, 1982; Blaxter, 1984) have also been challenged by evidence that suggests that poorer people receive as much if not more healthcare than richer people for equal need (Haynes, 1991; O'Donnell and Propper, 1991; Whitehead et al, 1997; van Doorslaer et al, 2000).

The fact that little is known about inequalities in the use of NHS services owes much to the methodological difficulties of establishing expected levels of health service need against which actual use can be compared. With the notable exception of studies based on individual data (Morrison et al, 1997; Payne and Saul, 1997), most attempts to develop indices of health need have involved the use of proxy measures. The most commonly used proxies for health service need are mortality (Ben-Shlomo and Chaturvedi, 1995; Black et al, 1995; Pain et al, 1996; Manson-Siddle and Robinson, 1998; Oliver and Thomson, 1999); socio-economic status (Carstairs and Morris, 1989; Pringle and Morton-Jones, 1994; Packham et al, 1999); and, for the study of particular procedures, admission rates (MacLoed et al, 1999; Hippisley-Cox and Pringle, 2000).

All of these have their merits and limitations (Gibson et al, 2002). Because mortality statistics fail to reflect the full extent of non-fatal morbidity, doubts remain as to their use as a measure of general health service need. Cause-specific mortality may be a valid proxy for morbidity where case fatality is high (Pickin and St Leger, 1993, p 27). However, statistical validity will be reduced as the clinical management of a disease becomes more effective (Curtis and Taket, 1996, p 47). The use of mortality as a need indicator is also complicated by the fact that survival rates for conditions such as cardiovascular disease and cancer exhibit statistically significant differences between the most and least affluent patients, the latter tending to experience more negative outcomes. While this may reflect poorer access and use of health services, factors unrelated to health service use may also determine survival outcomes. Care should therefore be taken in using mortality statistics that are weighted towards deprived groups as a simple indicator of health service need.

As noted in Chapter One, profound social gradients have been observed in the prevalence of a wide range of diseases. This has led to the suggestion that deprivation may act as a valid proxy for health service need. However, it cannot necessarily be assumed that strong social gradients in disease prevalence mean that, overall, populations in deprived *areas* have higher health service needs. Many conditions, although clearly exhibiting significant social gradients, are dominated by an underlying demographic gradient. As a result, a reliance on social status alone as a surrogate for poor health is likely to overestimate levels of poor morbidity in lower-status populations and, conversely, make underestimates for more elderly populations (Asthana et al, 2004a). This makes the simple comparison by deprivation scores against crude intervention rates, as in the influential 1998 Acheson Report (Acheson, 1998, p 113), highly problematic.

A third approach widely adopted in estimating health needs has been to draw on health service statistics. For example, cause-specific admission rates are sometimes used as a baseline against which to compare the subsequent use of particular procedures (MacLoed et al, 1999; Hippisley-Cox and Pringle, 2000). This is only valid if all patients with a given level of morbidity access health services to a uniform extent. If, as some evidence suggests, deprived groups are more likely to be admitted to hospital in the first place (Black et al, 1995; Majeed et al, 2000), differences between socio-economic groups in the uptake of hospital procedures relative to admission rates may reflect subsequent clinical evaluation rather than discriminatory clinical practice.

In view of the foregoing critiques, it is hardly surprising that Le Grand's conclusion that the jury is still out on the question of whether the NHS is characterised by inequalities in access and utilisation (Le Grand, 1991) still holds true today. For example, primary care utilisation does not appear to be characterised by a consistent socio-economic gradient. Yet, income effects in general practitioner (GP) consulting behaviour have been detected between different gender and age groups and the direction of these varies between demographic categories (Evandrou et al, 1992). This means that significant but opposing trends may be cancelled out when age and sex are aggregated across income groups. Similarly, aggregate utilisation of inpatient and outpatient care controlling for self-reported health status appears to favour the lowest income groups (O'Donnell and Propper, 1991). However, some studies of *specific* conditions and procedures suggest that there are marked inequalities in rates of utilisation according to need (for example, Payne and Saul, 1997). Particularly strong claims have been made for systematic inequalities in access to investigation and treatment for specialist cardiac services and socio-economic inequity in survival after cancer treatment (Goddard and Smith, 1998, cited by Jacobson, 1999).

The most recent research on inequalities in health service use also yields conflicting results. Using individual-level data from successive rounds of the HSE, Morris et al (2005) conclude that lower-income individuals and minority ethnic groups are more likely to consult their GP but less likely to receive secondary care. However, Gibson et al (2002), who use the HSE to derive community-level prevalence rates, found that relative to estimated need, deprived populations made *greater* use of inpatient cardiology services. It is important to emphasise that this does not necessarily reflect the equity orientation of the NHS. While previous studies of inverse care have interpreted lower rates of hospital use as evidence of poor access, it does not follow that higher rates are 'a good thing'. The fact that deprived groups may be accessing inpatient cardiac services to a greater extent than predicted could reflect a failure of primary and community management. This would be consistent with long-standing concerns about the *quality* of primary care services in deprived areas and particularly in inner London (Benzeval et al, 1995).

In summary, although claims that the accessibility and use of NHS services are subject to an 'inverse care effect' (Tudor Hart, 1971) have become received wisdom, research evidence that demonstrates systematic inequities in relation to deprivation is equivocal. The strongest evidence has come from primary care, where concerns have been expressed about the higher proportion of single-handed GPs, the lack of availability of GPs out of hours, the poor quality of GP premises in areas of high deprivation and the relatively low uptake of preventive services (for example, cancer screening programmes, health promotion and immunisation) in the poorest communities (Benzeval et al, 1995; Goddard and Smith, 1998). Against this, practice-level variations in referral patterns and prescribing do not appear to be related to differences in the social class composition of patient populations (Coulter, 1992; Wilkin, 1992; Gibson et al, 2002).

As already noted, claims that the utilisation of hospital care is subject to systematic bias against poor people have been challenged with evidence that, if anything, deprived groups are accessing inpatient services at a higher rate than implied by morbidity alone. As NHS resources are allocated in a way that reflects utilisation, this raises questions about which demographic and socio-economic groups are receiving less than their fair share. Some evidence suggests that, far from suffering from systematic inequalities, urban deprived populations receive resources for hospital and community services over and above levels of underlying morbidity. As it is debatable whether *hospital* resources have much to contribute towards the reduction of health inequalities compared to other sources of variation such as income distribution, housing, education and lifestyle, the extent to which this policy addresses the goals of health equity is in some doubt. At the same time, the targeting of resources to urban deprived areas introduces a new form of inequity by underestimating the needs of more elderly but less deprived populations (Asthana et al, 2003, 2004b), a possibility that we examine further in Chapter Twelve.

The policy implications

Adulthood is a highly significant period in the lifecourse with respect to the *manifestation* of health inequalities, those in lower socio-economic groupings being more at risk of premature death and disease than their more affluent counterparts. Recognition of this burden of premature disease together with the development of evidence in the postwar period linking smoking, poor diet and so on with cancers and heart disease, meant that for much of the 20th century, risk was largely associated with lifestyle factors in adult life. This was to change in the 1980s, which saw a revival of interest in the role of early life circumstances and signs that the pendulum would swing away from a concern with adult risk factors to an excess concentration on early life. In this chapter, we have emphasised the need to avoid treating these models as mutually exclusive paradigms. Lifecourse research suggests that the intrauterine environment, childhood circumstances, the life trajectories of children and young people and adult circumstances can all have a bearing on adult health, although the relative strengths of these effects may vary across different cohorts and different health outcomes.

Although it is now generally accepted that socio-economic circumstances during adulthood contribute to the production of health inequalities, the relative influence of different factors remains a subject of debate. Because individual-level exposures and behaviours lend themselves more easily to epidemiological research linking risk to adverse health outcomes, by far the strongest evidence base relates to the role of lifestyle factors. The association between measures of psychosocial health at an individual level and various health outcomes is also increasingly accepted. What is less clear, however, is the way in which lifestyle and psychosocial mechanisms work in conjunction with material conditions to increase vulnerability to disease. For the most part, research continues to treat these factors as *causes* of health inequalities. However, they should also be viewed as *outcomes* of socio-economic disadvantage.

As discussed in Chapter Two, because the single-risk approach spells out clear biological pathways that can be targeted for intervention, research that highlights the role of individual factors in the production of health inequalities has tended to receive the greatest media and policy attention. In the case of adult risk factors, this is unfortunate. Evidence presented in this chapter suggests that socio-economic differences in health behaviours are shaped by wider circumstances in ways that are currently poorly understood. Thus, unhealthy lifestyles cannot be simply attributed to a lack of knowledge or a lack of money, but may reflect a more complex response to the way in which people manage their experience of poverty. Against this background, inequalities in health behaviours may be less effectively addressed by the information campaigns or interventions targeting access to and affordability of healthy choices than by policies that explicitly address the way in which individual behaviours relate to interactions between the psychosocial environment and material deprivation.

In addition to mediating health behaviours, there is sufficient evidence to suggest that psychosocial and material factors can present health risks in their own right. As noted earlier, the strongest evidence of an association between reduced psychological well-being, increasing illness and higher mortality has been established at an individual level. The claim that variation in economic circumstances at a community level produces adverse psychosocial effects for those of low social status that in turn contributes to poor health outcomes is more controversial. Despite its enormous popularity in the late 1980s and 1990s, Richard Wilkinson's psychosocial hypothesis has been attacked on a number of grounds, including the empirical. The suggestion that an independent relationship exists between income inequality and mortality at a country level was for a time accepted as conventional wisdom, institutions such as the World Health Organization (WHO) citing the example of countries/states such as Costa Rica, Sri Lanka and Kerala as evidence of how high levels of health could be achieved at relatively low levels of wealth. Today, this very relationship is in some doubt, at least for more developed countries, some researchers claiming that the association at population level is artefactual.

Assessing this debate in Chapter Two, we concluded that it would be premature to dismiss the psychosocial hypothesis which, we believe, is not only plausible but has been supported by some empirical evidence. Nor do we interpret the hypothesis as a conservative model that ignores the importance of material living conditions. Ironically, the focus and policy implications of work that examines the role of material deprivation are very similar to that which supports the psychosocial hypothesis. Both highlight the deleterious effects of factors such as unemployment, low incomes, poor housing and poor neighbourhood conditions. Both research traditions also point to the need for income redistribution and a strong role for the state in supporting welfare provision. It is therefore ironic that the academic critique that has been levelled at the psychosocial hypotheses (and that in part appears to be driven by an objection to its supposed ideology) may have undermined its own case for health inequalities to be tackled through more structural reforms.

In fact, as Chapter Eleven suggests, although government policy has responded positively to the psychosocial hypothesis, it has done so through the use of localised community initiatives rather than far-reaching structural reforms. Thus, several initiatives that have been geared towards neighbourhood regeneration have explicitly identified positive effects on social support, social capital and mental health as intended outcomes. As many such schemes have suffered from both short-termism and a tendency to incorporate a very disparate range of targets, the extent to which a focus on psychosocial health has been sustained is debatable. It is nevertheless noteworthy that theories relating to the psychosocial hypothesis have been acknowledged in policies targeting neighbourhood regeneration and, to a lesser extent, crime.

By contrast, policies addressing key aspects of material deprivation (for example, income, employment, housing) have not, until the government's 2003 Cross-cutting Review, been explicitly linked to health inequalities and, as we discussed in Chapter Three, the impact of government policies in these sectors has been greater with respect to absolute than relative needs. Nor, with the possible exception of housing, has much evidence been produced on the impact of such policies on health outcomes (see Chapter Eleven). While this partly reflects the difficulties of designing and evaluating upstream initiatives to tackle health variations, the government's tolerance of a lack of evidence in this area sits uncomfortably with its professed commitment to subjecting the policy-making process and its impact to robust evaluation. The unfortunate consequence of the lack of evidence concerning the role and impact of so-called 'upstream initiatives' is a real fuzziness in the language of policy when discussing some of the more far-reaching issues. For example, the 2004 Public Health White Paper *Choosing health: Making healthier choices easier* acknowledges the fact that people's ability to make healthy behavioural choices is constrained by factors such as unemployment, lack of money, poor education, living in poor or temporary housing or in an area of high crime (HM Government and DH, 2004, p 13). Yet, rather than demonstrating how the government's policies are directly targeting the operation of such constraints, the Paper makes vague mention of the fact that the government is "promoting social justice and tackling the wider causes of ill-health and inequality in health ... [by] acting in a number of areas including social exclusion, neighbourhood renewal and childhood poverty" (HM Government and DH, 2004, p 14).

Such fuzziness makes adult risk factors a key area in which the policies designed to eradicate health inequalities do not map easily onto the factors that give rise to health variations. Chapter Eleven nevertheless refers to the pathways and sources of vulnerability that have been identified in this chapter. To this end, it examines evidence of the impact of interventions targeting lifestyle factors, psychosocial health and material deprivation. Again, the limitations of the evidence base are highlighted, particularly with respect to an understanding of the role that context plays in shaping the formation, implementation and effectiveness of policies and interventions. We return to this issue in Chapter Fourteen, which, criticising the current approach to the gathering of evidence in public health, proposes an alternative methodological framework.

References

Acheson, D. (1998) *Independent Inquiry into Inequalities in Health* (The Acheson Report), London: The Stationery Office.

Adler, N. and Snibbe, A. (2003) 'The role of psychosocial processes in explaining the gradient between socio-economic status and health', *Current Directions in Psychological Science*, vol 12, pp 119-23.

Andres, A. (2004) 'Determinants of self-reported mental health using the British Household Panel Survey', *The Journal of Mental Health Policy and Economics*, vol 7, pp 99-106.

Arber, S. (1996) 'Integrating nonemployment into research on health inequalities', *International Journal of Health Services*, vol 26, pp 445-81.

Arber, S. and Lahelma, E. (1993) 'Inequalities in women's and men's ill-health: Britain and Finland compared', *Social Science and Medicine*, vol 37, pp 1055-68.

Asthana, S., Gibson, A., Moon, G. and Brigham, P. (2003) 'Allocating resources for health and social care: the significance of rurality', *Health and Social Care in the Community*, vol 11, pp 486-93.

Asthana, S., Gibson, A., Moon, G., Brigham, P. and Dicker, J. (2004a) 'The demographic and social class basis of inequality in self-reported morbidity: an exploration using the Health Survey for England', *Journal of Epidemiology and Community Health*, vol 58, pp 303-7.

Asthana, S., Gibson, A., Moon, G., Dicker, J. and Brigham, P. (2004b) 'The pursuit of equity in NHS resource allocation: should morbidity replace utilisation as the basis for setting health care capitations?', *Social Science and Medicine*, vol 58, pp 539-51.

Aylin, P., Morris, S., Wakefield, J., Grossinho, A., Jarup, L. and Elliott, P. (2001) 'Temperature, housing, deprivation and their relationship to excess winter mortality in Great Britain, 1986-1996', *International Journal of Epidemiology*, vol 30, pp 1116-18.

Baker, A. and Rooney, C. (2003) 'Recent trends in alcohol-related mortality, and the impact of ICD-10 on the monitoring of these deaths in England and Wales', *Health Statistics Quarterly*, vol 17, pp 5-14.

Bartley, M., Sacker, A. and Clarke, P. (2004a) 'Employment status, employment conditions, and limiting illness: prospective evidence from the British Household Panel Survey 1991-2001', *Journal of Epidemiology and Community Health*, vol 58, pp 501-6.

Bartley, M., Fitzpatrick, R., Firth, D. and Marmot, M. (2000) 'Social distribution of cardiovascular disease risk factors: chance among men in England 1984-1993', *Journal of Epidemiology and Community Health*, vol 54, pp 806-14.

Bartley, M., Martikainen, P., Shipley, M. and Marmot, M. (2004b) 'Gender differences in the relationship of partner's social class to behavioural risk factors and social support in the Whitehall II study', *Social Science and Medicine*, vol 59, pp 1925-36.

Ben-Shlomo, Y. and Chaturvedi, N. (1995) 'Assessing equity in access to health care provision in the UK: does where you live affect your chances of getting a coronary artery bypass graft?', *Journal of Epidemiology and Community Health*, vol 49, pp 200-4.

Benzeval, M., Judge, K. and Whitehead, M. (1995) 'The role of the NHS', in M. Benzeval, K. Judge and M. Whitehead (eds) *Tackling inequalities in health: An agenda for action*, London: King's Fund, pp 95-121.

Berney, L., Blane, D., Davey Smith, G. and Holland, P. (2000a) 'Lifecourse influences on health in early old age', in H. Graham (ed) *Understanding health inequalities*, Buckingham: Open University Press, pp 79-95.

Berney, L., Blane, D., Davey Smith, G., Gunnell, D., Holland, P. and Montgomery, S. (2000b) 'Socioeconomic measures in early old age as indicators of previous lifetime exposure to environmental hazards to health', *Sociology of Health and Illness*, vol 22, pp 415-30.

Bethune, A. (1997) 'Unemployment and mortality', in F. Drever and M. Whitehead (eds) *Health inequalities: Decennial supplement*, London: ONS, pp 156-67.

Billson, H., Pryer, J.A. and Nichols, R. (1999) 'Variation in fruit and vegetable consumption among adults in Britain: an analysis from the dietary and nutritional survey of British adults', *European Journal of Clinical Nutrition*, vol 53, pp 946-52.

Black Report (1980) *Inequalities of health*, Report of a Research Working Group, Chair, Sir Douglas Black, London: DHSS.

Black, N., Langham, S. and Petticrew, M. (1995) 'Coronary revascularisation: why do rates vary geographically in the UK?', *Journal of Epidemiology and Community Health*, vol 49, pp 408-12.

Blane, D. (1999) 'Adults of working age (16/18 to 65 years)', in D. Gordon, M. Shaw, D. Dorling and G. Davey Smith (eds) *Inequalities in health: The evidence presented to the Independent Inquiry into Inequalities in Health, chaired by Sir Donald Acheson*, Bristol: The Policy Press, pp 23-32.

Blane, D., Mitchell, R. and Bartley, M. (2000) 'The "inverse housing law" and respiratory health', *Journal of Epidemiology and Community Health*, vol 54, pp 745-9.

Blane, D., Berney, L., Davey Smith, G., Gunnell, D. and Holland, P. (1999) 'Reconstructing the lifecourse: health during early old age in a follow up study based on the Boyd Orr cohort', *Public Health*, vol 113, pp 117-24.

Blaxter, M. (1984) 'Equity and consultation rates in general practice', *British Medical Journal*, vol 288, pp 1963-7.

Blaxter, M. (1990) *Health and lifestyles*, London: Routledge.

Boniface, D. and Tefft, M. (2002) 'Dietary fats and 16-year coronary heart disease mortality in a cohort of men and women in Great Britain', *European Journal of Clinical Nutrition*, vol 56, pp 786-92.

Bosma, H., Marmot, M., Hemingway, H., Nicholson, A., Brunner, E. and Stansfeld, S. (1997) 'Low job control and risk of coronary heart disease in Whitehall II (prospective cohort) study', *British Medical Journal*, vol 314, pp 558-65.

Bunker, S., Colquhoun, D., Esler, M., Hickie, I., Hunt, D., Jelinek, V., Oldenburg, B., Peach, H., Ruth, D., Tennant, C. and Tonkin, A. (2003) '"Stress" and coronary heart disease: psychosocial risk factors', *Medical Journal of Australia*, vol 178, pp 272-6.

Campbell, K., Waters, E., O'Meara, S., Kelly, S. and Summerbell, C. (2004) 'Interventions for preventing obesity in children (Cochrane Review)', *The Cochrane Library, issue 1, 2004*, Chichester: John Wiley & Sons Ltd.

Carstairs, V. and Morris, R. (1989) 'Deprivation, mortality and resource allocation', *Community Medicine*, vol 11, pp 364-72.

Chandola, T., Head, J. and Bartley, M. (2004a) 'Socio-demographic predictors of quitting smoking: how important are household factors?', *Addiction*, vol 99, pp 770-7.

Chandola, T., Kuper, H., Singh-Manoux, A., Bartley, M. and Marmot, M. (2004b) 'The effect of control at home on CHD events in the Whitehall II study: gender differences in psychosocial domestic pathways to social inequalities in CHD', *Social Science and Medicine*, vol 58, pp 1501-9.

Chandola, T., Martikainen, P., Bartley, M., Lahelma, E., Marmot, M., Michikazu, S., Nasermoaddeli, A. and Kagamimori, S. (2004c) 'Does conflict between home and work explain the effect of multiple roles on mental health? A comparative study of Finland, Japan, and the UK', *International Journal of Epidemiology*, vol 33, pp 884-93.

Church, J. and Whyman, S. (1997) 'A review of recent social and economic trends', in F. Drever and M. Whitehead (eds) *Health inequalities: Decennial Supplement*, London: ONS, pp 29-43.

Claussen, B., Davey Smith, G. and Thelle, D. (2003) 'Impact of childhood and adulthood socioeconomic position on cause specific mortality: the Oslo Mortality Study', *Journal of Epidemiology and Community Health*, vol 57, pp 40-5.

Copeland, L. (2003) 'An exploration of the problems faced by young women living in disadvantaged circumstances if they want to give up smoking: can more be done at general practice level?', *Family Practice*, vol 20, pp 393-400.

Coulter, A. (1992) 'The interface between primary and secondary care', in M. Roland and A. Coulter (eds) *Hospital referrals*, Oxford: Oxford University Press, pp 1-14.

Crofton, J. and Simpson, D. (2002) *Tobacco: A global threat*, Oxford: Macmillan Education.

Curtis, S. and Taket, A. (1996) *Health and societies: Changing perspectives*, London: Edward Arnold.

Curtis, S., Southall, H., Congdon, P. and Dodgeon, B. (2004) 'Area effects on health variation over the life-course: analysis of the longitudinal study sample in England using new data on area of residence in childhood', *Social Science and Medicine*, vol 58, pp 57-74.

Darmon, N., Briend, A. and Drewnowski, A. (2004) 'Energy-dense diets are associated with lower diet costs: a community study of French adults', *Public Health Nutrition*, vol 7, pp 21-7.

Darmon, N., Ferguson, E. and Briend, A. (2003) 'Do economic constraints encourage the selection of energy dense diets?', *Appetite*, vol 41, pp 315-22.

Davey Smith, G. (2003) 'Introduction: lifecourse approaches to health inequalities', in G. Davey Smith (ed) *Health inequalities: Lifecourse approaches*, Bristol: The Policy Press, pp xii-lix.

Davey Smith, G. and Kuh, D. (1996) 'Does early nutrition affect later health? Views from the 1930s and 1980s', in D. Smith (ed) *The history of nutrition in Britain in the twentieth century: Science, scientists and politics*, London: Routledge, pp 214-37 [reproduced in G. Davey Smith (ed) (2003) *Health inequalities: Lifecourse approaches*, Bristol: The Policy Press, pp 411-35].

Davey Smith, G., Hart, C., Blane, D. and Hole, D. (1998) 'Adverse socio-economic conditions in childhood and cause-specific adult mortality: prospective observational study', *British Medical Journal*, vol 316, pp 1631-5.

DETR (Department of the Environment, Transport and the Regions) (1999) *Unpopular housing: Report of the Policy Action Team 7*, London: DETR.

Dibsdall, L., Lambert, N., Bobbin, R. and Frewer, L. (2003) 'Low income consumers' attitudes and behaviour towards access, availability and motivation to eat fruit and vegetables', *Public Health Nutrition*, vol 6, pp 159-68.

Doll, R. and Hill, A.B. (1954) 'The mortality of doctors in Britain in relation to their smoking habits: a preliminary report', *British Medical Journal*, 1954 ii, pp 1451-5, reprinted in *British Medical Journal*, vol 328, pp 1529-33.

Doll, R., Peto, R., Boreham, J. and Sutherland, I. (2004) 'Mortality in relation to smoking: 50 years' observations on male British doctors', *British Medical Journal*: doi 10.1136/bmj.38142.554479.AE.

Drever, F. and Whitehead, M. (eds) (1997) *Health inequalities: Decennial Supplement*, London: ONS.

Drewnowski, A. (2004) 'Obesity and the food environment: dietary energy density and diet costs', *American Journal of Preventive Medicine*, vol 27, suppl 3, pp 154-62.

d'Souza, R., Strazdins, L., Lim, L., Broom, D. and Rodgers, B. (2003) 'Work and health in a contemporary society: demands, control, and insecurity', *Journal of Epidemiology and Community Health*, vol 57, pp 849-54.

Dunn, J.R. (2000) 'Housing and health inequalities: review and prospects for research', *Housing Studies*, vol 15, pp 341-66.

Dunn, J.R. (2002) 'Housing and inequalities in health: a study of socioeconomic dimensions of housing and self reported health from a survey of Vancouver residents', *Journal of Epidemiology and Community Health*, vol 56, no 9, pp 671-81.

Easterlow, D., Smith, S.J. and Mallinson, S. (2000) 'Housing for health: the role of owner occupation', *Housing Studies*, vol 15, pp 367-86.

Eriksson, J., Forsen, T., Osmond, C. and Barker, D. (2003) 'Obesity from cradle to grave', *International Journal of Obesity Related Metabolic Disorders*, vol 27, pp 722-7.

Evandrou, M., Falkingham, J., Le Grand, J. and Winter, D. (1992) 'Equity in health and social care', *Journal of Social Policy*, vol 21, pp 489-523.

Evans, J., Hyndman, S., Stewart-Brown, S., Smith, D. and Petersen, S. (2000) 'An epidemiological study of the relative importance of damp housing in relation to adult health', *Journal of Epidemiology and Community Health*, vol 54, pp 677-86.

Frankel, S., Davey Smith, G. and Gunnell, D. (1999) 'Childhood socioeconomic position and adult cardiovascular mortality: the Boyd Orr Cohort', *American Journal of Epidemiology*, vol 150, pp 1081-4.

French, S. (2003) 'Pricing effects on food choices', *Journal of Nutrition*, vol 133, pp 841S-843S.

Gibson, A., Asthana, S., Brigham, P., Moon, G. and Dicker, J. (2002) 'Geographies of need and the new NHS: methodological issues in the definition and measurement of the health needs of local populations', *Health and Place*, vol 8, pp 47-60.

Gimeno, D., Benavides, F., Amick, B., Benach, J. and Martinez, J. (2004) 'Psychosocial factors and work related sickness absence among permanent and non-permanent employees', *Journal of Epidemiology and Community Health*, vol 58, pp 870-6.

Goddard, M. and Smith, P. (1998) *Equity of access to health care*, York: Centre for Health Economics, University of York.

Graham, H. (1993) *When life's a drag: Women, smoking and disadvantage*, London: HMSO.

Graham, H. (2002) 'Building an inter-disciplinary science of health inequalities: the example of lifecourse research', *Social Science and Medicine*, vol 55, pp 2005-16.

Green, G., Gilbertson, J. and Grimsley, M. (2002) 'Fear of crime and health in residential tower blocks: a case study in Liverpool, UK', *European Journal of Public Health*, vol 12, pp 10-15.

Griffin, J., Fuhrer, R., Stansfeld, S. and Marmot, M. (2002) 'The importance of low control at work and home on depression and anxiety: do these effects vary by gender and social class?', *Social Science and Medicine*, vol 54, pp 783-98.

Grifiths, C. (2003) 'Deaths related to drug poisoning: results for England and Wales, 1997-2001', *Health Statistics Quarterly*, vol 17, pp 65-71.

Gunnell, D., Frankel, S., Nanchahal, K., Braddon, F. and Davey Smith, G. (1996) 'Life-course exposure and later disease: a follow-up study based on a survey of family diet and health in pre war Britain (1937-1939)', *Public Health*, vol 110, pp 85-94.

Gunnell, D., Davey Smith, G., Frankel, S., Nanchahal, K., Braddon, F., Pemberton, J. and Peters, T. (1998) 'Childhood leg-length and adult mortality: follow up of the Carnegie (Boyd Orr) survey of diet and health in pre-war Britain', *Journal of Epidemiology and Community Health*, vol 52, pp 142-52.

Hajat, S., Kovats, R., Atkinson, R. and Haines, A. (2002) 'Impact of hot temperatures on death in London: a time series approach', *Journal of Epidemiology and Community Health*, vol 56, pp 367-72.

Hallqvist, J., Lynch, J., Bartley, M., Land, T. and Blane, D. (2004) 'Can we disentangle life course processes of accumulation, critical period and social mobility: an analysis of disadvantaged socio-economic positions and myocardial infarction in the Stockholm Heart Epidemiology Program', *Social Science and Medicine*, vol 58, pp 1555-62.

Hardy, R., Wadsworth, M. and Kuh, D. (2000) 'The influence of childhood weight and socioeconomic status on change in adult body mass index in a British national birth cohort', *International Journal of Obesity Related Metabolic Disorders*, vol 24, pp 725-34.

Hardy R., Wadsworth, M., Langenberg, C. and Kuh, D. (2004) 'Birthweight, childhood growth, and blood pressure at 43 years in a British birth cohort', *International Journal of Epidemiology*, vol 33, pp 121-9.

Harper, S., Lynch, J., Hsu, W., Everson, S., Hillemeier, M., Raghunathan, T., Salonen, J. and Kaplan, G. (2002) 'Life course socioeconomic conditions and adult psychosocial functioning', *International Journal of Epidemiology*, vol 31, pp 395-403.

Hart, C. and Davey Smith, G. (2003) 'Relationship between number of siblings and adult mortality and stroke risk: 25 year follow up of men in the Collaborative Study', *Journal of Epidemiology and Community Health*, vol 57, pp 385-91.

Haynes, R. (1991) 'Inequalities in health and health service use: evidence from the general household survey', *Social Science and Medicine*, vol 33, pp 361-8.

Healy, J. (2003) 'Excess winter mortality in Europe: a cross country analysis identifying key risk factors', *Journal of Epidemiology and Community Health*, vol 57, pp 784-89.

Hemingway, H. and Marmot, M. (1999) 'Psychosocial factors in the aetiology and prognosis of coronary heart disease: systematic review of prospective cohort studies', *British Medical Journal*, vol 318, pp 1460-7.

Hertzman, C., Power, C., Matthews, S. and Manor, O. (2001) 'Using an interactive framework of society and lifecourse to explain self-related health in early adulthood', *Social Science and Medicine*, vol 53, pp 1575-85.

Hippisley-Cox, J. and Pringle, M. (2000) 'Inequalities in access to coronary angiography and revascularization: the association of deprivation and location of primary care services', *British Journal of General Practice*, vol 50, pp 449-54.

HM Government and DH (Department of Health) (2004) *Choosing health: Making healthy choices easier*, London: HM Government and DH.

Holland, P., Berney, L., Blane, D., Davey Smith, G., Gunnell, D. and Montgomery, S. (2000) 'Life course accumulation of disadvantage: childhood health and hazard exposure during adulthood', *Social Science and Medicine*, vol 50, pp 1285-95.

Hopton, J. and Hunt, S. (1996) 'Housing conditions and mental health in a disadvantaged area in Scotland', *Journal of Epidemiology and Community Health*, vol 50, pp 56-61.

Howden-Chapman, P. (2004) 'Housing standards: a glossary of housing and health', *Journal of Epidemiology and Community Health*, vol 58, pp 162-8.

Jacobson, B. (1999) 'Tacking inequalities in health and health care: the role of the NHS', in D. Gordon, M. Shaw, D. Dorling and G. Davey Smith (eds) *Inequalities in health: The evidence presented to the Independent Inquiry into Inequalities in Health, chaired by Sir Donald Acheson*, Bristol: The Policy Press, pp 100-17.

Jarvis, M. and Wardle, J. (1999) 'Social patterning of individual health behaviours: the case of cigarette smoking', in M. Marmot and R. Wilkinson (eds) *Social determinants of health*, Oxford: Oxford University Press, pp 240-55.

Jebb, S. (2002) 'Dietary strategies to prevent and treat obesity', in T. Carr and K. Descheemaeker (eds) *Nutrition and health*, Oxford: Blackwell Science, pp 48–54.

Johnson, I. (2002) 'Micronutrients, phytoprotectants and mechanisms of anticancer activity', in T. Carr and K. Descheemaeker (eds) *Nutrition and health*, Oxford: Blackwell Science, pp 89-104.

Jonsson, D., Rosengren, A., Dotevall, A., Lappas, G. and Wilhelmsen, L. (1999) 'Job control, job demands and social support at work in relation to cardiovascular risk factors in MONICA 1995', *Journal of Cardiovascular Risk*, vol 6, pp 379-85.

Kilpelainen, M., Terpo, E., Helenius, H. and Koskenvuo, M. (2001) 'Home dampness, current allergic diseases and respiratory infections among young adults', *Thorax*, vol 56, pp 462-7.

Korpi, T. (2001) 'Accumulating disadvantage: longitudinal analyses of unemployment and physical health in representative samples of the Swedish population', *European Sociological Review*, vol 17, pp 255-73.

Koskinen, O., Husman, T., Meklin, T. and Nevalainen, A. (1999) 'The relationship between moisture or mould observations in houses and the state of health of their occupants', *European Respiratory Journal*, vol 14, pp 1363-7.

Kuh, D. and Davey Smith, G. (1997) 'The life course and adult chronic disease: an historical perspective with particular reference to coronary heart disease', in D. Kuh and Y. Ben-Shlomo (eds) *A life course approach to chronic disease epidemiology*, Oxford: Oxford University Press, pp 15-41.

Kuh, D., Hardy, R., Langenberg, C., Richards, M. and Wadsworth, M. (2002a) 'Mortality in adults aged 26-54 years related to socioeconomic conditions in childhood and adulthood: postwar birth cohort study', *British Medical Journal*, vol 325, pp 1076-80.

Kuh, D., Hardy, R., Chaturvedi, N. and Wadsworth, M.E. (2002b) 'Birth weight, childhood growth and abdominal obesity in adult life', *International Journal of Obesity Related Metabolic Disorders*, vol 26, pp 40-7.

Kuh, D., Ben-Shlomo, Y., Lynch, J., Hallqvist, J. and Power, C. (2003) 'Life course epidemiology', *Journal of Epidemiology and Community Health*, vol 57, pp 778-83.

Lahelma, E., Arber, S., Rahkonen, O. and Silventoinen, K. (2000) 'Widening or narrowing inequalities in health? Comparing Britain and Finland from the 1980s to the 1990s', *Sociology of Health and Illness*, vol 22, pp 110-36.

Laitinen, J., Power, C. and Jarvelin, M. (2001) 'Family social class, maternal body mass index, childhood body mass index, and age at menarche as predictors of adult obesity', *American Journal of Clinical Nutrition*, vol 74, pp 287-94.

Lallukka, T., Sarlio-Lahteenkorva, S., Roos, E., Laaksonen, M., Rahkonen, O. and Lahelma, E. (2004) 'Working conditions and health behaviours among employed women and men: the Helsinki Health Study', *Preventive Medicine*, vol 38, pp 48-56.

Lang, R., Thane, C.W., Bolton-Smith, C. and Jebb, S.A. (2003) 'Consumption of whole-grain foods by British adults: findings from further analysis of two national dietary surveys', *Public Health Nutrition*, vol 6, pp 479-84.

Langenberg, C., Hardy, R., Kuh, D., Brunner, E. and Wadsworth, M. (2003) 'Central and total obesity in middle aged men and women in relation to lifetime socioeconomic status: evidence from a national birth cohort', *Journal of Epidemiology and Community Health*, vol 57, pp 816-22.

Lawlor, D., Ebrahim, S. and Davey Smith, G. (2002) 'Socioeconomic position in childhood and adulthood and insulin resistance: cross sectional survey using data from British women's heart and health study', *British Medical Journal*, vol 325, pp 805-10.

Le Grand, J. (1991) 'The distribution of health care revisited', *Journal of Health Economics*, vol 10, pp 239-45.

Leeflang, R., Klein-Hesselink, D. and Spruit, I. (1992) 'Health effects of unemployment – II. Men and women', *Social Science and Medicine*, vol 34, pp 351-63.

Leon, D. and Davey Smith, G. (2000) 'Infant mortality, stomach cancer, stroke and coronary heart disease: ecological analysis', *British Medical Journal*, vol 320, pp 1705-6.

Lewis, G., Bebbington, P., Brugha, T., Farrell, M., Gill, B., Jenkins, R. and Meltzer, H. (2003) 'Socio-economic status, standard of living, and neurotic disorder', *International Review of Psychiatry*, vol 15, pp 91-6.

Macintyre, S., Maciver, S. and Soomans, A. (1993) 'Area, class and health: should we be focusing on places or people?', *Journal of Social Policy*, vol 22, pp 213-34.

Macintyre, S., Ellaway, A., Hiscock, R., Kearns, A., Der, G. and McKay, L. (2003) 'What features of the home and the area might help to explain observed relationships between housing tenure and health? Evidence from the West of Scotland', *Health and Place*, vol 9, pp 207-18.

MacLeod, M., Finlayson, C., Pell, J. and Findlay, I. (1999) 'Geographic, demographic and socio-economic variations in the investigation and management of coronary heart disease in Scotland', *Heart*, vol 81, pp 252-6.

Maheswaran, R. and Elliott, P. (2003) 'Stroke mortality associated with living near main roads in England and Wales: a geographical study', *Stroke*, vol 34, pp 2776-80.

Majeed, A., Bardsley, M., Morgan, D., O'Sullivan, C. and Bindman, A. (2000) 'Cross-sectional study of primary care groups in London: association of measures of socio-economic and health status with hospital admission rates', *British Medical Journal*, vol 321, pp 1057-60.

Manson-Siddle, C. and Robinson, M. (1998) 'Superprofile analysis of socio-economic variations in coronary investigation and revascularization rates', *Journal of Epidemiology and Community Health*, vol 52, pp 507-12.

Marmot, M. and Feeney, A. (1996) 'Work and health: implications for individuals and societies', in D. Blane, E. Brunner and R. Wilkinson (eds) *Health and social organisation: Toward a health policy for the 21st century*, London: Routledge, pp 235-54.

Marmot, M., Shipley, M., Brunner, E. and Hemingway, H. (2001) 'Relative contribution of early life and adult socio-economic factors to adult morbidity in the Whitehall II study', *Journal of Epidemiology and Community Health*, vol 55, pp 301-7.

Marmot, M., Siegrist, J., Theorell, T. and Feeney, A. (1999) 'Health and the psychosocial environment at work', in M. Marmot and R.G. Wilkinson (eds) *Social determinants of health*, Oxford: Oxford University Press, pp 105-31.

Matthews, S., Power, C. and Stansfeld, S. (2001) 'Psychological distress and work and home roles: a focus on socio-economic differences in distress', *Psychological Medicine*, vol 31, pp 725-36.

Medina, S., Plasencia, A., Ballester, F., Mücke, H. and Schwartz, J. on behalf of the Apheis Group (2004) 'Apheis: public health impact of PM_{10} in 19 European cities', *Journal of Epidemiology and Community Health*, vol 58, pp 831-6.

Mindell, J. and Joffe, M. (2004) 'Predicted health impacts of urban air quality management', *Journal of Epidemiology and Community Health*, vol 58, pp 103-13.

Montgomery, S., Cook, D., Bartley, M. and Wadsworth, M. (1999) 'Unemployment pre-dates symptoms of depression and anxiety resulting in medical consultation in young men', *International Journal of Epidemiology*, vol 28, pp 95-100.

Morris, S., Sutton, M. and Gravelle, H. (2005) 'Inequity and inequality in the use of health care in England: an empirical investigation', *Social Science and Medicine*, vol 60, pp 1251-66.

Morrison, C., Woodward, M., Leslie, W. and Tunstall-Pedoe, H. (1997) 'Effect of socioeconomic group on incidence of, management of, and survival after myocardial infarction and coronary death: analysis of community coronary event register', *British Medicine Journal*, vol 314, p 541.

Næss, Ø., Claussen, B., Thelle, D. and Davey Smith, G. (2004) 'Cumulative deprivation and cause specific mortality: a census based study of life course influences over three decades', *Journal of Epidemiology and Community Health*, vol 58, pp 599-603.

New, S. (2002) 'Diet and osteoporosis: where are we now?', in T. Carr and K. Descheemaeker (eds) *Nutrition and health*, Oxford: Blackwell Science, pp 121-9.

Niedhammer, I., Goldberg, M., Leclerc, A., David, S., Bugel, I. and Landre, M. (1998) 'Psychosocial work environment and cardiovascular risk factors in an occupational cohort in France', *Journal of Epidemiology and Community Health*, vol 52, pp 93-100.

North, F., Syme, S., Feeney, A., Shipley, M. and Marmot, M. (1996) 'Psychosocial work environment and sickness absence among British civil servants: the Whitehall II study', *American Journal of Public Health*, vol 86, pp 332-40.

NSNR (National Strategy for Neighbourhood Renewal) (2000) *Report of the Policy Action Team 8: Anti-social behaviour*, London: The Stationery Office.

O'Donnell, O. and Propper, C. (1991) 'Equity and the distribution of NHS resources', *Journal of Health Economics*, vol 10, pp 1-19.

ODPM (Office of the Deputy Prime Minister) (2003) *English Housing Condition Survey 2001: Building the picture*, London: The Stationery Office.

ODPM (2004) *Mental health and social exclusion: Social Exclusion Unit report*, London: ODPM Publications.

ODPM (2005) *Sustainable communities: Settled homes, changing lives*, London: ODPM Publications.

Oliver, S.E. and Thomson, R.G. (1999) 'Are variations in the use of carotid endarterectormy explained by population need? A study of health service utilization in two English Health Regions', *European Journal of Endovascular Surgery*, vol 17, pp 501-6.

O'Neill, M., Jerrett, M., Kawachi, I., Levy, J., Cohen, A., Gouveia, N., Wilkinson, P., Fletcher, T., Cifuentes, L. and Schwartz, J. with input from participations of the Workshop on Air Pollution and Socioeconomic Conditions (2003) 'Health, wealth and air pollution: advancing theory and methods', *Environmental Health Perspectives*, vol 111, pp 1861-70.

ONS (Office for National Statistics) (2001) *Psychiatric morbidity among adults, 2000*, London: ONS.

ONS and DH (Department of Health) (2003) *Statistics on smoking: England, 2003*, Statistical Bulletin 2003/21, London: ONS and DH.

Packer, C., Stewart-Brown, S. and Fowle, S. (1994) 'Damp housing and adult health: results from a lifestyle study in Worcester', *Journal of Epidemiology and Community Health*, vol 48, pp 555-9.

Packham, C., Robinson, J., Morris, J., Richards, C., Marks, P. and Gray, D. (1999) 'Statin prescribing in Nottingham general practices: a cross-sectional study', *Journal of Public Health Medicine*, vol 21, pp 60-4.

Pain, C., Frankovitch, F. and Cook, G. (1996) 'Setting targets for CABG survey in the North Western Region', *Journal of Public Health Medicine*, vol 18, pp 449-56.

Parrott, S. and Godfrey, C. (2004) 'Economics of smoking cessation', *British Medical Journal*, vol 328, pp 947-9.

Payne, N. and Saul, C. (1997) 'Variations in the use of cardiology services in a health authority: comparison of coronary artery revascularization rates with prevalence of angina and coronary mortality', *British Medical Journal*, vol 314, pp 257-61.

Peat, J., Dickerson, J. and Li, J. (1998) 'Effects of damp and mould in the home on respiratory health: a review of the literature', *Allergy*, vol 53, pp 120-8.

Pelfrene, E., Leynen, F., Mak, R., de Bacquer, D., Kornitzer, M. and De Backer, G. (2003) 'Relationship of perceived job stress to total coronary risk in a cohort of working men and women in Belgium', *European Journal of Cardiovascular Prevention and Rehabilitation*, vol 10, pp 345-54.

Pensola, T. and Martikainen, P. (2004) 'Life-course experiences and mortality by adult social class among young men', *Social Science and Medicine*, vol 58, pp 2149-70.

Pickin, C. and St Leger, S. (1993) *Assessing health need using the life cycle framework*, Buckingham: Open University Press.

Pollack, C., van dem Knesebeck, O. and Siegrist, J. (2004) 'Housing and health in Germany', *Journal of Epidemiology and Community Health*, vol 58, pp 216-22.

Pollard, J., Greenwood, D., Kirk, S. and Cade, J. (2001) 'Lifestyle factors affecting fruit and vegetable consumption in the UK Women's Cohort Study', *Appetite*, vol 37, pp 71-9.

Powell, M. (1990) 'Need and provision in the National Health Service: an inverse care law?', *Policy & Politics*, vol 18, pp 31-7.

Power, C., Stansfeld, S., Matthews, S., Manor, O. and Hope, S. (2002) 'Childhood and adulthood risk factors for socio-economic differentials in psychological distress: evidence from the 1958 British birth cohort', *Social Science and Medicine*, vol 55, pp 1989-2004.

Pringle, M. and Morton-Jones, A. (1994) 'Using unemployment rates to predict prescribing trends in England', *British Journal of General Practice*, vol 44, pp 53-6.

RCP (Royal College of Physicians) (1994) *Homelessness and ill health*, Suffolk: The Lavenham Press.

Reilly, J.J., Methven, E., McDowell, Z.C., Hacking, B., Alexander, D., Stewart, L. and Kelnar, C.J.H. (2003) 'Health consequences of obesity', *Archives of Disease in Childhood*, vol 88, pp 748-52.

Robinson, D. (1998) 'Health selection in the housing system: access to council housing for homeless people with health problems', *Housing Studies*, vol 13, pp 23-41.

Robinson, S., Crozier, S., Borland, S., Hammond, J., Barker, D. and Inskip, H. (2004) 'Impact of educational attainment on the quality of young women's diets', *European Journal of Clinical Nutrition*, vol 58, pp 1174-80.

Rosvall, M., Ostergren, P., Hedblad, B., Isacsson, S., Janzon, L. and Berglund, G. (2002) 'Work-related psychosocial factors and carotid atherosclerosis', *International Journal of Epidemiology*, vol 31, pp 1169-78.

Rushton, D., Hoare, J., Henderson, L., Gregory, J., Bates, C., Prentice, A., Birch, M., Swan, G. and Farron, M. (2004) *The national diet and nutrition survey: Adults aged 19-64. Volume 4: Nutritional status (anthropometry and blood analyses), blood pressure and physical activity*, London: The Stationery Office.

SEU (Social Exclusion Unit) (1998) *Rough sleeping: Report by the Social Exclusion Unit*, London: SEU.

Siegrist, J. and Marmot, M. (2004) 'Health inequalities and the psychosocial environment – two scientific challenges', *Social Science and Medicine*, vol 58, pp 1463-73.

Shaw, M., Dorling, D., Gordon, D. and Davey Smith, G. (1999) *The widening gap: Health inequalities and policy in Britain*, Bristol: The Policy Press.

Smith, C., Smith, C., Kearns, R. and Abbott, M. (1993) 'Housing stressors, social support and psychological distress', *Social Science and Medicine*, vol 37, pp 603-12.

Smith, S.J. (1990) 'Health status and the housing system', *Social Science and Medicine*, vol 31, pp 753-62.

Somerville, M., Mackenzie, I., Owen, P. and Miles, D. (2000) 'Housing and health: does installing heating in their homes improve the health of children with asthma?', *Public Health*, vol 114, pp 434-9.

Stansfeld, S., Head, J., Fuhrer, R., Wardle, J. and Cattell, V. (2003) 'Social inequalities in depressive symptoms and physical functioning in the Whitehall II study: exploring a common cause explanation', *Journal of Epidemiology and Community Health*, vol 57, pp 361-7.

Stead, M., Macaskill, S., Mackintosh, A., Reece, J. and Eadie, D. (2001) '"It's as if you're locked in": qualitative explanations for area effects on smoking in disadvantaged communities', *Health and Place*, vol 7, pp 333-43.

Stronks, K., van de Mheen, H., van den Bos, J. and Mackenbach, J. (1995) 'Smaller socioeconomic inequalities in health among women: the role of employment status', *International Journal of Epidemiology*, vol 24, pp 559-68.

Thomas, C., Benzeval, M. and Stansfeld, S. (2005) 'Employment transitions and mental health: an analysis from the British Household Panel Survey', *Journal of Epidemiology and Community Health*, vol 59, pp 243-9.

Tod, A. (2003) 'Barriers to smoking cessation in pregnancy: a qualitative study', *British Journal of Community Nursing*, vol 8, pp 56-64.

Townsend, P. and Davidson, N. (1982) *Inequalities in health*, Harmondsworth: Penguin.

Tudor Hart, J. (1971) 'The inverse care law', *The Lancet*, vol 297, 27 February, pp 405-12.

Uren, Z. (2001) 'Geographical variations in deaths related to drug misuse in England and Wales, 1993-99', *Health Statistics Quarterly*, vol 11, pp 25-35.

Vahtera, J., Kivimaki, M., Pentti, J. and Theorell, T. (2000) 'Effect of change in the psychosocial work environment on sickness absence: a seven year follow up of initially healthy employees', *Journal of Epidemiology and Community Health*, vol 54, pp 484-93.

van Doorslaer, E., Wagstaff, A., van der Burg, H., Christiansen, T., de Graeve, D., Duchesne, I., Gerdtham, U.-G., Gerfin, M., Geurts, J., Gross, L., Häkkinen, U., John, J., Klavus, J., Leu, R.E., Nolan, B., O'Donnell, O., Propper, C., Puffer, F., Schellhorn, M., Sundberg, G. and Winkelhake, O. (2000) 'Equality in the delivery of healthcare in Europe and the US', *Journal of Health Economics*, vol 19, pp 553-83.

Wadsworth, M. (1997) 'Health inequalities in the life course perspective', *Social Science and Medicine*, vol 44, pp 859-69.

Wadsworth, M. and Kuh, D. (1997) 'Childhood influences on adult health: a review of recent work from the British 1946 national birth cohort study, the MRC National Survey of Health and Development', *Paediatric and Perinatal Epidemiology*, vol 11, pp 2-20.

Wardle, J. and Griffith, J. (2001) 'Socioeconomic status and weight control practices in British adults', *Journal of Epidemiology and Community Health*, vol 55, pp 185-90.

Wardle, J. and Steptoe, A. (2003) 'Socioeconomic differences in attitudes and beliefs about healthy lifestyles', *Journal of Epidemiology and Community Health*, vol 57, pp 440-3.

Wardle, J., Parmenter, K. and Waller, J. (2000) 'Nutrition knowledge and food intake', *Appetite*, vol 34, pp 269-75.

Weich, S., Blanchard, M., Prince, M., Burton, E., Erens, B. and Sproston, K. (2002) 'Mental health and the built environment: cross-sectional survey of individual and contextual risk factors for depression', *British Journal of Psychiatry*, vol 180, pp 428-33.

West, R. and Lowe, C. (1976) 'Regional variations in need for and provision and use of child health services', *British Medical Journal*, vol 272, pp 843-6.

Whincup, P., Gilg, J., Emberson, J., Jarvis, M., Feyerabend, C., Bryant, A., Walker, M. and Cook, D. (2004) 'Passive smoking and risk of coronary heart disease and stroke: prospective study with cotinine measurement', *British Medical Journal* doi:10.1136/bmj.38146.427188.55.

Whitehead, M. and Diderichsen, F. (2001) 'Social capital and health: tip-toeing through the minefield of evidence', *The Lancet*, vol 358, pp 165-6.

Whitehead, M., Evandrou, M., Haglund, B. and Diderichsen, F. (1997) 'As the health divide widens in Sweden and Britain, what's happening to access to care', *British Medical Journal*, vol 315, pp 1006-9.

Whitley, R. and Prince, M. (2005) 'Fear of crime, mobility and mental health in inner-city London, UK', *Social Science and Medicine*, vol 61, pp 1678-88.

Wilkin, D. (1992) 'Patterns of referral: explaining variation', in M. Roland and A. Coulter (eds) *Hospital referrals*, Oxford: Oxford University Press, pp 76-91.

Wilkinson, D. (1999) *Poor housing and ill health: A summary of research evidence*, Edinburgh: Scottish Office, Central Research Unit.

Williamson, G. (2002) 'A brief review of the impact of dietary polyphenols on cardiovascular disease', in T. Carr and K. Descheemaeker (eds) *Nutrition and health*, Oxford: Blackwell Science, pp 20-6.

Williamson, I., Martin, C., McGill, G., Monie, R. and Fennerty, A. (1997) 'Damp housing and asthma: a case control study', *Thorax*, vol 52, pp 229-34.

Wright, C., Parker, L., Lamont, D. and Craft, A. (2001) 'Implications of childhood obesity for adult health: findings from thousand families cohort study', *British Medical Journal*, vol 323, pp 1280-4.

ELEVEN

Health inequalities during adulthood: policy and practice

Introduction

Chapter Ten showed how socio-economic conditions during adulthood continue to exert a powerful impact on health and behaviour. This chapter retains the focus on the key sources of vulnerability, lifestyle, psychosocial health and material living conditions, as we seek to examine the evidence base for what works and its relationship to the policy environment. We note, however, that the boundaries are increasingly indistinct. Housing, for example, has a significant material dimension reflected in housing costs, the generation of wealth, a controlled physical environment and protection from the elements. It also has a significant psychosocial dimension, reflecting self-identity, social status and autonomy (Dunn, 2002).

The material determinants of health are also linked themselves in a multiple, complex and contingent manner. This was recognised in policy terms by *The health of the nation* (DH, 1992), where the Conservative government argued the need to inject a health dimension into all public policies (Smith and Mallinson, 1997), and the Department of the Environment (DoE) agreed that health improvements should be an aim of urban regeneration. The White Paper *Saving lives: Our healthier nation* (DH, 1999a) similarly stressed the need to address the social, economic and environmental determinants of health as well as lifestyle choices, and stressed the importance attaching to integrated policy making.

Such concern, while relatively recent, makes the task of distinguishing effective interventions and appropriate policy ever more hard. It highlights the dissonance between downstream and upstream policy, between the evidence-based agenda with its focus on individualised interventions and the continuing requirement for structural solutions (see Chapter Fourteen). It also illuminates the difficulties of the midstream, where attempts to achieve national policy objectives via local area-based initiatives (ABIs) reveal the tension between place-based and people-based policies (Joshi, 2001). Additionally, it challenges attempts at classification by demanding a holistic approach to health inequalities and, as in so many other instances, finds the actual evidence to be limited.

One contributory reason is that, despite the rhetoric, health remains on the margins of the regeneration agenda and the effects of changing or ameliorating deprivation on population health have received relatively little attention, partly

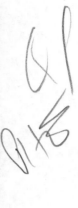

because it is managed by organisations that are not part of the health sector (Curtis et al, 2002). Another is that the holistic emphasis makes it a challenge to focus on the impact of policy on a particular age group, even one as wide as adulthood, because many of the area-based policies aim to be intergenerational with a particular emphasis, for example, on families with young children or older people. A third is that it is increasingly difficult to design and evaluate effective interventions. Randomised controlled trials (RCTs), key references for early years and childhood, albeit with limitations, are almost impossible to undertake in areas such as housing. There tends to be, therefore, increased reliance on self-reported health and psychosocial measures.

Health and lifestyle: diet and physical activity

Social inequalities have always been reflected in food consumption patterns (Leather, 1996). There are currently two key drivers to the healthy eating agenda in adulthood. The first is the association between diet and nutrition and coronary heart disease (CHD), stroke and some cancers. It is thus a salient feature of the government's National Service Frameworks (NSFs) for these areas. This has a clear inequalities (and lifecourse) dimension. Second, despite the reservations raised in Chapter Ten as to the relative contribution of material poverty as opposed to psychosocial responses to poverty, food is seen as part of a holistic approach to supporting those on a low income. It is thus integral to many regeneration projects funded by initiatives such as the Single Regeneration Budget (SRB) and the New Deal for Communities (NDC). Physical activity is closely linked to the healthy eating agenda. It is not only a key component in weight loss but one of the major modifiable risk factors for CHD. As we have seen, it also offers indirect protection from other risk factors such as high blood pressure, high cholesterol and diabetes mellitus (Press et al, 2003), yet sedentary lifestyles dominate in adulthood.

What works? Evidence and practice

Nutritional interventions

The issues of obesity and overweight have been introduced in Chapters Eight and Nine with many of the problems for overweight or obese children known to be deferred to later life. There is also an economic cost and one that is projected to rise to £3.6 billion by 2010 if the prevalence of obesity continues to rise at present rates (NAO, 2001). This is accounted for primarily in terms of lost output as a result of sickness.

Evidence supports the efficacy of low calorie and low fat/low energy diets as the focus for treatment regimes for adults. A 10% reduction in saturated fat intake by the UK population, for example, has been equated with a reduction in

CHD mortality of between 20% and 30% (DH, 2002b). Increased physical activity and CBT have proved effective adjuncts to such diets, supporting changes in eating habits and lifestyle, with physical activity known to have benefits above and beyond any possible impact on weight (Mulvihill and Quigley, 2003).

Maintenance of weight loss is easier if support structures, including support from health professionals, are in place, yet lack of information, lack of appropriate support services and negative perceptions of the client group are all likely to reduce the efficacy of weight loss interventions in health settings. Despite the significance of the issue there has been little research yet into how obesity might be better managed through changes in health practitioners' practice or the organisation of care (Harvey et al, 2001). Once again, there is a "general dearth of evidence in relation to public health interventions that address health inequality issues" (Mulvihill and Quigley, 2003, p 8), with little evidence as to what works best for the most disadvantaged and vulnerable. The Health Development Agency (HDA), locating a number of public health interventions where it suggests evidence is strong and the likelihood of success great, advocates brief interventions in primary care as a routine part of all medical consultations, adult–only services that include diet, physical activity and behaviour modification, and specialist obesity services able to deliver to the disadvantaged and vulnerable (Kelly, 2004, p 4).

Workplace interventions have the advantage of regular and sustained participation as well as supervision. The lack of evidence to endorse self-help peer groups and community-based interventions is thus surprising and is as likely to be an artefact of the structure and quantity of available research as a commentary on efficacy. The HDA, drawing on the evidence base, argues that tax incentives to employers to encourage exercise and physical activity both at work and travelling to work should be introduced, alongside a statutory requirement for local authorities to carry out health impact assessments of planning proposals, including the promotion of physical activity and healthy food choices (Kelly, 2004).

Consumption of fruit and vegetables has been shown to significantly reduce the risk of early death from heart disease, stroke and some cancers. Drawing on the minimum recommended daily consumption of 400g established by the WHO (World Health Organization) in 1991 and the US *5 A Day for Better Health Program* established the same year, the Department of Health (DH) funded five Five-a-day pilot sites across the country in 2000 designed to promote fruit and vegetables within the community setting (DH, 2002a). Evaluation found changes in people's knowledge and access to and intake of fruit and vegetables, with the initiatives stemming a fall in consumption against the national trend.

Critically, the programmes had the biggest impact on those people with the lowest intakes (DH, 2002a). However, there is a continued discrepancy between awareness and practice. Two key barriers are logistical and contextual. The practicalities of shopping, transporting and storing fruit and vegetables are considered key by many. The support of family and friends is also required, reflecting the social function of eating, workplace and recreational choices and the need to accommodate children's likes and dislikes (Anderson and Cox, 2000). Financial constraints are also important, with many believing fresh fruit and vegetables to be an expensive nutritional option.

Attempts to counter such barriers have similarly focused primarily at the community level. Aston–Mansfield (2001), addressing food poverty in the London Borough of Newham, found that a spectrum of food projects not only provided access to a healthier diet, but were successful on a number of other levels as well, meeting the specific needs of a diverse community, bolstering community networks and social cohesion and providing opportunities for local people to be involved in creating local solutions. Similar attributes are suggested in Box 11.1 by two examples from the Beacon Programme, introduced by the DH in 2000 with the aim of sharing information on successful local National Health Service (NHS) initiatives covering key areas of the NHS modernisation plans.

The politics of nutrition have, in the past, largely remained within the sphere of nutritional education or 'healthy eating'. This has resulted in a lack of consideration of the macro influences and workings of poverty, wealth and inequality. Food poverty has a number of characteristics: low–income households

---

Box 11.1: Community approaches to nutrition

Sandwell Community Food Project in the West Midlands has been established for over 10 years to tackle food access problems. The base (with a turnover of £70,000-£80,000 per annum) is a home delivery service focusing on fresh fruit and vegetables which serves the tuck shops at 13 local schools as well as local nursing homes and private homes (mainly with elderly occupants). It received a £120,000 annual grant from the National Lotteries Charity Board and an additional £97,000 to July 2001 from the Sandwell Health Authority as a Five-a-day pilot. The latter funds a double decker bus (fitted out as a kitchen and nutritional display) to visit the five most deprived areas as well as local schools providing fruit, cookery demonstrations and information.

The Asian cookery club was established in Luton in 1995. By 2000 it had reinvented itself as a grassroots project recruiting, training and employing cookery leaders to run cookery clubs within their local community with the emphasis on cooking traditional food in a healthier way, reducing the quantities of fat and salt used (in an attempt to counter the genetic predisposition to CHD and higher than average rates of diabetes). Our House, for example, hosts a cookery club alongside a crèche and English lessons. Critical to the project's success are lessons delivered in the home neighbourhood where students both know one another and the course leaders. The cost of £9,500 per annum has been funded by the Luton Health Action Zone (HAZ), with the programme lead funded by the Community NHS Trust.

spend proportionally more of their disposable income on food, find a healthy diet more expensive, cannot benefit from economies of scale and have difficulty accessing affordable healthier foods due to transport difficulties and lack of storage space. Access to knowledge is also a feature of food poverty, including knowledge about how to balance a budget, what constitutes a healthy diet, how to cook a healthy diet and how to make healthy choices in the face of a plethora of convenience foods. Evidence from a European-wide food and nutrition project that attempted to use the WHO health promotion approach suggests that both considerable time and political and organisational support are required if such an approach is to move from rhetoric (and a continued focus on nutritional education) to one that actively addresses the broader social, cultural and structural barriers to health. In this instance this would involve the appointment of lay food workers (who were able to address issues such as welfare benefits, education and employment alongside culturally relevant nutritional advice) and the allocation of mainstream funding (Kennedy, 2001).

The term '*food desert*' has been coined to describe areas of relative exclusion where people experience physical and economic barriers to accessing healthy food. Questions have been raised as to the degree to which such areas actually exist and the degree to which the nutritional quality of low-income consumers' diets is actually related to retail provision (see Chapter Four and Box 11.2). Research under the European Prospective Investigation into Cancer (EPIC) banner does suggest, however, that residential area can exert an independent effect on fruit and vegetable consumption through a variety of mechanisms such as cost, availability and local norms and thus supports measures to reduce community-level barriers as well as individual behavioural interventions (Shohaimi et al, 2004).

Box 11.2: Food access as a determinant of consumption

Wrigley et al (2003) used the redevelopment of a district shopping centre on a deprived housing estate in Leeds to look at the impact of a non-healthcare intervention on food consumption patterns. Their study confirmed food access as a local problem and suggested the "malleability of some of these problems to large scale area-based interventions" (p 179). The opening of the new Tesco store had a limited impact on diet overall but increased fruit and vegetable consumption post-intervention among those switching to the new store. The change was small in absolute terms (less than half a serving a day), and the average resident still consumed at least two portions a day below government recommended levels. However, the improvements included some of those most at risk, including those with the poorest diets pre-intervention and those switching from limited or budget stores.

Physical activity

The potential health gains consequent on regular physical activity are well established (see Chapter Ten). The prevalence of inactivity is also known to be high and to follow the now familiar distribution along lines of class, income and education. There is, therefore, a clear health inequalities agenda and one where targeted interventions should be expected to pay dividends. Yet, "far less is known about effective interventions for increasing physical activity" (Hillsdon et al, 2004, p 2), particularly among disadvantaged sectors of the population.

Most public health interventions, such as the primary care-based exercise on prescription schemes and media campaigns, have focused on individual behaviour change. At best these tend to raise activity levels among a small proportion of the population for a limited period of time (Eaton and Menard, 1998; Riddoch et al, 1998; Eakin et al, 2000). A review of reviews found controlled studies were also generally conducted with well-motivated and educated volunteers. Among such groups, brief individual-centred interventions in healthcare or community settings (focusing, for example, on advice and information) can produce modest short-term changes across 6-12 weeks, with referral to an exercise specialist resulting in longer-term changes (Hillsdon et al, 2004). Ongoing support (and social support in community settings) is a further facilitating factor. Moderately intensive interventions such as walking, which are independent of facilities, are also likely to be effective, at least in the short term, with studies in the community suggesting they could form the focus of sustained change. Similar findings applied to programmes designed specifically for those aged over 50.

The development of physical activity facilitators in primary care has thus been advocated alongside individually adapted health behaviour change programmes (Kelly, 2004). However, despite the popularity of primary care interventions in the UK, it is still not known, for example, "whether individual advice from a person's usual general practitioner may lead to significant increases in physical activity that can be sustained beyond three months" (Hillsdon et al, 2004, p 12). Some research suggests that the potential for lifestyle change emanating from primary care has not yet been achieved in practice (Lawlor et al, 1999); others suggest it may never be sufficient to counter the actual and perceived obstacles to change (Hillsdon et al, 2002), and that an initial focus on physical activity needs to be supported over time by other risk factor interventions (Eakin et al, 2000).

There is also a lack of review evidence of effectiveness in other areas such as environmental, community, policy or fiscal interventions such as cycling lanes or green travel plans and no admissible evaluations of commonly pursued interventions such as exercise referrals, the effectiveness of sports and physical activity development officers in the community or even participation in sport. This is not to say, of course, that such interventions are necessarily ineffective, merely that they have not been the subject of nor are readily amenable to systematic review. Box 11.3 outlines some early evidence drawn from users' surveys and routine traffic data as to the efficacy of the national cycle network.

It has also been suggested that taking exercise may help people give up smoking by moderating a number of the effects of nicotine withdrawal, such as mood and sleep disturbance, the incidence of stress, cravings for nicotine and weight gain. Levels of physical activity are also inversely related to smoking rates, with the suggestion that becoming more physically active can increase confidence to stop smoking and maintain abstinence (Ussher et al, 2002). Exercise is thus routinely recommended as an aid to smoking cessation, yet evidence at RCT level is again minimal, with several small trials showing trends towards a higher rate of abstinence in treatment groups but only one large trial in the US reporting significant benefits three months and 12 months after the end of the programme (Ussher et al, 2002). From an inequalities perspective it is also important to note that none controlled for socio-economic status, age or occupation.

A similar picture emerges as to the role of exercise in the management of depression. Research strongly supports the link between exercise and psychological well-being and exercise on prescription is becoming increasingly popular in the UK, often including depression as one of the referral criteria. Meta-analysis of

---

Box 11.3: Environmental intervention to support physical activity

Cycle ownership in the UK increased from 14% in 1975/76 to 32% in 1995/97, yet only 2% of routine journeys in the UK are made by bicycle compared to 18% in Denmark where a more cycle-friendly transport system exists (DoT, 1996). The UK National Cycle Network was initiated by the charity Sustrans with the aim of promoting non-motorised forms of transport as environmentally friendly alternatives to the car. Its remit has since broadened to include the promotion of healthy physical activity. The first 8,000 kilometres (km) phase has been completed at an estimated cost of £210 million and it is planned to extend the network to 16,000 km by 2005.

Routes are designed to run through population centres and, where possible, connect them to schools, shopping areas, and centres of employment. They therefore have the potential to facilitate short journeys that can be incorporated into everyday activity, as well as catering for recreational cycling and walking (Lawlor et al, 2003) User surveys on over 40 routes in 2000/01 suggest this aim is being met, with 43% of respondents using the network for a specific journey. However, the profile indicates a predominantly male (66%), white (98%) base, with almost half aged 45 years or older. A substantial proportion thought that the Network had helped them to increase the amount of regular physical activity they undertook by a large (42%) or small (28%) amount (Lawlor et al, 2003, p 99). Meanwhile, the importance attached to pleasant surroundings, safety and convenience all suggest the importance of the environment in facilitating physical activity.

exercise interventions suggests people who exercise are less depressed than non-exercisers. Yet, "the effectiveness of exercise in reducing symptoms of depression cannot be determined because of a lack of good quality research on clinical populations with adequate follow-up" (Lawlor and Hopker, 2001, p 1). However, exercise programmes are known to face similar problems of compliance to medication, with reported compliance rates of 20% to 50% as opposed to 20% to 59% for antidepressants.

Policy

The NHS Plan (DH, 2000a), *The NHS Cancer Plan* (DH, 2000b) and the corresponding *National Service Framework for Coronary Heart Disease* (DH, 2000c) all highlight diet, nutrition and physical activity as key areas for action. *The NHS Cancer Plan*, for example, accords diet the status of the second most important preventative tactic after reducing smoking, while the NSF for CHD demands that all NHS bodies, working in tandem with local authorities, establish programmes to increase physical activity, supported by 'green' transport plans and employee-friendly policies, and that every hospital should have clinical audit data that describe the total number and percentage of those recruited to cardiac rehabilitation who are physically active one year after discharge (Hillsdon et al, 2004). The *National Service Framework for Mental Health* does not include such targets but does advocate that "exercise, relaxation and stress management have a beneficial effect on mental health"(DH, 1999b).

The links between transport and health were also made explicit by the White Paper *A new deal for transport* (DETR, 1998), which stressed the access needs of the community as a whole. As a consequence, walking and cycling strategies now form part of Local Transport Plans (LTPs) and School Travel Plans (STPs), with accompanying targets to increase healthy transport choices, and it has been suggested these should be further encouraged through local authority grants (Kelly, 2004). Chapter Seven has, however, already highlighted the tensions between such policies and the continued reliance on the car for short journeys. It has also been noted that while a reduction of urban speed limits to 20 miles per hour (mph) might change cyclists' (and pedestrians') perceptions of safety, responsibility for speed reduction has been passed to local authorities without any extra resources and existing 30 mph speed limits are enforced only at 37 mph (Carnall, 2000). A study of 110 20 mph zones introduced in Kingston upon Hull suggests, however, that reluctance to invest might be a product of a typically limited approach to cost-benefit analysis. Here an investment of £4 million was estimated as having produced benefits of £40 million (IPPR, 2002, cited in Davis et al, 2005).

Similar tensions surround nutrition. The government's own health strategy, summarised within *Our healthier nation* (DH, 1999a), acknowledges that diet is central to our health throughout life and is therefore integral to balancing health inequalities. As noted previously the national Five-a-day programme is a cornerstone of this policy. Yet, as Chapter Fourteen later illustrates, the advertising spend on food by industry is of a vastly different order to spend by government on initiatives such as Five-a-day.

The Food Standards Authority (FSA) was established in 2000 as a consequence of the lack of confidence in the food industry. Its priorities encompass the improvement of dietary health (including the enforcement of food laws) and the reduction of inequalities by encouraging the disadvantaged and vulnerable to improve their diet (FSA et al, 2002). This includes an increasing role for local government who, in addition to traditional activity in areas such as allotments, meals on wheels and community dieticians can now, as a function of their well-being powers, use social and economic regeneration to improve eating habits. Local food policies are increasingly integrated into the community planning process, Health Improvement and Modernisation Plans and Local Agenda 21 strategies, as well as linking to anti-poverty strategies in many areas. The government's Policy Action Team 13 also explored geographical access to food as part of the government's National Strategy for Neighbourhood Renewal (NSNR). This similarly recommended local community-based and small-scale retailer-orientated solutions. Community cafes handling and preparing food and providing healthy, low-cost food to the local community have been a common response.

An important source of funds is the New Opportunities Fund (now the Big Lottery Fund), established by the 1998 National Lottery Act. It covers the areas of health, education and the environment, and aims to target Lottery funding on areas of social exclusion and disadvantage. A budget of £300 million from the Fund was allocated to Healthy Living Centres across the UK with the intention of improving health through community action and reducing inequalities in health in deprived areas. Funding for the Centres, which aimed to be accessible to some 20% of the UK's population and to take a holistic approach to health, was allocated by September 2002 with most Centres supported until 2006.

The Public Health White Paper *Choosing health* (HM Government and DH, 2004) prompted work with the farming and food industries to promote a Food and Health Action Plan to develop 'corporate social responsibility' (around, for example, the development, labelling, promotion and pricing of healthy foods) (DH, 2005). A model already existed in Scotland where *Eating for health* (Scottish Office, 1996) was shaped by a two-year inquiry, involving stakeholders from agriculture, the retail industry, public health and consumer interest groups and the publication in 1994 of a series of targets for dietary improvement. The main recommendations, confirmed subsequently by the White Paper *Towards a healthier Scotland* (Scottish Office, 1999), are to shape consumer tastes through information, advice and practical skills, to supply food for a healthier diet and to understand food better, including a model contract for catering specifications for wide use by public agencies and workplaces. The inequalities and preventive dimension is highlighted by an emphasis on targeting residents in low-income areas and the professionals who work with them, parents, young children and schools.

Overall, however, *Choosing health* maintains the focus on interventions that address lifestyle factors at an individual level. Two of the six overarching priorities are reducing obesity and improving diet and nutrition, and encouraging exercise. This, it suggests, is about marketing health, supporting individuals, as consumers, to make healthier choices, including the use of NHS trainers as a personal health resource, advising individuals on how to improve their lifestyle and the development of personalised health guides. It also suggest that inequalities in health can be addressed by "getting information across to people in different groups and securing better access to healthier choices for people in disadvantaged groups or areas" (HM Government and DH, 2004, p 6).

Policy as advocated by the DH adheres closely to the focus of the evidence base, advocating counselling and support for behaviour change, the identification of individual strategies and the promotion of an active workforce alongside exercise referral into a recognised system with appropriately qualified staff and participation in community-based activities such as 'health walks' (DH, 2002b). Thus, like the evidence base, the emphasis is very much on individualised interventions. Although discussion in the White Paper of the introduction of voluntary codes, for example, in food advertising, at least acknowledges the wider context in which food 'choices' are made, questions have been raised as to whether the government's strategy for public health goes far enough in targeting this wider context (see Chapter Fourteen).

Health and lifestyle: smoking and alcohol

The critical role played by smoking in health inequalities in the UK has been stressed throughout this book. It impinges on early life through smoking in pregnancy and in the home, and is a part of many children's own lifestyle by late childhood. The key interventions as they relate to pregnant women and children and adolescents have, therefore, already been outlined (see Chapters Five and Nine), and a large part of that discussion also pertains to the adult arena. There is, however, one important difference. Whereas many of the cessation programmes aimed at these groups contain question marks as to efficacy, the review-level evidence for smoking cessation in adulthood is both more extensive and positive.

What works? Evidence and practice

In a clinical setting with a clinician even minimal contact (less than three minutes per session) can increase abstinence rates, with effectiveness increasing with contact until a threshold is reached at between 31 and 90 minutes. Such evidence for effectiveness spans a range of health practitioners from physicians to general practitioners (GPs), nurses, dentists, psychologists and counsellors and a variety of format types (Naidoo et al, 2004), suggesting "the involvement of all health professional in smoking cessation interventions ... should be encouraged" and GPs should maintain and enhance brief interventions on smoking as part of their routine consultations (Kelly, 2004, p 2). Counselling and behavioural therapies such as stress management can further increase abstinence, as can follow-up support (including the telephone support provided by smokers' helplines), social support such as buddy systems, help with the cost of therapies, high-profile mass media and public education campaigns and an increase in the price of tobacco (Naidoo et al, 2004). Similar smoking cessation strategies are reported as effective for different target groups such as men and women, minority ethnic groups and older people. In contrast, self-help materials are found to have only a small effect, improving if they are tailored specifically to the individual.

Significantly, while many such interventions target vulnerable groups, they tend not to address their differential effectiveness and thus contribute little to the health inequalities agenda. A range of studies demonstrates, however, that successful quitting is related to older age, higher education or social status, low prior tobacco consumption and a non-smoking partner. Hence the burden of higher tobacco prices, for example, is likely to be felt disproportionately by those on lower incomes who tend to have the greatest difficulty in stopping smoking (Secker-Walker et al, 2004). The same association has been demonstrated for long-term quitting with, for example lower success rates among unemployed people. Unsuccessful quitters are thus likely to remain clustered among the disadvantaged, suggesting those below the median income require special attention in terms of smoking cessation services and treatments (Kelly, 2004). Not surprisingly, success among older smokers has been attributed to the emergence of health problems, with recent hospitalisation and the development of CHD appearing predictive (Osler and Prescott, 1998). This suggests individualisation of risk remains a potent force for change. Somewhat paradoxically, health promotion interventions are often not provided for those with mental illness, despite high rates of smoking, obesity, a poor diet and lack of exercise.

It is also important to note that while community interventions are advocated because of their multifaceted nature and their ability to address the broad societal context in which the decision to smoke is made, the most rigorous studies show limited evidence of an effect on prevalence at the community level, with a range of studies suggesting a net decline in intervention communities of between −1% and +3% per annum (Secker-Walker et al, 2004). Only two such community interventions have been the subject of an RCT in the UK, the Action Heart Project and Heartbeat Wales (Baxter et al, 1997; Tudor Smith et al, 1998). The latter, despite embracing mass media, health professionals, businesses and schools across the country, and utilising smoking cessation counsellors, stop-smoking groups and self-help groups, found no intervention effect across five years.

This was attributed in part to the rapid diffusion of many of the interventions beyond Wales while the programme was still in progress. However, it has also been stressed that health promotion for the prevention of CHD in adults consistently shows only small changes to the risk factor and no significant reduction in mortality except when applied to populations at high risk (such as people with hypertension or pre-existing cardiovascular disease) (Ebrahim and Davey Smith, 1997, 1998). As Box 11.4 shows, wider application, particularly when allied to a community development approach, may still be considered effective in the context of a more holistic definition of health gain. Attitudinal research would also tend to support a geographical focus, particularly one that is linked to regeneration, because of the lack of culture of quitting among the most deprived and the low priority typically accorded to the health risks associated with smoking compared to the enormity of other difficulties of daily living,

---

Box 11.4: Women, low income and a smoking initiative

It has long been recognised that smoking plays a complex role in the daily lives of women on a low income (Graham, 1993). Between 1996 and 1999, ASH (Action on Smoking and Health) Scotland was awarded funding from the Health Education Board for Scotland for a three-year project designed to facilitate community initiatives on women, low income and smoking (Gaunt-Richardson et al, 1998). Twenty diverse community-based initiatives were funded under the scheme, with a total project budget of £37,000. These included educational and recreational opportunities and emotional support for women with mental health problems (McKie et al, 1999), a dance and drama group for a rural community development on an isolated island (Barlow et al, 1999), and work with women who had experienced homelessness (Amos et al, 1999) – all groups with high levels of smoking.

A series of project evaluations proposed that the key indicator of success was not the number of people who had quit (typically limited), but process measures such as the confidence to address smoking behaviour, consideration of the wider implications of lifestyle, enhanced access to a range of services and continuation of discussion, activity and exercise groups beyond project funding. Constraints to community-based work included practical, psychosocial, process and infrastructure barriers including a lack of transport and childcare. The programme also found that community-based work "in tobacco control, and health promotion more generally, requires considerable support not only in terms of long-term funding but also appropriate advice, expertise and resources" (Gaunt-Richardson et al, 1998, p 311).

A more recent Scottish initiative, Breathing Space, founded on community development principles, aims to produce a significant shift in community norms towards non-toleration and non-practice of smoking in a low-income area in Edinburgh by focusing on four main health promotion settings (community, primary care, youth and schools, and the workplace [Ritchie et al, 2004]).

such as poor housing, unemployment, limited education, debt, crime and social isolation (Jackson and Prebble, 2002).

A recent review of initiatives to reduce the prevalence of exposure to second-hand smoke shows that bans (and to a lesser degree restrictions) on smoking in the workplace reduce exposure to second-hand smoke. This applies not only to employees. It also appears to be associated with community-wide reductions in self-reported exposure. Similarly, comprehensive institutional bans, if resourced and supported, are effective in reducing smoking in public places, with less intensive strategies such as signage allied to restrictions being partially effective (Taylor et al, 2005).

Heavy alcohol consumption is implicated in the key NSF areas of mental health, cancer and cardiovascular disease. It is also a source of concern in the regeneration agenda with links, as outlined later, with crime, violence and neighbourhood management. Most evidence, certainly at systematic review level, relates to the hospital or primary care setting. Here there is some evidence that heavy drinkers are twice as likely to moderate their drinking over the next 6-12 months as a result of a brief 5-20 minute intervention, with extended brief interventions (including several visits, counselling or motivational work) increasing effectiveness still further. This is particularly true for women (Waller et al, 2002; Kelly, 2004). Even very brief opportunistic interventions can be effective for those not seeking treatment, as can alcohol screening interventions in hospital emergency departments. However, despite the fact that it is the workplace that is a key location for much occupational and professional socialisation among people in the heavier drinking groups, there is a dearth of systematic review-level evidence about either workplace or community interventions (Waller et al, 2002). High-quality server training, accompanied by management support, is one exception, highlighted by the Health Development Agency (HDA) as a national intervention where the likelihood of success is high (Kelly, 2004, p 2). It has also been shown that blood–alcohol concentration laws and allied breath testing are effective against alcohol-related crashes and injuries (Mulvihill et al, 2005).

Policy

The policy background relating to smoking cessation has largely been outlined earlier in this book. Standard One of the NSF for CHD established that the NHS and partner agencies should develop, implement and monitor policies that reduce the prevalence of coronary risk factors in the population, and reduce inequalities in risks of developing heart disease. Standard Two argues that they should contribute to a reduction in the prevalence of smoking in the local population. In practice, this translates into recording the current smoking status of patients, providing opportunistic advice to smokers during routine consultations, including the prescription of nicotine replacement therapy (NRT) or bupropion in appropriate cases, and referring smokers onwards to a cessation service with health professionals such as nurses, health visitors, midwives and pharmacists trained to act as smoking cessation advisors. It also demands a focus on risk groups such as smokers in manual socio-economic groups and pregnant smokers, implying accessible services and behavioural support, usually on a group therapy basis, and one-to-one counselling in accessible settings such as GP surgeries and pharmacies (DH, 2002b).

The NHS Cancer Plan sets out to reduce the risk of cancer through reducing smoking and promoting a healthier diet and to raise public awareness with better, more accessible information. Tackling inequalities is one of the aims. Increased *Smoking kills* targets (see Chapter Five) aim to reduce smoking among manual groups from 32% in 1998 to 26% by 2010 and to make this explicit in the 20 health authorities with the highest smoking rates by producing local targets for these areas. A key component of this strategy, as already noted, is the NHS smoking cessation services, with results from the evaluation suggesting they have been effective in reaching smokers from the most disadvantaged areas (Chesterman et al, 2005). Of course, risk is not just associated with active smoking. It has been suggested that, across the lifecourse, second-hand smoke is the third leading cause of preventable death (Hovell et al, 2000, cited in Taylor et al, 2005). Consequently, bans in public places and workplaces to reduce involuntary exposure to tobacco smoke are moving rapidly from the local to the national scale, led again by action in Scotland.

The communities most at risk tend also to have poor access to preventative health services including cancer screening programmes. The £23.25 million Living with Cancer initiative thus directs New Opportunities Fund money for palliative care to deprived communities, targeting the socially deprived and ethnic groups, while by 2002 each primary care trust (PCT) is expected to have a trained healthcare professional to support smokers wanting to quit. A small national initiative with major employers also aims to help develop smoking policies for the workplace (DH, 2000b). Under the auspices of *Choosing health* (HM Government and DH, 2004), proposed restrictions on the advertising of tobacco will be tighter. However, only a partial ban on smoking in pubs and restaurants will be made, again leading to charges that the government's White Paper does not go far enough in addressing the wider context of health-damaging behaviours.

Policy with respect to alcohol encapsulates the same basic tensions as that relating to smoking. Legislation, allied to media and information campaigns and random breath testing, has long focused on de-normalising and reducing drink driving. It prohibits the sale of alcohol to those already drunk and increasingly criminalises the antisocial behaviour induced by alcohol. At the same time, alcohol is widely used (by an estimated 90% of adults in the UK), and licensing laws have been progressively relaxed over an extended period. Alcohol also makes a substantial contribution (estimated at £30 billion per annum) to the UK economy (with the drinks market estimated to support about one million jobs) and £7 billion per annum raised in excise duties. Policy has been criticised, therefore, for being unduly influenced by the drinks industry rather than public health or safety.

As noted above, the effects of legislation (other than drink driving), fiscal measures, education and the mass media, and the creation of a safer drinking environment (more seating and more information on safer drinking) have not been evaluated. With respect to the former, the Royal Colleges and the British Medical Association have called for a lowering of the blood-alcohol concentration for driving to 50mg per 100 ml in line with both most European countries and the evidence base. The potential for workplace policies to exert an impact on attitudes and drinking behaviour similarly remains neglected (Mulvihill et al, 2005). The *Alcohol harm reduction strategy for England* (Cabinet Office, 2004), outlined in Chapter Nine, does, however, focus on reducing the harm caused by crime and antisocial behaviour as well as that caused to health because of binge and chronic drinking. Measures include better education and communication, improved health and treatment services, action to combat alcohol-related crime and disorder and working with the alcohol industry. It advocates, for example, more extensive use of police powers against problem drinkers and a contribution by pubs and clubs to the costs of policing alcohol-related crime and disorder. It also expects the drinks industry to make a financial contribution to schemes that address misuse at the national and local level, and NHS staff to be trained to identify alcohol-related problems earlier.

The psychosocial environment: community regeneration

Psychosocial factors offer, as Chapter Two notes, a possible explanation for neighbourhood effects, potentially acting through social cohesion, position in the social hierarchy and the quality of social networks to influence health status. The significance of the local environment varies across the lifecourse, assuming more importance for young families and older people as well as those on a low income and those who are less mobile. The decline of locally based community relationships and resources can, therefore, systematically disadvantage those of lower socio-economic status. While there is relatively little evidence for a neighbourhood effect on mental health (Propper et al, 2004), there is a significant, albeit small association between the experience of poor mental health and the characteristics of the neighbourhood for certain groups, notably women, those who are not white, and those who are less educated. These compound the modest effects of the social and physical environment on wider health status (see Chapter Two). The neighbourhood is thus a potentially important site for health-related interventions yet, paradoxically, "offers least to those for whom it has the greatest significance" (Forrest and Kearns, 1999, p 21). Increased interest is thus being displayed in the relationship between community regeneration and health.

What works? Evidence and practice

Skifter Andersen suggests efforts to regenerate communities can be classified under 10 headings. These include physical renovation, active marketing, community empowerment and efforts to counter crime, increase social support and access to education and job training (Skifter Andersen, 2002). In practice, however, he found little evidence of such an analytical approach or that content was informed by a clear strategy. Parkinson (1998) similarly synthesising European practice found increasing use of area-based approaches but little conclusive evidence of identifiable improvements in socio–economic circumstances. Evaluation from a health perspective is made more difficult by the fact that such reviews do not often explicitly consider health (Stewart and Taylor, 1995; Forrest and Kearns, 1999). However, as Ambrose forcibly notes, the "looseness of specification of both 'causes' and 'effects', and the unknown influences of the obvious confounding variables" should not be accepted as argument against the manifest links between poor living conditions and health status (Ambrose, 2001, p 9).

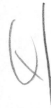

Physical renovation

There is a moderately strong suggestion that the spectrum of housing improvements encompassed under the community regeneration banner can improve mental health (Curtis et al, 2002; Macintyre et al, 2003; Thomson et al, 2003). Physical improvements appear central to such improvement. A Scottish survey encompassing nearly 3,000 households in different housing circumstances found that the home had psychosocial benefits as a haven, a locus of autonomy and a source of status. "More than any other feature … the presence of problems … such as dampness, lack of warmth and space, too much noise and general disrepair detracts from the acquisition of psycho–social benefits from the home" (Kearns et al, 2000, pp 405-6).

Rehousing and regeneration projects also appear capable of improving social outcomes (see Box 11.5). This includes perceptions of community participation and safety, as indicated, for example, by reduced fear of crime and increased incidence of social support (Thomson et al, 2001).

> **Box 11.5: The health gain associated with the Single Regeneration Budget**
>
> The research programme 'Cost-effectiveness in Housing Investment' has been working since 1993 to establish the exported costs to services such as health, education and policing which result from poor living conditions. A chronological study of the health gain associated with improvements to two run-down estates as part of the Central

Stepney SRB found a sevenfold improvement in illness days between 1996 and 2000. The main causes of ill health had been coughs and colds, aches and pains, asthma, bronchial problems, digestive disorders and depression. Comparison with the annual healthcare costs in an area of improved housing in Paddington with the Stepney estates pre-improvement similarly found a sevenfold difference, suggesting significant costs exported from the housing sector to the NHS.

The positive changes in health were considered clearly associated with improvements carried out under the SRB programme. Overcrowding, and levels of damp, cold and infestation all improved, alongside repairs and housing management. There was also a better sense of personal security and less fear of crime, higher satisfaction levels with local schools and a strengthened sense of belonging (Ambrose, 2001).

Russell and Killoran (2000) similarly draw on a redevelopment project in Hackney, where consultants found visits to the doctor and demand on the NHS dropped by one third, and improvements were recorded across a range of well-being indicators such as reduced calls to the police and fire brigade. Subsequent to the redevelopment there was also increased confidence to open the door to unexpected visitors and to let children play outside without supervision and reduced incidence of bullying. As with mental health, physical improvements appear central to social outcomes. Halpern (1995) found the introduction of community safety measures, traffic calming and children's play facilities reduced anxiety, depression and fear of crime while improving self-esteem and the perceived friendliness of an area.

The Joseph Rowntree Foundation's Area Regeneration Research Programme (see Box 11.6) found that housing design and estate layout also influenced the socialisation of children and the degree of informal interaction among residents (Forrest and Kearns, 1999). High-rise housing, for example, has been frequently identified in the UK context as more vulnerable to damage than traditional streets and lacking in environmental interest for children and possibilities for their informal supervisory care. The combination of density and physical isolation may also place particular demands on those who have below average social assets (Freeman, 1993).

Box 11.6: Community-led environmental improvements

The inner-city areas of Hyson Green and Forest Fields in Nottingham were two of the eight study areas included in the Joseph Rowntree Foundation's Area Regeneration Research Programme. Both had received Urban Task Force monies since the late 1980s, and at the time of the study were part of the Nottingham Partnership Council and in receipt of funds from the European Urban Programme. Across the study as a whole, residents rejected the hyperbole of large-scale regeneration and, in addition to jobs, requested small-scale local amenities and good public services with a local presence (Forrest and Kearns, 1999, p 48). Environmental improvements instigated by residents and local traders such as security gates, traffic calming measures, a business planning service and Hyson Green in Bloom project were found to have both enhanced the environment and led to social development. The latter was the result of improving communication and intergenerational assistance among residents as a result of project implementation, greater use of the neighbourhood, increased community confidence and security. Facilitating factors included community ownership, dedicated leadership, a responsive and flexible local authority with decentralised area management and a dense street pattern within which to implement improvements (Forrest and Kearns, 1999).

Substantive change on the ground appears related to significant investment. It has been estimated that the regeneration of the Castle Vale estate in Birmingham involved an expenditure of £145 million, the North Edinburgh Regeneration Partnership £76 million and the Meadow Well Estate on Tyneside £37 million (Hastings and Dean, 2003). Another key variable is the importance of partners agreeing a long-term strategy and raising tenants' capacity to play active roles as stakeholders (Evans, 1998).

Local reputation

Stigma exacerbates neighbourhood decline. It affects the population balance of an estate via selective out-migration while high levels of mobility are detrimental to the ability of people to access primary healthcare and education. Stigma also affects "the confidence of other groups which play key roles in determining neighbourhood trajectories" (Hastings and Dean, 2003, p 172). Businesses are thus reluctant to locate in the area, employers are felt to discriminate against estate residents, private sector services withdraw and the quality of public services can be undermined.

There has been an assumption in the past that reputation will improve alongside material conditions. However, it has proved more difficult to tackle the stigma associated with a neighbourhood via estate regeneration (Cole and Smith, 1996; Forrest and Kearns, 1999). The persistence of a problem image is now known to create barriers to the spread of knowledge and change (Hastings and Dean, 2003), while living in an area with a poor reputation or containing problem neighbours can mean residents are unable to derive any psychosocial benefits from their home (Kearns et al, 2000). Effective communication about change, including the employment of public relations staff and the attitudes of the local media, can be crucial, as are the visibility of change and provision of reasons to visit including, for example, sports or cinema complexes.

One of the most salient socio-economic features of problem estates is the high density of children (Cole and Smith, 1996), which, compounded by limited adult supervision, results in increased vandalism and wear and tear. Other common characteristics are a high percentage of lone parents and high unemployment rates. Curtis et al (2002) point to the importance of factors such as a community lettings policy to encourage key workers to stay in the area and a community investment fund to support improved community facilities. Other contributory factors to an effective social mix are considered to be layout and density (with implications for community safety), tenant involvement and ownership (the use of local labour, for example). Problems of image are often, however, intractable. The NSNR discusses the role of problem reputation but proposes no specific measures to address the problem (Hastings and Dean, 2003).

Community empowerment

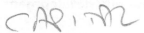

The much debated notions of *community* (based around shared characteristics of place, interest or attachment [Crow and Allan, 1994]) and *social capital* appear important to considerations of psychosocial health. Social capital has been variously defined as the social resources, norms and networks, processes or conditions that are central to healthy and economically viable communities (Mackian, 2002; Morrow, 2002). It is likely to be a scarce resource in areas where community has been eroded through population churning. It is also likely to be scarce in areas identified for regeneration given that social interaction is underpinned by attributes of the neighbourhood such as safety, familiarity and engagement and shared places. Yet, it is a potentially critical resource for partnership and a key component of governance, allowing individuals or groups to increase their capacity to interact with and influence other loci of government. It is argued to be created through civic participation and thus capable of being fostered by policy interventions. From a health perspective it is measurable via, for example, an increased sense of community and well-being and engagement in a health-promoting activity (Swann and Morgan, 2002).

It is also a highly elastic concept (Lynch et al, 2000), and one which is both difficult to operationalise and inadequately contextualised (Morrow, 1999). Recent contributions have argued forcibly that in order to maximise relevance, the concept of social capital must focus not just on what can be described as engendering social support at the community level (informal, horizontal networks), but "the most fundamental aspects of our political, legal and institutional structures" (Lynch et al, 2000, p 407). That is, it must include the broader context of vertical structures that limit the way knowledge, power and resources can be used across these networks and the role of state agency in facilitating the development of social capital. Scott (2004), for example, describes how changes in organisational culture and the creation of what he terms relational resources (such as a desire to cooperate rather than a duty to cooperate), proved an important step in creating mutual respect and trust and hence increasing social capital within the context of rural regeneration. Without sufficient social capital, it is argued, regeneration policies will not take root or be sustainable (Forrest and Kearns, 1999, p 9).

Curtis et al (2002) outline the theoretical justification for health gain consequent on renovation and associated community empowerment. Here, information leads to involvement, changes in behaviour and an increased ability to access services. Providers are better able to deliver services to a population that is less transient and alienated and improved demographics are achieved by virtue of more people staying in the area. To this can be added collective action to build/improve infrastructure and an emphasis on preventative action. Box 11.7 illustrates some of the ways in which community development can result in health gain.

Box 11.7: Community development as a source of health gain

In 1986 a community development project in Edinburgh prompted research into the relationship between damp housing and health status (Platt et al, 1989). A double-blind design established links between damp and particular streets and structures and with emotional distress in women and gastrointestinal problems and infections in children (Hunt, 1993). Spin-offs extended beyond housing improvements both locally and in other deprived communities to embrace other health-related initiatives such as a stress centre, exercise clubs, a fruit and vegetable cooperative and the securing of urban aid funding to improve access to services for older people (Whitehead, 1995, p 35).

In contrast, the Wise People's Project on the Cowgate Estate in Newcastle upon Tyne is still in its pilot phase. It had its origins in the high level of stress-related problems identified by a group of local women (in an area with a visible drug problem and no full-time dedicated health worker). Volunteer counsellors received training in stress management, depression, anxiety and anger management and, with support from the city council and mental health trust, are now based in a local community school (Cameron et al, 2003, p 41).

A qualitative study of health in two relatively deprived communities by the Health Education Authority similarly found better health to be associated with the trust of other community members, widespread informal networks encompassing friendship, leisure and work and the perceived power of citizens as measured by local activism and lobbying (Russell and Killoran, 2000). Facilitating factors are well-rehearsed in the literature on partnership. In addition to information they include commitment by key stakeholders, trust, reciprocity and respect, accountability, agreed vision, adequate timescales, support and training and access to resources that can be controlled locally (see, for example, Dowling et al, 2004). At the same time there is considerable stress in the literature on the "value of small schemes as opposed to mega schemes from outside" (Stewart and Taylor, 1995, p 62), not least because they are able to respond flexibly to changing circumstances. Research suggests, however, that while social capital and social support have positive effects on mental health and self-reported health, they "do not mediate (and only moderate some of) the effects of the basic structural factors" such as education and social class (Pevalin and Rose, 2003, p 1).

Constraints to effective regeneration

The potential for health gain in both material and psychosocial terms may be limited by the short-term nature of many regeneration schemes (as opposed to the time required to create partnerships and community involvement), their tendency to address symptoms rather than the structural factors causing inequality, to focus on limited aspects of deprivation and encompass but localised areas and selected populations. Work on the Neighbourhood Renewal Programme, for example, identified six key barriers that had restricted progress: failure to address the problems of local economies, to promote safe and stable communities, improve poor core services and involve communities, together with a lack of effective leadership and partnership, and lack of information (SEU, 2001). The Stepney case study highlighted in Box 11.5 found that the health gain associated with the SRB programme was being undermined by reductions in mainstream spending on health, education and law and order both in situ and in adjacent areas not eligible for area-based funding (Ambrose, 2001).

It is also acknowledged that redevelopment can cause stress and alienation and has the potential to increase health inequalities. The most impoverished and deprived tenants may, for example, be unable to afford the refurbished housing even at controlled rents, increased rent levels can have consequent negative impacts on job-seeking behaviour and nutrition (Thomson et al, 2003), and extended families may be separated by occupancy restrictions (Ambrose, 2001).

Policy

There is an already long and varied history of regeneration programmes in the UK, reflecting changing political beliefs and priorities (Stewart and Taylor, 1995; Foley and Martin, 2000; Russell and Killoran, 2000; Curtis et al, 2002). These range from the 1968 Urban Programme, which focused on just 12 community development projects in inner cities (but encouraged significant local involvement and challenged assumptions about the causes of deprivation), through to the economic and property-based schemes of the 1980s (formulated largely by local and central government but requiring private sector involvement and relying on the 'trickle-down' effects of economic growth), before reflecting renewed concern with the social and community aspects of regeneration in the 1990s and an emphasis on ABIs. Social exclusion, the involvement of the community and the need for interdepartmental working thus all have a long pedigree. The resulting programmes have not, however, significantly influenced mainstream service delivery or expenditure (Rhodes et al, 2003).

Many of the ABIs such as the New Deals for Employment, Employment Action Zones and SRB5 maintained a focus on the traditional regeneration agenda and did not place health high on their list of priorities despite, as Cameron et al (2003) point out, with reference to mental health, the fact that the issue has a "fundamental and continuing impact on the success of the local initiatives they fund" (Cameron et al, 2003, p 13). In contrast, HAZs, the NDC and Healthy Living Centres have served to introduce health and community safety to this wider regeneration agenda but have not found it an easy task. Contributory factors include the proliferation of ABIs in the most deprived areas, the rapidity with which they have succeeded one another and their often overlapping agendas (all areas that the Regional Coordination Unit now aims to address). The disparate nature of the HAZ agenda (see Chapter Three) also meant that less than 5% of programmes were directed at housing or the physical environment with a further 12% focusing on community empowerment (Judge et al, 1999, p 35).

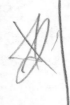

The key influences on the community regeneration and inequalities agenda and the place where health has had to make a mark have, therefore, been the Social Exclusion Unit, established in 1997 and two of its key policy responses (again see Chapter Three): the NDC (the most intensely resourced ABI in 30 years of urban policy in the UK, with funds of approximately £50 million per partnership or circa £5,000 per resident [Ralph and Peterman, 2004]) and the NSNR (supported by the Neighbourhood Renewal Unit or NRU). Both extend beyond housing and the physical fabric of neighbourhoods to encompass "the fundamental problems of worklessness, crime and poor public services" (SEU, 2001, p 5), with health forming one of five key outcome areas alongside employment, crime, education and housing, and programmes expected to encourage joined-up working between these key domains. The key difference is that the NSNR dose not rely on area-based funding (although some neighbourhood initiatives are included); instead, national policies are expected specifically to target the poorest neighbourhoods (Lupton and Power, 2005). Change is therefore centrally driven by a range of floor targets or Public Service Agreements (PSAs) established by the 2000 Spending Review. Enforced by the Treasury, these mean that, for the first time, government departments will be evaluated according to their performance in the most disadvantaged neighbourhoods (rather than with respect to national norms) (Hall and Hickman, 2002). Health inequalities, according to the New Commitment to Neighbourhood Renewal should, for example, be a key criterion for allocating NHS resources, and there are additional incentives to recruit and retain primary care staff in deprived areas alongside 200 Personal Medical Service Pilots designed to improve primary care (SEU, 2001).

Change is also supported by a new local delivery mechanism, Local Strategic Partnerships (LSPs). These are charged with bringing together the public, private, voluntary and community sectors, to improve the delivery of public services and the quality of life of people at the local level (DETR, 2001), and have been a condition of the Neighbourhood Renewal Fund (NRF) (the additional funding made available under the NSNR to the most deprived 88 local authorities in England) since 2002. LSPs are also considered to provide a way of local areas taking ownership of targets and setting their own targets, particularly if these are incorporated in local PSAs or Best Value Performance Plans.

The Social Exclusion Unit also advocates greater community involvement alongside a focus on reducing inequalities. This was reflected in revisions to earlier programmes such as the SRB where there was an increase in community and voluntary sector-led bids (Foley and Martin, 2000) prior to the scheme's dissolution by the Urban White Paper. It has also been reflected in NRF areas by the introduction of the Community Empowerment Fund (£35 million to enable community involvement in the LSP process) and the Community Chest which support local initiatives. The need for local ownership is also expected to be facilitated by Neighbourhood Management (£45 million in at least two rounds of Neighbourhood Management Pathfinders [2001-03]), which places a single person, team or organisation in charge at neighbourhood level – to help focus services on residents' needs by making service-level agreements, running local services, managing a devolved budget and putting pressure on higher tiers of government (NSNR, 2000a).

However, the implementation of such policies has not, as Chapter Three noted, been without its critics. The community-orientated approach to regeneration has proved a challenging one (not least because of the short-term nature of many of the initiatives with which it has been allied and the tensions between centrally defined targets and locally defined need). Significantly, a systematic review of the literature relating to community involvement in ABIs detected more change in the promotion of policy on community involvement than in practice (Burton et al, 2004). The evaluation of the NDC programme, for example, highlighted how floor targets had shifted the emphasis away from residents' concerns with vandalism and teenagers on the streets towards the reduction of burglaries (Lawless, 2004). The need for rapid and demonstrable improvements (and the pressures of partnership) can also distort intervention. Action in NDC areas, despite the wide-ranging agenda, has, for example, tended to focus on areas such as environmental clean-ups to the neglect of more challenging themes such as education and health. Indeed, an analysis of spending by outcome theme revealed that health had attracted the least commitment in 2001/02 (Lawless, 2004). Performance management has also been associated with a reluctance to allow experimentation that risks failure and hence a reluctance for regeneration managers to acknowledge the possibility of negative health impacts (Curtis et al, 2002). Most significantly, despite aggregate improvements in the poorest local authority areas and some convergence with respect to employment, education and teenage pregnancy, targets are unlikely to be met at the current level of intervention (Lupton and Power, 2005).

The psychosocial environment: crime

Crime is heavily concentrated in poorer areas and hence areas of ill health. Russell and Killoran (2000) report that 40% of crime is committed in just 10% of areas, locations where people are 10 times more likely to be a victim of personal crime and five times more likely to be a victim of property crime than in low-crime areas. Antisocial behaviour is also perceived to be twice as high in deprived areas as nationally (NSNR, 2000b). Perceptions of crime and fear of crime are not necessarily related to absolute levels. However, regeneration studies consistently find that being *a safe place* is the most highly rated neighbourhood attribute and that fear of break-ins and street crime is one of the main sources of mental stress and sometimes physical injury (Ambrose, 2001). Crime has been estimated to cost the UK £50 billion per annum (NSNR, 2000c).

The effects of crime on ill health extend beyond direct victims. It also affects non-victims (via fear, for example) and causes adjustments to lifestyle and behaviour. Both crime and fear of crime thus have implications for quality of life. Examples include not going out after dark or alone, avoiding particular areas and using public transport. Both victims and non-victims suffer from stress, depression, difficulties in sleeping, increased resort to cigarettes, alcohol and drugs and a drop in self-confidence. Women, people living alone and minority ethnic groups are disproportionately affected, while alcohol is often implicated in violent crime, particularly domestic violence.

What works? Evidence and practice

Stewart and Taylor (1995, p 47), reviewing the literature, find a number of collective approaches to crime prevention: reducing fear, improving security, improving environmental design, housing management and policing measures and preventing criminal behaviour through family, community and school-based activities. The Building Research Establishment, investigating the effect on health of building fabric, for example, suggested crime was one of the leading hazards in the home capable of mitigation by improvements to design and infrastructure (Raw and Hamilton, 1995, cited in Wilkinson, 1999). Another is reclaiming public space by engaging young people who are often the centre of concern over crime. Measures advocated include anti-truancy initiatives, youth and play provision and the inclusion of issues such as sexual harassment and bullying in the curriculum.

One initiative that potentially combines several of these features is the Neighbourhood Warden Schemes, defined as an official, visible and accessible presence in a residential area intended to assist in the maintenance of order. Policy Action Team 6 identified 50 such schemes across Britain, typically local authority-led with police involvement and supported by mainstream funding. Key functions were found to be crime prevention (often via a security patrol) and environmental improvements, together with housing management and community development. Evaluation was restricted to 16 of the schemes and limited in scope, but suggested that neighbourhood management could reduce crime, particularly juvenile disorder, and reduce residential mobility and the tensions caused by large numbers of voids. Estate visits found people "whose quality of life had palpably improved, whose self-esteem and confidence in themselves, their neighbours and their local services had risen greatly" (NSNR, 2000c, p 20). Successful schemes were seen to have clear objectives, resident, local authority and police involvement, good communications and training and continuity of wardens. They seemed to be particularly successful at reducing fear of crime among older people (Phillipson and Scharf, 2004).

An area of criminal activity where the health implications are even more explicit is domestic violence (see Box 11.8). The 2002 British Crime Survey suggested that domestic violence was a major crime in the country experienced by one in four women, and the government's *Living without fear* (Home Office and Cabinet Office, 1999) made it clear that Crime and Disorder Reduction Partnerships should identify the levels of domestic violence in their area and develop a strategy

---

Box 11.8: Tackling domestic violence

The Wakefield Domestic Violence Initiative sought to tackle the issue of domestic violence and put it on the public health agenda. The Initiative was one of five health projects in England in the Home Office's Crime Reduction Programme: Violence against Women, and was a partnership between Eastern Wakefield PCT, Support and Survival (a voluntary sector domestic violence organisation), the Police, Probation and Crown Prosecution Services and the Magistrates' Court.

Building on the known tendency for women to go to their GP surgery following a domestic violence incident, the aim was to enable GPs in 11 practices to identify domestic violence and to refer women appropriately. Participating GPs felt that they were able to provide a better standard of healthcare to women, and the project is to be extended across GP practices in the PCT. New funding has also been secured from the Home Office to fund a domestic violence project from October 2003. This will provide training and service delivery for the male perpetrators of domestic violence and a Strategy on Domestic Violence that is concerned with both survivors and perpetrators is being considered by the LSP (Harris, 2002, cited in Raj, 2003).

> Similar work, including a voluntary programme for perpetrators in the community and the screening of antenatal and postnatal women for domestic violence by health visitors and midwives, has been conducted in Cornwall, initially with support from the Cornwall and Isles of Scilly HAZ (Porter, 2002).

for addressing it as part of their broader strategy on crime reduction. Over 200 multiagency Domestic Violence Forums are now in place across the UK.

Research also suggests a strong link between heroin and crack cocaine use and some forms of crime. Indeed, a study of the retail drug market in eight deprived residential neighbourhoods in England suggests that regeneration per se will remain difficult without tackling drugs markets (Lupton et al, 2002). However, this is an area where multiagency strategies at the local level remain uncoordinated, enforcement has a limited impact, treatment is under-resourced and drugs education is not usually accredited in line with the new national standards (see Chapter Nine).

Policy

The 1998 Crime and Disorder Act aims to tackle youth crime, racially motivated crime, and antisocial behaviour. One product has been the creation of statutory Crime and Disorder Reduction Partnerships across England and Wales, with the police and local authorities having a duty to conduct a crime and disorder audit together with the local community and to implement a crime reduction strategy. Provisions include child safety orders (providing for curfews) and community safety orders. Ironically, however, the allied target under Neighbourhood Renewal returns the focus to crime rather than antisocial behaviour by aiming to reduce domestic burglary by 25% with no local authority district having a rate more than three times the national average by 2005.

The *Communities Against Drugs Initiative*, announced in April 2001, gave £220 million to Crime and Disorder Reduction Partnerships across three years to tackle drug-related crime in high-crime areas with significant drug problems. Suggested strategies included visible policing, neighbourhood wardens and support for community and parents' groups. The aim was to focus on local priorities, with local partnerships deciding how the money should be spent. Research has suggested that partnerships under the NDC be required to adopt a more strategic role to drug market activity, with Drug Action Teams (DATs) fulfilling the role in other areas (Lupton et al, 2002).

Community Safety Partnerships have also been introduced under the Safer Cities Programme, with the aim of reducing crime, reducing the fear of crime and encouraging a sound local economy as a means of generating a sense of well-being and safety. Specific measures include home security surveillance, CCTV and improvements to estate layout, schools and housing management.

The aim is to plan out crime as part of new build. This is supported, as noted earlier, by the £18.5 million Neighbourhood Wardens Scheme 2000-04.

Material deprivation: income and employment

"Tackling poverty is the most direct route to combating health inequalities" (Russell and Killoran, 2000, p 23). A low income affects where people live, their lifestyle, nutrition, access to credit and ability to heat their home, in other words, both access to the conditions necessary for health and choices in terms of healthy behaviour. Fuel poverty, for example, is defined as needing to spend more than 10% of household income on fuel in order to maintain a satisfactory heating regime (Fuel Poverty Advisory Group, 2003). In 2002 it was estimated that 1.9 million vulnerable households were fuel-poor, with 6.1 million families reporting some difficulties meeting debt repayments (FSA, 2004, p 72). Living in poverty can also cause stress and anxiety, adding a psychological dimension to the physiological and behavioural ones. Around one eighth of Citizens' Advice Bureau (CAB) debt advice clients, for example, are estimated to be receiving treatment for stress or depression consequent on their debt problems (CAB, 2003).

As Chapter Ten outlined, low income is not solely a feature of those who are not in employment. Those on a low-earned income or in insecure employment are also likely to experience poorer psychosocial working conditions, with a lack of individual control and limited social support, and to be exposed to more physical hazards. Unemployment itself causes deterioration in health not only for the person out of work but also their families. Unemployment rates are particularly high for minority ethnic groups and disabled people. While redundancy and unemployment are associated with an increased risk of mortality and morbidity, re-employment may not necessarily be associated with an improvement in security, income or health status (Glenn et al, 1998), and even positive changes in income are not rapidly followed by health improvement (Benzeval and Judge, 2001). Interventions focus on job creation and training, increasing available income and improving conditions at work.

What works? Evidence and practice

Job creation and training

It is now widely accepted that job creation alone "does not make a good basis for a regeneration strategy" (Chanan et al, 1999, p 12). Similarly, it is unlikely to provide a strong foundation for redressing health inequalities. Traditional regeneration programmes have been criticised for allocating a large proportion of their budget to employment yet creating jobs only for a minority of unemployed people. The non-employed, meanwhile, form an even larger population, estimated (even among those of working age) to be four times greater than the unemployed.

Nevertheless, the first five rounds of the SRB were estimated to have created or safeguarded some 690,000 jobs (Rhodes et al, 2003). Long-term capacity building is often also limited, linked to the regeneration programme itself, requiring skills lacking in local residents and possessing few local multipliers (Armstrong et al, 2001). An allied trend to displacement has also been noted, with those who are trained and employed tending to move on or, if they remain, squeezing out the most vulnerable as the local demographics change and house values rise (Chanan et al, 1999).

Research suggests that discrete efforts to improve employment prospects by allying job creation with training are similarly unlikely to secure a general improvement in the problems of an area (Skifter Andersen, 2002) and hence sustainable health gain. In some SRBs, for example, only 2% of working-age residents were found to have participated in government training schemes even though the majority (61%) of working-age households were headed by someone who was unemployed or otherwise economically inactive. Few residents were, therefore, "job-ready" (Rhodes et al, 2003, p 1420). A number of studies of active labour market interventions, where training is targeted to the local supply of jobs associated with regeneration, have suggested immediate and beneficial health effects arising from participation, including reductions in levels of anxiety and depression and improvements in social adjustment, self-esteem and satisfaction with life (Curtis et al, 2002). However, such findings are not consistent across interventions and tend to be variable with respect to long-term impact.

For many, when it comes to getting a job, it has been suggested that social contacts are more important than job-related skills, hence the importance of initiatives such as mentoring and job clubs (Fines and Griffiths, 2001). Step-by-step return to the formal labour market has also been attempted via intermediate labour market (ILM) initiatives, the creation of jobs in third sector (not-for-profit) organisations and managed workspace provision. Properly managed, research suggests the ILM model of waged work in specially created temporary jobs may deliver a more sustained progression from welfare to work than other programmes for the long-term employed (Marshall and Macfarlane, 2000) as well as contributing to neighbourhood regeneration via the provision of local services (see Box 11.9).

Box 11.9: Intermediate labour market (ILM) programmes

ILM programmes originated in Glasgow with subsequent growth stimulated by government programmes such as the New Deal. The core feature is paid work on a temporary contract. The aim is to embed long-term unemployed people in the labour market by providing not just supervised work experience but also training, confidence building and job search. It has been argued that this may require six to nine months of sustained support (Marshall and Macfarlane, 2000). Work typically focuses on additional economic activities, ideally of community benefit, in order not to replace existing jobs.

The Wise Group, for example, originated as a series of not-for-profit businesses in Glasgow providing home insulation, efficient heating systems, home security and safety together with environmental upgrading. Their activities thus had the additional benefit of raising the purchasing power of lower-income households by reducing fuel bills (McGregor et al, 1997).

A survey of current ILM jobs shows they are mostly held by 18- to 25-year-olds. Evaluation suggests over 60% can leave for employment compared to below 40% in other programmes. Where participants have been followed up, over 90% who gain a job are still in work after six months compared with less than 40% in other programmes. Drop-out rates are also lower than comparative programmes and long-term earnings higher. Operators have, however, faced problems with the security of funding from New Deal and European sources (Marshall and Macfarlane, 2000). Other weaknesses include a focus on men and a narrow range of commercial activities, hence training and employment opportunities (McGregor et al, 1997)

A specific case of supported return relates to those with a severe mental disorder. Levels of unemployment are high in this group in the UK, typically falling in the 61–73% range. Here, in helping obtain competitive employment, supported employment, where ongoing support is provided in a normal work setting, appears to be more effective than prevocational training following, for example, the sheltered workshop model. This applies whether success is measured by numbers in such employment, hours worked or wages earned. It is, however, less widely available (Crowther et al, 2004).

Another approach to job creation is to maximise local economic activity via the social or informal economy, thus increasing the circulation of money within the locality. Examples of the social economy include Local Exchange Trading Schemes (LETS), time banks and credit unions, self-help groups, training and job search schemes, community cooperatives and businesses such as childcare, community cafes, transport and recycling and development trusts. Community reinvestment trusts, for example, offer loans not only to individuals such as self-employed people and small businesses but to voluntary organisations and community enterprises.

A study of 20 community regeneration organisations in 10 UK cities found that effective community regeneration was associated with the permanence, financial independence and entrepreneurial skills contained within the organisation. Its sustainability was thus integral to the creation of regenerative capacity, measured in the short term by the ability to generate new projects and to withdraw from existing projects, and in the long term relative to jobs and enterprises created (Thake, 1995). In the Netherlands the concept of a social return, together with neighbourhood budgets, ensures that there is a spin-off from any major development for deprived neighbourhoods and that linkages are systematically developed with the wider economy, training and transport so that employment policy and community involvement work in tandem.

Increasing available income

Income can also be increased by tackling the problems of low benefit uptake. The provision of welfare advice in non-traditional settings, most particularly within primary healthcare, has been seen as one solution. It has a clear health inequalities dimension with many schemes targeting either older people or chronically disabled people, groups known to have low levels of benefit take-up and high levels of poverty.

A literature review of welfare advice in primary care identified 37 projects in the UK, mostly dating from the 1990s (Greasley and Small, 2002). Very few projects were subject to an experimental design but a number of important outcomes were outlined. First, accessibility to advice was increased because of raised awareness among patients and staff, the use of accessible locations, home visits and a reduction in stigma as a result of legitimisation by health workers. Second, the services functioned as a resource for health professionals, enabling more effective use of time, particularly in deprived areas where many consultations had a psychosocial basis. Third, there was some evidence, as Box 11.10 highlights,

---

Box 11.10: Welfare benefits advice in primary care

The CAB made welfare benefits advice available to seven GP practices in a deprived part of Liverpool, supported by home visits where necessary. A total of 68 participants were interviewed at referral and again six months later, with 40 of these interviewed again at 12 months. Most (76%) were able to apply for a new benefit, with 71% receiving an increase in income as a result of benefits advice. For the latter there was a statistically significant improvement six months later in levels of energy and tiredness, emotional role functioning, and mental health. This was attributed to factors such as improvements to diet and social activities because of increased income and an ability to pay household bills promptly. However, this was not maintained at a statistically significant level at the end of the 12-month period. One explanation was the high level of chronic morbidity among the claimants, the majority of whom had a physical disability. There was also a trend towards reduced GP consultations and the prescription of new drugs as opposed to an increase in the comparator group (Abbot and Hobby, 2000).

Similar results, although not at a statistically significant level, have been found in other studies and this is supported by a wealth of anecdotal evidence (Burton and Diaz de Leon, 2002; Greasley and Small, 2002). Lack of statistical significance is attributed to small studies and the circumscribed nature of the intervention in terms of the wider health context.

---

that the availability of such advice may lead to an improvement in the health and quality of life of patients and reduced use of NHS resources (Greasley and Small, 2002). Such services may also reduce the mental stress and frustration of dealing with the benefits system.

A second strategy is to increase available income by reducing outgoings. This has several potential strands such as increasing energy efficiency, reducing the cost of food through food purchasing cooperatives, community allotments and community cafes, tackling the issue of debt, most particularly the scarcity of loan products that are appropriate and affordable, and increasing financial literacy. Between 1979 and 2001, non-mortgage consumer credit increased by 1,248% to £131,883 million (CAB, 2001, p 10) and we witnessed a revolution in financial services in the UK. Yet, it has been estimated that seven million consumers in the UK have difficulties with literacy and numeracy, meaning they are unable to make the best use of financial services or the tax and benefit systems, are vulnerable to abusive practice and frequently take decisions that compound their indebtedness (CAB, 2001).

A minority of those in debt seek advice, so attention has focused on the development of advice services, signposting by front-line staff and the development of a financial literacy curriculum (see Box 11.11). Again few such initiatives have been formally evaluated or synthesised in the published literature. However, a survey of over 60 CAB projects designed to improve financial literacy defined effective practice as: community-based schemes; delivered in collaboration with key partners such as the Basic Skills Agency, health, the Probation Service, or schools; extending beyond debt prevention to encompass financial literacy issues such as insurance, savings and pensions; and focusing on advice around life-changing events (CAB, 2001).

Box 11.11: Debt advice

DAWN provides Debt Advice Within Northumberland, and started as a partnership between Northumberland Social Services, Northumberland Mental Health Trust, Northumberland HAZ and Northumberland College. It explicitly acknowledges the links between health and debt, aiming to improve the health of local people by reducing the stress of vulnerable individuals suffering the effects of debt. Four debt support workers are employed with peers trained to deliver financial assertiveness workshops in a variety of different locations such as community and Sure Start centres. A survey of psychological therapists suggested, however, that the most common cause of debt was the inadequate amount of money service users had to live on (Sharpe and Bostock, 2002).

The disadvantage of debt for poor people is typically widened by high interest rates and lack of access to cheap payment methods. Credit unions (of which there are some 700 in Britain) are owned and controlled by members and provide access to credit at affordable rates, enabling people to reassert control over their finances, while LETS potentially allow all residents to contribute to the local economy (North, 2000). Basic bank accounts have also been available since 2001, providing financial credibility and security without access to credit or cheque guarantee cards, while small loans can be arranged between, for example, housing associations and community banks. As part of their requirement to produce a social action plan, the energy regulators Ofgem have now proposed a series of one-stop shops based on developing the credit union model to provide energy advice, budgetary and monetary advice, energy efficiency measures and facilities for bill payments (NEA et al, 2002).

Improving conditions at work

A third option is to focus on the creation of health-enhancing working conditions and social and financial support during and after training. As Chapter Ten has shown, the health benefits of any job are not the same as those of a good job. There is a suggestion that only those re-employed in secure jobs show better levels of mental health than unemployed people, while temporary alternative employment may produce worsening physiological changes.

There are a limited number of evaluations of workplace interventions to reduce stress, as opposed to individual-orientated interventions such as stress management (Hogstedt and Lundberg, 2002). Whitehead (1995, p 42) reviewed initiatives attempting to improve psychosocial conditions in the workplace, and found that organisational changes (such as shift patterns and communication, including the involvement of workers in the identification of problems and their solution), can reduce stress. Improvements in productivity were often identified as a secondary gain. However, a systematic review of organisational interventions designed to reduce stress in the workplace found such interventions to be generally ineffective (van der Klink et al, 2001). High or improving supervisory support may nevertheless act as a buffer to the health risks associated with low or decreasing job control (Vahtera et al, 2000, p 492). Work in Stockholm with bus drivers suggests more attention should be given to the wider work environment. Here, physical design changes and technological innovation to reduce traffic congestion and lessen passenger demands on drivers were found to significantly reduce stress levels (Evans et al, 1999).

Policy

Policies have recognised the need to focus on reducing the risk of persistent poverty as this has been demonstrated to be the most damaging for health, hence the emphasis on education and the creation of work opportunities (Benzeval and Judge, 2001). There is also a case for taking preventative action by identifying those at risk of remaining unemployed long term (Campbell et al, 1998). In the early 1990s formal regeneration, through a series of Task Forces, City Action Teams, Training and Enterprise Councils, Business in the Community and City Challenge, focused on getting people into jobs and targeting the most deprived estates (Stewart and Taylor, 1995). The Priority Estates Programme meanwhile expanded from a focus on housing management and tenant involvement to employment creation, with one-stop shops aiming to integrate training and business development opportunities for estate residents.

A more recent response has been the establishment of 32 Action Teams for Jobs, set up in the highest unemployment areas in order to focus on locally identified barriers to work and to help deliver PSA targets set for the Departments for Education and Employment (DfEE) and Social Security (DSS) under the Neighbourhood Renewal banner. These aim to raise employment rates in the 30 local authority districts with the worst labour market position, generate more sustainable employment and increase employment rates of disabled people, lone parents, minority ethnic groups and those aged over 55. Policy relating to one such barrier, childcare, has been discussed in Chapter Five. At the same time Neighbourhood Renewal aims to increase adult skills in order to increase employability, with a particular emphasis on community-based learning

There has also been a renewed interest in community cooperatives, with good practice emphasising the importance of community cohesion and the existence of a community base before conditions are conducive to economic initiatives. Capacity building was introduced experimentally into the European Social Fund training programmes for unemployed people in the UK from 1997. The aim is to boost the capacity of local community organisations so that they can act as a bridge, drawing the most difficult to reach into activities that will increase their employability. Funding is also available for complementary activities such as counselling, mentoring and job searching (Chanan et al, 1999). The Home Office Active Community Unit now coordinates community activity, aiming to raise the numbers involved, remove the barriers to volunteering including those relating to benefits and availability for work and increase funding. The report from Policy Action Team 9, for example, proposed establishing a community resource fund and technical assistance vouchers together with a Neighbourhood Endowment Fund.

One obvious problem is that the community businesses thus created tend to reflect the employment profile of the estate, dominated by unskilled, low-paid and largely male jobs. Managerial failure is high, small business support often lacking, and it is difficult to make links with a hostile external environment. The £96 million Phoenix Fund, administered by the Small Business Service, aims to increase enterprise in deprived areas, while the Social Investment Task Force has proposed a community investment tax credit to bring investment and expertise into local economic renewal.

A parallel strand is the individualisation of responsibility. The New Deal programmes for young people, lone parents, long-term unemployed over 25, partners of the unemployed, disabled people and those over 50 have been introduced progressively since 1997 and have now been made permanent. A key innovation was to assign a Personal Advisor to every participant. Employment Zones (EZs), operational since 2000, have a broadly similar approach (see Chapter Three) but are located in areas with persistent problems of long-term unemployment, with providers selected by competitive tender (Hales et al, 2003). Such options focus, however, on those able to be economically active and make very little impression on those who are unable to enter paid employment on a full-time basis, a sector which can make up half of the adult population in the regeneration area. Not surprisingly, the New Deals have been better at helping those who need a little help rather than those with multiple disadvantage and special needs, with pressures on staff time combined with targets increasing the focus on the job-ready rather than intermediate outcomes such as social support and rehabilitation (Walker, 2001). For example, over half of those aged 50-65 who are out of work are on sickness and disability benefit yet between July 2001 and November 2003 only 1.9% of the population eligible for New Deal for Disabled People had registered with the programme (DWP, 2003).

Some programmes are attempting to address such deficits and help people into sustained employment, such as Work-based Learning for Adults, a voluntary training programme for adults without work and with poor employability skills, and StepUP, which provides a guaranteed job and support, including workplace buddies, for clients with extremely low employability after completion of a New Deal option. Nevertheless, evaluation of EZs, another initiative aimed at persistent long-term unemployment in 15 disadvantaged areas of Britain, found that in both these zones and a number of New Deal for 25 plus comparators almost half the participants had not been helped into work over two years (Hales et al, 2003).

Health damage is also associated with sudden drops in income, demanding protection at key transition points such as unemployment, retirement and divorce (Benzeval and Judge, 2001). The need to increase benefit uptake among entitled groups was one of the recommendations of the Acheson Report (1998), with the suggestion that welfare counsellors be located in primary care centres in deprived areas. This recommendation, together with changes in primary care, most particularly the creation of PCTs with responsibilities both for commissioning care and responding to local health needs (DH, 1997, 2000a), has given considerable impetus to the provision of welfare advice in primary care (Greasley and Small, 2002). In 1999, for example, health authorities were provided with £2 million to fund CABx to provide welfare advice in health settings. Community strategies with their integrated approach to economic, social, and environmental well-being, are similarly seen as a good place to address issues of debt.

Many of the recommendations made by the NRF Policy Action Team 14 on financial inclusion, such as support for basic bank accounts and credit unions, have now been implemented. Significant policy responses in terms of financial literacy include the *Skills for Life* and *Confident Consumers* programmes, both introduced in 2001. The former, with a £1.5 billion budget, aimed to reduce the number of adults with weak literacy or numeracy skills by 750,000 across the next three years, while the latter (through the Basic Skills Agency and Consumers' Association) was aimed at young adults with low numeracy or literacy. The establishment of the Community Legal Service has also been important, supporting, for example, dedicated debt advisors in many CABx (CAB, 2003). CAB has also called for a national strategy to improve financial literacy (including information, access, education and evaluation) and the financial literacy proofing of all government policies.

Material deprivation: housing

A first potent link between housing and health was severed by public health legislation in the late 19th and early 20th centuries. Yet, as Chapter Ten has shown, the enduring association between poor health and housing remains the subject of continuing epidemiological study, spanning the effects of housing quality, health selection, housing conditions and stress and homelessness. Generally, home ownership is associated with practical and psychosocial gains, reflecting not just the existence of fewer environmental health risks but also the possession of a financial asset, locational freedom and the flexibility to adapt to changing requirements across the lifecourse (Easterlow and Smith, 2004).

What works? Evidence and practice

There has been a long tradition of using housing interventions to meet social aims, including the provision of allied services and support, while up until the Second World War the Minister of Health was responsible for the nation's housing (Best, 1995). Yet there is a marked lack of studies, particularly prospective controlled studies, designed to establish the health effects of housing interventions (Ellaway and Macintyre, 1998). One systematic review of interventions relating to rehousing based on medical priority, population-wide rehousing, refurbishment and renovation, and improvements in energy efficiency, identified only 18 despite a search strategy that extended back to 1887. Just 11 of these were prospective and only nine included a control (Thomson et al, 2001). Most studies suggested some health gain as a result of the intervention. However, as the authors suggest, small size, a lack of control for confounding variables and high rates of attrition all limit generalisability.

The small number of studies also means that the range of potential health gains has not been adequately explored. They tend to focus on self-reported health rather than use of health services or the incidence of medical symptoms, although

Carr-Hill and colleagues (1993, cited in Morton et al, 2000) found that people in poor housing conditions consumed 50% more health services than expected, while in 1991 Boardman estimated the cost to the NHS of cold housing alone to be £800 million per year. Further shortfalls relate to the narrow definitions of housing and health, a focus on single-issue studies, a concern with children and older people and a neglect of context or content (Saegert et al, 2003).

Housing quality

As Chapter Ten noted, housing quality is most directly linked to individual health outcomes through the two related factors of cold and damp (Best, 1995; Morton et al, 2000). There is some evidence to suggest that energy efficiency measures and measures to prevent damp penetration can improve general health and well-being and reduce respiratory symptoms (Ambrose, 2001; Thomson et al, 2003). This combines with the inverse housing law to suggest that the targeting of poor-quality housing in areas of harsh climate is "likely to be an effective means of improving respiratory health and narrowing health inequalities" (Blane et al, 2000, p 748). Such housing improvements also reduce fuel bills and may be more effective, given population mobility, than targeting particular client groups (Somerville et al, 2000).

Hopton and Hunt (1996) found that the installation of heating in a low-income housing area reduced the incidence of damp, mould and cold, but their focus was only on child health where they found heating was able to prevent further deterioration but unable to improve symptomatic health, possibly as a consequence of rising unemployment and financial problems. For adults, symptoms due to housing conditions are more likely to be masked by previous health history (Hunt, 1993), and to be the subject of parallel influence by other concerns with a significant health dimension such as work and money worries (Evans et al, 2000). As Box 11.12 shows, even in the mild South West housing improvements designed to reduce condensation and dampness may have a health impact beyond respiratory gain.

Research investigating the excess winter deaths attributable to heart attacks and strokes similarly finds that improvements to the thermal efficiency of dwellings and the affordability of heating them would be of potential substantial public health benefit (Wilkinson et al, 2001), particularly if targeted at older households and dwellings with poor space heating. Targeted investment in new and improved housing could also "improve health by reducing the risks of accidents and fire, as well as overcrowding and cold, damp conditions" (Best, 1995, p 66).

As Box 11.12 suggests, there is increasing evidence to indicate that housing improvements need to be paralleled by initiatives to improve quality of life and enhance community life if they are to be sustainable (Evans, 1998; Skifter Andersen, 2002). Tackling health inequalities by targeting housing deprivation is not, therefore, just about improving amenities or reducing overcrowding but about

Box 11.12: The Watcombe Housing Project

At the time of intervention the largely local authority-owned Watcombe estate in Torquay was marked by high levels of unemployment and lone-parent households. It was also distinguished by high call-out and visiting rates from the local GP practice and poor housing conditions, including limited or non-existent central heating, poor ventilation and inadequate insulation. Dampness, condensation and mould were common problems. A quasi-random housing improvement programme was introduced with insulation, double glazing, re-roofing, heating, ventilation and rewiring installed in two distinct phases in 1999 and 2000. Surveys of the indoor environment were carried out before and after the improvement programme alongside health questionnaires which distinguished high levels of asthma and arthritis (Somerville et al, 2002). The subsequent health gain related not just to reduced respiratory distress but issues of mental health and domestic and social behaviour. Heating has enabled children, for example, to do homework upstairs rather than remain in the one heated room downstairs. Success is attributed not just to the physical improvements but also to the pre-existing Health Gain Initiative, which had employed a community development worker and raised community awareness on the estate.

the ways in which residents perceive their accommodation and neighbourhood, the degree of control they exercise over their home environment and the demands it places on them (Marsh et al, 2000; Dunn, 2002).

Housing stress and health selection

The potential to address health inequalities via the housing sector is increasingly prejudiced by the fact that home ownership has become the dominant tenure and accepted household norm whereas it was the public sector that was designed to be health selective and provide an element of healthcare (Smith and Mallinson, 1997; Easterlow et al, 2000; Easterlow and Smith, 2004). It is more difficult, therefore, to maintain the health component by focusing simply on a sector that now functions increasingly as a residualised safety net. It is also more difficult to ensure that the market does not discriminate against those with health problems or a disability.

Research suggests that those with poor health find it hard to attain owner-occupation not just because of their health but because of a lack of stable employment and increased reliance on benefits (Easterlow and Smith, 2004). They face similar difficulties sustaining their position in the housing market and maintaining the use and exchange value of their properties (Smith et al, 2004). Similar reservations surround the ability of the market to accommodate those on low or fluctuating incomes, with owner–occupation at the margins causing poverty, debt and health problems, particularly among those with no previous experience of debt (Nettleton and Burrows, 1998).This is not just a marginal problem – 1.3 million adults and children in Britain experienced mortgage repossession between 1990 and 1998 (Nettleton and Burrows, 2000).

Dunn (2000), reviewing the literature on medical priority rehousing found 'scant and equivocal' evidence of health improvement. In large part this stems from a paucity of studies. Generally, he suggests those rehoused on mental grounds improve (see also Thomson et al, 2003), while more equivocal results are obtained for those with physical health problems. This is largely supported by Smith et al (1997), who find that while medical rehousing is most commonly used to address physical health problems, particularly mobility or visual problems, the most notable health gains come from rehousing people with mental health problems. This is borne out by Box 11.13. Ironically, households with health and other housing needs may find themselves refused medical priority.

Box 11.13: The benefits associated with medical priority rehousing

A longitudinal study in Newcastle upon Tyne interviewed 253 households before and after determination and implementation of a medical priority rehousing application.

Medical priority rehousing was associated with net improvements in housing and environmental conditions. It was also associated with improvements in mental health and mobility. Respondents who were rehoused reported significant net improvements in depression, tiredness, sleeplessness, use of prescribed medication and use of medical services. Improvements were not equally distributed with respondents aged 50 and under more likely to report significant benefits. Nor was medical priority rehousing able to influence the incidence of acute respiratory problems or the prevalence of long-term illness and disability (Blackman et al, 2003).

Research also suggests less weight is attached to quality of life issues, access to formal services and to informal care, although these are key components of health need and amenable to improvement by relocation. Medical rehousing and community care tend, therefore, to be "seen as two quite distinct operations, rather than as two sides of a single coin" (Smith and Mallinson, 1997, p 193). The potential for greater alignment is explored in Chapter Thirteeen with specific reference to older people and the drift into residential and nursing care.

Provision for people with learning difficulties and people with mental health problems is more likely to be found in the special needs provision of housing associations. The lack of evidence as to what works in this area is strikingly reinforced by a Cochrane Review designed to establish the effects of supported housing, outreach support and standard care for people with severe mental disorders. Although setting out to establish service utilisation, mental state, social functioning and satisfaction with such varying models of care, the review was unable to find any studies that met the inclusion criteria (Chilvers et al, 2004).

As we have noted with respect to community regeneration, housing stress may also be a corollary of renovation, whether focused on the accommodation itself or the wider neighbourhood. The perceived adequacy of tenant information, involvement and control may be critical variables, particularly given the literal proximity to home of the intervention and the fact that many of those affected will have little opportunity to exercise control in other areas of life. Specifically, research has suggested that tenants who felt they were well *enough* informed about renewal were significantly less likely to experience adverse health effects as a result of the process (Allen, 2000). The empowerment of front-line staff is held to be an important first step in the empowerment of service users.

Successive surveys have found the decentralisation of housing management services similarly gives increased tenant satisfaction (Stewart and Taylor, 1995, p 21), with the series of estate visits conducted by Policy Action Team 5 as part of the NSNR suggesting that local management and tenant participation, as part of a holistic package of measures, had reduced crime and secured a significant improvement in health (NSNR, 1999). Box 11.14 shows one example of how this has been embedded in good practice.

Box 11.14: Increasing tenant information and control – Bell Farm

The Bell Farm Estate in York was built by the local authority in the 1930s. Estate Action funding from the DoE was secured from 1992-95 to improve the area and image of the estate. Particular emphasis was given not only "to multi-service involvement in plans for the neighbourhood, and to encouraging different forms of resident participation in the regeneration process" (Cole and Smith, 1996, p 2) but also to ways in which this involvement could be maintained after the programme had finished.

Internal modernisation covering heating and hot water systems together with replacement bathrooms and kitchens was organised according to the Tenants' Choice model used by York City Council for all such schemes. This was supplemented by environmental improvements and a community hall, which also provided a base for local services and the Residents' Association. A model estate contract was developed by consultants working in partnership with local residents. This maintained the multiagency approach to regeneration by securing service-level agreements (provided in residents' packs) covering housing, social services, police, health, environmental health, leisure and community education. Evaluation found members of the Household Panel "unequivocal about the better prospects for living on Bell Farm" (Cole and Smith, 1996, p 66). This was attributed to changed allocation priorities and physical improvements on the estate. However, the highest rates of dissatisfaction were found among single mothers whose marginalisation and isolation were unaffected by the project.

Homelessness

A further dimension to health selection is arguably that which moves people out of housing and onto the streets. Here there tends to be a dichotomy between the 'officially homeless' (usually families and older people) and the unregistered 'single homeless people'. Despite the significant increase in youth homelessness in recent years the majority of the 'visible' latter are still aged between 25 and 59 (Kemp, 1997, cited in Fitzpatrick et al, 2000). Graham-Jones et al (2004), reviewing appropriate models of care for the groups as a whole, find an emphasis on the health needs of single homeless people, as opposed to families. They also find a neglect of the issue in the UK literature compounded by the difficulties of working with such highly mobile and vulnerable clients (see also Power et al, 1999a). The needs of older homeless people are also often neglected (Crane and Warnes, 2000).

The range of issues facing homeless people (such as access to family, accommodation, money and food), alongside specific health promotion issues (such as first aid training, substance misuse, hypothermia and malnutrition), underlines the need for broad-based interventions that extend beyond health (Power and Hunter, 2001). A review of good practice by the Health Education Authority's expert group on homelessness and health promotion emphasises the potential of tailoring national campaigns in areas such as sexual and mental health to homeless people, training staff working with the homeless to increase sensitivity, and using Health Fairs and existing networks to raise awareness of health and social services (Power et al, 1999b). Research conducted by the *Big Issue* in the North, for example, led to a pilot nurse-run mobile clinic to address the health-related problems of *Big Issue* vendors and the *Big Issue* has similarly worked in conjunction with the Samaritans to address the high suicide rates among the homeless and on an action research project to enable *Big Issue* vendors to fill an information-giving role to support the health needs of other homeless people (Hunter and Power, 2000; Power and Hunter, 2001). Evaluation is limited.

It is also argued that inadequate access to health services is a key health determinant, particularly for those with a *dual diagnosis*, that is, mental health problems and a drug or alcohol dependency (Fitzpatrick et al, 2000). Evidence from the US, while scarce, suggests the potential of intensive case management, assertive outreach and transitional housing to produce improvements in the quality of life of homeless people. This is borne out by evidence from the one controlled trial to report from 35 projects funded in the early 1990s to improve access to primary care for homeless people (Graham-Jones et al, 2004; see Box 11.15).

Interventions designed to prevent the initiation of homelessness at the individual level can also be expected to be beneficial in redressing health inequalities. For adults these include housing advice and aid services, support for tenants with mental health and substance misuse problems, support for people at risk of losing their homes through relationship breakdown, antisocial behaviour or debt, and

Box 11.15: The health potential of advocacy for homeless people

A quasi-experimental trial of centre-based and outreach advocacy, focused on a large inner-city practice in Liverpool, found significant short-term psychosocial improvements among people receiving support in accessing services and advocacy from a family health worker as opposed to usual care. Outreach, they suggested, was more effective than centre-based advocacy. Benefits included a reduction in emotional distress and improvements in ability to sleep and self-esteem. Early and proactive intervention was similarly found to be beneficial (Graham-Jones et al, 2004).

The study also suggested that a dedicated health advocacy service could reduce the workload of GPs and other health workers (Reilly et al, 2004). Assertive outreach was unable to influence the workload associated with symptomatic homeless patients requiring medication, but could reduce recourse to the health system for psychosocial needs, the primary health need of the studied group. This had the effect of making the intervention cost-neutral despite the fact that the availability of the health advocate created a considerable demand for the service among the outreach population and arguably a more appropriate pattern of help seeking. Investigation into the skill mix required may suggest that this is also a role that could be adopted by lay workers.

resettlement programmes for people leaving prison and the armed forces (Fitzpatrick et al, 2000). Early results from Shelter's Inclusion Project, which aims to address the high support needs and antisocial behaviour that put households at risk of eviction and homelessness, are encouraging (Shelter, 2005a). This more holistic approach to homelessness mirrors the shift in emphasis away from the health-related characteristics of the housing stock towards Neighbourhood Renewal.

Policy

There is a dose–response relationship between poor housing and health and one, moreover, in which history matters (Marsh et al, 2000). Early experience of housing deprivation increases the likelihood of ill health in adulthood, while current conditions are also critical. Such pathways suggest direct health benefits would accrue from tackling housing conditions per se but most particularly from focusing on housing for families with children.

Policy of this nature obviously has considerable historical precedents in earlier sanitary and public health reforms together with philanthropic housing projects (Burridge and Ormandy, 1993). More recent history is more varied. The Priority Estates Project was introduced, for example, by the DoE in 1979 in recognition of the problems of difficult-to-let areas of council housing (including management, service delivery and physical condition). The UK Health for All Network, inspired by the WHO's European Healthy Cities Programme and Health for All by the Year 2000, sought to pursue city-wide healthy strategies with an inequalities dimension and including the provision of a high-quality physical environment and housing quality. At the same time, the Right to Buy legislation introduced by the 1980 Housing Act, the inability to build new houses with capital receipts and the deregulation of the credit market were typical of a larger movement which saw responsibility for basic welfare provision, most particularly housing and health, pass into the hands of individual householders, along with an individualisation of risk. In general terms the social housing policy established by the Conservative government (and the prevailing trends) has continued, with responsibility for the provision of social housing shifting from local authorities to registered social landlords and investment in social housing stock allied to better management and reforms to personal housing support (Crane and Warnes, 2000).

Housing investment has been cut more than other forms of public expenditure in the recent past, with total investment in social housing programmes falling from £7 billion to £3 billion between 1993 and 1998 (Evans, 1998). The government's Strategy for Homelessness proposes increasing the supply of new social housing by 50% (75,000 houses by 2008), but Shelter has suggested expenditure needs to be trebled, currently standing at just 0.2% of the Gross Domestic Product (GDP) (Shelter, 2005b). The housing renewal programme has, however, increasingly become subsumed within the wider regeneration programmes. Estate Action, for example, admitted economic development initiatives from 1988 and encouraged crime reduction measures from 1992 before being incorporated into the SRB process in 1994. Housing Plus, introduced in 1995, similarly aimed to make investment in social housing more sustainable by funding housing associations to invest in social and economic measures (such as the social infrastructure, crime prevention, reductions in the jobs and skills gap and the retention of more money locally) alongside improvements to the housing stock.

The link between health and housing has, however, "moved up the UK policy agenda" (Marsh et al, 2000, p 411). The Acheson Report (1998) served to highlight housing and environment as key areas for future policy development if health inequalities were to be reduced, and this was furthered by the White Paper *Saving lives* (DH, 1999a), which similarly recognised housing as one of the key environmental factors that affects health. A floor target also aims (see Chapter Three) to bring all social housing into decent condition by 2010 and to increase the proportion of private housing in decent condition occupied by vulnerable groups. Tenant participation compacts establishing standards for involving and empowering tenants were also introduced in April 1999 and one of the Policy Action Teams set up in 1998 to contribute to the NSNR formally identified housing management as a key factor in stabilising fragile communities. In this context *Best Value* is seen as the key to securing a service provider presence on estates, with one-stop shops giving access to a range of agencies including health providers, and super caretakers or concierges providing an identifiable link between landlords and tenants, including again the ability to liaise with and deliver other services. Costs tend, however, to fall on housing accounts irrespective of the fact that savings should be evident in areas as diverse as environmental and social services (NSNR, 1999).

Criticism has also been directed at the lack of intervention to counter the problems posed by the poor condition of private housing stock, with owner-occupation now accommodating more than half the poor and a growing number of other vulnerable households who are responsible for their own repairs, maintenance and improvements. Renovation and disabled facilities grants have, for example, been reduced, and the distribution of housing improvement agencies remains uneven, highlighting the lack of a substitute for the straitened medical priority rehousing system. Floor targets are, however, now being extended to cover private housing as well, accompanied by £1.6 billion investment in housing, including £80 million extra for housing management and measures to tackle low demand and abandonment via local housing strategies (SEU, 2001). There has also been some recognition of the significance of cold and damp housing. One of four energy policy goals established by the Energy White Paper (DTI, 2003) was the eradication of fuel poverty, with vulnerable households (such as those containing children and older people) expected to have been removed from fuel poverty by 2010. Alongside improvements to the energy efficiency of social housing, the Home Energy Efficiency Scheme and its successor Warm Front have provided grants for the installation of a range of energy efficient measures. A total of 900,000 households benefited from more affordable heating as a result of Warm Front in the period 2001-04, at a cost of £600 million (DEFRA, 2004).

The 1977 Housing (Homeless Persons) Act clarified the responsibilities of local authorities towards homeless people, and transferred these responsibilities from social services to housing departments. It also reinforced the traditional division between single and family homelessness, focusing the statutory response to homelessness on families and children, while many of the services available to the single homeless remain the province of the voluntary sector (Fitzpatrick et al, 2000). The bifurcation of policy with respect to homelessness was furthered by a number of other key initiatives such as the 1990 Rough Sleepers' Initiative (RSI), which funded the project-based provision of accommodation, outreach and resettlement work by the non-statutory statutory sector, while the 1996 Housing Act directed support to voluntary sector organisations for projects to help single people in housing need. One obvious drawback is that services tended to develop on an ad hoc basis, and tended to follow the availability of funding rather than need (Crane and Warnes, 2000). This has, however, been challenged by the 2002 Homelessness Act, which widened eligibility for local authority help to many of the vulnerable groups over-represented among rough sleepers and the subsequent requirement for local authorities to have a homelessness prevention strategy in place by 2003 (ODPM, 2005a).

The Social Exclusion Unit established rough sleeping as one of its first priorities and set an initial target of reducing numbers of people sleeping rough in England by two thirds by 2002, drawing on a combination of resettlement, coordination and prevention. The ensuing Homeless Action Programme, which replaced the RSI in 1999, has been described as a policy of continuity rather than change, with a continuation of the triennial cycle of project funds (£145 million for London and £34 million for the rest of England in the period 1999-2002), and a reliance on the social care market (Crane and Warnes, 2000). However, the establishment of the Rough Sleepers Unit and Youth Homelessness Action Partnership to coordinate pre-existing government programmes and to manage the various project funds through a single budget has also extended the philosophy of strategic, multiagency working to the homeless arena (Fitzpatrick et al, 2000). Funding has also become available for services under the Drug and Alcohol Specific Grant and from the DSS (for hostel beds and move-on accommodation), while the need to change the health behaviour of socially excluded groups and for community-based health promotion has become a pervasive political theme since the publication of *Our healthier nation* in 1998 (Power and Hunter, 2001).

Critics would suggest real progress depends on changes at the structural level to counter adverse housing and labour market trends, cuts in social security benefits, rising levels of poverty and family restructuring. This has been embraced by the recent five-year plan, *Sustainable communities: Homes for all* (ODPM, 2005b) and the subsequent strategy for tackling homelessness (ODPM, 2005a). This aims to reduce homelessness by expanding housing opportunities (including £90 million for the Hostels Improvement Programme), providing support for vulnerable people, tackling the wider causes and symptoms of homelessness (including benefit reforms, unemployment, domestic violence, antisocial behaviour and improved access to a range of services such as drug, alcohol, mental health and legal services), and reducing rough sleeping and the reliance on temporary accommodation. A corollary is a new target aimed at halving the number of households in temporary accommodation by 2010.

Conclusion

This chapter has struggled to maintain the link established in the early part of the lifecourse between the factors that give rise to health variations and the political and practical response. Table 11.1 shows that the strongest evidence base continues to relate to lifestyle factors and interventions at the individual and community level. The number of trials underpinning the table also suggests that the evidence base is stronger for adulthood than the earlier periods of the lifecourse, a possible function of the temporal extent of this stage and the incidence of morbidity and mortality. However, just two areas account for this: diet and physical

Table 11.1: Interventions during adulthood: summary of the evidence base

	Source
HOUSING AND COMMUNITY REGENERATION	
Limited interventions relating to rehousing, renovation, energy efficiency measures and damp prevention suggest some health gain but generalisability is limited	Systematic review
Medical priority rehousing appears more likely to result in improved mental rather than physical health	Literature review
Lack of review-level evidence	
Community regeneration	
Housing interventions in general	
Homelessness	
Supported housing, outreach support	
INCOME AND EMPLOYMENT	
For those with a severe mental disorder supported employment appears to be more effective than pre-vocational training in helping obtain competitive employment	Cochrane Review
There is limited evidence to suggest organisational interventions to reduce stress in the workplace are effective	Systematic review
Lack of review-level evidence	
Welfare advice	
Job creation and training	
DIET AND PHYSICAL ACTIVITY	
There is evidence to support the effectiveness of low calorie and low fat/low energy diets for the treatment of obesity and overweight in adults	Review of reviews
Physical activity is effective in producing a modest total weight loss and is an effective adjunct (as is CBT) to diet	Review of reviews
Brief individual-centred interventions in healthcare or community settings (focusing, for example, on advice and information) can produce modest short-term changes in physical activity across 6-12 weeks	Review of reviews
Referral to an exercise specialist in the community and interventions that promote moderate-intensity physical activity such as walking, which are not facility dependent, are associated with longer-term changes in behaviour	Review of reviews
Lack of review-level evidence	
Interventions for the prevention of obesity and overweight	
Maintenance of long-term weight loss	
Upstream interventions for both diet and physical activity	
The efficacy of exercise referral and sport development officers	
The role of exercise in smoking cessation and depression	

(continued)

Table 11.1: Interventions during adulthood: summary of the evidence base (continued)

	Source
SMOKING AND ALCOHOL	
Smoking	
In a clinical setting with a clinician even minimal contact can increase abstinence rates, with effectiveness increasing with contact until a threshold is reached at between 31 and 90 minutes	Review of reviews
Counselling and behavioural therapies such as stress management can further increase abstinence, as can follow-up support, social support such as buddy systems, help with the cost of therapies, high-profile mass media and public education campaigns and an increase in the tobacco price	Review of reviews
Bans and to a lesser degree reductions on smoking in the workplace reduce exposure to second-hand smoke	Review of reviews
Comprehensive institutional smoking bans are effective in reducing smoking in public places	Review of reviews
Alcohol	
Some evidence that heavy drinkers are twice as likely to moderate their drinking over the next 6-12 months as a result of a brief 5-20 minute intervention in a hospital or primary care setting	Review of reviews
Extended brief interventions (including several visits, counselling or motivational work) increase effectiveness further, particularly for women	Review of reviews
Blood-alcohol concentration laws reduce alcohol-related crash fatalities with breath testing reducing associated fatal and non-fatal injuries	Review of reviews
High-quality server training together with management support can reduce intoxication in patrons	Review of reviews
Lack of review-level evidence	
Interventions at the community level and the workplace	
Alcohol consumption in pregnancy	

activity; and smoking and alcohol. This is reflected in the emphasis of the recent Public Health White Paper, where personalisation of approach, tailored information and access to services are all seen as key to enabling people to make healthier choices in areas such as diet and nutrition, physical activity, smoking and sensible drinking. Paradoxically, however, the continued neglect of socio-economic and ethnic variations in many studies means there is a lack of understanding of the very features that might make such intervention appropriate for vulnerable groups and those with multiple risks – what would increase smoking cessation among heavy smokers and women of lower socio-economic class, for example? Significantly, the links between such behavioural choice and the structural determinants of health also remain attenuated.

When attention is turned instead to psychosocial health or material deprivation (and the more holistic interventions such as housing, crime and employment), the evidence base is far more tenuous, and good practice examples and critiques can frequently only be found in government-sponsored evaluations. There is a particular paucity of evidence relating to the broader social determinants of health and upstream interventions that seek, for example, to counter unemployment, redistribute income or inject economic investment (Davey Smith et al, 2001). Indeed, the government's response in both areas has tended to focus on ABIs rather than far-reaching structural reform or adjustments in mainstream spend. Even here, despite the rhetoric of integrated policy making, health has tended to remain on the margins of the regeneration agenda. Its inclusion as an explicit outcome area in both the NDC programme and the Neighbourhood Renewal programme has not yet, for example, ensured corresponding investment and evaluation.

In Chapter Fourteen we focus on this dissonance between the existing evidence base for public health, with its focus on individualised interventions, and the continuing requirement for structural solutions to health inequalities. Here, alternatives to the over-reliance on systematic reviews are discussed, and we suggest that a 'gold standard' for public health research should be one that involves comparison and contextualisation. Meanwhile, Chapters Twelve and Thirteen attempt to unpick the consequences of poverty and income polarisation for health inequalities in later life. They find it an often neglected research area, beset with definitional challenges.

References

Abbot, S. and Hobby, L. (2000) 'Welfare benefit advice in primary care: evidence of improvements in health', *Public Health*, vol 114, no 5, pp 324-7.

Acheson, D. (1998) *Independent Inquiry into Inequalities in Health*, London: The Stationery Office.

Allen, T. (2000) 'Housing renewal – doesn't it make you sick?', *Housing Studies*, vol 15, no 3, pp 443-61.

Ambrose, P.J. (2001) 'Living conditions and health promotion strategies', *Journal of the Royal Society for the Promotion of Health*, vol 121, no 1, pp 9-15.

Amos, A., Gaunt-Richardson, P., McKie, L. and J.B. (1999) 'Addressing smoking and health among women living on low income iii. Ayr Barnardo's Homelessness Service and Dundee Women's Aid', *Health Education Journal*, vol 58, pp 329-40.

Anderson, A.S. and Cox, D. (2000) 'Five a day – challenges and achievements', *Nutrition and Food Science*, vol 30, no 1, pp 30-4.

Armstrong, H.W., Kehrer, B. and Wells, P. (2001) 'Initial impacts of community economic development initiatives in the Yorkshire and Humber Structural Funds programme', *Regional Studies*, vol 35, no 8, pp 673-88.

Aston-Mansfield (2001) *The right to a healthy diet: Sustaining the fight against food poverty*, London: Aston-Mansfield.

Barlow, J., Gaunt-Richardson, P., Amos, A. and McKie, L. (1999) 'Addressing smoking and health among women living on a low income ii. TAPS Tiree: a dance and drama group for rural community development', *Health Education Journal*, vol 58, pp 321-8.

Baxter, T., Milner, P., Wilson, K., Leaf, M., Nichol, J., Freeman, J., Cooper, N. and Nicholl, J. (1997) 'A cost effective, community based heart health promotion project in England: prospective comparative study', *British Medical Journal*, vol 315, no 7108, pp 582-5.

Benzeval, M. and Judge, K. (2001) 'Income and health: the time dimension', *Social Science and Medicine*, vol 52, no 9, pp 1371-90.

Best, R. (1995) 'The housing dimension', in M. Benzeval, K. Judge and M. Whitehead (eds) *Tackling inequalities in health: An agenda for action*, London: King's Fund, pp 53-68.

Blackman, T., Anderson, J. and Pye, P. (2003) 'Change in adult health following medical priority rehousing: a longitudinal study', *Journal of Public Health Medicine*, vol 25, no 1, pp 22-8.

Blane, D., Mitchell, R. and Bartley, M. (2000) 'The "inverse housing law" and respiratory health', *Journal of Epidemiology and Community Health*, vol 54, no 10, pp 745-9.

Boardman, B. (1991) *Fuel poverty: From cold homes to affordable warmth*, London: Belhaven.

Burridge, R. and Ormandy, D. (1993) 'Introduction', in R. Burridge and D. Ormandy (eds) *Unhealthy housing: Research, remedies and reform*, London: E & FN Spon, pp xv-xxxv.

Burton, P., Goodlad, R., Croft, J., Abbott, J., Hastings, A., Macdonald, G. and Slater, T. (2004) *What works in community involvement in area-based initiatives? A systematic review of the literature*, Online Report 53/04, London: Home Office.

Burton, S. and Diaz de Leon, D. (2002) 'An evaluation of benefits advice in primary care: Camden and Islington Health Action Zone', in L. Bauld and K. Judge (eds) *Learning from Health Action Zones*, Chichester: Aeneas, pp 241-9.

CAB (Citizens' Advice Bureau) (2001) *Summing up: Bridging the financial literacy divide*, London: CAB.

CAB (2003) *In too deep*, London: CAB.

Cabinet Office (2004) *Alcohol harm reduction strategy for England*, London: The Stationery Office.

Cameron, M., Edmans, T., Greatley, A. and Morris, D. (2003) *Community renewal and mental health*, London: King's Fund.

Campbell, M., Sanderson, I. and Walton, F. (1998) *Local responses to long-term unemployment*, York: York Publishing Services for the Joseph Rowntree Foundation.

Carnall, D. (2000) 'Cycling and health promotion', *British Medical Journal*, vol 320, p 888.

Carr-Hill, R., Coyle, D. and Ivens, C. (1993) 'Poor housing, poor health', Unpublished report funded by the DoE.

Chanan, G., West, A., Garratt, C. and Humm, J. (1999) *Regeneration and sustainable communities*, London: Community Development Foundation.

Chesterman, J., Judge, K., Bauld, L. and Ferguson, J. (2005) 'How effective are the English smoking treatment services in reaching disadvantaged smokers?', *Addiction*, vol 100, suppl 2, pp 36–45.

Chilvers, R., Macdonald, G. and Hayes, A. (2004) 'Supported housing for people with severe mental disorders (Cochrane Review)', *The Cochrane Library*, Chichester: John Wiley & Sons Ltd.

Cole, I. and Smith, Y. (1996) *From estate action to estate agreement: Regeneration and change on the Bell Farm Estate, York*, Bristol/York: The Policy Press/Joseph Rowntree Foundation.

Crane, M. and Warnes, A. (2000) 'Policy and service responses to rough sleeping among older people', *Journal of Social Policy*, vol 29, no 1, pp 21–36.

Crow, G. and Allan, G. (1994) *Community life: An introduction to local social relations*, Hemel Hempstead: Harvester Wheatsheaf.

Crowther, R., Marshall, M., Bond, G. and Huxley, P. (2004) 'Vocational rehabilitation for people with severe mental illness (Cochrane Review)', *The Cochrane Library, issue 3, 2004*, Chichester: John Wiley & Sons Ltd.

Curtis, S., Cave, B. and Coutts, A. (2002) 'Is urban regeneration good for health? Perceptions and theories of the health impacts of urban change', *Environment and Planning C: Government and Policy*, vol 20, no 4, pp 517–34.

Davey Smith, G., Ebrahim, S. and Frankel, S. (2001) 'How policy informs the evidence', *British Medical Journal*, vol 322, no 7280, pp 184–5.

Davis, A., Cavill, N., Rutter, H. and Crombie, H. (2005) *Making the case: Improving health through transport*, London: Health Development Agency.

DEFRA (Department for the Environment, Food and Rural Affairs) (2004) *Fuel poverty in England: The government's plan for action*, London: DEFRA.

DETR (Department of the Environment, Transport and the Regions) (1998) *A new deal for transport: Better for everyone*, London: The Stationery Office.

DETR (2001) *Local strategic partnerships government guidance. March 2001*, London: DETR.

DH (Department of Health) (1992) *The health of the nation: A strategy for health in England and Wales*, London: HMSO.

DH (1997) *The new NHS: Modern and dependable*, Cm 3807, London: The Stationery Office.

DH (1999a) *Saving lives: Our healthier nation*, London: The Stationery Office.

DH (1999b) *National Service Framework for Mental Health*, London: DH.

DH (2000a) *The NHS Plan*, London: The Stationery Office.

DH (2000b) *The NHS Cancer Plan*, London: DH.

DH (2000c) *National Service Framework for Coronary Heart Disease*, London: DH.

DH (2002a) *Five-a-day pilot initiatives: Executive summary of the pilot initiative evaluation plan*, London: DH.

DH (2002b) *Health improvement and prevention: National service frameworks: A practical aid to implementation in primary care*, London: DH.

DH (2005) *Choosing a better diet: A food health action plan*, London: DH.

DoT (Department of Transport) (1996) *National cycling strategy*, London: DoT.

Dowling, B., Powell, M. and Glendinning, C. (2004) 'Conceptualising successful partnerships', *Health and Social Care in the Community*, vol 12, no 4, pp 309-17.

DTI (Department of Trade and Industry) (2003) *Our energy future: Towards a low carbon economy*, London: DTI.

Dunn, J.R. (2000) 'Housing and health inequalities: review and prospects for research', *Housing Studies*, vol 15, no 3, pp 341-66.

Dunn, J.R. (2002) 'Housing and inequalities in health: a study of socioeconomic dimensions of housing and self reported health from a survey of Vancouver residents', *Journal of Epidemiology and Community Health*, vol 56, no 9, pp 671-81.

DWP (Department for Work and Pensions) (2003) *New Deal for Disabled People (NDDP): First synthesis research report*, London: DWP.

Eakin, E., Glasgow, R. and Riley, K. (2000) 'Review of primary care-based physical activity intervention studies', *The Journal of Family Practice*, vol 49, no 2, pp 158-68.

Easterlow, D. and Smith, S.J. (2004) 'Housing for health: can the market care?', *Environment and Planning A*, vol 36, no 6, pp 999-1017.

Easterlow, D., Smith, S.J. and Mallinson, S. (2000) 'Housing for health: the role of owner occupation', *Housing Studies*, vol 15, no 3, pp 367-86.

Eaton, C. and Menard, L. (1998) 'A systematic review of physical activity promotion in primary care office settings', *British Journal of Sports Medicine*, vol 32, no 1, pp 11-16.

Ebrahim, S. and Davey Smith, G. (1997) 'A systematic review and meta-analysis of randomised controlled trials of health promotion for prevention of coronary heart disease in adults', *British Medical Journal*, vol 314, no 7095, pp 1666-74.

Ebrahim, S. and Davey Smith, G. (1998) 'Effects of the heartbeat Wales programme: effects of government policies on health behaviour must be studied', *British Medical Journal*, vol 317, no 7162, p 886.

Ellaway, A. and Macintyre, S. (1998) 'Does housing tenure predict health in the UK because it exposes people to different levels of housing related hazards in the home and its surroundings?', *Health and Place*, vol 4, no 2, pp 141-51.

Evans, G., Johansson, G. and Rydstedt, L. (1999) 'Hassles on the job: a study of job intervention with urban bus drivers', *Journal of Organizational Behavior*, vol 20, no 2, pp 199-208.

Evans, J., Hyndman, S., Stewart-Brown, S., Smith, D. and Petersen, S. (2000) 'An epidemiological study of the relative importance of damp housing in relation to adult health', *Journal of Epidemiology and Community Health*, vol 54, pp 677–86.

Evans, R. (1998) 'Tackling deprivation on social housing estates in England: an assessment of the housing plus approach', *Housing Studies*, vol 13, no 5, pp 713–26.

Fines, A. and Griffiths, J. (2001) *Literature review on employability*, London: Health Development Agency.

Fitzpatrick, S., Kemp, P. and Klinker, S. (2000) *Single homelessness: An overview of research in Britain*, Bristol/York: The Policy Press/Joseph Rowntree Foundation.

Foley, P. and Martin, S. (2000) 'A new deal for the community? Public participation in regeneration and local service delivery', *Policy & Politics*, vol 28, no 4, pp 479–92.

Forrest, R. and Kearns, A. (1999) *Joined-up places? Social cohesion and neighbourhood regeneration*, York: York Publishing Services for the Joseph Rowntree Foundation.

Freeman, H. (1993) 'Mental health and high-rise housing', in R. Burridge and D. Ormandy (eds) *Unhealthy housing: Research, remedies and reform*, London: E & FN Spon, pp 168–90.

FSA (Financial Services Authority) (2004) *Financial risk outlook*, London: FSA.

FSA, LACORS (Local Authorities Coordinating Body on Food and Trading Standards) and LGA (Local Government Association) (2002) *Food: The local vision: A joint statement by the LGA, LACORS and the FSA*, London: LACORS/LGA/FSA.

Fuel Poverty Advisory Group (2003) *First annual report*, London: DTI.

Gaunt-Richardson, P., Amos, A. and Moore, M. (1998) 'Women, low income and smoking: developing community-based initiatives', *Health Education Journal*, vol 57, pp 303–12.

Glenn, L., Beck, R. and Burkett, G. (1998) 'Effect of a transient, geographically localised economic recovery on community health and income studied with longitudinal household cohort interview method', *Journal of Epidemiology and Community Health*, vol 52, pp 749–57.

Graham, H. (1993) *When life's a drag: Women, smoking and disadvantage*, London: HMSO.

Graham-Jones, S., Reilly, S. and Gaulton, E. (2004) 'Tackling the needs of the homeless: a controlled trial of health advocacy', *Health and Social Care in the Community*, vol 12, no 3, pp 221–32.

Greasley, P. and Small, N. (2002) 'Welfare advice in primary care', Nuffield portfolio programme report no 17 (www.nuffield.leeds.ac.uk/downloads/portfolio/welfare.pdf), accessed 14 October 2004.

Hales, J., Taylor, R., Mandy, W. and Miller, M. (2003) *Evaluation of Employment Zones: Report on a cohort survey of long-term unemployed people in the zones and a matched set of comparison areas*, London: National Centre for Social Research.

Hall, S. and Hickman, P. (2002) 'Neighbourhood renewal and urban policy: a comparison of new approaches in England and France', *Regional Studies*, vol 36, no 6, pp 691-707.

Halpern, D. (1995) *Mental health and the built environment: More than bricks and mortar*, London: Taylor and Francis.

Harris, V. (2002) *Domestic abuse screening pilot in primary care 2000-2002*, Wakefield: Support and Survival.

Harvey, E., Glenny, A.-M., Kirk, S. and Summerbell, C. (2001) 'Improving health professionals' management and the organisation of care for overweight and obese people (Cochrane Review)', *The Cochrane Library, issue 3, 2004*, Chichester: John Wiley & Sons Ltd.

Hastings, A. and Dean, J. (2003) 'Challenging images: tackling stigma through estate regeneration', *Policy & Politics*, vol 31, no 2, pp 171-84.

Hillsdon, M., Foster, C., Naidoo, B. and Crombie, H. (2004) *The effectiveness of public health interventions for increasing physical activity among adults*, London: Health Development Agency.

Hillsdon, M., Thorogood, M., White, I. and Foster, C. (2002) 'Advising people to take more exercise is ineffective: a randomized controlled trial of physical activity promotion in primary care', *International Journal of Epidemiology*, vol 31, no 4, pp 808-15.

HM Government and DH (Department of Health) (2004) *Choosing health: Making healthy choices easier*, London: HM Government and DH.

Hogstedt, C. and Lundberg, I. (2002) 'Work-related policies and interventions', in J. Mackenbach and M. Bakker (eds) *Reducing inequalities in health*, London: Routledge, pp 85-103.

Home Office and Cabinet Office (1999) *Living without fear: An integrated approach to tackling violence against women*, London: Home Office.

Hopton, J. and Hunt, S. (1996) 'The health effects of improvements to housing: a longitudinal study', *Housing Studies*, vol 11, no 2, pp 271-86.

Hovell, M.F., Zakarian, J.M., Matt, G.E., Hofstetter, R., Bernert, J.T. and Pirkle, J. (2000) 'Effect of counselling mothers on their children's exposure to environmental tobacco smoke: a randomised trial', *British Medical Journal*, vol 321, pp 337-42.

Hunt, S. (1993) 'Damp and mouldy housing: a holistic approach', in R. Burridge and D. Ormandy (eds) *Unhealthy housing: Research, remedies and reform*, London: E & FN Spon, pp 69-93.

Hunter, G. and Power, R. (2000) *Assessing the feasibility of peer education among homeless people: Summary bulletin*, London: Health Development Agency.

IPPR (Institute for Public Policy Research) (2002) *Streets ahead*, London: IPPR.

Jackson, N. and Prebble, A. (2002) *Perceptions of smoking cessation products and services among low income smokers*, London: Health Development Agency.

Joshi, H. (2001) 'Is there a place for area-based initiatives?', *Environment and Planning A*, vol 33, no 8, pp 1349-52.

Judge, K., Barnes, M., Bauld, L., Benzeval, M., Killoran, A., Robinson, R., Wigglesworth, R. and Zeilig, H. (1999) 'Health Action Zones: earning to make a difference', Report submitted to the DH, June (www.ukc.ac.uk/pssru), accessed 15 March 2002.

Kearns, A., Hiscock, R., Ellaway, A. and Macintyre, S. (2000) '"Beyond four walls": the psycho-social benefits of home: evidence from west central Scotland', *Housing Studies*, vol 15, no 3, pp 387-410.

Kelly, M. (2004) *The evidence of effectiveness of public health interventions – and the implications*, London: Health Development Agency.

Kemp, P. (1997) 'The characteristics of single homeless people', in R. Burrows, N. Pleace and D. Quilgars (eds) *Homelessness and social policy*, London: Routledge, pp 69-87.

Kennedy, L. (2001) 'Community involvement at what cost? Local appraisal of a pan-European nutrition promotion programme in low income neighbourhoods', *Health Promotion International*, vol 16, no 1, pp 35-45.

Lawless, P. (2004) 'Locating and explaining area-based urban initiatives: New deal for communities in England', *Environment and Planning C: Government and Policy*, vol 22, no 3, pp 383-99.

Lawlor, D. and Hopker, S. (2001) 'The effectiveness of exercise as an intervention in the management of depression: systematic review and metaregression analysis of randomised controlled trials', *British Medical Journal*, vol 322, no 7277, pp 1-8.

Lawlor, D., Keen, S. and Neal, R. (1999) 'Increasing levels of physical activity through primary care: GPs' knowledge, attitudes and self-reported practice', *Family Practice*, vol 16, no 3, pp 250-4.

Lawlor, D., Ness, A., Cope, A., Davis, A., Insall, P. and Riddoch, C. (2003) 'The challenges of evaluating environmental interventions to increase population levels of physical activity: the case of the UK national cycle network', *Journal of Epidemiology and Community Health*, vol 57, no 2, pp 96-101.

Leather, S. (1996) *The making of modern malnutrition: An overview of food poverty in the UK*, London: Caroline Walker Trust.

Lupton, R. and Power, A. (2005) 'Disadvantaged by where you live? New Labour and neighbourhood renewal', in J. Hills and K. Stewart (eds) *A more equal society?*, Bristol: The Policy Press, pp 119-42.

Lupton, R., Wilson, A., May, T., Warburton, H. and Turnbull, P. (2002) *A rock and a hard place: Drug markets in deprived neighbourhoods*, Home Office Research Study 240, London: Home Office Research, Development and Statistics Directorate.

Lynch, J., Due, P., Muntaner, C. and Davey-Smith, G. (2000) 'Social capital – is it a good investment strategy for public health?', *Journal of Epidemiology and Community Health*, vol 54, pp 404-8.

McGregor, A., Ferguson, Z., Fitzpatrick, I., McConnachie, M. and Richmond, K. (1997) *Bridging the jobs gap: An evaluation of the wise group and the intermediate labour market*, York: York Publishing Services for the Joseph Rowntree Foundation.

Macintyre, S., Ellaway, A., Hiscock, R., Kearns, A., Der, G. and McKay, L. (2003) 'What features of the home and the area might help to explain observed relationships between housing tenure and health? Evidence from the west of Scotland', *Health and Place*, vol 9, no 3, pp 207-18.

Mackian, S. (2002) 'Complex cultures: rereading the story about health and social capital', *Critical Social Policy*, vol 22, no 2, pp 203-25.

McKie, L., Gaunt-Richardson, P., Barlow, J. and Amos, A. (1999) 'Addressing smoking and health among women living on a low income i. Dean's community club: a mental health project', *Health Education Journal*, vol 58, pp 311-20.

Marsh, A., Gordon, D., Heslop, P. and Pantazis, C. (2000) 'Housing deprivation and health: a longitudinal analysis', *Housing Studies*, vol 15, no 3, pp 411-28.

Marshall, B. and Macfarlane, R. (2000) *The intermediate labour market: A tool for tackling long-term unemployment*, York: York Publishing Services for the Joseph Rowntree Foundation.

Morrow, V. (1999) 'Conceptualising social capital in relation to the well-being of children and young people: a critical review', *Sociological Review*, vol 47, no 4, pp 744-65.

Morrow, V. (2002) 'Children's experiences of "community": implications of social capital discourses', in C. Swann and A. Morgan (eds) *Social capital: Insights from qualitative research*, London: Health Development Agency, pp 10-28.

Morton, S., Myers, P. and Walton, E. (2000) *Health update: Environment and health: Housing*, London: Health Education Authority.

Mulvihill, C. and Quigley, R. (2003) *The management of obesity and overweight: An analysis of reviews of diet, physical activity and behavioural approaches*, London: Health Development Agency.

Mulvihill, C., Taylor, L., Waller, S. with Naidoo, B. and Thom, B. (2005) *Prevention and reduction of alcohol misuse*, London: Health Development Agency.

Naidoo, B., Warm, D., Quigley, R. and Taylor, L. (2004) *Smoking and public health: A review of reviews of interventions to increase smoking cessation, reduce smoking initiation and prevent further uptake of smoking*, London: Health Development Agency.

NAO (National Audit Office) (2001) *Tackling obesity in England: Report by the Comptroller and Auditor General*, London: The Stationery Office.

NEA (National Energy Action), NEF (New Economics Foundation) and PFRC (Personal Finance Research Centre) (2002) *Ending fuel poverty and financial exclusion: A factor four approach: Summary report*, London: NEA, NEF, Ofgem, PFRC and npower.

Nettleton, S. and Burrows, R. (1998) 'Mortgage debt, insecure home ownership and health: an exploratory analysis', *Sociology of Health and Illness*, vol 20, no 5, pp 731-53.

Nettleton, S. and Burrows, R. (2000) 'When a capital investment becomes an emotional loss: the health consequences of the experience of mortgage possession in England', *Housing Studies*, vol 15, no 3, pp 463-79.

North, P. (2000) 'Is there space for organisation from below within the UK government's action zones? A test of "collaborative planning"', *Urban Studies*, vol 37, no 8, pp 1261-78.

NSNR (National Strategy for Neighbourhood Renewal) (1999) *Report of Policy Action Team 5: Housing management*, London: The Stationery Office.

NSNR (2000a) *Report of Policy Action Team 4: Neighbourhood management*, London: The Stationery Office.

NSNR (2000b) *Report of Policy Action Team 8: Anti-social behaviour*, London: The Stationery Office.

NSNR (2000c) *Report of Policy Action Team 6: Neighbourhood wardens*, London: The Stationery Office.

ODPM (Office of the Deputy Prime Minister) (2005a) *Sustainable communities: Settled homes; changing lives: A strategy for tackling homelessness*, London: ODPM.

ODPM (2005b) *Sustainable communities: Homes for all*, Cm 6424, London: The Stationery Office.

Osler, M. and Prescott, E. (1998) 'Psychosocial, behavioural, and health determinants of successful smoking cessation: a longitudinal study of Danish adults', *Tobacco Control*, vol 7, no 3, pp 262-7.

Parkinson, M. (1998) *Combating social exclusion: Lessons from area-based programmes in Europe*, Bristol: The Policy Press.

Pevalin, D. and Rose, D. (2003) *Social capital for health: Investigating the links between social capital and health using the British Household Panel Survey*, London: Health Development Agency.

Phillipson, C. and Scharf, T. (2004) *The impact of government policy on social exclusion among older people: A review of the literature for the Social Exclusion Unit in the breaking the cycle series*, London: ODPM.

Platt, S., Martin, C. and Hunt, S. (1989) 'Damp housing, mould growth and symptomatic health state', *British Medical Journal*, vol 298, pp 1673-8.

Porter, R. (2002) *Cornwall domestic violence co-ordination project: Evaluation report*, Plymouth: University of Plymouth.

Power, R. and Hunter, G. (2001) 'Developing a strategy for community based health promotion targeting homeless populations', *Health Education Research*, vol 16, no 5, pp 593-602.

Power, R., French, R., Connelly, J., George, S., Hawes, D., Hinton, T., Klee, H., Robinson, D., Senior, J., Timms, P. and Warner, D. (1999a) 'Health, health promotion, and homelessness', *British Medical Journal*, vol 318, no 7183, pp 590-2.

Power, R., French, R., Connelly, J., George, S., Hawes, D., Hinton, T., Klee, H., Robinson, D., Senior, J., Timms, P. and Warner, D. (1999b) *Promoting the health of homeless people: Setting a research agenda*, London: Health Education Authority.

Press, V., Freestone, I. and George, C.F. (2003) 'Physical activity: the evidence of benefit in the prevention of coronary heart disease', *Quarterly Journal of Medicine*, vol 96, pp 245-51.

Propper, C., Jones, K., Bolster, A., Burgess, S., Johnston, R. and Sarker, R. (2004) *Local neighbourhood and mental health: Evidence from the UK*, Bristol: University of Bristol.

Raj, P.T. (2003) *Tackling health inequalities: Compendium*, London: Health Development Agency.

Ralph, D. and Peterman, W. (2004) 'Community-led urban regeneration: early lessons from the New Deal for Communities' (www.uic.edu/cuppa/cityfutures/papers/webpapers/cityfuturespapers/session6_1/6_1communityledurban.pdf), accessed 10 June 2005.

Raw, G. and Hamilton, R. (eds) (1995) *Building regulation and health*, Watford: Building Research Establishment.

Reilly, S., Graham-Jones, S., Gaulton, E. and Davidson, E. (2004) 'Can a health advocate for homeless families reduce workload for the primary healthcare team? A controlled trial', *Health and Social Care in the Community*, vol 12, no 1, pp 63-74.

Rhodes, J., Tyler, P. and Brennan, A. (2003) 'New developments in area-based initiatives in England: the experience of the Single Regeneration Budget', *Urban Studies*, vol 40, no 8, pp 1399-26.

Riddoch, C., Puig-Ribera, A. and Cooper, A. (1998) *The effectiveness of physical activity promotion schemes in primary care: A systematic review*, London: Health Education Authority.

Ritchie, D., Parry, O., Gnich, W. and Platt, S. (2004) 'Issues of participation, ownership and empowerment in a community development programme: tackling smoking in a low-income area in Scotland', *Health Promotion International*, vol 19, no 1, pp 51-9.

Russell, H. and Killoran, A. (2000) *Public health and regeneration: Making the links*, London: Health Education Authority.

Saegert, S., Klitzman, S., Freudenberg, N., Cooperman-Mroczek, J. and Nassar, S. (2003) 'Healthy housing: a structured review of published evaluations of US interventions to improve health by modifying housing in the United States, 1999-2001', *American Journal of Public Health*, vol 93, no 9, pp 1471-7.

Scott, M. (2004) 'Building institutional capacity in rural Northern Ireland: the role of partnership governance in the LEADER II programme', *Journal of Rural Studies*, vol 20, pp 49-59.

Scottish Office (1996) *Eating for health: A diet action plan for Scotland*, Edinburgh: Scottish Office.

Scottish Office (1999) *Towards a healthier Scotland: A White Paper on health*, Cm 4269, Edinburgh: The Stationery Office.

Secker-Walker, R., Gnich, W., Platt, S. and Lancaster, T. (2004) 'Community interventions for reducing smoking among adults (Cochrane Review)', *The Cochrane Library, issue 3, 2004*, Chichester: John Wiley & Sons Ltd.

SEU (Social Exclusion Unit) (2001) *A new commitment to neighbourhood renewal: National strategy action plan*, London: Cabinet Office.

Sharpe, J. and Bostock, J. (2002) *Supporting people with debt and mental health problems: Research with psychological therapists in Northumberland*, Northumberland HAZ and Newcastle, North Tyneside and Northumberland Mental Health NHS Trust.

Shelter (2005a) *Shelter inclusion project: Two years on*, London: Shelter.

Shelter (2005b) 'Housing department must treble GDP on social housing says Shelter after major investigation', Shelter Press Release, 17 March.

Shohaimi, S., Welch, A., Bingham, S., Luben, R., Day, N., Wareham, N. and Khaw, K. (2004) 'Residential area deprivation predicts fruit and vegetable consumption independently of individual educational level and occupational social class: a cross sectional population study in the Norfolk cohort of the European Prospective Investigation into Cancer (EPIC-Norfolk)', *Journal of Epidemiology and Community Health*, vol 58, no 8, pp 686-91.

Skifter Andersen, H. (2002) 'Can deprived housing areas be revitalised? Efforts against segregation and neighbourhood decay in Denmark and Europe', *Urban Studies*, vol 39, no 4, pp 767-90.

Smith, S.J. and Mallinson, S. (1997) 'Housing for health in a post-welfare state', *Housing Studies*, vol 12, no 2, pp 173-200.

Smith, S.J., Alexander, A. and Easterlow, D. (1997) 'Rehousing as a health intervention: miracle or mirage?', *Health and Place*, vol 3, no 4, pp 203-16.

Smith, S.J., Easterlow, D. and Munro, M. (2004) 'Housing for health: does the market work?', *Environment and Planning A*, vol 36, no 4, pp 579-600.

Somerville, M., Mackenzie, I., Owen, P. and Miles, D. (2000) 'Housing and health: does installing heating in their homes improve the health of children with asthma?', *Public Health*, vol 114, pp 434-9.

Somerville, M., Basham, M., Foy, C., Ballinger, G., Gay, T., Shute, P. and Barton, A. (2002) 'From local concern to randomized trial: the Watcombe Housing Project', *Health Expectations*, vol 5, no 2, pp 127-35.

Stewart, M. and Taylor, M. (1995) *Empowerment and estate regeneration*, Bristol: The Policy Press.

Swann, C. and Morgan, A. (2002) 'Introduction', in C. Swann and A. Morgan (eds) *Social capital for health: Insights from qualitative research*, London: Health Development Agency, pp 3-8.

Taylor, L., Wohlgemuth, C., Warm, D., Taske, N., Naidoo, B. and Millward, L. (2005) *Public health interventions for the prevention and reduction of exposure to second-hand smoke: A review of reviews*, London: National Institute for Health and Clinical Excellence.

Thake, S. (1995) *Staying the course: The role and structure of community regeneration organisations*, York: York Publishing Services for the Joseph Rowntree Foundation.

Thomson, H., Petticrew, M. and Morrison, D. (2001) 'Health effects of housing improvement: systematic review of intervention studies', *British Medical Journal*, vol 323, no 7306, pp 187-90.

Thomson, H., Petticrew, M. and Douglas, M. (2003) 'Health impact assessment of housing improvements: incorporating research evidence', *Journal of Epidemiology and Community Health*, vol 57, no 1, pp 11-16.

Tudor Smith, C., Nutbeam, D., Moore, L. and Catford, J. (1998) 'Effects of the heartbeat Wales programme over five years on behavioural risks for cardiovascular disease: quasi-experimental comparison of results from Wales and a matched reference area', *British Medical Journal*, vol 316, no 7134, pp 818-22.

Ussher, M., West, R., Taylor, A. and McEwen, A. (2002) 'Exercise interventions for smoking cessation (Cochrane Review)', *The Cochrane Library, issue 3, 2004*, Chichester: John Wiley & Sons Ltd.

Vahtera, J., Kivimäki, M., Pentti, J. and Theorell, T. (2000) 'Effect of change in the psychosocial work environment on sickness absence: a seven year follow up of initially healthy employees', *Journal of Epidemiology and Community Health*, vol 54, pp 484-93.

van der Klink, J., Blonk, R. and Schene, A. (2001) 'The benefits of interventions for work-related stress', *American Journal of Public Health*, vol 91, pp 270-6.

Walker, R. (2001) 'Great expectations: can social science evaluate New Labour's policies?', *Evaluation*, vol 7, no 3, pp 305-30.

Waller, S., Naidoo, B. and Thom, B. (2002) *Prevention and reduction of alcohol misuse: Review of reviews*, London: Health Development Agency.

Whitehead, M. (1995) 'Tackling inequalities: a review of policy initiatives', in M. Benzeval, K. Judge and M. Whitehead (eds) *Tackling inequalities in health: An agenda for action*, London: King's Fund Publishing, pp 22-52.

Wilkinson, D. (1999) *Poor housing and ill health: A summary of the research evidence*, Edinburgh: Scottish Office.

Wilkinson, P., Landon, M., Armstrong, B., Stevenson, S., Pattenden, S., Fletcher, T. and McKee, M. (2001) *Cold comfort: The social and environmental determinants of excess winter deaths in England, 1986-96*, Bristol: The Policy Press.

Wrigley, N., Warm, D. and Margetts, B. (2003) 'Deprivation, diet, and food-retail access: findings from the Leeds "food deserts" study', *Environment and Planning A*, vol 35, no 1, pp 151-88.

TWELVE

Health inequalities during older age: research evidence

Introduction

Due to the overwhelming use of occupational class in health inequalities research, rather less attention has been paid to health differences between socio-demographic than socio-economic groups. In addition to leading to the relative neglect of important characteristics such as ethnicity, the use of occupational status as a basis for classification has had the unfortunate consequence of rendering invisible those who do not participate in paid work by virtue of their older age. Yet, as we discussed in Chapter Three, old age is a period of significant income poverty. Moreover, divisions in wealth are pronounced in older age and the gap between rich and poor pensioners has continued to grow. This growth in socio-economic variation may have important implications for the level of health variation within this age group.

This chapter explores the consequences of poverty and income polarisation for health inequalities in later life. This is in itself no simple task. According to Khaw (1999), inequalities in health in older people have been neglected for a number of reasons. First, as already noted, the use of occupational status means that health inequalities have been easily identified in younger cohorts but not in groups that are past retirement. Yet, as we observe in the first part of this chapter (which examines variations in mortality and morbidity), previous occupation can be captured both in longitudinal studies that follow up subjects before and after retirement, and in surveys that explicitly collect information on last main occupation, and this has been found to have a major effect on the health of older people (Arber, 1996). Studies using alternative indicators of socio-economic status (for example, housing tenure and educational qualifications) also show that health inequalities persist throughout life.

A second factor identified by Khaw (1999) that explains the relative dearth of health variations literature on this age group is the misconception that health inequalities in older people are less amenable to successful intervention. She challenges this assumption, suggesting "there is abundant evidence that modifying life-styles and environment, or treatment of conditions at older ages have a substantial effect on elderly people's health. If anything, many interventions may in fact have greater absolute impact for elderly people" (Khaw, 1999, p 40). We explore this idea in greater depth in the second part of the chapter, which examines the significance of lifestyle factors (diet/nutrition, smoking and physical exercise) and the environment (housing and neighbourhood conditions) to inequalities in health in later life.

Third, Khaw argues that health inequalities among older people have been neglected because they are seen as of less benefit to society and hence of lower priority. The implication here is that older people in general have been devalued. In fact, concerns about ageism have been an important research theme, particularly in respect to differential access to health services. Indeed, in 2001 the Department of Health (DH) launched a *National Service Framework (NSF) for Older People*, in which the need to root out age discrimination in access to National Health Service (NHS) or social care services was established as a core standard. Thus, the lack of information on health inequalities in later life in part reflects the tendency for research on older people to focus more on inequalities *between* different age groups than on variations *within* older age bands. In the third part of the chapter, which focuses in particular on inequalities in access to health services, we discuss the extent to which age is a more important source of health exclusion for older people than socio-economic status per se.

Inequalities in mortality and morbidity

As noted in Chapter One, social class differences in premature death are greatest during early adulthood and become narrower with age. This may partly reflect the fact that deaths at younger ages are comparatively rare and can be attributed to a more limited set of risk factors. Changes in the validity of socio-economic measures with increasing age may also account for the relative narrowing of social gradients (Marang-van de Mheen et al, 2001). For example, in the 25-year follow-up of civil servants from the first Whitehall Study, social differentials in mortality based on an occupational status measure (pre-retirement employment grade) decreased with age, whereas those based on a non-work measure (car ownership) seemed to decline less. This may reflect the fact that pre-retirement work-based measures do not adequately capture current socio-economic circumstances. Alternatively, the narrowing of social differences in mortality post-retirement may reflect the importance of work in generating health inequalities (Marmot and Shipley, 1996).

Although health inequalities are subject to age-related decline, social gradients in health among older people have been demonstrated using a wide range of indicators of socio-economic status. These include occupation, education, housing tenure, car ownership and ownership of resources. For example, in the 1971 Longitudinal Study cohort, Standardised Mortality Ratios (SMRs) (1971-92) of those aged 60-74 years ranged from 77 among owner-occupiers to 115 among local authority tenants (the respective range for those aged 74+ was 91-104). The SMR of those owning two or more cars was 77 compared to 115 for those without a car (91-104 for 74+ years) (Smith and Harding, 1997). Subsequent analysis of this Longitudinal Study cohort found that being in rented accommodation and in a household without access to a car carried a 35-45% higher mortality rate over 21 years (Breeze et al, 1999). In a recent study, mortality differences according to educational level were found in both middle-aged and older men in England and Wales, challenging previous evidence that relative inequalities among older people are invariably smaller than among younger groups (Huisman et al, 2004). Like other research, this work highlighted the fact that, because mortality and morbidity are concentrated in older age groups, *absolute* differences in mortality between less and more advantaged groups increase at older ages, even when relative differences decline (Marmot and Shipley, 1996; Smith and Harding, 1997; Grundy and Sloggett, 2003). This makes health inequalities in the older population a major public health problem (Bowling, 2004).

In addition to examining mortality inequalities among older people, an increasing number of studies have focused on morbidity inequalities. Using data from the Health Survey for England (HSE) (1993-95) to analyse differentials in the health of adults aged 65-84 years, Grundy and Sloggett (2003) found the receipt of Income Support was significantly associated with bad/very bad self-reported health, the presence of a long-standing illness, the presence of two or more specific long-standing conditions, the number of prescribed medications and psychiatric morbidity. Some associations were also found between housing tenure (particularly among women), educational qualifications and health status. However, none of the indicators used were as consistently associated with poor health outcomes as receipt of Income Support.

The 2000 HSE, which explicitly focused on the health of people aged 65+, also found differences in health according to socio-economic status, but for a far more limited set of health indicators. Among those living in private households, those who had been in non-manual occupations were significantly more likely than previous manual workers to say that their health was good or very good (Falaschetti et al, 2002). However, no difference was found in the prevalence of long-standing illness or, among men, psychiatric morbidity. Indeed, among women, those in non-manual social classes were more likely to report poor psychological morbidity than their manual counterparts (Tait and Fuller, 2002). Differences in findings between this and previous HSEs may reflect choice of socio-economic measure. As research suggests that indicators relating to previous circumstances (for example, occupationally defined social class or educational qualifications) best predict variations in self-reported health among older adults when paired with a current deprivation indicator (Grundy and Holt, 2001), it is possible that the use of social class data in the reported analysis of the 2000 HSE meant that some differentials in health were overlooked.

This is certainly suggested by studies that find significant social gradients in psychiatric morbidity among older people. For example, in a survey of patients aged 65+ in two London general practices, those with no occupational pension were at significantly higher risk of having high depression scores, an association that held after adjusting for higher disability levels in this group (Harris et al, 2003). Following up subjects of the original Whitehall Study, men who had low-grade jobs in middle age had double the odds of poor mental health of senior administrators, although those who had moved from low to middle grades before retirement had a reduced risk of poor mental health (Breeze et al, 2001). In the Medical Research Council (MRC) Trial of Assessment and Management of Older People in the Community, people in a manual social class who had been in a rented home both during working age and old age had a 75% increase in risk of poor morale compared to people in a non-manual class who had been owner-occupiers at both times (Breeze et al, 2004a). The Office for National Statistics (ONS) Survey of Psychiatric Morbidity among adults in Britain carried out in 2000 lends strong weight to such findings. This found that, in adults aged 60-74 years, neurotic disorders (including depression) were more prevalent in the manual social classes, 18% of those in Social Class V being affected, compared to 6% in Social Classes I and II. There was a steady increase in disorder with decreasing household income. Risk was also associated with receipt of state benefits. Decreasing social class and household income, lower educational qualifications and increased dependence on state benefits were also associated with reduced cognitive function, which in turn increased the risk of mental health problems (Evans et al, 2003).

Associations between mental health and socio-economic status in old age appear to be mediated by a number of factors. As indicated earlier, there is a strong association between mental and physical health, particularly disability. Questions have been asked about the extent to which the association between disability and mental health may reflect a reverse causal relationship, depression leading to disablement rather than vice versa. Longitudinal studies show a strong association between disablement at baseline and subsequent onset of depression, confirming that disability is a significant risk factor for poor mental health in old age (Evans et al, 2003, p 31). However, evidence also suggests that persistent depression has its own disabling effects (Ormel et al, 2002). With some exceptions such as the 2000 HSE (Hirani and Malbut, 2002), most studies suggest that the prevalence of disability varies significantly according to socio-economic status (Grundy and Glaser, 2000; Grundy and Holt, 2000; Melzer et al, 2000, 2001; Huisman et al, 2003). Thus, higher rates of disability among poor people account for at least some of the socio-economic variation in the mental health status of older people. Heavy involvement in care giving has also been associated with symptoms of anxiety and psychological distress (Hirst, 2003) and, because of the higher prevalence of disability among poor people, the working-class retired are more likely to be caring for a spouse than their middle-class counterparts (Glaser and Grundy, 2002).

Socio-economic differences in patterns of social interaction may also influence health inequalities in older age (Grundy and Sloggett, 2003). A number of studies indicate that a lack of social networks increases risk of depression (Blazer et al, 1991; Prince et al, 1997; Osborn et al, 2004) as well as impaired immune function (Bouhuys et al, 2004) and poor physical health (Janevic et al, 2004). Recent research conducted as part of the ONS Omnibus Survey found that 7% of older people described themselves as often or always lonely. Respondents identified three sets of factors as influences on loneliness: impaired social networks, functional or environmental impairments and personality factors (Victor et al, 2004). At least some of these factors vary according to socio-economic status. For example, in the Omnibus Survey, older people who possessed fewer educational qualifications and who had poor mental health ratings were found to be particularly vulnerable to loneliness. Because older people tend to spend more time than younger people in their immediate neighbourhood and to derive a strong sense of emotional investment from their home and surrounding community, individual risk for loneliness can be exacerbated by neighbourhood factors such as high population turnover, fear of crime and a lack of public and private spaces. An Economic and Social Research Council (ESRC)-funded study that focused on older people in nine deprived wards confirmed a strong relationship between social exclusion and poverty – 41% of respondents were excluded in some way from social relations, and 16% were severely or very severely lonely, a significantly higher rate than in the more representative Omnibus Survey (Scharf et al, 2004).

The 2000 HSE also found large differences in social support according to socio-economic status. A severe lack of perceived social support was experienced more by men and women in manual social classes and by those in the lower-income groups. For example, 10% of men in the highest income group reported severe lack of perceived social support, compared with 29% of men in the lowest income group. Those in non-manual social classes and higher income groups had more contact with friends, but there was no clear relationship between contact with family and either social class or income. Perceived social support was significantly associated with self-reported health status, as men with severe lack of perceived social support were twice as likely to report poor health as men with no lack of support. There was also a strong relationship between perceived social support and mental health, the odds ratio for men with severe lack of support (in relation to no lack of support) being 3.41 (Boreham et al, 2002).

In addition to socio-economic inequalities, pronounced health inequalities have been observed in old age according to gender and ethnicity. Although data from the British General Household Survey (GHS) suggests that there is little difference between the sexes in the reporting of self-assessed health and limiting long-standing illness, older women are substantially more likely to experience functional impairment in mobility and personal self-care than men of the same age (Arber and Cooper, 1999). Older women are also at significantly higher risk of mental health problems than older men. In the ONS Survey of Psychiatric

Morbidity, 13% of men and women aged 60-64 had a neurotic disorder. Among men, prevalence rates fell to 5% for those aged 65-69 and 6% for those aged 70-74. Among women, by contrast, 12% aged 65-69 and 11% aged 70-74 were affected (Evans et al, 2003, p 9). In contrast to men, where marriage offers a protective effect against depressive symptoms, marriage is a risk factor for depression among older women. Divorce/separation increases risk of mental disorder in both sexes. Differences in mental health according to sex are sufficiently profound to suggest that gender mediates the association between mental health and other risk factors. For example, although social support is understood to be beneficial to psychological well-being, the fact that women typically have more extensive and supportive social networks does not protect them against poor psychological health. It is therefore possible that key factors associated with the increased risk of depression in women include higher rates of poverty, disability and living alone.

Ethnicity also emerges as a significant determinant of health inequalities in old age. In contrast to social class variations, ethnic variations in health become more pronounced with age. Drawing on the 1999 HSE and the Fourth National Survey (FNS) of minority ethnic groups, profiles of self-reported health among Caribbean and Indian people were found to be similar to each other and to show a worsening in health in comparison with the white English group from the mid-thirties to the mid-forties onwards, while the Pakistani and Bangladeshi groups had the worse profiles of all (Nazroo et al, 2004). Again, ethnicity is likely to mediate the relationship between ill health and certain risk factors. For example, in the HSE/FNS study, respondents' ratings of the quality of their local area in terms of crime and physical activity, and scores for community participation, did not show a clear advantage for white people. The profound ethnic differences that exist in access to financial resources – particularly among older cohorts – may thus be playing a more significant role.

Although there is strong evidence of health inequalities among older groups with respect to psychological health and, to a lesser extent, self-reported health, evidence for social gradients in physical health is rather mixed. Analysis of the US National Health Interview Survey found that older people with higher socio-economic status experienced lower numbers of chronic conditions and less limitation of activity even in their last years of life (Liao et al, 1999). By contrast, although cognitive functioning and mental health were positively correlated with socio-economic resources in the Berlin Aging Study, functional physical health was not (Mayer and Wagner, 1993). Other studies that focus on more specific indicators of physical health also yield mixed findings. Lower socio-economic status has been associated with an earlier age at menopause (Lawlor et al, 2003), and poorer rehabilitation outcomes following an acute myocardial infarction (Lacey and Walters, 2003). However, vulnerability to winter mortality in older people in Britain does not appear to vary according to socio-economic status (Maheswaran et al, 2004; Wilkinson et al, 2004). Similarly, although a low rate of childhood growth has been identified as a risk factor for later hip fracture

(Cooper et al, 2001), and significant associations have been found between fracture incidence and ward-level deprivation among younger adults, this effect is not observed in older age groups (Jones et al, 2004; West et al, 2004).

Such findings support the conclusion drawn by most researchers that differentials in health status decline after middle age (Mishra et al, 2004). This reflects the impact of excess premature mortality among lower socio-economic groups, the narrowing of socio-economic differentials in older age (a trend that has reversed with the recent growth of affluent older people) and the growing importance of demography relative to socio-economic status as a determinant of health with increasing age. As already noted, however, although relative health differences decrease in later life, absolute health differences between more and less advantaged groups increase. This means that health inequalities in the older population remain a major public health challenge.

Health risk factors in older age

It is generally accepted that health variations among this age group in part reflect the lifecourse accumulation of advantage or disadvantage. In recent years, however, growing interest has been expressed in the role of current socio-economic circumstances in shaping the health of older people. For example, the Longitudinal Survey in Europe on Nutrition and the Elderly: A Concerted Action Study found that a healthy lifestyle at older ages (measured in terms of diet, physical activity and smoking status) was related to a delay in the deterioration of health status and a reduced mortality risk (de Groot et al, 2004). This suggests that the health of older people is not set in stone by previous lifecourse influences but is amenable to improvement through lifestyle and environmental interventions.

Lifestyle factors

Diet and nutrition

The idea that lifestyle factors may play a critical role in preserving and promoting health in older age has long been popular with supporters of the free radical theory of ageing. According to this theory, ageing is the cumulative result of oxidative damage to the cells and tissues of the body. Increased oxidative stress has been linked to several major age-associated diseases, including atherosclerosis and cancer, to damage to the immune system and, through mitochondrial DNA mutations which result in a progressive reduction in energy output, to general signs of ageing such as loss of memory, hearing, vision and stamina. Dietary antioxidants are regarded as being important in modulating the oxidative stress of ageing and age-associated diseases. These include vitamin C, vitamin E, selenium, dietary folate, alpha-lipoic acid and carotenoids (Dreosti, 1998; Richard and Roussel, 1999; Meydani, 2001, 2002; Miquel, 2001).

Supporters of the free radical theory also advocate restricting calorie intake. In Britain, however, the main cause for concern in older people tends to be under-nutrition rather than over-nutrition. This is particularly true for those who are hospitalised or institutionalised, with 55% of older hospitalised patients undernourished on admission and many deteriorating further across their stay (Milne et al, 2002). Malnourishment is associated with poor health, including impaired immune response and cardiac function, muscle wastage and reduced mobility (Avenell and Handoll, 2004). It is also associated with poor outcomes from illness (including longer hospital stays, a longer period of rehabilitation and increased mortality), but can be reversed by nutritional support.

If oxidative stress plays a major role in ageing and in the development of age-related degenerative disease, then the consumption of adequate levels of antioxidants in the diet could be a key strategy for preserving health and protecting against the development of major diseases in old age. In dietary terms, the implications of the free radical theory are that intake of red meat, margarine and vegetable oils high in polyunsaturated fats should be restricted, consumption of foods rich in antioxidants (for example, dark leafy vegetables, fruits, nuts and green tea) increased and nutritional supplements used. As we have noted in Chapter Ten, there is consistent evidence that diets rich in fruit and vegetables and other plant foods are associated with moderately lower overall mortality rates and lower death rates from cardiovascular disease and some types of cancer. However, randomised intervention trials to date have failed to show any consistent benefit from the use of antioxidant supplements on cardiovascular disease or cancer risk (Stanner et al, 2004). Relatively few studies have also been conducted in older age groups, although people aged 75+ are at particular risk of poor nutrition and increased oxidative stress. One exception, part of the MRC Trial of Assessment and Management of Older People in the Community, found that low blood vitamin C concentrations were strongly predictive of mortality in people aged 75-84 years (Fletcher et al, 2003). Among older people in the US Cardiovascular Health Study, which involved a 10-year follow-up of older adults with different dietary patterns, those with higher than expected (relative to their calorie intake) consumption of vitamins and minerals and below expected consumption of fats and alcohol enjoyed more years of life and years of healthy life than older people in other dietary groups, although they did not have better outcomes with respect to cardiovascular health (Diehr and Beresford, 2003).

Although the role of specific antioxidants and vitamin supplementation (which, it is argued, is a poor substitute for a diet rich in antioxidants) remains subject to debate, observational studies of the links between oxidative stress and adverse health outcomes are convincing. Thus, the free radical theory may provide one explanation for social gradients in health among older people. According to the Over 65 UK National Diet and Nutrition Survey (NDNS), important social and geographical inequalities exist with respect to micronutrient intakes, older people of lower socio-economic status and those living in the North of Britain having significantly lower intakes of vitamin C, B-vitamins, selenium and carotenoids, a pattern that reflects lower consumption of vegetables by these groups (Bates et al, 1999, 2001, 2003; Thane et al, 2002). Within the sample, lower intakes of key micronutrients were associated with poorer health status (Margetts et al, 2003).

Similar trends in dietary patterns were observed in the MRC Trial of Assessment and Management of Older People in the Community (Fletcher et al, 2003), and in a study of older people in Nottingham which found that older age and lower educational qualifications predicted low vegetable intake, while low income and low social class were associated with low intake of fruit. Among men, living alone also appeared to reduce fruit and vegetable consumption (Donkin et al, 1998). Lower socio-economic status was also found to be significantly associated with low fruit and vegetable consumption by older men in the Caerphilly and Speedwell Collaborative Heart Disease Study. In this sample, only 4.3% of the men met the recommended target of five daily portions, while 33.3% of the men consumed one or fewer portions of fruit and vegetables per day. Fruit and vegetable intake reflected plasma concentrations of antioxidants, which showed a dose–response relationship to the frequency of consumption (Strain et al, 2000).

Lower intakes of fruit and vegetable consumption among older people of lower socio-economic status are likely in large part to reflect earlier dietary patterns. As we observed in Chapters Eight and Ten, a strong relationship between social advantage and 'healthy' diets is evident from childhood and persists into adulthood. However, other factors may also play a role in determining diets in older age, including access and affordability of healthy foods, loss of appetite and taste, lack of motivation (affecting older people living alone, for example) and dental status. In the Over 65 UK NDNS, for example, levels of vitamin C in the blood were significantly related to the presence, number and distribution of natural teeth. Over half of the respondents with dentures found difficulty eating foods such as nuts, apples and raw carrots. Among those with natural teeth, one in five experienced difficulty, chewing ability strongly reflecting numbers of teeth (Sheiham and Steele, 2001). In total, 50% of people over 65 living in the community had some natural teeth, compared to 21% of those living in institutions. Dental status declined with age, with only 35% of those over 75 in the total sample being dentate (Whynne, 1999). There are social and geographical variations in oral health status, loss of teeth being more common in the North of England than the South, and among those of lower social class (Steele et al, 1996).

Finally, the very low incomes available to the poorest pensioners suggest that affordability may be a significant barrier to the purchasing of healthy foods. In-depth interviews carried out as part of a recent ESRC-funded study of socially excluded older people found that the challenges of managing on a fixed low income meant that respondents regarded as luxuries what would be considered standard items by many. According to two interviewees:

"You can only buy the cheapest of food. Besides bread and fresh milk, sometimes I buy what you call a shank, you know a gammon shank, and I boil that because they are only about £1.24 and I do cabbage and we have that with some other veg...."

"I go in for the cheap stuff.... The only time I have a really decent meal is a Sunday. I love my Sunday dinner." (Scharf et al, 2005, pp 17-18)

Concerns have also been raised about the quality of food provided in institutional homes caring for older people. However, compared to the movement that is gathering in the UK to improve meals for schoolchildren, this issue has received relatively little attention.

Physical activity

In addition to improvements in nutrition, evidence supports the beneficial role of *moderate* physical activity (for example, walking, cycling, and gardening) in promoting health in older age. Because older people are generally more susceptible to oxidative stress, the beneficial and harmful effects of *strenuous* exercise (which is associated with increased production of free radicals) is more in balance (Polidori et al, 2000; Ji, 2001). However, it is recognised that moderate exercise plays an important part in the quality of life of older people. It can slow down age-related decline in muscle strength and bone density, promote weight loss, improve mental well-being and modify risk factors for coronary heart disease (CHD) and diabetes.

As loss of muscle strength and stability makes people vulnerable to falls, physical activity (with calcium and vitamin D supplementation) has been identified as a key intervention for falls prevention (see Chapter Thirteen). According to the NSF for Older People, falls are the leading cause of mortality in older people aged over 75 in the UK. Over 400,000 older people in England attend Accident and Emergency Departments following an accident and up to 14,000 a year die in the UK as a result of an osteoporotic hip fracture. Most falls do not result in a serious injury but they can lead to a loss of confidence and mobility, an increase in dependence and disability and eventual admission into long-term care. In 2000, it was estimated that hip fractures resulted in an annual cost to the NHS of £1.7 billion in England alone (DH, 2001, pp 76-7).

There remains debate about the type and amount of activity needed to promote optimal health and function in older people (Houde and Melillo, 2002). Among women, for example, a lack of participation in formal exercise is often compensated for by involvement in heavy housework (Lawlor et al, 2002). Nevertheless, older Britons are likely to be more sedentary than is good for their health. A survey of activity levels in Scotland found that over one third of respondents aged 65-84 years did no leisure-time physical activity and a further 17% did less than two hours a week (Crombie et al, 2004). In the British Women's Heart and Health Study, participation in physical exercise was found to be lowest in those living in the North of the country and from lower socio-economic classes. Socio-economic differences in physical activity thus appear to persist into older age. Despite this, studies examining influences on the incidence of osteoporosis and osteoporotic fractures offer conflicting results. Pearson et al (2004) report that, among older women recruited from a general practice register, those living in the most deprived areas had a significantly higher likelihood of osteoporosis and were significantly more likely to have had a history of previous fracture. Other research, however, has failed to identify a significant association between deprivation and risk for fracture in older people (Jones et al, 2004; West et al, 2004).

Smoking

As observed in Chapter Ten, cigarette smoking is the leading avoidable cause of premature death in middle age. The scope for extending years of life through avoidance of smoking reduces with age (Taylor et al, 2002). According to the long-term study of smoking-related mortality among British doctors, giving up at the age of 30 gains around 10 years of life expectancy, compared to three years when a 60-year-old smoker stops (Doll et al, 2004). Thereafter, however, the relative health risks of smoking in older age and the benefits that can be gained from smoking cessation in later life have been subject to debate. On the one hand, cumulative damage from long-term smoking may be so great that its effects are irreversible. On the other hand, because smoking contributes to oxidative damage and is associated with lower blood concentrations of vitamin C, giving up in older age may yield the same kinds of benefits that have been hypothesised for antioxidant-rich diets.

Uncertainty about the health effects of smoking cessation in older age reflects the lack of research that is conducted on this age group, methodological difficulties (for example, in isolating the effects of contemporary from previous factors and adjusting for the 'ill quitter effect') and differences in the relative effect of current lifestyle according to specific conditions. For example, there appears to be less scope in later life for reducing risks of dying from smoking-related cancers than for lowering risk of cardiovascular mortality (LaCroix et al, 1991; LaCroix and Omenn, 1992). Indeed, several studies suggest that the cardiovascular health of older people can be significantly improved by encouraging them to give up smoking (Paganini-Hill and Hsu, 1994; Iso et al, 2005). For other conditions, evidence of the effects of cessation in later life has been more inconsistent. In one prospective US study, smokers who quit even after the age of 60 years had better pulmonary function than continuing smokers (Higgins et al, 1993). In another, the pulmonary function of older people who had quit between the ages of 40 and 60 years was better than current smokers, but there was an apparent lack of benefit if cessation was delayed to the age of 60 (Frette et al, 1996).

Similarly, while early case control studies found that smoking might protect against Alzheimer's disease, recent prospective studies suggest that older people who smoke may be at increased risk for dementia (Ott et al, 2004).

On balance, it seems that, although stopping smoking as early as possible is important, gains can still be made by giving up in older age. As noted in Chapter Ten, because people from poorer, more disadvantaged social groups are less likely to quit than those from more advantaged groups, the social divide in smoking prevalence increases with age. Since 1974, the greatest percentage decrease in the proportion smoking has been among people aged 60 and over, where the prevalence has more than halved from 34% to 15% in 2002 (data derived from the ONS). The minority who continue to smoke are drawn disproportionately from lower socio-economic groups. Thus, the fact that smoking continues to present a significant health hazard in later life suggests that this is likely to be a contributor to health inequalities in old age.

Housing and environmental factors

Because older people spend between 70% and 90% of their time in their home (Baltes et al, 1990, cited by ODPM, 2005), housing is a particularly important factor influencing health and well-being in this age group. Research exploring the relationships between housing and health was outlined in Chapter Ten. In brief, studies have emphasised the links that exist between substandard housing and poor respiratory health, excess winter mortality, exposure to contaminants, risk of accidents, and poor psychological well-being. Concerns have been particularly expressed about the vulnerability of older people to cold conditions in the home. This may act as a risk factor for respiratory problems, increasing the severity of asthma and chronic obstructive pulmonary disease (COPD), and potentially delaying recovery on discharge from hospital (Howden-Chapman, 2004). The World Health Organization (WHO) recommends that the indoor temperature for older people should not fall below 18-20°C. However, according to the 2001 English Housing Condition Survey (ODPM, 2003), 29.3% of people over 60 years and 31.1% of those aged over 75 live in houses that do not provide a reasonable degree of thermal comfort. Every year there are more than 20,000 excess winter deaths among older people (www.helptheaged.org.uk).

Older people living in the private rented sector appear to be particularly vulnerable to poor housing conditions (Izuhara and Heywood, 2003). Due to legislative changes since the 1980s, however, the role of this sector has changed, and the number of older people who are renting on a long-term basis has declined. Owner-occupation among older households is thus increasing. In 2001, 72% of people aged 65-74 and 61% of people aged 85 and over were owner-occupiers (data derived from the ONS), and by 2011 nearly 80% of households headed by 60- to 74-year-olds are expected to own their own homes (RCLTC, 1999). While housing tenure is often used as a proxy for socio-economic status, owner-occupation in old age does not necessarily mean a high income or good housing conditions (Breeze et al, 2004a). According to the 2001 English House Condition Survey, 39% of older households (that include someone aged 75 years or more) in the private sector (owner-occupied and rented) live in non-decent homes. Overall, single people are more vulnerable to housing problems than those living as a couple. Among people aged 60 and over, 31% of couples and 38% of single households lived in non-decent housing, mostly due to the lack of thermal comfort (ODPM, 2003).

Although the poor are significantly more likely to live in substandard housing than more advantaged groups, empirical evidence of a relationship between socio-economic deprivation, poor housing and poor health in older age is lacking (see, for example, Aylin et al, 2001; Maheswaran et al, 2004). This partly reflects a degree of protection offered by social sector housing. Local authority and housing association properties of relatively recent construction are more likely to possess central heating than older owner-occupied properties in highly deprived neighbourhoods. This may partly explain why winter mortality in older British people is not associated with socio-economic deprivation. However, people in local authority or housing association dwellings do appear to be vulnerable to low indoor temperatures during cold periods if their heating costs are high (Wilkinson et al, 2001).

Aspects of home design can also present hazards to older people. There is particular concern about the numbers of accidents and falls that occur within the homes of older people. As noted earlier, falls may not only result in serious injury, but even death in older people. They can lead to a loss of mobility and independence and eventual admission to a care home. Inadequate lighting, inappropriate stair coverings and a lack of hand supports and/or grab rails increases older people's chances of falling (Easterbrook et al, 2001). However, while affordability could plausibly prevent older people from seeking to implement home improvements, the incidence of osteoporotic fractures among older people does not appear to be associated with socio-economic deprivation (Jones et al, 2004; West et al, 2004). By contrast, pedestrian-related injuries in older people are significantly associated with socio-economic status (Lyons et al, 2003). This relationship partly reflects individual factors (that is, access to personal transport). It also results from the higher volumes of traffic that occur in urban deprived areas. Traffic-related accidents in older age are an important public health problem. Nearly half of pedestrian fatalities caused by road accidents are people aged 60 years and over (Brook Lyndhurst Ltd, 2004, p 45).

As already discussed, depression and psychological problems among older people are strongly associated with socio-economic status, and research suggests that housing and environmental design may play a role in this. Fear of crime and antisocial behaviour can be exacerbated by concerns about home security, poor lighting in the local neighbourhood, a tendency for groups of people to hang around (which can itself reflect environmental design) and high local crime rates. Safe and easy access to basic services such as local shops, post offices, general pharmacies and banks are also very important to older people, as is the ability to maintain social networks and avoid isolation. For several reasons, poor people are more likely to be vulnerable to 'unhealthy' neighbourhoods than well-off people (Breeze et al, 2005). First, as discussed in Chapter Ten, concerns about crime, vandalism, hooliganism and troublesome teenagers are most prevalent in poor, predominantly council-built areas. Disproportionately high levels of fear of crime among older people contrast with persistently lower levels of victimisation. However, area-specific studies suggest that fear of crime among poorer old people may be largely justified. Scharf et al's (2002) research found that 40% of the older people interviewed had been the victim of crime in the last year or two, rising to nearly half of those in poverty. The significant trauma associated with crime for frail people and the adoption of a risk minimisation lifestyle, where safety is bought at the expense of personal freedoms, also contribute to higher levels of fear.

A second factor that increases the vulnerability of the older poor is service deprivation. Although this is a problem most commonly associated with rural living, a lack of access to basic services has also been highlighted as an issue in peripheral council estates. Finally, the ability of older people to develop and maintain social networks can be undermined by a lack of access to safe public places, high population turnover (which can undermine familiarity with one's neighbourhood) and the lack of personal transport. Because the poorest, oldest and most frail are more dependent on public transport, their activities tend to be the most spatially constrained. Against this, affluent older people are less likely to have close family members such as children living nearby, which may increase vulnerability to social isolation and a lack of social support.

Proximity to family and a desire to maintain existing social contacts are key factors influencing the stated desire of most older people, even those with considerable disabilities, to stay in their own homes. Despite this, around one in 20 people over the age of 65 years are in care homes. Since 1970, there has been a general increase in the numbers of people in long-term institutional care, and the locus of that care has shifted from hospital long-stay wards and local authority residential homes to privately operated nursing and residential homes. Thus, between 1970 and 2000, the number of local authority residential home places fell from 108,700 to 59,000 and long-stay hospital places from 52,000 to 20,400, while the number of places in privately operated nursing and residential homes increased from 44,000 to 390,000 (Laing and Buisson, 2000, 2001, cited by Johnson, 2002).

As Johnson (2002) suggests, home is closely associated with privacy, security, independence and autonomy and a move to residential care can threaten this. However, options for older people have been limited by cost considerations, meaning that many have had little choice but to enter care homes. Changes in the pattern of home care support have been of significance here. Help with meeting so-called 'low-level needs' (for example, help with self-care, domestic tasks, the provision of aids and adaptations and transport and other assistance to enable them to get out of the house) is not only highly valued by older people, it can make a critical difference to maintaining independence. Yet between 1992 and 2000, the number of households receiving home care support decreased by 25% (Tanner, 2003). This decline in domiciliary care reflected increasing pressure on social services budgets and differences in the ways in which home care and residential care were paid for. While charging procedures for residential care took account of benefits, pensions, capital (including the value of a person's home) and savings, charges for home care services were discretionary and could not be set against a person's property. As a result, the provision of care at home to home owners who were asset-rich but income-poor was more costly to social services departments than placing them in residential homes where they had to realise their assets (Johnson, 2002). Several researchers have expressed concern about the degree to which such perverse incentives have resulted in inappropriate placements. For example, one study in North West England found that 71% of new admissions to residential homes were of low dependency, many of whom could be supported with home-based care (Challis et al, 2000).

Significantly, the impact of perverse incentives may not have been uniform across the socio-economic spectrum. Affluent older people can either organise their own private domestic help or pay for (means-tested) packages of home care provided by social services departments. However, many pensioners on average and lower incomes are unable to afford the domiciliary care that they need. Unless they can rely on informal personal care provided by family, relatives and friends (Deeming and Keen, 2002), older people of low to moderate means may have been vulnerable to being steered by social services departments into residential care instead of receiving care in the community. Differences in the care pathways developed for different socio-economic groups have been demonstrated by empirical evidence, although the relationship between income and the use of long-term care services is not straightforward. An earlier review of the limited literature suggested there was an association between low income levels and higher rates of service utilisation, but with some indications that statistical significance would be lost if disability was taken into account (Almond et al, 1999). Almond et al's own survey found that, once variables such as disability, health status and the availability of informal care were controlled, those in the lowest income quintile were both least likely to use private domestic help and to receive the lowest levels of publicly funded home help (alongside those in the top income quintile). The Evaluating Community Care for Elderly People Study of 400 users of long-term care also suggested that there was a statistically significant and negative association between low income and the volume of use of community-based services, suggesting some users may be deterred from using services because of the existence of charges, a possibility reinforced by the fact that district nursing services, for which no charge is made, showed no relationship to income (Almond et al, 1999). By contrast, Hancock et al (2002) looked explicitly at whether older people's economic resources affected their likelihood of care home entry and found no significant effect for income. Moreover, although there was a financial incentive to place home owners into institutional settings, this group were less likely to be admitted into long-term care.

Not surprisingly, the system of community care described earlier was heavily criticised for its bias towards residential care, the lack of emphasis on prevention and for adopting a service-based rather than a client-based approach. Under New Labour, changes have been made to charging procedures. Thus, since 2002/03, the component of Income Support that was paid directly to residential and nursing home establishments is now distributed to local authorities who are encouraged to use home-based alternatives to residential care. Other developments such as Intermediate Care guidance and the provision of community equipment (see Chapter Thirteen) also support the maintenance of older people's independence through, for example, the use of active rehabilitation to prevent admission to long-term care. Given many older people's preference to stay at home, these developments are to be welcomed, although some doubts have been expressed regarding the extent to which new policies will reach out preventively to older people with 'lower-level' needs (Tanner, 2003). Moreover, current attempts to modernise social services will principally benefit the recently retired. Nearly half a million people aged 65 and over are already living in long-term care, and changes in policy may have exacerbated the rate of care home closures. Being evicted from their care homes can be so disorientating and distressing for older people that the experience amounts to 'transfer trauma' (Murtiashaw, 2001, cited by Scourfield, 2004). If older people on lower incomes were more likely to be admitted into residential care in the first place, then they are the main victims of increased volatility in the system.

Access to health services

The resources that have been invested in initiatives such as Intermediate Care reflect a wider policy concern with strengthening services for older people. In 2001, the DH launched an NSF for Older People that explicitly acknowledged that services had previously failed to meet older people's needs, sometimes by discriminating against them. Indeed, the first of eight standards incorporated into the Framework drew on evidence from a range of services including cardiac care and non-cancer palliative care services to highlight the need to root out age discrimination in accessing NHS or social care services.

The NSF usefully identified the extent to which access to healthcare varies *between* different age groups. However, with the exception of the disadvantage faced by older people from black and minority ethnic groups (DH, 2001, pp 17, 90), it had relatively little to say about variations *within* older age bands. A number of factors have hampered the collection of evidence in this area. First, as noted in

Chapter Ten, there are methodological difficulties in establishing expected levels of health service need against which actual use can be compared, so less is generally known about inequalities in access to services than inequalities in health status. Second, what we do know about equity in healthcare tends to concern the population as a whole rather than specific age groups. Again, methodological factors play a role. Age standardisation is so common in epidemiological and health services research that important interactions between age, gender and social status are often overlooked. Research of this nature also tends towards narrowly defined aims. Thus, studies examining ageism will adjust for socio-economic variables when analysing data pertaining to the wider population, while researchers exploring inequities by deprivation will adjust for age. As a result, direct evidence of socio-economic inequalities in the use of healthcare by older people is lacking.

Examination of the few UK studies of healthcare equity that have focused on people aged 65+ suggests that those of lower socio-economic status may be less likely to access hospital, primary and community-level services. Inequity by deprivation has been found with respect to knee joint replacements (Milner et al, 2004); screening for abdominal aortic aneurysms (Kim et al, 2004); emergency hospital admissions (Bernard and Smith, 1998); and influenza vaccinations (Breeze et al, 2004b) among older people. Older people of higher socio-economic status have a greater chance of dying at home, perhaps because they are better able to access home care (Grande et al, 1998; Higginson et al, 1999; Grundy et al, 2004). Concerns have also been raised about accessibility to mental health services for which there are high levels of unmet need. In the ONS Survey of Psychiatric Morbidity, only 41% of respondents with the revised Clinical Interview Schedule (CIS-R) scores of 18 or above (that is, with levels of neurotic symptoms likely to require treatment) had visited a general practitioner (GP) with a mental health complaint in the previous year: 4% had seen a community psychiatric nurse, 3% a psychiatrist and 2% a psychologist. Although 78% of these respondents reported having difficulties with activities of daily living, only 17% had received any form of community care (Evans et al, 2003, pp 50-1).

With respect to support for mental health difficulties, older people who are living in institutions do not fare significantly better than older people living in the community. Although psychiatric illness is common among older people in general hospitals, a postal questionnaire survey of old-age psychiatrists providing psychiatric services to older people in general hospital wards found that 89% were unhappy with the service, which was slow, reactive and, due to problems of coordination between general hospital and psychiatric staff, led to the poor management of comorbid psychiatric and physical illness in older people (Holmes et al, 2003). A postal survey of managers of care homes in the UK similarly identified a range of problems with regard to the provision of mental heathcare – 41% of care home managers felt that at least 50% of their residents needed psychiatric evaluation, 38% reported that their homes 'never' received any visits from old-age psychiatrists and only half described the current frequency of visits as adequate (Purandare et al, 2004). As noted earlier, the prevalence of psychiatric morbidity among older people is characterised by significant social gradients. Thus, those of lower socio-economic status are likely to bear the brunt of inadequacies in service provision in this area. Evidence suggests that older people from black and minority ethnic populations are also poorly served. For example, Bowes and Wilkinson (2003) suggest that dementia services are culturally insensitive to the views and experiences of dementia among older South Asian people and their families and carers. Compared to non-South Asian people, this group are more likely to have negative views about residential care, make limited use of non-NHS support and deal with the later stages of dementia at home. Yet they experience considerable difficulty in accessing appropriate home-based support.

Several studies that have not explicitly focused on older people but that have examined patterns of healthcare use for conditions that disproportionately affect this age group have also searched for evidence of socio-economic inequality. For example, among patients newly diagnosed with glaucoma (67% of whom were aged 61+), those of lower occupational class, of African-Caribbean origin, with no access to a car, fewer educational qualifications and in rented accommodation, were more likely to be late presenters, an important risk factor for subsequent blindness (Fraser et al, 2001). Comparing access to care for adults undergoing stroke rehabilitation in two Welsh authorities, Allen et al (2004) found that ability to access private finance made a significant difference to service quality. In the less deprived authority, where three out of four families were able to make a financial contribution to their care package, patients benefited from more timely discharge, a greater choice in their discharge arrangements and better joined-up working between their health and social care agencies.

Although cancer survival rates are improving in the UK, outcomes for deprived patients are poorer than those of more affluent patients and, between the late 1980s and late 1990s, the deprivation gap in survival grew (Coleman et al, 2004). This has raised questions as to whether poor people suffer from differential access to treatment. Pollack and Vickers (1998) suggest that, with respect to effective diagnosis of and referral for cancers of the colorectum, lung and breast, primary care is failing patients from deprived areas. Their study, which analysed over 140,000 hospital admissions in South East England in the early 1990s, found that patients from deprived areas were more likely to be admitted as emergencies and ordinary inpatients than their counterparts from more affluent areas. Patients with lung and breast cancers from deprived areas were less likely to receive surgery; and patients with colorectal cancer from deprived areas were less likely to be admitted to specialised units. The authors suggest that these findings could indicate that patients from deprived areas were presenting at a later stage in the course of their disease (Pollack and Vickers, 1998). Whynes et al (2003) report that those from more deprived areas are less likely to accept an invitation to be screened for colorectal cancer, suggesting that socio-economic gradients may exist in disease progression at prognosis. Similarly, among women aged 65 and over attending a South London practice, non-manual social class, higher school leaving age, home ownership and higher income all predicted uptake of mammography (Harris et al, 2002).

Against these findings, several studies question whether socio-economic differences in survival rates in patients with cancer can be attributed to more advanced disease at presentation (Schrijvers et al, 1995; Hole and McArdle, 2002) or differences in treatment. Among over 4,000 patients diagnosed with colorectal cancer in the former Wessex Health Region, 75% of whom were aged 65 and over, there was no evidence of differences in either stage of disease at presentation or treatment by deprivation (Wrigley et al, 2003). Nor was socio-economic status associated with length of time between first referral and treatment or treatment for colorectal cancer in a study of patients in North and North East Scotland (Campbell et al, 2002). Greater survival from breast cancer among women from more affluent parts of Glasgow could not be explained by pathological stage at presentation (Macleod et al, 2000), and no significant differences were detected with respect to radiotherapy, chemotherapy or endocrine therapy. According to all of these studies, access to care in the NHS appears to be fairly equitable with respect to socio-economic status.

As it is commonly believed that both deprived and older people are disadvantaged with regard to access to health services, people who are old and deprived might be expected to be the most disadvantaged of all. Unfortunately, very little research has examined inequalities in access among this age group and that that exists is equivocal. There is, however, strong evidence to suggest that, regardless of their socio-economic status, older people suffer discrimination in health services on the basis of their age (Bowling, 1999; Dudley et al, 2002; Bond et al, 2003; DeWilde et al, 2003; Brown, 2004; Hacker and Stanistreet, 2004). Age also appears to interact with gender in creating differentials in treatment between men and women. For example, women who present with symptoms of CHD tend to be older than men. While this has a bearing on the severity of symptoms and comorbidity, it may also make women more vulnerable to age-based discrimination (Wenger, 1997; Williams et al, 2004).

Despite the good intentions of the NSF for Older People and the additional investment that has been made into new services such as Intermediate Care (see Chapter Thirteen), the scope for eradicating ageism in the provision and use of NHS services may be limited by the possibility that age discrimination is built into the current approach to distributing healthcare resources. The English formula for allocating funds for Hospital and Community Health Services (HCHS) adopts a utilisation-based model to assess need for healthcare. This assumes that historical patterns of service uptake between different care groups (as revealed by utilisation) are appropriate (Mays, 1995), a problematic assumption given the concerns that are regularly expressed about ageism, sexism, racism and socio-economic bias in access to healthcare, and one that allows any bias in healthcare utilisation to become self-perpetuating. For example, if it is accepted that older patients can and should gain from more intensive treatment, then use-based per capita allocations for older age bands could be regarded as conservative. There is some empirical support for this. Comparing morbidity-based capitations for the inpatient treatment of CHD with target HCHS allocations, Asthana et al (2004) found that the morbidity-based model would result in a significant shift of resources towards areas serving older demographic populations. By contrast, the utilisation-based formula allocated resources to areas with younger demographic profiles to a higher level than implied by morbidity alone.

There is a geographical dimension to this as in much of England, particularly to the West of the country, rural areas have demographically older profiles than urban deprived areas. Most health inequalities researchers and policy makers in Britain are concerned to direct more resources towards the urban poor. Thus, the fact that the current formula allocates resources to areas that would be expected to benefit from a health inequalities budget may appear at first sight to be unproblematic. However, the goals of healthcare equity and health equity require very different policy responses and, as we discussed in Chapter Ten, it is generally agreed that the NHS (and particularly national *hospital* services) has relatively little to contribute towards the reduction of health inequalities compared to other sources of variation such as income distribution, education, housing and lifestyle. The central aim of the current resource allocation system is to allocate resources to geographical areas in order to secure equal opportunity of access for equal healthcare needs. Thus, the targeting of core services to urban deprived populations over and above levels of underlying morbidity is likely to be an ineffective (and perhaps co-opting) response to health inequalities. It is one, moreover, that introduces a new form of inequity by underestimating the needs of more elderly but less deprived populations (Asthana et al, 2004).

The policy implications

It is not insignificant that this is one of the shortest chapters in this book. In contrast to other periods of the lifecourse, there has been a relative dearth of research on health inequalities in older age. Yet poverty levels among older people are comparable to those among children, and many of the factors that present health risks for younger age groups also impact on health inequalities among older people. Evidence from this chapter suggests that, while differentials in health status in part reflect differences in the lifecourse accumulation of advantage and disadvantage, the health of older people is not set in stone by previous lifecourse influences. Healthy lifestyles have been related to a delay in the deterioration of health status, suggesting that there is scope for improving health, even at later ages. However, while there is considerable interest in the concept of 'slowing down the ageing process' in the US, where there is a strong elderly lobby, this idea has received very little attention in the UK. Further research is thus needed on the role that lifestyle factors play in influencing health status in this age group in order to establish the risks presented by known socio-economic variations in factors such as diet, physical activity and smoking.

In contrast to the relative lack of interest in lifestyle factors, research has focused on the role of housing and the environment in shaping health and well-being in older people, although empirical evidence of a relationship between socio-economic deprivation, poor housing and poor health in older age is not strong. Given the high levels of depression and psychological problems among older people, however, this focus on housing is undoubtedly appropriate. Older people spend most of their time at home and in their communities and are therefore particularly likely to be affected by factors such as neighbourhood decline. Fear of crime, for example, can lead to the adoption of a risk minimisation lifestyle, which, as well as increasing social isolation, reduces opportunities for physical activity. However, most older people want to remain in their own homes. There is some evidence that those of low to moderate means have been more likely to have been steered into residential care rather than receiving care in the community as they have not had the resources to pay for domiciliary care. It is therefore important to ensure that measures to support independent living reach members of all socio-economic groups. Similar concerns have been raised with respect to access to health services, although here the needs for rural older people must be considered alongside those of their urban counterparts.

Chapter Thirteen examines evidence of the interventions designed to address the issues highlighted in this chapter and, interestingly, notes a strong policy response to the needs of older people. Perhaps this is one area in which health inequalities researchers, who have paid very little attention to older age, could learn much from policy makers. In addition to formulating a number of positive initiatives with respect to housing, the provision of health and social services and access to services, the latter have been explicit about the need to adopt an anti-ageist stance and a more inclusionary approach to this age group. These developments are discussed in more detail in the following chapter.

References

Allen, D., Griffiths, L. and Lyne, P. (2004) 'Accommodating health and social care needs: routine resource allocation in stroke rehabilitation', *Sociology of Health and Illness*, vol 26, pp 411-32.

Almond, S., Bebbington, S., Judge, K., Mangalore, R. and O'Donnell, O. (1999) 'Poverty, disability and the use of long-term care services', in Royal Commission on Long-Term Care (ed) *With respect to old age: Long term care – Rights and responsibilities. The context of long-term care policy. Research volume 1*, London: The Stationery Office, pp 115-56.

Arber, S. (1996) 'Integrating nonemployment into research on health inequalities', *International Journal of Health Services*, vol 26, pp 445-81.

Arber, S. and Cooper, H. (1999) 'Gender differences in health in later life: the new paradox?', *Social Science and Medicine*, vol 48, pp 61-76.

Asthana, S., Gibson, A., Moon, G., Dicker, J. and Brigham, P. (2004) 'The pursuit of equity in NHS resource allocation: should morbidity replace utilisation as the basis for setting health care capitations?', *Social Science and Medicine*, vol 58, pp 539-51.

Avenell, A. and Handoll, H. (2004) 'Nutritional supplementation for hip fracture aftercare in the elderly', *The Cochrane Database of Systematic Reviews 2004, issue 1*, Art. No: CD001880.

Aylin, P., Morris, S., Wakefield, J., Grossinho, A., Jarup, L. and Elliott, P. (2001) 'Temperature, housing, deprivation and their relationship to excess winter mortality in Great Britain, 1986-1996', *International Journal of Epidemiology*, vol 30, pp 1100-18.

Baltes, M., Wahl, H.-W. and Schmid-Furstoss, U. (1990) 'The daily life of the elderly at home: activity patterns, personal control and functional health', *Journal of Gerontology: Social Sciences*, vol 45, pp 173-9.

Bates, C., Thane, C., Prentice, A. and Delves, H. (2003) 'Selenium status and its correlates in a British national diet and nutrition survey: people aged 65 years and over', *Journal of Trace Elements in Medicine and Biology*, vol 16, pp 1-8.

Bates, C., Cole, T., Mansoor, M., Pentieva, K. and Finch, S. (2001) 'Geographical variations in nutrition-related vascular risk factors in the UK: National Diet and Nutrition Survey of people aged 65 years and over', *Journal of Nutrition, Health and Aging*, vol 5, pp 220-5.

Bates, C., Prentice, A., Cole, T., van der Pols, J., Doyle, W., Finch, S., Smithers, G. and Clarke, P. (1999) 'Micronutrients: highlights and research challenges from the 1994-5 National Diet and Nutrition Survey of people aged 65 years and over', *British Journal of Nutrition*, vol 82, pp 7-15.

Bernard, S. and Smith, L. (1998) 'Emergency admissions of older people to hospital: a link with material deprivation', *Journal of Public Health Medicine*, vol 20, pp 97-101.

Blazer, D., Burchett, B., Service, C. and George, L. (1991) 'The association of age and depression among the elderly: an epidemiologic exploration', *Journal of Gerontology*, no 46, pp 201-5.

Bond, M., Bowling, A., McKee, D., Kennelly, M., Banning, A., Dudley, N., Elder, A. and Martin, A. (2003) 'Does ageism affect the management of ischaemic heart disease?', *Journal of Health Services Research and Policy*, vol 8, pp 40-7.

Boreham, R., Stafford, M. and Taylor, R. (2002) *Health Survey for England 2000: Social capital and health*, London: The Stationery Office.

Bouhuys, A., Flentge, F., Oldehinkel, A. and van den Berg, M. (2004) 'Potential psychosocial mechanisms linking depression to immune function in elderly subjects', *Psychiatry Research*, vol 127, pp 237-45.

Bowes, A. and Wilkinson, H. (2003) '"We didn't know it would get that bad": South Asian experiences of dementia and the service response', *Health and Social Care in the Community*, vol 11, pp 387-96.

Bowling, A. (1999) 'Ageism in cardiology', *British Medical Journal*, vol 319, pp 1353-5.

Bowling, A. (2004) 'Socioeconomic differentials in mortality among older people', *Journal of Epidemiology and Community Health*, vol 58, pp 438-40.

Breeze, E., Sloggett, A. and Fletcher, A. (1999) 'Socioeconomic and demographic predictors of mortality and institutional residence among middle aged and older people: results from the Longitudinal Study', *Journal of Epidemiology and Community Health*, vol 53, pp 765-74.

Breeze, E., Fletcher, A., Leon, D., Marmot, M., Clarke, R. and Shipley, M. (2001) 'Do socioeconomic disadvantages persist into old age? Self-reported morbidity in a 29-year follow-up of the Whitehall Study', *American Journal of Public Health*, vol 91, pp 277-83.

Breeze, E., Jones, D., Wilkinson, P., Latif, A., Bulpitt, C. and Fletcher, A. (2004a) 'Association of quality of life in old age in Britain with socioeconomic position: baseline data from a randomised controlled trial', *Journal of Epidemiology and Community Health*, vol 58, pp 667-73.

Breeze, E., Mangtani, P., Fletcher, A., Price, G., Kovats, S. and Roberts, J. (2004b) 'Trends in influenza vaccination uptake among people aged over 74 years, 1997-2000: survey of 73 general practices in Britain', *BMC Family Practice*, vol 5, pp 8-14.

Breeze, E., Jones, D., Wilkinson, P., Bulpitt, C., Grundy, E., Latif, A. and Fletcher, A. (2005) 'Area deprivation, social class, and quality of life among people aged 75 years and over in Britain', *International Journal of Epidemiology*, vol 34, no 2, pp 276-83.

Brook Lyndhurst Ltd (2004) *Sustainable cities and the ageing society: The role of older people in an urban renaissance*, Report for the ODPM, London: Brook Lyndhurst Ltd.

Brown, D. (2004) 'A literature review exploring how healthcare professionals contribute to the assessment and control of postoperative pain in older people', *Journal of Clinical Nursing*, vol 13, pp 74-90.

Campbell, N., Elliott, A., Sharp, L., Ritchie, L., Cassidy, J. and Little, J. (2002) 'Impact of deprivation and rural residence on treatment of colorectal and lung cancer', *British Journal of Cancer*, vol 87, pp 585-90.

Challis, D., Mozley, C., Sutcliffe, C., Bagley, H., Price, L., Burns, A., Huxley, P. and Cordingley, L. (2000) 'Dependency in older people recently admitted to care homes', *Age and Ageing*, vol 29, pp 255-60.

Coleman, M., Rachet, B., Woods, L., Mitry, E., Riga, M., Cooper, N., Quinn, M., Brenner, H. and Esteve, J. (2004) 'Trends and socioeconomic inequalities in cancer survival in England and Wales up to 2001', *British Journal of Cancer*, vol 90, pp 1367-73.

Cooper, C., Eriksson, J., Forsen, T., Osmond, C., Tuomilehto, J. and Barker, D. (2001) 'Maternal height, childhood growth and risk of hip fracture in later life: a longitudinal study', *Osteoporosis International*, vol 12, pp 623-9.

Crombie, I., Irvine, L., Williams, B., McGinnis, A., Slane, P., Alder, E. and McMurdo, M. (2004) 'Why older people do not participate in leisure time physical activity: a survey of activity levels, beliefs and deterrents', *Age and Ageing*, vol 33, pp 287-92.

Deeming, C. and Keen, J. (2002) 'Paying for old age: can people on lower incomes afford domiciliary care costs?', *Social Policy & Administration*, vol 36, pp 465-81.

de Groot, L., Verheijden, M., de Henauw, S., Schroll, M., van Staveren, W. and the Seneca Investigators (2004) 'Lifestyle, nutritional status, health, and mortality in elderly people across Europe: a review of the longitudinal results of the SENECA study', *The Journals of Gerontology Series A: Biological Sciences and Medical Sciences*, vol 59, pp 1277-84.

DeWilde, S., Carey, I., Bremner, S., Richards, N., Hilton, S. and Cook, D. (2003) 'Evolution of statin prescribing 1994-2001: a case of agism but not of sexism?', *Heart*, vol 89, pp 417-21.

DH (Department of Health) (2001) *National Service Framework for Older People*, London: DH.

Diehr, P. and Beresford, S.A. (2003) 'The relation of dietary patterns to future survival, health and cardiovascular events in older adults', *Journal of Clinical Epidemiology*, vol 56, pp 1224-35.

Doll, R., Peto, R., Boreham, J. and Sutherland, I. (2004) 'Mortality in relation to smoking: 50 years' observations on male British doctors', *British Medical Journal*, doi 10.1136/bmj.38142.554479.AE.

Donkin, A., Johnson, A., Morgan, K., Neale, R., Page, R. and Silburn, R. (1998) 'Gender and living alone as determinants of fruit and vegetable consumption among the elderly living at home in urban Nottingham', *Appetite*, vol 30, pp 39-51.

Dreosti, I. (1998) 'Nutrition, cancer, and aging', *Annals of the New York Academy of Sciences*, vol 854, pp 371-7.

Dudley, N., Bowling, A., Bond, M., McKee, D., McClay, S., Banning, A., Elder, A., Martin, A. and Blackman, I. (2002) 'Age- and sex-related bias in the management of heart disease in a district general hospital', *Age and Ageing*, vol 31, pp 37-42.

Easterbrook, L., Horton, K., Arber, S. and Davidson, K. (2001) *International review of interventions in falls among older people*, London: DTI.

Evans, O., Singleton, N., Meltzer, H., Stewart, R. and Prince, M. (2003) *The mental health of older people*, London: The Stationery Office.

Falaschetti, E., Malbut, K. and Primatesta, P. (2002) *Health Survey for England 2000: The general health of older people and their use of health services*, London: The Stationery Office.

Fletcher, A., Breeze, E. and Shetty, P. (2003) 'Antioxidant vitamins and mortality in older persons: findings from the nutrition add-on study to the Medical Research Council Trial of Assessment and Management of Older People in the Community', *American Journal of Clinical Nutrition*, vol 78, pp 999-1010.

Fraser, S., Bunce, C., Wormald, R. and Brunner, E. (2001) 'Deprivation and late presentation of glaucoma: case control study', *British Medical Journal*, vol 322, pp 639-43.

Frette, C., Barrett-Connor, E. and Clausen, J. (1996) 'Effect of active and passive smoking on ventilatory function in elderly men and women', *American Journal of Epidemiology*, vol 143, pp 757-65.

Glaser, K. and Grundy, E. (2002) 'Class, caring and disability: evidence from the British Retirement Survey', *Ageing and Society*, vol 22, pp 325-42.

Grande, G., Addington-Hall, J. and Todd, C. (1998) 'Place of death and access to home care services: are certain patient groups at a disadvantage?', *Social Science and Medicine*, vol 47, pp 565-79.

Grundy, E. and Glaser, K. (2000) 'Socio-demographic differences in the onset and progression of disability in early old age: a longitudinal study', *Age and Ageing*, vol 29, pp 149-57.

Grundy, E. and Holt, G. (2000) 'Adult life experiences and health in early old age in Great Britain', *Social Science and Medicine*, vol 51, pp 1061-74.

Grundy, E. and Holt, G. (2001) 'The socio-economic status of older adults: how should we measure it in studies of health inequalities?', *Journal of Epidemiology and Community Health*, vol 55, pp 895-904.

Grundy, E. and Sloggett, A. (2003) 'Health inequalities in the older population: the role of personal capital, social resources and socio-economic circumstances', *Social Science and Medicine*, vol 56, pp 935-47.

Grundy, E., Mayer, D., Young, H. and Sloggett, A. (2004) 'Living arrangements and place of death of older people with cancer in England and Wales: a record linkage study', *British Journal of Cancer*, vol 91, pp 907-12.

Hacker, J. and Stanistreet, D. (2004) 'Equity in waiting times for two surgical specialties: a case study at a hospital in the North West of England', *Journal of Public Health*, vol 26, pp 56-60.

Hancock, R., Arthur, A., Jagger, C. and Matthews, R. (2002) 'The effect of older people's economic resources on care home entry under the United Kingdom's long-term care financing system', *Journals of Gerontology Series B: Psychological Sciences and Social Sciences*, vol 57, pp S285-93.

Harris, T., Cook, D., Shah, S., Victor, C., DeWilde, S., Beighton, C. and Rink, E. (2002) 'Mammography uptake predictors in older women', *Family Practice*, vol 19, pp 661-4.

Harris, T., Cook, D., Victor, C., Rink, E., Mann, A., Shah, S., DeWilde, S. and Beighton, C. (2003) 'Predictors of depressive symptoms in older people – a survey of two general practice populations', *Age and Ageing*, vol 32, pp 510-18.

Higgins, M., Enright, P., Kronmal, R., Schenker, M., Anton-Culver, H. and Lyles, M. (1993) 'Smoking and lung function in elderly men and women: the Cardiovascular Health Study', *Journal of the American Medical Association*, vol 269, pp 2741-8.

Higginson, I., Jarman, B., Astin, P. and Dolan, S. (1999) 'Do social factors affect where patients die: an analysis of 10 years of cancer deaths in England', *Journal of Public Health Medicine*, vol 21, pp 22-8.

Hirani, V. and Malbut, K. (2002) *Health Survey for England 2000: Disability among older people*, London: The Stationery Office.

Hirst, M. (2003) 'Caring-related inequalities in psychological distress in Britain during the 1990s', *Journal of Public Health Medicine*, vol 25, pp 336-43.

Hole, D. and McArdle, C. (2002) 'Impact of socioeconomic deprivation on outcome after surgery for colorectal cancer', *British Journal of Surgery*, vol 89, pp 586-90.

Holmes, J., Bentley, K. and Cameron, I. (2003) 'A UK survey of psychiatric services for older people in general hospitals', *International Journal of Geriatric Psychiatry*, vol 18, pp 716-21.

Houde, S. and Melillo, K. (2002) 'Cardiovascular health and physical activity in older adults: an integrative review of research methodology and results', *Journal of Advanced Nursing*, vol 38, pp 219-34.

Howden-Chapman, P. (2004) 'Housing standards: a glossary of housing and health', *Journal of Epidemiology and Community Health*, vol 58, pp 162-8.

Huisman, M., Kunst, A. and Mackenbach, J. (2003) 'Socioeconomic inequalities in morbidity among the elderly: a European overview', *Social Science and Medicine*, vol 57, pp 861-73.

Huisman, M., Kunst, A., Anderson, O., Bopp, M., Borgan, J.-K., Borrell, C., Costa, G., Deboosere, P., Desplanques, G., Donkin, A., Gadeyne, S., Minder, C., Regidor, E., Spadea, T., Valkonen, T. and Mackenbach, J. (2004) 'Socioeconomic inequalities in mortality among elderly people in 11 European populations', *Journal of Epidemiology and Community Health*, vol 58, pp 468-75.

Iso, H., Date, C., Yamamoto, A., Toyoshima, H., Watanabe, Y., Kikuchi, S., Koizumi, A., Wada, Y., Kondo, T., Inaba, Y., Tamakoshi, A. and JACC (Japan Collaborative Cohort Study for Evaluation of Cancer Risk) Study Group (2005) 'Smoking cessation and mortality from cardiovascular disease among Japanese men and women: the JACC Study', *American Journal of Epidemiology*, vol 161, pp 170-9.

Izuhara, M. and Heywood, F. (2003) 'A life-time of inequality: a structural analysis of housing careers and issues facing older private tenants', *Ageing and Society*, vol 23, pp 207-24.

Janevic, M., Janz, N., Dodge, J., Wang, Y., Lin, X. and Clark, N. (2004) 'Longitudinal effects of social support on the health and functioning of older women with heart disease', *International Journal of Aging and Human Development*, vol 59, pp 153-75.

Ji, L. (2001) 'Exercise at old age: does it increase or alleviate oxidative stress?', *Annals of the New York Academy of Sciences*, vol 928, pp 236-47.

Johnson, J. (2002) 'Taking care of later life: a matter of justice', *British Journal of Social Work*, vol 32, pp 739-50.

Jones, S., Johansen, A., Brennan, J., Butler, J. and Lyons, R. (2004) 'The effect of socioeconomic deprivation on fracture incidence in the United Kingdom', *Osteoporosis International*, vol 15, pp 520-4.

Khaw, K. (1999) 'Inequalities in health: older people', in D. Gordon, M. Shaw, D. Dorling and G. Davey Smith (eds) *Inequalities in health: The evidence presented to the Independent Inquiry into Inequalities in Health, chaired by Sir Donald Acheson*, Bristol: The Policy Press, pp 33-44.

Kim, L., Thompson, S., Marteau, T., Scott, R. and Multicentre Aneurysm Screening Study Group (2004) 'Screening for abdominal aortic aneurysms: the effects of age and social deprivation on screening uptake, prevalence and attendance at follow-up in the MASS trial', *Journal of Medical Screening*, vol 11, pp 50-3.

Lacey, E. and Walters, S. (2003) 'Continuing inequality: gender and social class influences on self perceived health after a heart attack', *Journal of Epidemiology and Community Health*, vol 57, pp 622-7.

LaCroix, A. and Omenn, G. (1992) 'Older adults and smoking', *Clinical Geriatric Medicine*, vol 8, pp 69-87.

LaCroix, A., Lang, J., Scherr, P., Wallace, R., Cornoni-Huntley, J., Berkman, L., Curb, J., Evans, D. and Hennekens, C. (1991) 'Smoking and mortality among older men and women in three communities', *New England Journal of Medicine*, vol 324, pp 1619-25.

Laing and Buisson (2000) *Care of elderly people market survey*, London: Laing and Buisson.

Laing and Buisson (2001) *Health care market review 2000-2001*, London: Laing and Buisson.

Lawlor, D., Ebrahim, S. and Davey Smith, G. (2003) 'The association of socio-economic position across the life course and age at menopause: the British Women's Heart and Health Study', *BJOG: An International Journal of Obstetrics and Gynaecology*, vol 110, pp 1078-87.

Lawlor, D., Taylor, M., Bedford, C. and Ebrahim, S. (2002) 'Is housework good for health? Levels of physical activity and factors associated with activity in elderly women. Results from the British Women's Heart and Health Study', *Journal of Epidemiology and Community Health*, vol 56, pp 473-8.

Liao, Y., McGee, D., Kaufman, J., Cao, G. and Cooper, R. (1999) 'Socioeconomic status and morbidity in the last years of life', *American Journal of Public Health*, vol 89, pp 569-72.

Lyons, R.A., Jones, S.J., Deacon, T. and Heaven, M. (2003) 'Socioeconomic variation in injury in children and older people: a population study', *Injury Prevention*, vol 9, pp 33-7.

Macleod, U., Ross, S., Twelves, C., George, W., Gillis, C. and Watt, G. (2000) 'Primary and secondary care management of women with early breast cancer from affluent and deprived areas: retrospective review of hospital and general practice records', *British Medical Journal*, vol 320, pp 1442-5.

Maheswaran, R., Chan, D., Fryers, P.T., McManus, C. and McCabe, H. (2004) 'Socio-economic deprivation and excess winter mortality and emergency hospital admissions in the South Yorkshire Coalfields Health Action Zone, UK', *Public Health*, vol 118, pp 167-76.

Marang-van de Mheen, P., Shipley, M., Whitley, J., Marmot, M. and Gunning Schepers, L. (2001) 'Decline of the relative risk of death associated with low employment grade at older age: the impact of age-related differences in smoking, blood pressure and plasma cholesterol', *Journal of Epidemiology and Community Health*, vol 55, pp 24-8.

Margetts, B., Thompson, R., Elia, M. and Jackson, A. (2003) 'Prevalence of risk of undernutrition is associated with poor health status in older people in the UK', *European Journal of Clinical Nutrition*, vol 57, pp 69-74.

Marmot, M. and Shipley, M. (1996) 'Do socio-economic differences in mortality persist after retirement? 25 year follow up of civil servants from the first Whitehall study', *British Medical Journal*, vol 313, pp 1177-80.

Mayer, K. and Wagner, M. (1993) 'Socioeconomic resources and differential aging', *Ageing and Society*, vol 13, pp 517-50.

Mays, N. (1995) 'Geographical resource allocation in the English National Health Service, 1974-1994: the tension between normative and empirical approaches', *International Journal of Epidemiology*, vol 24, pp S96-102.

Melzer, D., Izmirlian, G., Leveille, S. and Guralnik, J. (2001) 'Educational differences in the prevalence of mobility disability in old age: the dynamics of incidence, mortality, and recovery', *Journals of Gerontology Series B: Psychological Sciences and Social Sciences*, vol 56, pp S294-301.

Melzer, D., McWilliams, B., Brayne, C., Johnson, T. and Bond, J. (2000) 'Socioeconomic status and the expectation of disability in old age: estimates for England', *Journal of Epidemiology and Community Health*, vol 54, pp 286-92.

Meydani, M. (2001) 'Nutrition interventions in aging and age-associated disease', *Annals of the New York Academy of Sciences*, vol 928, pp 226-35.

Meydani, M. (2002) 'The Boyd Orr lecture: nutrition interventions in aging and age-associated disease', *Proceedings of the Nutrition Society*, vol 61, pp 165-71.

Milne, A., Potter, J. and Avenell, A. (2002) 'Protein and energy supplementation in elderly people at risk from malnutrition', *The Cochrane Database of Systematic Reviews 2002, issue 2*, Art. No. CD003288.

Milner, P., Payne, J., Stanfield, R., Lewis, P., Jennison, C. and Saul, C. (2004) 'Inequalities in accessing hip joint replacement for people in need', *European Journal of Public Health*, vol 14, pp 58-62.

Miquel, J. (2001) 'Nutrition and ageing', *Public Health Nutrition*, vol 4, pp 1385-8.

Mishra, G., Ball, K., Dobson, A. and Byles, J. (2004) 'Do socioeconomic gradients in women's health widen over time and with age?', *Social Science and Medicine*, vol 58, pp 1585-95.

Murtiashaw, S. (2001) *The role of long-term care ombudsmen in nursing home closures and natural disasters*, Washington, DC: National Long-Term Care Ombudsmen Resource Centre.

Nazroo, J., Bajekal, M., Blane, D. and Grewal, I. (2004) 'Ethnic inequalities', in A. Walker and C. Hennessy (eds) *Growing older: Quality of life in old age*, Buckingham: Open University Press, pp 35-59.

ODPM (Office of the Deputy Prime Minister) (2003) *English Housing Condition Survey 2001: Building the Picture*, London: The Stationery Office.

ODPM (2005) *Excluded older people: Social Exclusion Unit interim report*, London: The Stationery Office.

Ormel, J., Rijsdijk, F., Sullivan, M., van Sonderen, E. and Kempen, G. (2002) 'Temporal and reciprocal relationship between IADL/ADL disability and depressive symptoms in late life', *Journals of Gerontology Series B: Psychological Sciences and Social Sciences*, vol 57, pp 338-47.

Osborn, D., Fletcher, A., Smeeth, L., Stirling, S., Bulpitt, C., Breeze, E., Ng, E., Nunes, M., Jones, D. and Tulloch, A. (2004) 'Factors associated with depression in a representative sample of 14,217 people aged 75 and over in the United Kingdom: results from the MRC trial of assessment and management of older people in the community', *International Journal of Geriatric Psychiatry*, vol 18, pp 623-30.

Ott, A., Andersen, K., Dewey, M., Letenneur, L., Brayne, C., Copeland, J., Dartigues, J.-F., Kragh-Sorensen, P., Lobo, A., Martinez-Lage, J., Stijnen, T., Hofman, A. and Launer, L. for the EURODEM Incidence Research Group (2004) 'Effect of smoking on global cognitive function in nondemented elderly', *Neurology*, vol 62, pp 920-4.

Nazroo, J., Bajekal, M., Blane, D. and Grewal, I. (2004) 'Ethnic inequalities', in A. Walker and C. Hennessy (eds) *Growing older: Quality of life in old age*, Buckingham: Open University Press, pp 35-59.

Paganini-Hill, A. and Hsu, G. (1994) 'Smoking and mortality among residents of a California retirement community', *American Journal of Public Health*, vol 84, pp 992-5.

Pearson, D., Taylor, R. and Masud, T. (2004) 'The relationship between social deprivation, osteoporosis, and falls', *Osteoporosis International*, vol 15, pp 132-8.

Polidori, M., Mecocci, P., Cherubini, A. and Senin, U. (2000) 'Physical activity and oxidative stress during aging', *International Journal of Sports Medicine*, vol 21, pp 154-7.

Pollack, A. and Vickers, N. (1998) 'Deprivation and emergency admissions for cancers of colorectum, lung and breast in South East England: ecological study', *British Medical Journal*, vol 317, pp 245-52.

Prince, M., Harwood, R., Blizard, R., Thomas, A. and Mann, A. (1997) 'Social support deficits, loneliness and life events as risk factors for depression in old age: The Gospel Oak Project VI', *Psychological Medicine*, vol 27, pp 323-32.

Purandare, N., Burns, A., Challis, D. and Morris, J. (2004) 'Perceived mental health needs and adequacy of service provision to older people in care homes in the UK: a national survey', *International Journal of Geriatric Psychiatry*, vol 19, pp 549-53.

RCLTC (Royal Commission on Long-Term Care) (1999) *With respect to old age: Long term care – rights and responsibilities*, London: The Stationery Office.

Richard, M. and Roussel, A. (1999) 'Micronutrients and ageing: intakes and requirements', *Proceedings of the Nutrition Society*, vol 58, pp 573-8.

Scharf, T., Phillipson, C. and Smith, A. (2004) 'Poverty and social exclusion – growing older in deprived urban neighbourhoods', in A. Walker and C. Hennessy (eds) *Growing older: Quality of life in old age*, Buckingham: Open University Press, pp 81-106.

Scharf, T., Phillipson, C. and Smith, A. (2005) *Multiple exclusion and quality of life among excluded older people in disadvantaged neighbourhoods*, London: ODPM.

Scharf, T., Phillipson, C., Smith, A. and Kingston, P. (2002) *Growing older in socially deprived areas: Social exclusion in later life*, London: Help the Aged.

Schrijvers, C., Mackenbach, J., Lutz, J., Quinn, M. and Coleman, M. (1995) 'Deprivation, stage at diagnosis and cancer survival', *International Journal of Cancer*, vol 63, pp 324-9.

Scourfield, P. (2004) 'Questions raised for local authorities when old people are evicted from their care homes', *British Journal of Social Work*, vol 34, pp 501-16.

Sheiham, A. and Steele, J. (2001) 'Does the condition of the mouth and teeth affect the ability to eat certain foods, nutrient and dietary intake and nutritional status amongst older people?', *Public Health Nutrition*, vol 4, pp 797-803.

Smith, J. and Harding, S. (1997) 'Mortality of women and men using alternative social classifications', in F. Drever, and M. Whitehead (eds) *Health inequalities: Decennial Supplement*, London: ONS, pp 168-83.

Stanner, S., Hughes, J., Kelly, C. and Buttriss, J. (2004) 'A review of the epidemiological evidence for the "antioxidant hypothesis"', *Public Health Nutrition*, vol 7, pp 407-22.

Steele, J., Walls, A., Ayatollahi, S. and Murray, J. (1996) 'Major clinical findings from a dental survey of elderly people in three different English communities', *British Dental Journal*, vol 180, pp 17-23.

Strain, J., Elwood, P., Davis, A., Kennedy, O., Coulter, J., Fehily, A., Mulholland, C., Robson, P. and Thurnham, D. (2000) 'Frequency of fruit and vegetable consumption and blood antioxidants in the Caerphilly cohort of older men', *European Journal of Clinical Nutrition*, vol 54, pp 828-33.

Tait, C. and Fuller, E. (2002) *Health Survey for England 2000: Psychosocial well-being among older people*, London: The Stationery Office.

Tanner, D. (2003) 'Older people and access to care', *British Journal of Social Work*, vol 33, pp 499-515.

Taylor, D., Hasselblad, V., Henley, S., Thun, M. and Sloan, F. (2002) 'Benefits of smoking cessation for longevity', *American Journal of Public Health*, vol 92, pp 990-6.

Thane, C., Paul, A., Bates, C., Bolton-Smith, C., Prentice, A. and Shearer, M. (2002) 'Intake and sources of phylloquinone (vitamin K1): variation with socio-demographic and lifestyle factors in a national sample of British elderly people', *British Journal of Nutrition*, vol 87, pp 605-13.

Victor, C., Scambler, S., Bond, J. and Bowling, A. (2004) 'Loneliness in later life', in A. Walker and C. Hennessy (eds) *Growing older: Quality of life in old age*, Buckingham: Open University Press, pp 107-26.

Wenger, N.K. (1997) 'Coronary heart disease: an older woman's major health risk', *British Medical Journal*, vol 315, pp 1085-90.

West, J., Hippisley-Cox, J., Coupland, C., Price, G., Groom, L., Kendrick, D. and Webber, E. (2004) 'Do rates of hospital admission for falls and hip fracture in elderly people vary by socio-economic status?', *Public Health*, vol 118, pp 576-81.

Whynes, D., Frew, E., Manghan, C., Scholefield, J. and Hardcastle, J. (2003) 'Colorectal cancer, screening and survival: the influence of socio-economic deprivation', *Public Health*, 117, pp 389-95.

Whynne, A. (1999) 'Nutrition in older people', *Nutrition and Food Science*, vol 5, pp 219-23.

Wilkinson, P., Landon, M., Armstrong, B., Stevenson, S., Pattenden, S., Fletcher, T. and McKee, M. (2001) *Cold comfort: The social and environmental determinants of excess winter deaths in England, 1986-1996*, Bristol: The Policy Press.

Wilkinson, P., Pattenden, S., Armstrong, B., Fletcher, A., Kovats, R., Mangtani, P. and McMichael, A. (2004) 'Vulnerability to winter mortality in elderly people in Britain: population based study', *British Medical Journal*, vol 329, p 647.

Williams, R., Fraser, A. and West, R. (2004) 'Gender differences in management after acute myocardial infarction: not "sexism" but a reflection of age at presentation', *Journal of Public Health*, vol 26, pp 259-63.

Wrigley, H., Roderick, P., George, S., Smith, J., Mullee, M. and Goddard, J. (2003) 'Inequalities in survival from colorectal cancer: a comparison of the impact of deprivation, treatment, and host factors on observed and cause specific survival', *Journal of Epidemiology and Community Health*, vol 57, pp 301-9.

THIRTEEN

Older age: policy and practice

Introduction

There is no consensus as to when old age starts or whether it should be defined by chronological age or frailty. Indeed, as policy initiatives such as Better Government for Older People (BGOP) include all those aged over 50, old age may embrace three generations. There is, however, an undisputed increase in the number of very elderly people and a growth in elderly-only households. These demographic and social trends have combined with factors such as the changing context of informal care and the cost of acute care to focus attention on the health and social care needs of older people, an area where research has traditionally been both undervalued and underfunded (Bowling and Ebrahim, 2001, p 223). The *Independent Inquiry into Inequalities in Health* (Acheson, 1998) also reinforced the message that older people have particular health needs.

The *National Service Framework for Older People* was published in March 2001 and was supported by an additional £1.4 billion for the development of health and social services (to 2004), with an extra £1 billion set aside for community-based services by 2006. Its aim was to promote the independence and well-being of older people, including the support for them to live at home or in community settings as far as possible. Towards this end it sets eight standards for improving health and social care across the spectrum, including access to Intermediate Care services at home or in designated care settings, a specialist falls service, integrated mental health services and, significantly from a preventative point of view, the promotion of health and well-being (DH, 2001a).

These standards are underpinned by four, now largely familiar, principles. The first is a partnership approach between the National Health Service (NHS), local government, the independent sector and older people themselves/their carers with the aim of producing integrated assessment, commissioning and service provision. The second focuses on a timely response to needs, including aspects such as information sharing and teams working across primary care, acute services and community. The third is the adoption of person-centred care regardless of age (including the devolution of budgets to front-line practitioners and service users and a diversity of service provision), while the fourth is the promotion of health and an active life.

The need to address the inequities that surround access to services and care for older people as a whole has largely directed attention away from the existence of increasing inequalities among older people themselves. The problems facing many black and minority ethnic elders and their carers, including low income, limited savings, lack of knowledge of benefits and services and the lack of recognition within health, housing and social care of the diversity of needs, is one possible exception (Katbamna et al, 1998; Patel, 1999; Evandrou, 2000). Nevertheless, as we have shown, there is a growing body of evidence that lack of education, low income, manual occupations and housing tenure are associated with greater mortality and the prevalence of disability among older people (Breeze et al, 2004).

Research strongly suggests that older people themselves are more concerned about their independence and quality of life, including their home environment and their ability to travel easily, rather than the availability or quality of care services. This chapter, while developing the health risk factors and environmental factors introduced in Chapter Twelve, thus focuses on the preventative agenda. Here the emphasis is on the promotion of quality of life and community engagement and on the prevention or delay of costly intensive services (Lewis et al, 1999). It also focuses on the key policy drivers that have combined to raise the profile of this agenda. These include an emphasis on preventing and delaying dependency, a greater understanding of the whole systems approach within health and social care and a concern to improve the general health and well-being of populations, rather than a focus solely on the management or cure of ill health. This is reflected more broadly in the government's recent strategy for an ageing society, which stresses the maintenance of independence and an active role in society (based on a decent income and housing), alongside the aim of higher employment rates (HM Government, 2005).

Diet and nutrition

As Chapter Twelve has shown, the protective role of antioxidants and other dietary factors suggests that there is scope for health gain if a diet rich in dark leafy vegetables, fruits, nuts, unrefined cereal, fish, and small quantities of quality vegetable oils could be more accessible to poor people. In contrast to the earlier stages of the lifecourse, under-nutrition is also a major cause for concern in older people. We now consider evidence of interventions designed to improve the quantity and quality of nutrition in older people.

What works? Evidence and practice

Research based in Scotland suggests that the diet of older people varies little from that of the population as a whole, with over-consumption of fats, sugars and salt, under-consumption of fruit and vegetables and a contradiction between beliefs and behaviour (McKie et al, 2000). There is a role, therefore, for targeted dietary advice in the community, including nutritional requirements and initiatives to reduce dietary risk. However, older people may have to invest more time in order to access food in a manageable way, overcoming structural barriers such as distance, mobility, portability and financial constraints, in order to continue to buy and prepare what they consider to be 'proper food' (McKie, 1999). The imperative is typically the importance attached to food in maintaining their independence, but food consumption and food shopping are also both recognised as playing a wider role in social networks and providing a structure to the day (Cooper et al, 1999).

A systematic review of healthy eating among older people found a paucity of evaluative studies, despite addressing adequate nutrition, nutritional deficiencies and disease reduction. These provided limited evidence of effective healthy eating strategies or policies for older people. There was, however, some (often weak) evidence to support small group programmes including nutrition alongside social and physical activities, health promotion programmes with a nutritional component and community programmes targeted at groups with a high risk of nutritional deficiency or coronary heart disease (CHD). Group participation, together with goal setting, appeared to be critical factors (Fletcher and Rake, 1998). Studies were typically limited by their tendency to treat older people as an homogenous group, with limited controls for age, dietary intake or energy expenditure. The range of preventative strategies, process and nutritional content also tended to be poorly described, with an overwhelming focus on interventions from the US.

Malnutrition is likely to be amenable to both dietary interventions (meals-on-wheels, for example) and non-dietary solutions (such as treatment of depression, correction of dental problems and exercise regimes) in the community. In hospital too, there may be a role for encouragement and assistance as much as for supplementation. A Cochrane systematic review of the effectiveness of oral dietary supplements for older people found that such supplements produced a small but consistent weight gain and had a statistically significant beneficial effect on mortality. There was also some evidence that they reduced the length of stay in hospital. However, the interventions tended to be too short to detect any improvements in morbidity, functional status or quality of life (Milne et al, 2002). Some of the trials also included some dietary advice as part of the intervention but its additive effect could not be evaluated. A Cochrane systematic review of dietary advice for illness-related malnutrition in adults similarly found insufficient evidence to establish whether dietary advice improved the outcomes of malnourished patients (Baldwin et al, 2001). However, it did suggest that weight gain was greater in people who also received nutritional supplements.

Older people with hip fractures are also often malnourished at the time of fracture, with evidence again suggesting that poor food intake in hospital may further hinder recovery. A systematic review of nutritional supplementation for elderly hip fracture patients found some evidence that oral protein and energy feeds may reduce unfavourable outcome (death or complications) and perhaps reduce long-term complications and time spent on a rehabilitation ward (Avenell and Handoll, 2004). Overall, however, the evidence was still weak due to defects in the reviewed studies, particularly inadequate size, methodology and outcome assessment. The limited evidence base also prevents any conclusion being drawn as to the efficacy of nutritional supplements for preventing or reducing pressure ulcers or bed sores, although there is a suggestion that people with poor nutrient status or dehydration are more vulnerable because of skin weakness (Langer et al, 2003).

Dietary deficiency of folates has been claimed to contribute to the aetiology both of Alzheimer's disease and vascular dementia. However, a limited number of trials of folic acid supplementation found no evidence of benefit on either cognitive function or mood among either healthy older people or those with dementia (Malouf et al, 2003). However, the trials did not focus just on those with metabolic deficiencies, and were conducted for a short time period only.

Policy

There seems to be a policy vacuum with respect to diet and nutrition specifically for older people. As noted in Chapter Eleven, *The NHS Plan* (DH, 2000a), *The NHS Cancer Plan* (DH, 2000b) and the corresponding NSFs for CHD and Diabetes (DH, 2000c, 2001b) all highlight diet and nutrition as key areas for action – yet make little or no mention of these issues in relation to older people. The same applies to *Saving lives: Our healthier nation* (DH, 1999a) and to the related national Five-a-day Programme. Similarly, *Choosing health* (HM Government and DH, 2004), while focusing on interventions that address lifestyle factors at an individual level and attaching priority to reducing obesity and improving diet and nutrition, does not explore these with reference to age (other than by a focus on obesity in children). Indeed, the Public Health White Paper has been criticised more widely for failing to include measures which particularly help older people (Age Concern, 2005, p 7). This has not been rectified by the subsequent delivery plan (DH, 2005a), which, with an emphasis on diet-related disease and obesity, contains just one reference to older people, as opposed, for example, to specific sections addressing children and young people, and nutrition in the workplace.

Within this agenda, some strategies have embraced older people, albeit largely by default. Local initiatives within the Five-a-day Programme have included older people and the problems they can encounter in accessing and preparing health foods. The NSFs for CHD and Diabetes will require primary care treatment regimes to include appropriate advice on diet alongside physical activity and smoking to patients with CHD and diabetes by 2006. Local Delivery Plans, established by the Department of Health's (DH) *Priorities and Planning Framework 2003-06*, are also expected to address active ageing, including diet and exercise (ODPM, 2003).

The issue of malnutrition, including poor nutrition while in institutional care, similarly appears to be ignored by the political agenda, despite being amenable to central intervention and guidance, whether within hospitals, residential care, day care or sheltered housing. The more specific area of supplementation also remains the subject of reservations. The National Institute for Clinical Excellence's (NICE) falls guidelines (NICE, 2004), for example, while pointing to the emerging evidence linking vitamin D deficiency with propensity for falling, finds this insufficient to recommend its use as an aid to fracture reduction. The Health Development Agency (HDA) suggests comprehensive pharmacological osteoporosis prevention programmes should be introduced in general practice and primary care, but again the preventative emphasis is not yet reflected in practice. NICE does not expect to publish clinical guidelines until 2006.

Physical activity

Exercise is recognised to play an important part in the quality of life of older people, improving physiological and psychological function, helping to maintain personal independence and reducing the demands for short-term and long-term care services. It is also one factor among many that can act to prevent falls. This section focuses in particular on the latter, prompted by the frequency of these events in older people's lives, their significance in triggering a requirement for hospitalisation and care and their multifactorial causation, all of which serve to illustrate the imperative for a more holistic preventative agenda.

What works? Evidence and practice

The benefits of physical activity are manifest (DH, 2004a), but it is often difficult to increase levels in practice (Munro et al, 2004), reinforcing the need (see Box 13.1) to integrate specific interventions with recommendations on daily physical activity and to consider the range of structural barriers such as transport, suitable exercise settings and social expectations.

As with younger adults, review-level evidence suggests that interventions designed specifically for adults aged 50 and over are effective in producing short-term changes in physical activity and are likely to be effective in producing mid- to long-term changes. The latter is most likely to be achieved by interventions that promote moderate and non-endurance physical activities (such as flexibility exercises), use behavioural or cognitive approaches combining group and home-based exercise sessions rather than a class or group-only format, and utilise telephone support and follow-up (King et al, 1998). Research from Australia has also built on the frequency with which older people consult their general practitioner (GP) to suggest that primary care could be an effective source of health promotion messages and to demonstrate significant improvements in

Box 13.1: Exercise for health and well-being

More Exercise for Seniors (*MBvO* in Dutch) is a weekly exercise programme designed specifically for people aged 65 and over. Widely adopted since 1980, 300,000 older people now participate in the programme, which aims to improve physical, mental and social functioning. However, attention has only recently been directed to the evaluation of health gain. Participants (aged 65-80 and living independently) were divided into two experimental groups who participated in a once or twice weekly 45-minute exercise group at a local community centre for 10 weeks. The control group received a health education programme. Improvements in health-related quality of life (including cognitive, social, physical and emotional functioning) was confined to people whose physical activity was below the median at baseline and who participated in the programme twice a week. No significant improvement in functional status (the ability to perform tasks and to fulfil social roles associated with daily living) was detected. The short timescale across which improvements were sought was considered to militate against the attribution of improvements but still suggested a need to combine exercise programmes with recommendations on daily physical activity (Stiggelbout et al, 2004).

walking, social contact and self-rated health over one year consequent on an initiative to educate GPs (Kerse et al, 1999).

There is a lack of review-level evidence as to effective interventions among disadvantaged groups, despite prevalence levels being lower in some minority ethnic groups, people in low-income households, those in lower social classes and people with low levels of education (DH, 2004a). Individual projects suggest, nevertheless, that exercise can improve the mental health and well-being of more disadvantaged people. An adaptation of a health promotion programme known to increase physical activity and knowledge of health and development as well as reducing loneliness in less active elderly groups was, for example, adapted to reach Turkish immigrants. It was found capable of improving mental health and mental well-being in the over-55s (although ironically, probably because of the limited duration, no statistically significant improvements in physical well-being or activity were recorded) (Reijneveld et al, 2003).

The role of exercise within a holistic approach to falls prevention

There is no consensus definition of a fall but approximately 30% of people over 65 years of age and living in the community fall each year. The number is higher in institutions (McClure et al, 2005). Although only one fall in 10 results in a fracture, a fifth of fall incidents require medical attention, often triggering (particularly in the case of hip fractures) a requirement for intermediate or long-term care (Avenell and Handoll, 2004). Considerable importance therefore attaches to the falls prevention agenda.

Many risk factors appear to interact in those who suffer falls and fall-related fractures, with environmental hazards interacting critically with individual behaviour. Research in Israel identified a set of five factors that increased the risk of both falls and depression (Biderman et al, 2002): poor self-rated health, poor cognitive status, functional disability, two or more clinic visits in the past month, and slow walking speed. This multifactorial causation suggests that the most appropriate interventions will be multidisciplinary, involving medical, functional, and psychosocial aspects of geriatric care.

Many preventative programmes based on these risk factors have been established and evaluated. These include exercise programmes, physiotherapy, the provision of walking aids, the management of medical problems (such as depression, vision and medication), environmental modification (particularly reduction in home hazards [Day et al, 2002]), nutritional or hormonal supplementation and education, often in combination. A systematic review of 62 trials suggests that such interventions are more likely to be effective when targeting known fallers, although even here the reductions in risk are small and the clinical significance and cost-effectiveness not always clear (Gillespie et al, 2003). Interventions that target multiple risk factors are, however, marginally effective, as are targeted exercise interventions or physical therapy, the modification of home hazards and the reduction of psychotropic medication.

A review of 11 trials of exercise programmes for older people concluded that exercise could reduce falls as long as certain conditions were met (Gardner et al, 2000). These included appropriate targeting (so that people were neither too fit nor too frail and perhaps at a threshold where loss of muscle strength and stability become critical), and an effective exercise regime with key variables including intensity, regularity, sustainability and a focus on balance as well as strength. Centre-based exercise was seen to confer additional benefits in terms of social interaction. None of the fall prevention initiatives studied, however, was sufficiently powerful to show a reduction in serious fall injuries such as fractures, although some reported a reduction in healthcare use as a result of the intervention and other benefits suggested included a reduction in fear and improvements in other health-related areas such as sleep, depression and cardiovascular health (see for example, Box 13.2).

A systematic review focusing on the modification of the home environment for the reduction of injuries found an overwhelming focus on falls data for older people. However, of the 15 studies considered, only two produced a statistically significant reduction in falls (despite evidence of improvements to homes), with none translating this into a significant reduction in actual injuries (Lyons et al, 2004). The counterintuitive results were largely explained by the small size of many of the samples, the short timescale over which the programmes were typically conducted, and the low penetration of many of the suggested improvements, with little available information on uptake or sustainability. One study did find a reduction in home hazards to have an additive impact when used alongside

Box 13.2: Exercise for the prevention of falls

A total of 233 women aged 80 years and older (a group at high risk for falling) were randomised to an exercise intervention designed to prevent falls and injuries. Here, they were prescribed strength and balance retraining exercises by a physiotherapist in the course of four home visits. A control group received the same number of social visits by a nurse, together with usual care. At six months there was a significant improvement in two measures of strength and balance in the intervention group but no significant differences between the two groups in six other tests of strength, gait, endurance and function. Despite only modest improvements in physical functioning, falls and moderate injuries were reduced in the exercise group compared with the control (Campbell et al, 1997).

Attrition was low and the majority (71%) of the 213 participants remaining at the end of year one agreed to continue for a second year, with the intervention group receiving bi-monthly telephone calls from the physiotherapist. Those who continued were more active and less afraid of falling at the end of year one, and took fewer medications at baseline compared with those who declined to take part. At the end of the second year, 31 (44%) of those remaining in the intervention group were still exercising at least three times a week and the lower fall rate achieved in year one was sustained. More frequent visiting from the physiotherapist and encouragement from the GP to continue exercising may have improved exercise compliance (Campbell et al, 1999).

A repeat trial in New Zealand demonstrated that the intervention was capable of translation into usual clinical practice when delivered by trained nurses and was effective for both men and women. Falls fell by 30% in the exercise groups and fewer falls resulted in injury. There was, however, no difference between groups with respect to serious injury (Robertson et al, 2001).

exercise training and improvements to vision (Day et al, 2002). A number of positive outcomes for fall reduction were also indicated by a systematic review of occupational therapy interventions for community-dwelling older people that had a largely similar focus: advice on assistive devices given as part of a home hazards assessment. Some evidence also supported the role of skills training, combined with a home hazard assessment, in decreasing the incidence of falls in older people at high risk of falling, with the suggestion that comprehensive occupational therapy could improve not just functional ability but social participation and quality of life (Steultjens et al, 2004).

It remains easier to prevent falls in cognitively normal older people living in the community, and those who present to Accident and Emergency Departments after falls, than it is to prevent falls among older people with cognitive impairment and dementia and those living in nursing homes, even though this is a group particularly prone to falling (Shaw et al, 2003). Exercise may, nevertheless, increase physical functioning among the institutional population although it is unable to reduce the incidence of falls because of the number of other risk factors (Gardner et al, 2000), while multifactorial programmes including staff education, attention to environmental safety and medication review are also supported (Oliver and Masud, 2004).

Informal care networks and individual psychology may make the difference in determining how older people approach and respond to therapeutic interventions designed to restore independence. A study of the care pathways of 100 older people following a fractured neck of femur by the Nuffield Institute for Health found that older people considered their own motivation and help from family and friends to be more important than professional help in regaining health and confidence. The same factors were perceived as critical to sustaining independent living post-discharge (Herbert et al, 2000).

Population interventions, where several falls prevention measures are introduced as a package across the community as a whole, have the potential advantage of mobilising change on a large scale and achieving a more sustained effect by becoming embedded in the social and physical structure of the community. Their applicability is also suggested by the multifactorial causation noted earlier and the commonality of the predisposing factors. However, a recent Cochrane Review with a focus on reducing fall-related injuries (McClure et al, 2005), identified only five studies of sufficient methodological rigour (including the use of a control community). With the exception of one Australian programme (see Box 13.3), these were all drawn from Scandinavia and based on the World

Box 13.3: Population-based interventions

The Stay on Your Feet Programme was a four-year-long population-based programme designed to prevent falls among older people (those aged 60 and over) living in a large rural coastal region of New South Wales, Australia (Kempton et al, 2000). The targeted population of approximately 80,000 received a multistrategy intervention addressing knowledge, attitudes, behaviours, the use of medication, footwear, home hazard reduction and other risk factors related to falls that utilised both community education and policy development. Outcomes, in terms of fall-related hospital visits, were compared with those in a distant rural coastal region (with approximately 62,000 inhabitants in the targeted age range) who agreed to remain intervention-free for the whole period.

The programme resulted in a significant 20% decrease in fall-related hospitalisations in the intervention area compared to the control community (after adjusting for baseline fall-related injury rates). It was estimated that about 77% of the targeted population was in contact with at least one aspect of the intervention over the duration of the programme. The intervention was funded by the government health department, with a total cost of approximately $AUS600,000.

Health Organization (WHO) safe community model. All showed a significant decrease in fall-related injuries ranging from 6% to 33%, suggesting they could form the basis for effective public health interventions.

Limitations to the evidence base

Common themes combine to restrict the utility of the evidence base. Once again (with the exception of community-based interventions) there is a focus on North American rather than European interventions (van Haastregt et al, 2000). There is no consensus definition of falls, no agreement as to the optimum length of an intervention and considerable variations in what may be defined as usual care. It is difficult to differentiate between interventions based on client characteristics, although both the falls-risk profile and the emphasis of individual interventions are specific to populations or settings. It is also hard to isolate the potential contribution of individual components within typically multifactorial interventions (more so given the paucity of details on the actual implementation), while randomisation and self-report is problematic given the high prevalence of cognitive impairment in care homes (Oliver and Masud, 2004).

Policy

Government policy on physical activity for adults (30 minutes a day of at least moderate intensity activity on five or more days a week) is considered to apply equally to older people (DH, 2004a). Particular stress is placed, however, on retaining mobility through daily activity and walking (reflecting the reality of many older people's lives, the fact that even low to moderate activity can produce health benefits among this age group and the need to avoid injury), and activities that promote strength and balance (reflecting the need to prevent falls). As already noted, the NSF for CHD also requires primary care treatment regimes to include appropriate advice on physical activity, diet and smoking to patients with CHD and diabetes by 2006, while a Physical Activity Plan is expected in support of *Choosing health* (HM Government and DH, 2004). Standard Eight of the NSF for Older People also focuses on the promotion of an active life in older age.

The specific prevention of falls has been a policy focus for over a decade. The Standard on Falls (Standard Six) within the NSF for Older People (DH, 2001a) has its origins in *The health of the nation* (DH, 1992) and in the 1999 White Paper, *Saving lives: Our healthier nation* (DH, 1999a), which cited accidents in the home among those over the age of 65 as a significant concern (Easterbrook, 2002). The NSF itself made prevention of further falls in older people who attend the Accident and Emergency Department after a fall a priority and recognised cognitive impairment as an important risk factor for falls. It also focused on fall prevention initiatives in residential or nursing homes, even though, as already noted, this is a challenging environment in which to reduce falls as opposed to improving physical functioning.

The range of contributory factors is recognised by the HDA, which, in identifying a number of public health interventions where evidence is strong and the likelihood of success is high, suggests that home, pharmacological, medical and occupational therapy assessment should be made compulsory for all patients over 65 treated at Accident and Emergency Departments for falls (Kelly, 2004). The HDA also reinforces the role of exercise by recommending that trained staff should routinely deliver home exercise programmes to all people over the age of 70 living in domestic or residential homes through the primary care system. At present, however, such comprehensive approaches, whether for primary or secondary prevention, are largely absent. Falls guidelines have also been recently produced. These draw on the evidence base to recommend routine case risk identification by healthcare professionals followed by a multifactorial risk assessment and multifactorial interventions focusing on strength and balance training together with an assessment of home hazards, vision and medication (NICE, 2004).

Smoking cessation

Smoking cessation initiatives and policy have been explored in Chapters Five, Nine and Eleven as they relate to the three key target groups: pregnant women, young people and disadvantaged adults. Older people, in contrast, were not identified as a priority either within the 1998 White Paper *Smoking kills* (DH, 1998) or subsequent guidance, and while a focus on economic disadvantage might have been expected to include older people, the focus in practice has been on deprived areas or smoking-related illnesses. Little explicit attention has therefore been given to the development of services specifically for older people, and evaluation has not generally sought to address the issue of age except for the young. Long-term drug and alcohol treatment for older adults has similarly been under-investigated (Satre et al, 2004).

Research has also suggested that doctors are less likely to provide smoking cessation advice to older people, despite the significance of smoking-related respiratory disabilities in old age (Maguire et al, 2000). However, where monitoring data from the English smoking cessation services does include age-related data, this shows smokers over the age of 60 to have higher cessation rates than their younger counterparts at both four weeks and one year – 65% of older smokers, for example, were reported as abstinent at four weeks, as opposed to 41% of those aged 16-30 (Raw et al, 2001).

Four generic lessons were identified from the evaluation of English smoking treatment services, considered capable of informing the development of services in other health systems. By implication these should also apply to smoking cessation for older people. This suggests that early guidance from government can encourage services to adhere to evidence-based treatment, that treatment needs to be accessible to smokers and hence locally flexible, that nicotine addiction and behavioural therapies should be coordinated and that fixed-term funding militates against staff recruitment and retention and hence the establishment of a sustainable service (Bauld et al, 2005). The importance of social networks, support groups and close family who support the decision also suggest that support to quit could be particularly important for the very elderly and isolated.

Housing

The effects of ageing and environmental barriers mean that older people spend more time in their home, which can be either an important source of independence or a cause for concern. As Chapter Twelve has noted, many elderly households live in substandard housing. An unsatisfactory living environment, together with fears and doubts about living at home, are among the factors that contribute to entry into residential care. Most older people, however, want to remain in their own homes. Measures that can support this range from assistive technology, to better heating, the prevention of accidents, and assistance with basic repairs and maintenance. The home is also the focus for the four models of care identified as alternatives to long-term care – intensive home support and coresident care (both considered later under social support) together with very sheltered housing and assistive technology (RCLTC, 1999a). Yet, despite its pivotal role, until recently there has been a neglect of housing in community care plans, policy and research (Tinker, 1999).

What works? Evidence and practice

Low-intensity services such as housing adaptations and home repair schemes are designed to enable older people to maintain independence in their own homes. A systematic review was able to find little or no research evidence that actually addressed the effectiveness of such initiatives with respect to older people, and no study addressing their effectiveness in reducing demand on other more costly services (Godfrey, 1999). Research does suggest, however, that housing interventions need to be multidimensional, spanning the physical environment, the provision of low-level preventative help and personal care and the development or maintenance of links to the local community and informal support networks (Parkinson and Pierpoint, 2000).

The Anchor Trust found that there was frequently little correlation between levels of disability and dependency if the physical environment was right with the building meeting the needs of the occupants. This requires the ability to respond to changing functional ability and the modification of key features such as kitchens and bathrooms, which often become disabling environments (Parkinson and Pierpoint, 2000). A recent study combined typical disability profiles for England and Wales with a range of care packages, adaptations and assumptions concerning the availability of informal care. This provided evidence that housing adaptations and assistive technology can substitute for and supplement formal care in a cost–effective manner. In most cases the initial investment was recouped via lower care costs within the average life expectancy of the user, although good practice adaptations and increasing disability across time increased the costs, often substantially (Lansley et al, 2004). A national study carried out for the Joseph Rowntree Foundation similarly supported increased investment in adaptations, finding that minor adaptations produced a range of positive and lasting consequences for nearly all recipients while major adaptations had the ability to transform people's lives (Heywood, 2001).

The installation of aids and adaptations can cause particular problems for people waiting to leave hospital. Around 6% of delayed discharges are attributed to patients waiting for an adaptation to be carried out to their own home and/or for a home care package to be arranged (DH, 2002), with the Audit Commission asserting that equipment services "have the potential to make or break the quality of life of many older or disabled people" (Audit Commission, 2000). Hospital Discharge Schemes (primarily in the voluntary sector) provide fast–track repairs and improvements specifically for people in hospital so that they can be sent home to a property that is warm, dry and adapted. A good practice review stresses not only the capacity of such schemes to reduce delayed discharge but the ability to identify and resource the real range of adaptations and repairs required for independence, with corresponding improvements in quality of life and reduced demands on occupational therapists (Adams, 2001). Such schemes are also considered successful at preventing readmission to hospital (Millar, 1996).

An appropriate physical environment not only depends on aids and adaptations, but also on the satisfactory fabric of the home itself. Local care and repair and handyperson schemes, many under the aegis of Home Improvement Agencies (HIAs), provide repairs and renovations as well as adaptations. Handyperson schemes were introduced from the late 1980s in order to provide assistance with small repairs (such as doors, guttering, plumbing and electrical work) and minor adaptations (such as hand rails, bath aids, tap levers and ramps) that would cause distress and discomfort if left undone. A survey of 63 handypersons' schemes in the mid–1990s found that the majority of clients were older women, living alone and on low incomes. Although much of the work done was minor (typically costing less than £150), it was a key component in enabling older people to stay at home and providing improvements that would otherwise remain undone (Appleton, 1996). However, despite demand exceeding supply, all the schemes reported feeling insecure about their long–term funding prospects, with mainstream funding difficult to secure.

A more holistic response to a similar scenario is the Should I Stay or Should I Go Programme, a national initiative coordinated by Care and Repair England (the coordinating body for HIAs) and funded by a range of national and local bodies including the Housing Associations Charitable Trust, The Housing Corporation, Countryside Agency and Help the Aged (see Box 13.4).

Box 13.4: Care and Repair

The aim of Should I Stay or Should I Go is to stimulate the development of housing options services – schemes that provide information, advice, support and practical help to older (primarily low-income) people who are living in poor or unsuitable housing and/or are considering moving. Housing options workers, located within a range of agencies, including HIAs, Age Concern projects and Housing Advice Centres, aim to help individuals reach a decision about their future housing needs (including adaptations, repairs, financial advice, security, falls prevention and a move to sheltered housing), and provide the practical help necessary to implement the decision. The national programme aims to identify good practice and replicable service models.

Evaluation of eight pilot projects selected to include a range of areas and populations found that the projects served a mainly elderly (average age 76), frail population with multiple health needs who valued the personal and informative approach. Almost half lived alone and over one fifth had no informal carers to turn to. Housing option workers were, however, limited by their inability to influence housing and social care policy (the need for a greater choice of accommodation or the availability of community care grants, for example), or the response of other providers on referral (including requests for home care or housing adaptations). The pilot suggested one worker could assist up to 100 older people per annum (Mountain and Buri, 2005).

Warmth is another integral component of an appropriate home. Affordable heating and improved thermal efficiency are both effective preventative interventions to curb excess deaths, and this is particularly true for older households, living in older dwellings, with no central heating, unsatisfactory or expensive heating (Wilkinson et al, 2001). Insulating existing homes, providing effective safe heaters, and where necessary subsidised power, has been shown to increase older people's health and well-being (Thomson et al, 2001).

Sheltered housing illustrates well the impossibility of separating the physical attributes of the home from the caring activities conducted within its walls. It is traditionally offered for rent and designed to provide accessible, private and easily maintained accommodation for older people. It also provides support from health and social services. Very sheltered housing typically offers extra-communal facilities such as laundry, meals and a 24-hour warden service. Standard sheltered housing schemes have also experimented with offering shopping and cleaning in the early stages of the tenancy, a time when there are often high levels of tenancy failure. One key problem is matching client profile with a rapidly changing need for support (see Box 13.5). Another is availability; only about 3.5% of the sheltered

Box 13.5: Sheltered housing

The Somerville very sheltered housing scheme in Lewisham aimed to extend the range of social care for those living in the community. Twenty-four-hour supervision and individual-based care is provided for 26 flats, occupied predominantly by women. Issues raised by evaluation included the difficulties of targeting the scheme at those for whom it was most suitable and cost-effective (hence the need for a full assessment), and confusion over the purpose of the scheme (with tenants in ordinary sheltered housing often receiving more care through the home help service than those in the extra care scheme). Nevertheless, the tenants were generally happy with the package provided and one third showed an improvement (Seymour, 1997, cited in Tinker et al, 1999, p 186).

A similar scheme in Wolverhampton found the quality of life for tenants to be higher than in residential homes, with the net cost to social services approximately half of a residential place or large care package in the community. The providers estimated substantial savings of £123,000 for the 36 tenants over the first two years of the scheme (none of whom have moved on to residential care) based on comparison with the care they would have otherwise continued to receive. There was little functional difference between tenants and their peers in the community; the former typically reported a more positive health rating but were less able to perform social activities (Tinker et al, 1999).

housing stock falls into this very sheltered category. It is also more expensive than staying at home in terms of resource costs.

There are indications that major housing providers such as Anchor Housing are now developing Intermediate Care schemes in existing and new sheltered housing projects (Wistow et al, 2002), and that sheltered housing is being linked to hospital discharge schemes so that discharge is not delayed while waiting for home adaptations or repairs (Adams, 2001). Supported housing may also provide a link to the regeneration agenda, promoting employment opportunities, a culture of community tolerance and combating discrimination and isolation. This may be particularly so where people are either welcomed into schemes for social activities, meetings, meals or the use of other communal facilities or where outreach services such as low-level home help (cleaning, laundry and personal care) are taken out to other vulnerable people in the area. Such outreach warden services may be funded as part of a housing management agreement and eligible for Housing Benefit if they become part of the rent and a condition of occupancy, with the property becoming, in effect, sheltered housing for the duration of the tenancy (Parkinson and Pierpoint, 2000).

Policy

The 2000 Local Government Act placed responsibility on local authorities to promote the economic, environmental and social well-being of their communities, including factors such as transport and supported housing, that have the potential to increase independence and better qualify of life of older people. At the same time their role (and to some extent that of health authorities) has shifted away from the direct provision of services towards the enablement and facilitation of service delivery across the whole range of agencies operating in the area (Lewis et al, 1999). This is reflected in their responsibility (also stemming from the Local Government Act) to develop Local Strategic Partnerships (LSPs) (to provide a framework for policies that cut across the range of organisational boundaries) and to promote an integrated approach to health, by overseeing the implementation of the NSFs (Audit Commission, 2002a). The Performance Assessment Framework for councils and the public health targets for the NHS offer additional scope for a coordinated approach to the promotion of well-being, independence and health in old age, and an opportunity to bring health inequalities and public health into community planning (DH, 2004c).

Such levers and incentives for communities to refocus services have been criticised as weak (ADSS et al, 2004), but the holistic approach continues and is now also found in the guidance relating specifically to housing for older people. The aim of *Quality and choice: A strategic framework for older people's housing* (DETR/DH, 2001) and its successor documents (ODPM, 2003) was to raise awareness of the importance of housing across the local government, social care and health agenda. It requires not only that all relevant strategies include a housing component in a consistent way (a previously much neglected dimension as shown by the Joseph Rowntree Foundation, 2000), but also that older people are included and involved in strategic planning and thinking. This process extends to Community and Community Safety Strategies, Best Value Reviews, Care and Support Service Plans and Local Transport Plans (LTPs). Five key areas have been identified for new policy and service developments, all areas that parallel the interventions described already: services that promote independence (diversity and choice); the availability of information and advice; improved flexibility to meet changing needs (such as community equipment services); quality housing that is warm, safe and secure; and joint working. The objectives are to sustain independence at home and support active and informed choices about accommodation.

One of the three Learning and Improvement Networks set up by the Health and Social Care Change Agent Team in the DH has also focused specifically on housing (the other two addressing intermediate care and discharge pathways) (DH, 2004b). Part of the Network's role has been to encourage and support bids for DH funding (£87 million for the period 2004-06) for the development of up to 1,500 new extra care units of accommodation (a very sheltered model that lies between sheltered housing and the accommodation and care provided in residential care homes). There are also signs that some primary care trusts (PCTs) are beginning to take an active interest in the potential role of HIAs, and starting to commit funding for joint initiatives, particularly those that address NSF Standard Six on falls (Easterbrook, 2002). Housing authorities are also being encouraged to work with health and social care partners when drawing up their new private sector renewal policies, which could include hospital discharge and accident prevention services (ODPM, 2003).

While concern has long been raised about the paucity of investment in the preventative health and social care agenda, and questions remain about the relationship between Intermediate Care and primary prevention, there is a suggestion, therefore, that real effort is beginning to be made to address the long neglected role of housing in promoting independence. In 2000, for example, case studies conducted by The Housing Corporation and Anchor Trust found their preventive role and scope had been limited by their uneven distribution across the country, meaning that many older people have no access to such help and continue to face difficulties in accessing or funding adaptations irrespective of tenure (Parkinson and Pierpoint, 2000). Funding for preventive services in housing, including adaptations and community alarms was, however, reviewed as part of the government's Interdepartmental Review on the Future Funding of Supported Accommodation. This recognised that preventive housing and support services are vital for maintaining independence in the home. From 2003, funding for support services has therefore been excluded from Housing Benefit and local authorities' Housing Revenue Account and funded instead from a locally managed Supporting People Fund, determined by joint planning mechanisms involving local partners including the health and social care sectors. The funding is likely, however, to be cash-limited and will therefore require performance measurements to demonstrate the cost–effectiveness and benefit of preventive approaches to service delivery. Grants specifically for owner-occupiers also ceased in July 2003, and have been replaced by a general discretionary power held by local authorities to provide help for repairs in this sector alongside the existing mandatory Disabled Facilities Grants. The intention to incorporate the Lifetime Home Standards into new builds and renovations by 2007 should also gradually reduce the need for modifications (HM Government, 2005).

There is also evidence that the issue of fuel poverty is being addressed on an increasingly integrated basis. As noted in Chapter Eleven, the government's aim is to eradicate fuel poverty among vulnerable households (including older people) by 2010. Key to this is the Warm Front Scheme. Established in 2000, this provides grants for the installation of a range of energy efficiency measures (such as central heating and insulation) for the private sector alongside energy advice. The scheme was criticised for not being sufficiently targeted at the fuel-poor and many vulnerable households (particularly older people) were not eligible because they were not claiming the passport benefits (Income Support, Housing Benefit or Council Tax Benefit). A benefit entitlement check has now, therefore, been added to the scheme in order to increase eligibility, and the scheme was extended in 2005 for a further seven-year period (DEFRA, 2004). Another drawback is its limited utility for hard-to-treat properties (those without a gas supply or with solid walls, for example, features of many fuel-poor homes) and its focus on urban areas. The Winter Fuel Payment, introduced as a universal benefit in 1997 for householders aged 60 and over, has been similarly criticised for failing to address the specific needs of older people who are fuel-poor (Phillipson and Scharf, 2004). Cold Weather Payments, in contrast, are still targeted at the heating costs of people on low incomes who receive a range of means-tested benefits, including Pension Credit.

Social support and personal care

The home is also the focus for social support and personal care, both at a low level and as an alternative to long-term care. There is, however, a lack of evidence concerning the effectiveness and outcomes of preventive strategies from the social care perspective (Godfrey, 1999). Indeed, many would argue that the medical model cannot be transferred to the social care arena, and that the individualised nature of social care militates against the construction of an evidence base (Baldock, 1997, p 82). A further confounding factor is the focus on people who are often disabled as well as elderly, and who grow older as the intervention proceeds. Actual physical improvements or substantial changes in their circumstances are thus unlikely (Bours et al, 1998, p 1084).

What works? Evidence and practice

Home visiting provides low-intensity support, capable of identifying a large number of unmet medical and social needs and mediates access to the larger health and social care system. A systematic review and meta-analysis of home visiting programmes focusing on the range of functions typically performed by a health visitor (surveillance, support, health promotion and the prevention of ill health) found that they were able to reduce significantly both mortality and admissions to intensive care among elderly and frail elderly people alike (Elkan et al, 2001), together with a clinically important reduction in the risk of admission to long-term institutional care (Egger, 2001). However, the multifaceted programmes reviewed provided little insight into the processes involved, and hence little indication as to what elements of the intervention were actually effective and which groups might benefit most. One possible key was the breadth of response, with successful home visiting programmes referring to a wide range of agencies (Elkan et al, 2001). Research has also suggested that home visiting may offer the most benefit to those who are at low risk at baseline.

More intensive home support depends on information (referral agents), assessment (invariably neither multidisciplinary nor comprehensive), management and coordination of care and the input of key service components. A literature review suggests it may not be the package of services themselves "but co-ordination, through integrated health and social care management" (RCLTC, 1999a, p 44) that reduces institutional admission rates (particularly hospital admission rates) and physical and cognitive functioning (see Box 13.6, also Box 13.10).

Research has also highlighted the important role played by low-level services such as housework and laundry in enhancing the quality of life of older people and helping them maintain their independence (Clark et al, 1998). Evidence suggests that home carers often provide a source of emotional as well as physical support, while the appearance of the home can have a positive impact on sense of well-being and social participation. Despite the community care agenda, however, home care services have been largely withdrawn since the 1980s as support from social services has come to focus largely on personal care for those with the highest needs. Within this generally restrictive context the 1996 Community Care (Direct Payments) Act has attempted to increase flexibility in the deployment of resources by allowing older people to receive payments for their care directly, and employing personal assistants themselves.

Box 13.6: Direct payments for social care

Research in three local authority areas in England found older people who received direct payments to be used for social care reported feeling happier, more motivated and having an improved quality of life than before. There was a positive impact on their social, emotional and physical health, which was attributed to greater choice, continuity and control over their support arrangements, including the ability to employ Personal Assistants who spoke the same language and who were culturally sensitive (Joseph Rowntree Foundation, 2004). Older people were also able to negotiate when the services were delivered, bank unused hours and use the service to meet the needs they deemed the most important (Joseph Rowntree Foundation, 2001).

An alternative model piloted by social services departments in Kent, Gateshead, Darlington and Lewisham, together with the NHS in Darlington, investigated the impact of devolving budgets to the *staff* directly responsible for enabling highly dependent older people (with high-risk institutional care) to remain living in the community. A budgetary limit restricted expenditure to two thirds of the cost of a place in residential care. Evaluation showed significant differences between intervention and control as far as quality of life, depression, dissatisfaction, felt ability to cope, morale, social activity, ability to manage basic tasks and reduction of need for basic services were concerned. When the routine development of this care management approach was evaluated in two contrasting areas, similar positive results were found (see Tinker et al, 1999).

A comprehensive survey of health authorities and local authorities in England in 1998/99 aimed to assess the development of preventive strategies. These were defined to include interventions both inside and outside the home, and interventions providing practical/physical support as well as those providing personal/social care (Lewis et al, 1999). This suggested that progress was associated with a number of common traits, including cross-agency goals, senior leadership, dedicated budgets and staff, incorporation within corporate objectives, the engagement of older people, a commitment to sustainability and the use of a community development approach, with staff able to act flexibly, responsively and relatively independently. Major barriers, however, continued in terms of reliance on soft or short-term monies rather than mainstream funding and ageist attitudes and low expectations among professionals, the general public and older people themselves.

Family care, particularly the presence in the home of a single main carer, often remains the most important support for an older person. Over half of all co-resident care is delivered by spouses, by definition mostly older people themselves. They are less likely than carers in separate households to share this care with health and social services and more likely than other carers to assume a heavier care burden, suffer from higher stress levels and associated illness (particularly when caring for partners with dementia), and to face injuries from care giving (lifting and so on). Again, there is very little systematic research about the effectiveness of such personal care, or strategies to support it such as respite care (Cotterill et al, 1997), only an acknowledgement that support whether in the form of respite care, day care, information and training is generally in short supply (see, for example, Katbamna et al, 1998; Jewson et al, 2003).

Finally, despite the acknowledged importance of social interaction, there are few studies of potential health benefits resulting from activities such as befriending, support groups or home sharing. Godfrey (1999) identified nine studies focusing on the reduction of social isolation with positive results in terms of user experience and satisfaction, but only one instance of a significant improvement in self-reported health status as a result of the intervention. Four further studies were identified relating to disparate self-help or mutual support groups, but positive results were found in only two, a bereavement group and a telelink support group, that appeared to have a significant impact on mental health among those who were most isolated and under greater stress because of recent loss/reduction of sight.

Policy

Since 1997, the government has repeatedly stressed the need for organisations and government departments to cooperate more closely in the delivery of public services, placing the emphasis on the needs of the service user. It has been paralleled by an increased stress on the whole systems approach within health and social care, and the need to redesign services that help people to maximise their independence. *Better services for vulnerable people* (DH, 1997) and the Audit Commission report *The coming of age* (Audit Commission, 1997), for example, both highlighted the importance of recognising the interdependence of health and social care agencies in delivering a full continuum of care for older people. The need to integrate services for older people then became a Labour Party manifesto commitment in 2001, with the declared aim of building on Care Direct to provide a better integration of health, housing, benefits and social care for older people. This notion is now being taken forward by the Department for Work and Pensions (DWP) in the form of the Link-Age Programme, which aims to provide user-focused information and advice together with community support, and is aimed at all older people who need support from social services (DWP, 2004). The intention is also to develop an integrated home visiting service (providing a full care, benefit, heating and housing check-up).

A number of other initiatives intend to move policy in the same direction. BGOP aimed to improve public services for older people by better meeting their needs, listening to their views, and encouraging and recognising their contribution, including simplified access to services, improved linkages between agencies and clearer and more accessible information on rights. Evaluation (of the 28 pilot projects) suggested that it had helped to put citizen–centred governance into practice and to develop community organisations and capacity (Haydon and Boaz, 2000). In addition, it pointed to the benefits of preventive approaches for promoting independence and an active old age itself. However, doubts have also been cast as to the desire among residents for more active citizenship and the existence of sufficient local autonomy or capacity to actually take citizens' needs into account (Martin and Boaz, 2000). The development of PCTs, particularly where these are coterminous with social services departments, also offers scope to deliver integrated care locally and redesign services across agency boundaries. The requirement to develop Health Improvement Programmes, for example, provided a focus for health and local authorities to work jointly to consider the impact on health of a wider range of factors, while the role of the Local Government Act has already been outlined and the development of Intermediate Care is discussed in more detail later.

In practice, however, the challenge of integrating health and social care and setting a preventive agenda to address lower-level needs remains considerable (Lewis, 2001). Social care has continued to be a residual service within the welfare state and need, which the 1990 NHS and Community Care Act promised to meet, has not been the major principle underpinning service delivery. Indeed, the number of households receiving home care from social services reduced by 18% from 1999 to 2002 as resources became increasingly focused on the most dependent (ADSS et al, 2004). Unmet need and the affordability of domiciliary care for lower-income groups are thus significant problems (Deeming and Keen, 2002), and the family has continued to be the main provider (Lewis, 1999). The

King's Fund commissioned the Wanless Social Care Review to investigate the long-term demand for and supply of social care for older people in England. This is due to report by Spring 2006 (King's Fund, 2005).

The 1998 White Paper *Modernising social services* (Secretary of State for Health, 1998) introduced a wide set of initiatives designed to promote independence. These included the Promoting Independence partnership and prevention grants, which, despite the relatively small amounts involved (£650 million on the former and £100 million on the latter over three years), were welcomed as representing an explicit shift in mainstream funding towards early intervention (Lewis et al, 1999, p 53). However, the definition of the target population with low-intensity needs as those receiving less than 10 hours per week domiciliary care or under six visits per week, suggested that the real focus remained on secondary rather than primary prevention (Wistow et al, 2002). This has been borne out by subsequent research, which has found little evidence of investment in, and few strategies for, developing low-level prevention and support services (see Phillipson and Scharf, 2004, p 59). This trend continues with the recent Social Care Green Paper. This similarly stresses the importance of the preventative agenda and more personalised social care provision and delegates a budget (£60 million for 2006-08) for partnership projects addressing prevention and the delivery of integrated health and social care. It also emphasises that the mainstream movement has to be met from existing funds (DH, 2001a).

The 1995 Carers (Recognition and Services) Act provided the scope for carers to ask social services for an assessment of their own needs in maintaining a caring relationship. Implementation was, however, patchy and *Modernising social services* returned to this agenda, introducing proposals for a national carers' support package and an increase in services to people who have an informal carer. *The national strategy for carers* (DH, 1999b) subsequently aimed to provide information, support and care for carers themselves, including the establishment of the Carers' Special Grant (with a budget of £140 million for 1999/2001) to facilitate short breaks for carers. Again, however, evidence suggests this has not been fully taken up by local authorities (Jewson et al, 2003). The 1996 Community Care (Direct Payments) Act was also extended to older people in February 2000, and the government has since placed a duty on local authorities in England to offer direct payments to all those eligible for them. Take-up by older people has been slow, but the government has signalled its commitment to increasing the number of older people using them (DH, 2005b).

Neighbourhood perceptions and mobility

Older people are particularly dependent on their immediate locality and often have a strong sense of local identity as a result of long-term residence (SEU, 2004a). They are thus particularly vulnerable to the process of economic decline and high population turnover at the neighbourhood level. A recent exercise to gather older people's views on neighbourhood renewal, for example, carried out for the Audit Commission by Age Concern, highlighted the importance of transport, community safety and housing repairs. Many also identified the importance of neighbourliness and community spirit and saw themselves as having a key role in fostering and maintaining this (Audit Commission, 2002a). Such factors tend to be considered more important to quality of life than the availability or quality of care services, and research suggests that such a sense of neighbourhood may also be associated with various measures of health and physical activity in older people (Stuck et al, 1999; Pollack and von dem Knesebeck, 2004).

What works? Evidence and practice

Recent research suggests that older people in the most deprived urban wards are at multiple risk of exclusion, stemming from poverty, social isolation, crime, lack of amenities and a hostile environment. This risk is significantly higher than that experienced elsewhere in Britain and is structured by age, gender and 'race', such that older women are more likely to be multiply deprived than men and older pensioners than younger, with very high concentrations of poverty among Somali and Pakistani elders (Scharf et al, 2002).

Many of the measures to reduce exclusion have already been outlined in Chapter Eleven. Income in particular is a key, with the (then) Minimum Income Guarantee (MIG) failing to reach many of those most in need (NAO, 2002), between £1.7 and £2.9 billion benefits (including Housing Benefit, Council Tax Benefit and a range of disability-related benefits) remaining unclaimed by older people in 2002/03 (SEU, 2005), and applications to the Social Fund from older people significantly depressed (Kempson et al, 2002). Welfare advice, as discussed in Chapter Eleven, is indicated with the National Audit Office identifying 23 different relevant benefits for this age group and pilots by the Benefits Agency under BGOP finding that a variety of models such as a one-stop office for older people, home visiting and outreach services (including a parish network of volunteers in rural areas) and dedicated telephone helplines had the potential not only to increase benefit take-up but also to meet needs across a range of areas (Sippings, 2000; Chang et al, 2001). Many would argue, however, that persistently low levels of uptake suggest the focus must move instead to higher incomes for pensioners, including preventive measures while in work and improved options for insurance and equity release (see ADSS et al, 2004; Joseph Rowntree Foundation Task Group, 2004; Phillipson and Scharf, 2004).

Other parts of the solution include improving the physical characteristics of the neighbourhood (street lighting and surveillance and a reduction in litter and graffiti, for example) and visible social controls such as neighbourhood or street wardens. These are initiatives that reduce fear of crime, and satisfaction with the local area and community although appearing to play but a minor role in the incidence of crime itself (Pain, 2000). The work of HIAs has a part to play, increasing security and confidence in the home. Research also confirms that the policy-making process has to focus explicitly on older people, actively engaging them in the process of renewal as a whole. The Homesafe Initiative, part of the Safer Cities Programme in Plymouth, for example, found the installation of additional security features in older people's homes made residents feels safer and more secure (with an apparent reduction in burglaries on the local scale), and decreased the likelihood they would move (see also Box 13.7). Older people remained fearful, however, of public spaces outside the home (Mawby, 1999).

Box 13.7: Regeneration and health

The Golborne Single Regeneration Budget (SRB) partnership within the London Borough of Kensington and Chelsea funds a number of projects provided (free) by Sixty Plus, a local charity which aims to enable older people to improve their health and independence. One of these, Garden Guardians, provides a package of measures to improve home security and reduce isolation aimed particularly at minority ethnic elders. A team of (mainly young) volunteers help older people to keep their gardens tidy, with the secondary aim of deterring bogus callers, who are more likely to visit homes with visible signs of neglect. The project also improves household security (the project leader is a handyman who carries out minor repairs and fits home safety and security equipment in the course of his day-to-day contact with older residents) and repairs gates and fences. Derelict patches of land in the neighbourhood have also been cleared, providing opportunities for healthy gardening activity for older people who do not have gardens themselves.

Identified benefits include increased enjoyment of the gardens, intergenerational contact, reduced fear of crime and raised awareness of services (for volunteers and clients alike). Garden Guardians also has links with the fire service, which supplies smoke alarms to the project's clients, and performs safety checks in their homes, and the project runs healthy eating information sessions jointly with Health Wise in Golborne (www.renewal.net/documents/RNET/case%20study/Sixtyplus.doc).

The ability to travel serves a number of important functions for older people, including involvement in the local community and leisure activities, independence (including the ability to shop), exercise, social interaction and access to services. Conversely, a lack of mobility can lead to low morale, depression and loneliness (Atkins, 2001). Ageing often brings greater reliance on others for transport due to declining driving ability, the loss of licence-holding partners and financial constraints. Affordable public transport thus assumes an important role in tackling isolation. However, many face barriers to such travel including poor accessibility, lack of travel information, high costs and lack of awareness of their needs by transport providers. Older people are, for example, often unaware of the available community and voluntary transport (frequently provided by older people themselves working in a voluntary capacity), including special transport schemes such as dial-a-ride and shop mobility, or the availability of concessionary fares. Atkins (2001) concluded that local authorities should aim to increase the availability of mainstream services in order to maximise social inclusion and reduce the demand for more expensive, targeted services.

Pedestrian safety is a further critical issue for older people, with (other than in rural areas) those aged over 70 in the UK making more journeys on foot than by car (Noble, 2000). Factors such as a decline in vision and hearing, physical mobility, cognitive processes and ill health all increase the risk (albeit slightly) of older pedestrians being involved in a pedestrian accident. However, physical frailty greatly increases their risk of being seriously or fatally injured and, as a result, has led some to suggest that older drivers should be encouraged to drive as long as possible (Mitchell, 2000). Unfortunately, such risk is most pronounced for the older-old, those aged 80 and over, the group for whom the risks attached to continued driving are also likely to be the greatest.

Dunbar et al (2004) reviewed a number of interventions designed to improve safety for older people with activities falling under two broad heads: information and training for older pedestrians and other drivers, and changes to the road environment. The review found few educational programmes for older pedestrians as a whole and, as with children and young people (see Chapter Seven), little evidence that such interventions (including those that focus on functional impairment, self-awareness and compensation) actually influence behaviour or reduce accident risk. Other road users, particularly drivers, can be more effectively targeted by coordinated programmes, and this has been demonstrated to reduce accident risk for pedestrians.

In contrast, changes to the road environment are, as with children, more effective, including interventions that reduce vehicle speed, separate vehicles and pedestrians, and afford protection when crossing roads. Improving the visibility of both pedestrians and vehicles is also effective. Two areas of particular importance for older people are the maintenance of a high-quality walking area to reduce tripping and increasing signal timing at crossings to allow for the lower walking speed of older people, including crossings that adapt the crossing time by detecting the presence and speed of pedestrians.

Dunbar et al (2004) also reviewed a number of interventions that sought community involvement in order to increase safety for older or disabled pedestrians. The focus, as in Box 13.8, has often been on fall prevention and the use of peer educators.

Policy

Lewis et al (1999, p 2) highlight how *Our healthier nation* (DH, 1999a) not only articulated a preventive philosophy, including increasing the length of people's

Box 13.8: Pedestrian safety – the potential for community interventions

In Australia a group of older people were trained in aspects of fall prevention and encouraged to survey local places. The hazards identified were brought to the attention of the relevant agencies, such as local businesses or local government, resulting in corrective action (Powell et al, 2000). The older people also acted as peer educators, visiting local groups to pass on information. Such activity could also function on an individual level. Research with focus groups in England suggested many older people wanted a central telephone line they could use to report potential hazards (Atkins, 2001) (a method that has been utilised in British Columbia [Dunbar et al, 2004]).

Evidence of success is still equivocal, however. Community involvement in Scandinavia, from where many of the interventions originate, tends to operate both for a prolonged period and on an holistic basis, with interventions spanning education, engineering, and enforcement measures (see Bjerre and Schelp, 2000), and evaluation failing to separate the relative efficacy of the individual components. Success may also be culture-specific, reflecting a tradition of collective action and broad participation which may not translate to a more individualistic culture (Lindqvist et al, 2001).

lives and the number of years people spend free from illness, but also focused on the creation of healthy neighbourhoods, with a particular emphasis on the living environments of older people, alongside themes of empowerment and community involvement. Greater emphasis was also placed on the societal factors affecting health and well-being, epitomised by the development of Health Action Zones (HAZs) and Healthy Living Centres, both of which have focused a considerable amount of their attention on the welfare of older people (albeit with a focus on age-related issues and age discrimination rather than on the impact of cumulative disadvantage throughout the life course) (Phillipson and Scharf, 2004, p 71).

This trend has been strengthened by the significance of the regeneration agenda, which, as noted in Chapter Eleven, has broadened to include health improvement and achieve greater alignment with the social exclusion agenda, and which involves considerable funds for the reshaping of the physical and social environment. However, older people are still often marginal to the process, with little systematic attention given to their needs (Phillipson and Scharf, 2004), and little evidence "that local, regional and national policy is coming to terms with the full implications of having an ageing society" (Riseborough and Jenkins, 2004, p 7). Recommendations for rectification span the range of issues discussed in this chapter, with suggestions for performance targets to increase the level of inclusion of older people in strategic planning and service design (including a broader range of accommodation, housing options and services to enable older people to avoid long-term care); employment and self-employment; decision making;

community capacity building; and the number of regeneration bids led by and including older people. Riseborough and Jenkins (2004) also suggest the removal of the perverse incentives in Income Tax arrangements and pension schemes that discourage older workers/people over retirement age from continuing in the paid workforce.

The government has now designated the DWP to take the lead on older people's issues and in 2002 established the Pensions Service to provide a dedicated benefits service for pensioners. This enabled a more proactive and tailored approach to be made to the take-up of benefits, addressing some of the many persistent barriers to benefit take-up such as complexity, lack of information, confusion over entitlements and relying on pensioners to initiate the process (NAO, 2002). Means testing, remains, however, a significant barrier, although the Pension Credit (introduced in October 2003 and subsuming the MIG) is designed to be seen as just another part of pension entitlement. This has allowed access to those with modest savings or additional income while also harmonising rules with those for Council Tax and Housing Benefit, and allowing expanded access to the Social Fund. A total of 2.65 million pensioner households now receive Pension Credit as opposed to the government target of 3 million by 2006 (Age Concern, 2005).

Policies that have targeted crime and the fear of crime among vulnerable groups such as older people include the Reducing Burglary Initiative (£32 million for neighbourhoods that experience high burglary rates), Neighbourhood Wardens (see Chapter Eleven), Locks for Pensioners (with £8 million from the Crime Reduction Programme directed at improving security for low-income pensioners in local authority areas that had burglary rates above the national average), and the Distraction Burglary Task Force (created by the Home Office in 2000) (Phillipson and Scharf, 2004). The DWP has also been monitoring the impact of fear of crime on the quality of life of older people as part of their programme for tackling poverty and social exclusion. In the short period for which statistics have been produced this has, however, remained unchanged, at 10% between 1998 and 2000 (Chivite-Matthews and Maggs, 2002).

The 1995 Disability Discrimination Act sought to increase access to Public Service Vehicles, via, for example, the introduction of low-floor buses. This was furthered by the White Paper *A new deal for transport: Better for everyone* (DETR, 1998), which noted that, as a matter of social justice, high-quality public transport should be designed for everyone to use (Atkins, 2001). This included issues such as accessibility, affordability and personal security, as well as gender, age, ethnicity and religion. *Transport 2010* (DETR, 2001) aims to help older people by delivering more accessible buses, trains and taxis, half-price local bus fares for pensioners, and providing support for a wide range of flexible, community transport projects, such as minibus and taxi-based schemes, and accessibility planning has been incorporated into the next round of LTPs (which also include provisions for community input) due in 2006 (SEU, 2004a). However, despite this recognition of the centrality of transport, older people still remain ineligible for the mobility component of the Disability Living Allowance if they claim for the first time aged 65 or over (Howard, 2002).

Access to services: intermediate care

The NSF for Older People required health organisations to review and justify any age-related policies on clinical grounds by October 2001. Previously, such discrimination had been evident in areas as diverse as GP referrals, access to coronary care units and cardiac rehabilitation and community health services such as podiatry (Roberts, 2002). Since then, age-related policies have become less common in the NHS but are still evident in areas such as health promotion (targeted primarily at young people), differential diagnosis (particularly with respect to mental health problems), inclusion in clinical trials (where multiple medication and chronic health problems still remove a large proportion of older people from the evidence base), onward referral from Accident and Emergency Departments and specialists in key areas such as arthritis. It has also been argued that little has changed since Help the Aged's Dignity on the Ward campaign, which stressed how hospital practice often failed to meet the basic needs of older people, including their mental health and rehabilitation.

For many older people it is the lack of access to services such as chiropody, dentistry, eye care and continence that affects them the most and can produce depression and isolation (SEU, 2005), as can lack of access to low-level preventative services discussed earlier. The current policy impetus to incorporate public, patient and carer perspectives into strategic planning may be an important driver for change if implemented well, although incremental evolution and rationing tend to militate against radical redistribution (Roberts, 2002). In this section we focus on the first of two particularly high-profile services: Intermediate Care.

Intermediate Care, as the name suggests provides a range of services at the interface between hospital and home. It can function either as a 'step up' from the community or a 'step down' from hospital, reducing both inappropriate admissions to acute inpatient care and long-term residential care and delayed discharge from hospital. As such it includes a number of community-based service models, ranging from rapid response schemes, hospital at home and residential rehabilitation and recuperation, to supported discharge and day rehabilitation (Roe et al, 2003). Each of these in turn may exist in many different forms, reflecting the needs of the local health and social care community (Martin et al, 2004), but guidelines expect them to be time-limited (not usually exceeding six weeks), to involve active therapy and cross-professional working and to maximise independence with the aim of allowing the patient to return home (DH, 2001c). A second implicit aim is to gate-keep the use of acute NHS resources (Wistow et al, 2002).

Nocon and Baldwin's (1998) analysis of policy trends in rehabilitation indicated that there is a growing consensus that the concept of rehabilitation involves not only the restoration of physical and/or mental functioning, but also of the individual's role within the community. Proponents of the social model of rehabilitation have, therefore, widened the debate to include the impact of social and physical environments on rehabilitation.

What works? Evidence and practice

A growing body of research has sought to evaluate the costs, quality and effectiveness of such schemes (for systematic reviews of such research, see Parker et al, 2000; Richards and Coast, 2003). However, in order to produce scientifically robust evidence of the effectiveness of Intermediate Care schemes, most published studies have compared inpatient outcomes with those of a single model of Intermediate Care, often through the use of randomised controlled trials (RCTs) (Steiner et al, 2001; Wilson et al, 2003), and with a focus on physical functioning within a medical model (Wistow et al, 2002).

The results of these are often equivocal, probably at least in part because of the variations within services, including dedicated and trained staff, levels of active rehabilitation and institutional location (Fleming et al, 2004). Hospital at home, for example, provides treatment by healthcare professionals in the patient's home for conditions that would normally require acute hospital inpatient care. Like intermediate care as a whole, it is time-limited. A generic systematic review found no significant difference in patient health outcomes where the scheme focused on elderly patients with a mix of medical conditions (partly because of the high nursing costs incurred irrespective of location), while those focusing on patients recovering from a stroke produced conflicting results (Shepperd and Iliffe, 2001). Patients allocated to hospital at home expressed greater satisfaction with care than those in hospital, but the reverse pertained for carers, and while hospital at home resulted in a reduction in hospital length of stay, reducing pressure on beds, it also increased overall length of care (Shepperd and Iliffe, 2001). Costs may also be transferred within the health system, particularly to primary care, while eligibility is often low (Shepperd et al, 1998).

One confounding factor, as far as stroke recovery is concerned, may be suboptimal care in the acute phase. A systematic review of stroke care has confirmed that reduced death, dependency and institutionalisation are all associated with specialised stroke units (reflecting coordinated multidisciplinary rehabilitation, programmes of education and training in stroke, and specialisation of medical and nursing staff) (Stroke Unit Trialists' Collaboration, 1997). A recent Norwegian RCT of early supported discharge following such specialised stroke unit care found that the intervention group (where support was given from a mobile team comprising a physiotherapist, occupational therapist and nurse together with the consulting services of a stroke physician) had significantly better functional outcomes at one year, together with a reduced hospital stay. Patients suffering from moderate or severe strokes were able to benefit the most (Fjærtoft et al, 2003).

A systematic review of the effectiveness of hospital at home for acute episodes of chronic obstructive pulmonary disease (COPD) (where six of the seven trials focused on people in their late sixties and early seventies) similarly found no significant differences in hospital readmissions or mortality at two to three months but cost savings and reduced pressure on beds (Ram et al, 2004). However, frequency and length of care varied, as did the characteristics of usual care and, as is so often the case, it was impossible to establish from the review process which components of the service were effective, which types of patients were able to benefit most or who should best deliver such interventions.

A systematic review of the ability of day hospitals to prolong independent living (Forster et al, 1999) similarly found no significant difference between them and alternative service provision, although there was a lower risk of death, functional deterioration and a poor outcome (such as the need for intensive care or severe disability) compared with those who received no comparative care. Day hospital patients were also less likely to be placed in institutional care than those without care packages, although results were compromised by the changes in policy and service delivery that had occurred over the 30-year review period and the considerable loss to follow-up among those not receiving comparative care.

A more recent RCT focused on stroke patients, the largest group receiving treatment in geriatric day hospitals, and compared this treatment with domiciliary rehabilitation. It found the latter to be as effective for patients, although social functioning and mental state remained low at six-month follow-up. It also found the interventions to be cost-neutral, with domiciliary rehabilitation reducing health service costs but increasing social services costs (Roderick et al, 2001). A mixed model of care was therefore suggested, depending on patient characteristics and the availability of personal support

Conclusions also vary with chosen measures of outcome. A systematic review of the effect of post-hospital discharge schemes on the chronically sick and elderly found little evidence to support nursing after-care, including a lack of positive impact on the quality of life or the risk of rehospitalisation and limited impact on compliance (such as attitudes and medicines), although costs were reduced in several studies (Bours et al, 1998). However, a more recent review claimed with 'relative certainty' that supported discharge was significantly associated with a greater proportion of patients living at home 6-12 months after hospital admission, as compared to patients receiving usual care, and a reduction in admission to long-stay care without differences in mortality between the treatment and control group. Other outcomes, such as hospital admissions during the follow-up period, and the effects on functional status or patient/carer satisfaction were, however, inconclusive or mixed (Hyde et al, 2000).

Evidence is also equivocal when it comes to admission avoidance. COPD, for example, is associated with significant morbidity, mortality and costs to healthcare systems. Nursing outreach programmes, where support with medication and coping strategies, education and monitoring can be administered at home, potentially offer scope for reduced utilisation of hospital services. However, a systematic review found that while patients with moderate COPD might benefit from the nursing outreach programme in terms of mortality and health-related quality of life gains, there was no available data on reductions in hospital utilisation and the gains did not apply to patients with severe COPD (Smith et al, 2001).

Paradoxically, this search for scientific clarity has also obscured "one of the central concepts of intermediate care: the extent to which it functions as part of a *whole system*" (Asthana and Halliday, 2003, p 15), and the ways in which different parts of the system relate to each other. Indeed, while the value of such an approach is acknowledged in the literature, it remains the exception in practice rather than the rule (Vaughan and Lathlean, 1999). One such exception is the model developed in Cornwall (see Box 13.9), which is not only multifaceted but links into the broader aspects of independent living (see also Herbert and Lake, 2004).

Box 13.9: Intermediate Care: a whole systems approach in Cornwall

Cornwall HAZ facilitated the development of a range of Intermediate Care services. These included a rapid response service to provide urgent nursing or therapy assessment at home, a holding service to contain a situation until an appropriate package of care was assembled and a range of rehabilitation options spanning home, residential Homeward Bound Units, community hospitals and nursing home placements.

Intermediate Care coordinators within each PCT ensure oversight of capacity and throughput, allowing patients to be allocated to the most appropriate point in the system according to their assessment and care plans. This client-centred approach involves establishing links not only with a range of healthcare professionals but also with key voluntary agencies, transport providers, equipment suppliers and related services such as sheltered housing and Care and Repair.

Evaluation evidence suggests the Homeward Bound Units yield positive outcomes with regards to costs, effectiveness and quality, improving the health and well-being of service users. This is mirrored across the Intermediate Care models as a whole, reflecting the local investment in the infrastructure and partnership working (Asthana and Halliday, 2003).

An allied dimension is integrated care and a case management approach (see Box 13.10). Both have been shown to reduce personal dependency and dependence on care, while meta-analysis, although dated, supports the contribution of comprehensive geriatric assessments to the process (Stuck et al, 1993, cited in Steiner, 2001). Results pooled across five different service models showed an overall decrease in mortality in geriatric evaluation and management (GEM) units and home assessment services (HAS), with GEM units also improving physical functioning at six and 12 months and GEM, HAS and hospital to home assessment services (essentially supported discharge) improving living location. No significant differences in outcomes were observed for outpatient or consultative assessments. A prospective trial over three years applied to people over the age of 75 concluded that comprehensive geriatric assessment can delay the development of disability and permanent admission to nursing home care.

Box 13.10: Integrated Care: an Italian example

A randomised trial was conducted in Northern Italy of 200 older people with multiple needs. Half were allocated to an intervention group, which received integrated social and medical care organised by trained case managers in conjunction with the community geriatric evaluation unit and GPs, while the control group continued to receive conventional community services.

Patients allocated to the intervention group were found to face a reduced risk of institutional admission (both to hospital and nursing homes) and a reduced length of stay. They also required less frequent home visits and less medication. There was also a statistically significant improvement in physical functioning alongside a reduced decline in cognitive status. Together these resulted in financial saving to the intervention (once staff costs were taken into account) of £1,125 per person per year (some 23% less than the healthcare costs per capita in the control group).

Success was attributed to the trained care managers who were able to integrate care and construct appropriate care plans, the use of the community geriatric evaluation unit as gatekeepers and the close collaboration achieved between this unit, care managers and GPs (Bernabei et al, 1998).

Policy

The National Beds Inquiry, *The NHS Plan* and the NSF for Older People all provided the impetus for the development of Intermediate Care (DH, 2002). The National Beds Inquiry was undertaken between 1998 and 2000 in response to growing political and media concern about the shortage of hospital beds to cope with winter crises (the number of acute hospital beds having been declining for over 30 years). The availability of winter pressures monies from 1997/98 to 2000/01 also meant that authorities were able to develop a range of services that attempted to maximise capacity in the acute sector by developing community alternatives to hospital admission.

Together, this produced a commitment to a significant shift in patterns of health services for older people. *The NHS Plan*, published in July 2000, explicitly acknowledged the problem of the growing intermediate group of older people who needed rehabilitation and non-institutionally based community care (Lewis, 2001). It announced an increase in acute hospital beds up to 2003/04 and a long-term increase in Intermediate Care places to facilitate a shift towards 'care closer to home'. This was backed by resources with the government's response to the Royal Commission on Long-Term Care pledging a total of £1.4 billion for investment in health and social care for older people, including an extra £900 million investment by 2003/04 in Intermediate Care. *The NHS Plan* also required health and social care agencies to put in place rapid response teams, which could provide emergency care for people at home to help prevent unnecessary hospital admissions, intensive rehabilitation services (to be situated normally in hospitals), recuperative facilities, closer working arrangements and possible co-location of social workers and GPs and integrated home care teams that emphasised the independence of older people.

The final step in the development of policy for Intermediate Care was the NSF for Older People (DH, 2001a). Access to Intermediate Care services at home or in designated care settings is the third of the eight standards within the Framework and required the development of 5,000 additional Intermediate Care beds and 1,700 non-residential Intermediate Care places in addition to the provision available in 1999/2000. It also required that an additional 150,000 people should receive Intermediate Care to promote their rehabilitation, after their discharge from hospital, while a further 70,000 people should receive Intermediate Care services to prevent unnecessary hospital admission. A parallel development was the establishment of the Health and Social Care Change Agent Team in 2001, initially to tackle the problems of delayed discharge (and to focus on those areas with the worst records), but more recently to support NSF implementation more widely, including the promotion of the single assessment process and shared care pathways (DH, 2004c).

Intermediate Care services now provide active convalescence for more than 333,000 people a year (as opposed to 132,000 in 1999), with 80% of these people being older people, and with Intermediate Care beds having almost doubled in the same period and delayed discharges reducing from 6,400 in December 2001 to 2,600 in June 2004 (Philp, 2004). The majority of England is also now covered by integrated community equipment services as opposed to the existence of 400 separate services in 2000. However, a number of question marks remain (Martin et al, 2004), not least around whether the process is primarily focused on the patient or the organisation (Steiner, 2001). Wistow et al (2002, p iii), for example, suggest there are "tensions between an holistic approach to the needs of older people, on the one hand, and some of the most forceful drivers of day-today policy and practice on the other", including a perception that older people will simply be 'warehoused' to free acute bed space.

Other reservations include the ability to achieve an appropriate degree of medical assessment and support and effective integration with other elements of the health and social care system. Concerns have been raised, for example, over the substitution of Intermediate Care for specialist geriatric rehabilitation units, the problems of access to acute services and diagnostic facilities for patients and the risk of duplicating provision or simply shifting scarce resources around the system (Grimley Evans and Tallis, 2001). There is also a need for rigorous administrative support in areas such as shared records, joint protocols, robust screening and assessment procedures and the lack of an evidence base for the types of interventions enshrined in Intermediate Care.

Such reservations have not been helped by the 2003 Community Care (Delayed Discharges) Act, which came into force in January 2004. This gives local authorities two days to assess needs and arrange care for any patient no longer requiring an acute hospital bed. Failure to comply will result in a fine of £100 per day that discharge is delayed beyond this limit and, given new tariffs for acute care episodes in the NHS, provides them "with a formal mechanism by which they can restrict their exposure to financial risk by transferring costs out of the system and back into the community" (Rowland and Pollock, 2004, p 5). At the same time the government has allocated £100 million each year to local authorities to enable them to reimburse the NHS as a result of delayed discharges. The expectation is that this will lead to investment in community-based services in order to avoid delayed discharges and provide the leverage to ensure senior managers and front-line staff are committed to the issue (Henwood, 2004). However, as Rowland and Pollock (2004) continue, this may underestimate the underfunding and current lack of capacity in the community care sector and ignore the fact that patients' wishes and needs are both likely to be underplayed in order to facilitate compliance.

Access to services: mental health

Access to mental health is the second high-profile service we consider. Mental health is a pervasive challenge, with 630,000 people having severe mental health problems at any one time, ranging from schizophrenia to deep depression. The reported prevalence of mild depressive symptoms among community-dwelling older people over the age of 65 is between 15% and 20%. A similar proportion is socially isolated (17% of those aged over 65 in the UK), with no daily social contact with another person (*The Observer*, 2005). The negative effect of depression and cognitive impairment on rehabilitation is well recognised but mental health problems themselves tend to be neglected and under-treated in primary care (Burns et al, 2001; Speer and Schneider, 2003), and the vast majority of older people who suffer from symptoms of depression will not receive any treatment

(Biderman et al, 2002). Research also suggests that the use of psychiatric services is still the subject of stigma among the elderly population (Livingston et al, 2002), with primary care offering both the preferred treatment setting and opportunities to reduce healthcare utilisation (Speer and Schneider, 2003).

What works? Evidence and practice

A first recommendation to emerge from the literature is that procedures for screening are improved and extended in both primary and secondary healthcare in order to increase recognition of mental health problems in general and access to appropriate services (Burns et al, 2001). A second is that these are supported by illness-specific guidelines on diagnosis, assessment and management (Trickey et al, 2000). Training would need to be an integral part of such a shift. A survey of primary care nurses responsible for the Over-75s Checks (a group who are likely to provide a substantial part of the routine care for patients with dementia) found, for example, only one fifth of respondents ever used formal validated cognitive tests as part of the Over-75s Check and responses to a vignette on dementia resulted in variable and often suboptimal response (Trickey et al, 2000).

If access to appropriate services is secured, one review found the evidence base supported the efficacy of a number of geriatric mental health interventions, most particularly those for major depression and dementia (Bartels et al, 2002). In the case of the former, it argued for both antidepressants and psychosocial interventions focusing on cognitive behavioural therapy (CBT), with the suggestion that pharmacological and psychosocial interventions were likely to be more effective in combination. However, it also noted that a recent meta-analysis had suggested that the administration of a placebo together with visits from the prescribing physician could account for 80% of the effects of medication (without the continuing controversies over side-effects) (see also Speer and Schneider, 2003). It also noted the limited attention given to minor depression, suicide and anxiety, despite their significance.

A literature review (Godfrey, 1999) found only three studies related to the prevention of depression in older people. Each of these studies considered a different type of service (a therapeutic group, primary care nurse intervention and music therapy). Positive results were, therefore, only suggestive and, with only small samples, there was insufficient evidence to support the beneficial effects of 'low-intensity' interventions for older people with depression. However, the literature did suggest a strong interrelationship between depression, physical disability and poor social networks. Two studies of interventions by psychiatric teams, one with elderly inpatients, one with older people at home, found such interventions could improve physical functioning, reduce readmissions to hospital or nursing home and reduce length of stay (Banerjee et al, 1996; Slaets et al, 1997).

Dementia is often found alongside physical frailty in hospitals and in residential and nursing homes, with the majority of residents of all kinds of care homes having dementia. Dementia is over-represented, for example, among people attending hospital after falls, and the consequences of falls are more severe for people with dementia, in that they stay longer in hospital and are less likely to return home afterwards (DH, 2002). In general, psychosocial treatments for the cognitive symptoms of dementia (such as problems with memory and language) are not effective other than on a temporary basis, and although an emerging evidence base suggests the potential of cholinesterase inhibitors to delay cognitive decline and enhance cognitive functioning for mild to moderate Alzheimer's dementia over six to 12 months with an allied delay in nursing home placements (Bartels et al, 2002), further trials are still required (Wild et al, 2003; Sink et al, 2005).

In contrast, empirical evidence supports the value of psychosocial interventions in addressing the behavioural symptoms of dementia (such as agitation and depression), particularly exercise, music and environmental modifications such as access to an outdoor area or surroundings that approximate home (see Box 13.11). There is less agreement on the effectiveness of antipsychotic, anticonvulsant or antidepressant treatments with only weak evidence as to the efficacy of a range of pharmacological agents currently used to treat the neuropsychiatric symptoms of dementia (Sink et al, 2005). The reviewers also

---

Box 13.11: Taking the community into the home

Moving people with dementia into residential care is unsettling and can cause further deterioration in their ability to cope. Hogewey, in Weesp near Amsterdam, caters for those with dementia who can no longer live in their own home by basing care on 'homes within homes'. These 'lifestyle groups' are based on seven different lifestyles reflecting prevailing socio-economic and cultural distinctions within the Netherlands. They include 'Amsterdamse', based on the type of life lived in crowded urban areas such as Amsterdam, and 'Indische', referring to people from the former colony of Indonesia as well as groups based on religion, wealth, home making, a working-class lifestyle and a cultural lifestyle based around the arts, classical music and history. Daily activities, food and custom vary between the different groups (Notter et al, 2004).

A second Dutch initiative aims to integrate mental healthcare for the chronically impaired into residential homes (broadly similar to sheltered homes in the UK in that residents live in publicly funded self-contained apartments with the housing function increasingly supplemented by social care). Alternative models range from the location of a psychiatric unit within the home, or the inclusion of psychiatric nurses (employed by the hospital and with direct access to resources), to the direct employment of psychiatric staff (Depla et al, 2003).

warn that attempts to generalise from the evidence base are constrained by the variability with which the interventions are specified, the variety of diagnoses included and the difficulty of rigorously assessing outcomes in this population. The use of antioxidant drugs has also not yet been the subject of adequate trials (Sauer et al, 2004).

A literature review of the use of therapeutic activities with people with Alzheimer's found findings were similarly confounded by the lack of emphasis on gender, ethnicity, racial and cultural differences, cognitive impairment, the use of convenience samples among captive populations and the lack of theories to guide the choice of activities such as lowering the stress threshold as a reason to support the use of music therapy (Marshall and Hutchinson, 2001).

Policy

Mental health was recognised in 1999 as one of government's top four priorities for the health service (DH, 1999a), and has been a recent focus for policy and resources. This has not always extended to older people. The NSF for Mental Health, one of the earliest NSFs, focused on the needs of working-age adults up to the age of 65, as did the subsequent report by the Social Exclusion Unit on mental health and social exclusion (SEU, 2004b). It has fallen to the NSF for Older People to address and resource the issue with respect to older people (DH, 1999c), with Standard Seven aiming to promote good mental health in older people and to treat and support those older people with dementia and depression. This requires that "older people who have mental health problems have access to integrated mental health services, provided by the NHS and councils to ensure effective diagnosis, treatment and support, for them and their carers" (DH, 2001a, p 13). Subsequent guidance recognises that the majority of older people do not come into contact with specialist mental health services and that local protocols to improve detection, assessment and treatment should thus cover primary care, general hospitals, care homes and social services.

A survey by the Audit Commission in 2001/02 (that is, before the NSF for Older People could be expected to have an impact) found shortfalls in the provision of services, their coordination and planning. Moreover, the three aspects tended to be correlated so that areas diverged considerably in the standard offered. In particular it was noted that many GPs did not attach sufficient weight to the early diagnosis of dementia, with protocols to aid diagnosis used only in the minority of cases of both depression and dementia. There were also shortfalls in specialist support and training for the latter, and fewer than half the areas had specialist mental health teams for older people fully available (despite the requirement for a single assessment process to be in place by April 2002) (Audit Commission, 2002b). There was also an identified requirement to shift the balance of care towards the community, reflecting again the wishes of older people, with often limited access to respite care, a shortage of culturally appropriate services, home care workers trained to support people with mental health problems and specialist homes for people with dementia. Hospital placements were therefore being used because of a lack of community services.

A more recent report suggests that despite both money and activity, there is still "a widespread sense of unease that improvements are not happening fast enough and not making a real difference to the lives of service users" (Rankin, 2004, p 5). Progress towards the involvement of carers, for example, is mixed, as is the involvement of service users with their own care, with representation of black and minority ethnic perspectives particularly poor (Phillipson and Scharf, 2004). A survey of carers in touch with Rethink found that while almost half believed that support for carers had improved, one in six said they had no local support in their area. It has also been suggested that conceptualisations of independence continue to place the emphasis on the physical safety and well-being of older people rather than on their emotional and psychological health (Henwood, 2002).

These issues do, however, continue to be addressed. The NSF requires PCTs to ensure that, by April 2004, every general practice is using a locally agreed protocol to diagnose, treat and care for patients with depression and dementia (Audit Commission, 2002b). The government has also argued that people with mental health problems, including cognitive impairment, should have access to Intermediate Care services, suggesting that they can benefit equally well, particularly perhaps from services provided at home (DH, 2002). The Health and Social Care Change Agent Team has also recently focused on integration, addressing ways in which mental health services for older people can be integrated with general hospital and community services (DH, 2004c). A first report on the implementation of the NSF for Older People is due at the end of 2005 (www.healthcarecommission.org.uk). However, preliminary findings suggest the focus on acute and primary care still remains too strong to allow sufficient resources to be directed to mental health, with continued staff shortages, a lack of Intermediate Care for older people with mental health needs and inconsistent use of protocols.

Conclusion

Table 13.1 summarises the evidence base as it relates to old age. It juxtaposes a few, often very specific, findings (relating to mental health, for example) with large areas where evidence remains scarce or non-existent. This reflects the paucity of research into effective interventions in old age. The focus on nutrition and physical activity evident in other stages of the lifecourse remains to a degree but, for example, there is a lack of review-level evidence relating to healthy eating in old age, the effectiveness of dietary advice, or interventions to reduce serious falls and injuries. Conversely, the focus on other health behaviours such as smoking, evident from childhood, disappears in old age, and areas where you would expect

Table 13.1: Interventions during old age: summary of the evidence base

	Source
DIET AND NUTRITION	
For older people at risk of malnutrition, oral dietary supplements produce a small but consistent weight gain and have a beneficial effect on mortality and (in the case of hospital patients) length of stay	Cochrane Review
Oral protein and energy feeds may similarly reduce death or complications for patients with hip fractures	Cochrane Review
Lack of review-level evidence	
Healthy eating interventions in general	
Dietary advice on illness-related malnutrition	
Folic acid supplementation on cognitive function and dementia	
PHYSICAL ACTIVITY	
Interventions that promote moderate and non-endurance physical activities can increase physical activity in the short term	Systematic review
Behavioural or cognitive approaches, home-based exercise and telephone support can increase adherence	Systematic review
Targeted exercise interventions are marginally effective in reducing the risk of falls	Cochrane Review
Multidisciplinary, multifactorial interventions, physical therapy, the modification of home hazards and the reduction of psychotropic medication are also likely to be beneficial	Cochrane Review
Such interventions are most effective when targeting known fallers BUT	Cochrane Review
A community-based approach to fall-related injuries also appears effective	Cochrane Review
Lack of review-level evidence	
Interventions to increase physical activity in the medium to long term	
Interventions to reduce serious falls and injuries	
SMOKING CESSATION	
Lack of review-level evidence	
Effective smoking cessation strategies for older people	
HOUSING	
Lack of review-level evidence	
The impact of housing adaptations and home repair schemes	
SOCIAL SUPPORT AND PERSONAL CARE	
Home visiting programmes can significantly reduce mortality, admissions to intensive care and admissions to long-term care among the elderly and frail elderly	Systematic review
Lack of review-level evidence	
Effective elements within home visiting packages	
The role played by low-level services (for example, housework and laundry) in maintaining independence	
The effectiveness of personal care and related supportive strategies such as respite care	
Initiatives to reduce social isolation	

(continued)

Table 13.1: Interventions during old age: summary of the evidence base (continued)

	Source
NEIGHBOURHOOD PERCEPTIONS AND MOBILITY	
Changes to the road environment (for example, to reduce vehicle speed, separate vehicles and pedestrians and afford protection when crossing roads) increase safety	Literature review
Improving the visibility of pedestrians and vehicles is also effective	Literature review
Lack of review-level evidence	
Interventions to increase social inclusion	
Community-based safety interventions	
INTERMEDIATE CARE	
Evidence for the effectiveness of individual components of intermediate care packages tend either to be equivocal or highly specific	Systematic review
Comprehensive geriatric assessment can reduce mortality with some models improving physical functioning and living location	Meta-analysis
Lack of review-level evidence	
A whole systems approach	
The effectiveness of individual components, the types of patients able to benefit most and appropriate modes of delivery	
Implications for quality of life and cost-effectiveness	
MENTAL HEALTH	
Antidepressants and psychosocial interventions focusing on CBT are effective against major depression	Review of reviews
Pharmacological and psychosocial interventions are likely to be more effective in combination	Review of reviews
The value of psychosocial interventions for the behavioural symptoms of dementia	Review of reviews
Evidence as to the effectiveness of pharmacological agents such as cholinesterase inhibitors remains modest and generalisability limited	Cochrane Review
Lack of review-level evidence	
Effective interventions for minor depression, suicide and anxiety	
The effectiveness of antioxidants in the treatment of dementia	
Psychosocial treatments for the cognitive symptoms of dementia	

to find a research focus specific to older people, such as housing, social support and a holistic approach to integrated care, are largely absent.

In contrast, this chapter has outlined a number of positive policy developments for older people. Key has been the NSF for Older People, with its explicit anti-ageist stance and the recognition accorded to independence and well-being. Other significant advances have included *The NHS Plan* and developments in the field of Intermediate Care, which have begun to address both the long-disputed health and social care boundary and the options available for people who require nursing or medical attention on other than a constant basis. Strategies such as *Quality and choice for older people's housing* have also acknowledged that older people define health in an holistic manner, and that a "radical change of perspective is needed if public services are to meet the challenges of our ageing society" (ADSS et al, 2004, p 1). This entails a broader approach that extends beyond health and social care services to involve issues such as transport, housing, education, leisure and advice (Audit Commission and BGOP, 2004). Increasing weight has also been attached to the engagement of older people themselves (ranging from BGOP to the extension of direct payments to older people needing care services) and to the shifting of patterns of expenditure away from crisis services and towards prevention.

The National Audit Office found that the government had also made progress towards better coordination, establishing a Cabinet Committee on Older People, appointing the Secretary of State for Work and Pensions as the government Champion for Older People, designating the DWP to take the lead on older people's issues and establishing the Pensions Service to provide a dedicated benefits service for pensioners (NAO, 2003). However, it also identified a requirement for further improvements in coordination, consultation and the use of evidence in formulating policy, including the need for an Older People's Strategy, to provide an overall framework for work across government. Others have similarly argued for a national framework for prevention, to include housing, health, social services and education, and urged that the promotion of well-being becomes a core function for all agencies, underlined by mainstream funding to promote successful ageing and a comprehensive performance assessment framework (Parkinson and Pierpoint, 2000; Wistow et al, 2003; ADSS et al, 2004; Joseph Rowntree Foundation Task Group, 2004).

In 2003 the Welsh Assembly introduced such a strategy, focusing on independence, citizenship and well-being (Welsh Assembly Government, 2003); Northern Ireland has a similar strategy at the consultation stage. The DWP subsequently introduced a national strategy for England in 2005, focusing on the establishment of a Commission for Equality and Human Rights to counter age discrimination and challenge attitudes to older workers, together with an Observatory on Ageing, with the aim of sharing knowledge. The tripartite objective, as noted in the introduction to this chapter, is to increase employment rates and career flexibility (including reform to incapacity benefits), to enable older people both to play a full and active role in society and to maintain independence and control (HM Government, 2005).

Concern has been expressed that financial constraints may continue to undermine aspirations. The devolution of commissioning to PCTs, for example, means that little money is ring-fenced for new priorities such as prevention, mental health or Intermediate Care, and waiting list pressures thus tend to cut across the whole systems approach to maintain the focus on acute services. The costs of long-term and domiciliary care also continue to be borne in large part by older people themselves and their families. The Royal Commission on Long-Term Care, for instance, argued forcibly that the need for long-term care was a risk and that this risk should be pooled across the population and underwritten by taxation based on need (RCLTC, 1999b). The government, however, rejected this recommendation (DH, 2000d), preferring to place the emphasis instead on Intermediate Care services and other preventive and rehabilitative services, such as community equipment. Factors such as pensions' policy, Pension Credit (essentially Income Support for pensioners) and the Attendance Allowance (which is non-contributory and non-means-tested) therefore become important but under-researched factors influencing access to preventative and long-term care as well as quality of life.

In conclusion, this chapter concurs strongly with Phillipson and Scharf's analysis (2004) for the Social Exclusion Unit. It finds that policy has begun to produce a cultural shift in the perception of older people and to tackle specific problems that cluster in old age, but has been less successful in addressing the focus of this book – health inequalities and the accompanying structural "inequalities which are carried through into old age and which reflect the experiences of particular birth cohorts and groups within these cohorts" (Phillipson and Scharf, 2004, p 8), most particularly poverty. Preventive services, despite the rhetoric, are also still underfunded and underdeveloped, with resources continuing to focus on the most vulnerable 15% rather than the wider older population (Joseph Rowntree Foundation Task Group, 2004).

References

Acheson, D. (1998) *Independent Inquiry into Inequalities in Health*, London: The Stationery Office.

Adams, S. (2001) *On the mend: Hospital discharge services and the role of home improvement agencies*, Nottingham: Care & Repair England.

ADSS (Association of Directors of Social Services), LGA (Local Government Association), Audit Commission, BGOP (Better Government for Older People), Nuffield Institute for Health and Joseph Rowntree Foundation (2004) 'Public services for tomorrow's older citizens: changing attitudes to ageing' (www.nuffield.leeds.ac.uk), accessed 1 June 2005.

Age Concern (2005) *The age agenda 2005: Public policy and older people*, London: Age Concern England.

Appleton, N. (1996) *Handyperson schemes: Making them work*, York: York Publishing Sevices for the Joseph Rowntree Foundation.

Asthana, S. and Halliday, J. (2003) 'Intermediate Care: its place in a whole-systems approach', *Journal of Integrated Care*, vol 11, no 6, pp 15-23.

Atkins, W. (2001) *Older people: Their transport needs and requirements – Summary report*, London: DETR.

Audit Commission (1997) *The coming of age: Improving care services for older people*, London: Audit Commission.

Audit Commission (2000) *Fully equipped*, London: Audit Commission.

Audit Commission (2002a) *Integrated services for older people: Building a whole system approach in England*, London: Audit Commission.

Audit Commission (2002b) *Forget me not 2002: Developing mental health services for older people in England*, London: Audit Commission.

Audit Commission and BGOP (Better Government for Older People) (2004) *Older people – Independence and well-being: The challenge for public services*, London: Audit Commission.

Avenell, A. and Handoll, H. (2004) 'Nutritional supplementation for hip fracture aftercare in the elderly', *The Cochrane Database of Systematic Reviews 2004, issue 1*, Art. No. CD001880.

Baldock, J. (1997) 'Social care in old age: more than a funding problem', *Social Policy and Administration*, vol 31, no 1, pp 73-89.

Baldwin, C., Parsons, T. and Logan, S. (2001) 'Dietary advice for illness-related malnutrition in adults', *The Cochrane Database of Systematic Reviews 2001, issue 2*, Art. No. CD002008.

Banerjee, S., Shamash, K., Macdonald, A.J.D. and Mann, A.H. (1996) 'Randomized controlled trial of effect of intervention by psychogeriatric team on depression in frail elderly people at home', *British Medical Journal*, vol 313, no 7064, pp 1058-61.

Bartels, S.J., Dums, A.R., Oxman, T.E., Schneider, L.S., Areen, P.A., Alexopoulos, G.S. and Jeste, D.V. (2002) 'Evidence-based practices in geriatric mental health care', *Psychiatric Services*, vol 53, no 11, pp 1419-31.

Bauld, L., Coleman, T., Adams, C., Pound, E. and Ferguson, J. (2005) 'Delivering the English smoking treatment services', *Addiction*, vol 100, suppl 2, pp 19-27.

Bernabei, R., Landi, F., Gambassi, G., Sgadari, J., Zuccala, G., Mor, V., Rubenstein, L.Z. and Carbonin, P. (1998) 'Randomised trial of impact of model of integrated care and case management for older people living in the community', *British Medical Journal*, vol 316, no 7141, pp 1348-51.

Biderman, A., Cwikel, J., Fried, A. and Galinsky, D. (2002) 'Depression and falls among community dwelling elderly people: a search for common risk factors', *Journal of Epidemiology and Community Health*, vol 56, no 8, pp 631-6.

Bjerre, B. and Schelp, L. (2000) 'The community safety approach in Falun, Sweden – is it possible to characterise the most effective prevention endeavours and how longlasting are the results?', *Accident Analysis and Prevention*, vol 32, no 3, pp 461-70.

Bours, G., Ketelaars, C., Frederiks, C., Abu-Saad, H. and Wouters, E. (1998) 'The effects of aftercare on chronic patients and frail elderly patients when discharged from hospital: a systematic review', *Journal of Advanced Nursing*, vol 27, no 5, pp 1076-86.

Bowling, A. and Ebrahim, S. (2001) 'Glossaries in public health: older people', *Journal of Epidemiology and Community Health*, vol 55, no 4, pp 223-6.

Breeze, E., Jones, D., Wilkinson, P., Latif, A., Bulpitt, C. and Fletcher, A. (2004) 'Association of quality of life in old age in Britain with socioeconomic position: baseline data from a randomised controlled trial', *Journal of Epidemiology and Community Health*, vol 58, no 8, pp 667-73.

Burns, A., Dening, T. and Baldwin, R. (2001) 'Care of older people: mental health problems', *British Medical Journal*, vol 322, no 7289, pp 789-91.

Campbell, A., Robertson, M., Gardner, M., Norton, R. and Buchner, D. (1999) 'Falls prevention over two years: a randomised controlled trial in women 80 years and older', *Age and Ageing*, vol 28, no 6, pp 513-18.

Campbell, A., Robertson, M., Gardner, M., Norton, R., Tilyard, M. and Buchner, D. (1997) 'Randomised controlled trial of a general practice programme of home based exercise to prevent falls in elderly women', *British Medical Journal*, vol 315, no 7115, pp 1065-9.

Chang, D., Spicer, N., Irving, A., Sparham, I. and Neeve, L. (2001) *Modernising service delivery: The Better Government for Older People prototypes*, DSS Research Report 136, Leeds: Corporate Document Services.

Chivite-Matthews, N. and Maggs, P. (2002) *Crime, policing and justice: The experience of older people: Findings from the British Crime Survey, England and Wales*, London: Home Office.

Clark, H., Dyer, S. and Horwood, J. (1998) *'That bit of help': The high value of low level preventative services for older people*, Bristol/York: The Policy Press in association with *Community Care* and the Joseph Rowntree Foundation.

Cooper, H., Arber, S., Fee, L. and Ginn, J. (1999) *The influence of social support and social capital on health: A review and analysis of British data*, London: Health Education Authority.

Cotterill, L., Hayes, L., Flynn, M. and Sloper, P. (1997) 'Reviewing respite services: some lessons from the literature', *Disability and Society*, vol 12, no 5, pp 775-8.

Day, L., Fildes, B., Gordon, I., Fitzharris, M., Flamer, H. and Lord, S. (2002) 'Randomised factorial trial of falls prevention among older people living in their own homes', *British Medical Journal*, vol 325, no 7356, pp 128-31.

Deeming, C. and Keen, J. (2002) 'Paying for old age: can people on lower incomes afford domiciliary care costs?', *Social Policy and Administration*, vol 36, no 5, pp 465-81.

DEFRA (Department for Environment, Food and Rural Affairs) (2004) *Fuel poverty in England: The government's plan for action*, London: DEFRA.

Depla, M., Pols, J., de Lange, J., Smits, C., de Graaf, R. and Heeren, T. (2003) 'Integrating mental health care into residential homes for the elderly: an analysis of six Dutch programs for older people with severe and persistent mental illness', *Journal of the American Geriatrics Society*, vol 51, pp 1275-9.

DETR (Department of the Environment, Transport and the Regions) (1998) *A new deal for transport: Better for everyone*, London: The Stationery Office.

DETR (2001) *Transport 2010: Meeting the local transport challenge*, London: DETR.

DETR/DH (Department of Health) (2001) *Quality and choice: A strategic framework for older people's housing*, London: DETR/DH.

DH (Department of Health) (1992) *The health of the nation: A strategy for health in England and Wales*, London: HMSO.

DH (1997) *Better services for vulnerable people*, London: The Stationery Office.

DH (1998) *Smoking kills*, London: The Stationery Office.

DH (1999a) *Saving lives: Our healthier nation*, London: The Stationery Office.

DH (1999b) *The national strategy for carers*, London: DH.

DH (1999c) *National Service Framework for Mental Health*, London: DH.

DH (2000a) *The NHS Plan*, London: The Stationery Office.

DH (2000b) *The NHS Cancer Plan*, London: DH.

DH (2000c) *National Service Framework for Coronary Heart Disease*, London: DH.

DH (2000d) *The NHS plan: The government's response to the Royal Commission on Long Term Care*, London: The Stationery Office.

DH (2001a) *National Service Framework for Older People*, London: DH.

DH (2001b) *National Service Framework for Diabetes*, London: DH.

DH (2001c) *Intermediate Care: Health service circular 2001/01, local authority circular (2001)1*, London: DH.

DH (2002) *National Service Framework for Older People – Supporting implementation Intermediate Care: Moving forward*, London: DH.

DH (2004a) *At least five a week: Evidence on the impact of physical activity and its relationship to health*, London: DH.

DH (2004b) *Local delivery plans 2005/08 – Technical note*, London: DH.

DH (2004c) *Changing times: Improving services for older people: Report on the work of the Health and Social Care Change Agent Team 2003/04*, London: DH.

DH (2005a) *Choosing a better diet: A food health action plan*, London: DH.

DH (2005b) *Independence, wellbeing and choice*, London: DH.

Dunbar, G., Holland, C.A. and Maylor, E.A. (2004) *Older pedestrians: A critical review of the literature*, Road safety research report no 37, London: DfT.

DWP (Department for Work and Pensions) (2004) *Link-Age: Developing networks of services for older people*, London: DWP.

Easterbrook, L. (2002) *Healthy homes, healthier lives: Health improvement through housing related initiatives and services*, Nottingham: Care & Repair England.

Egger, M. (2001) 'Commentary: when, where, and why do preventive home visits work?', *British Medical Journal*, vol 323, no 7303, pp 8-9.

Elkan, R., Kendrick, D., Dewey, M., Hewitt, M., Robinson, J., Blair, M., Williams, D. and Brummell, K. (2001) 'Effectiveness of home based support for older people: systematic review and meta analysis', *British Medical Journal*, vol 323, no 7303, pp 1-8.

Evandrou, M. (2000) 'Social inequalities in later life: the socio economic position of older people from ethnic minority groups in Britain', *Population Trends*, vol 101, autumn, pp 11-17.

Fjærtoft, H., Indredavik, B. and Lydersen, S. (2003) 'Stroke unit care combined with early supported discharge: long-term follow-up of a randomized controlled trial', *Stroke*, vol 34, no 11, pp 2687-92.

Fleming, S., Blake, H., Gladman, J., Hart, E., Lymbery, M., Dewey, M., McCloughry, H., Walker, M. and Miller, P. (2004) 'A randomised controlled trial of a care home rehabilitation service to reduce long-term institutionalisation for elderly people', *Age and Ageing*, vol 33, no 4, pp 384-90.

Fletcher, A. and Rake, C. (1998) *Effectiveness of interventions to promote healthy eating in elderly people living in the community: A review*, London: Health Education Authority.

Forster, A., Young, J. and Langhorne, P. (1999) 'Systematic review of day hospital care for elderly people', *British Medical Journal*, vol 318, no 7187, pp 837-41.

Gardner, M.M., Robertson, M.G. and Campbell, A.J. (2000) 'Exercise in preventing falls and fall related injuries in older people: a review of randomised controlled trials', *British Journal of Sports Medicine*, vol 34, no 1, pp 7-17.

Gillespie, L., Gillespie, W., Robertson, M., Lamb, S., Cumming, R. and Rowe, B. (2003) 'Interventions for preventing falls in elderly people', *The Cochrane Database of Systematic Reviews 2003, issue 4*, Art. No. Cd000340.

Godfrey, M. (1999) *Preventive strategies for older people: Mapping the literature on effectiveness and outcomes*, Kidlington: Anchor Trust.

Grimley Evans, J. and Tallis, R. (2001) 'A new beginning for care for elderly people?', *British Medical Journal*, vol 322, no 7290, pp 807-8.

Haydon, C. and Boaz, A. (2000) *Making a difference: Better Government for Older People evaluation report*, Warwick: Local Government Centre, University of Warwick.

Henwood, M. (2002) 'Age discrimination in social care', in Help the Aged (ed) *Age discrimination in public policy: A review of evidence*, London: Help the Aged, pp 72-88.

Henwood, M. (2004) *Reimbursement and delayed discharges: Discussion paper for the Integrated Care Network*, Leeds: Integrated Care Network.

Herbert, G. and Lake, G. (2004) *Developing the intermediate tier: Sharing the learning*, Leeds: Nuffield Institute for Health.

Herbert, G., Townsend, J., Ryan, J., Wright, D., Ferguson, B. and Wistow, G. (2000) *Rehabilitation pathways for older people after fractured neck of femur*, Leeds: Nuffield Institute for Health and York Economics Consortium.

Heywood, F. (2001) *Money well spent: The effectiveness and value of housing adaptations*, Bristol/York: The Policy Press/Joseph Rowntree Foundation.

HM Government (2005) *Opportunity age: Meeting the challenges of ageing in the 21st century*, London: DWP.

HM Government and DH (Department of Health) (2004) *Choosing health: Making healthy choices easier*, London: HM Government and DH.

Howard, M. (2002) 'Age discrimination in social security', in Help the Aged (ed) *Age discrimination in public policy: A review of evidence*, London: Help the Aged, pp 90-109.

Hyde, C., Robert, I. and Sinclair, A. (2000) 'The effects of supporting discharge from hospital to home in older people', *Age and Ageing*, vol 29, no 4, pp 271-9.

Jewson, N., Jeffers, S. and Kalra, V. (2003) *Family care, respite services and Asian communities in Leicester*, Leicester: Ethnicity Research Centre, University of Leicester.

Joseph Rowntree Foundation (2000) *Findings: Planning for older people at the health/housing interface*, York: Joseph Rowntree Foundation.

Joseph Rowntree Foundation (2001) *Piloting choice and control for older people: An evaluation*, York: Joseph Rowntree Foundation.

Joseph Rowntree Foundation (2004) *Findings: 'It pays dividends': Direct payments and older people*, York: Joseph Rowntree Foundation.

Joseph Rowntree Foundation Task Group (2004) *From welfare to well-being: Planning for an ageing society: Summary conclusions of the Joseph Rowntree Foundation Task Group on housing, money and care for older people*, York: Joseph Rowntree Foundation.

Katbamna, S., Bhakta, P., Parker, G., Ahmad, W., Baker, R. and Lilly, E. (1998) *Experiences and needs of carers from the south Asian communities*, Leicester: Nuffield Community Care Studies Unit, University of Leicester.

Kelly, M. (2004) *The evidence of effectiveness of public health interventions – and the implications*, London: Health Development Agency.

Kempson, E., Collard, S. and Taylor, S. (2002) *Social fund use amongst older people*, DWP Research Report 172, Leeds: Corporate Document Services.

Kempton, A., van Beurden, E., Sladden, T., Garner, E. and Beard, J. (2000) 'Older people can stay on their feet: final results of a community–based falls prevention programme', *Health Promotion International*, vol 15, pp 27-33.

Kerse, N., Flicker, L., Jolley, D., Arroll, B. and Young, D. (1999) 'Improving the health behaviours of elderly people: randomised controlled trial of a general practice education programme', *British Medical Journal*, vol 319, pp 683-7.

King, A., Rejeski, W. and Buchner, D. (1998) 'Physical activity interventions targeting older adults: a critical review and recommendations', *American Journal of Preventive Medicine*, vol 15, no 4, pp 316-33.

King's Fund (2005) 'Wanless Social Care Review' (www.kingsfund.org.uk/healthpolicy/wanless.html), accessed 31 March 2005.

Langer, G., Schloemer, G., Knerr, A., Kuss, O. and Behrens, J. (2003) 'Nutritional interventions for preventing and treating pressure ulcers', *The Cochrane Database of Systematic Reviews 2003*, issue 4, Art. No. CD003216.

Lansley, P., McCreadie, C. and Tinker, A. (2004) 'Can adapting the homes of older people and providing assistive technology pay its way?', *Age and Ageing*, vol 33, no 6, pp 571-6.

Lewis, H., Fletcher, P., Hardy, B., Milne, A. and Waddington, E. (1999) *Promoting well-being: Developing a preventive approach with older people*, Kidlington: Anchor Trust.

Lewis, J. (1999) 'The concepts of community care and primary care in the UK: the 1960s to the 1990s', *Health and Social Care in the Community*, vol 7, no 5, pp 333-41.

Lewis, J. (2001) 'Older people and the health–social care boundary in the UK: half a century of hidden policy conflict', *Social Policy and Administration*, vol 35, no 4, pp 343-59.

Lindqvist, K., Timpka, T. and Schelp, L. (2001) 'Evaluation of a traffic injury prevention program in a WHO Safe community', *Accident Analysis and Prevention*, vol 33, no 5, pp 599-607.

Livingston, G., Leavey, G., Kitchen, M., Manela, M., Sembhi, S. and Katona, C. (2002) 'Accessibility of health and social services to immigrant elders: the Islington study', *British Journal of Psychiatry*, vol 180, no 4, pp 369-73.

Lyons, R., Sander, L., Weightman, A., Patterson, J., Jones, S., Lannon, S., Rolfe, B., Kemp, A. and Johansen, A. (2004) 'Modification of the home environment for the reduction of injuries (Cochrane Review)', *The Cochrane Library*, Chichester: John Wiley & Sons Ltd.

McClure, R., Turner, C., Peel, N., Spinks, A., Eakin, E. and Hughes, K. (2005) 'Population-based interventions for the prevention of fall-related injuries in older people (review)', *The Cochrane Database of Systematic Reviews 2005, issue 1*, Art. No. CD004441.

McKie, L. (1999) 'Older people and food: independence, locality and diet', *British Food Journal*, vol 101, no 7, pp 528-36.

McKie, L., MacInnes, A., Hendry, J., Donald, S. and Peace, H. (2000) 'The food consumption patterns and perceptions of dietary advice of older people', *Journal of Human Nutrition and Dietetics*, vol 13, pp 173-83.

Maguire, C., Ryan, J. and Kelly, A. (2000) 'Do patient age and medical condition influence medical advice to stop smoking', *Age and Ageing*, vol 29, no 3, pp 264-6.

Malouf, R., Grimley Evans, J. and Areosa Sastre, A. (2003) 'Folic acid with or without vitamin b12 for cognition and dementia', *The Cochrane Database of Systematic Reviews 2003, issue 4*, Art. No. CD004514.

Marshall, M. and Hutchinson, S. (2001) 'A critique of research on the use of activities with persons with Alzheimer's disease: a systematic literature review', *Journal of Advanced Nursing*, vol 35, no 4, pp 488-96.

Martin, G., Peet, S., Hewitt, G. and Parker, H. (2004) 'Diversity in intermediate care', *Health and Social Care in the Community*, vol 12, no 2, pp 150-4.

Martin, S. and Boaz, A. (2000) 'Public participation and citizen-centred local government: lessons from the Best Value and Better Government for Older People pilot programmes', *Public Money and Management*, April-June, pp 47-53.

Mawby, R. (1999) 'Providing a secure home for older residents: evaluation of an initiative in Plymouth', *The Howard Journal*, vol 38, no 3, pp 313-27.

Millar, B. (1996) 'Staying power', *Health Service Journal*, vol 11, January, pp 14-15.

Milne, A., Potter, J. and Avenell, A. (2002) 'Protein and energy supplementation in elderly people at risk from malnutrition', *The Cochrane Database of Systematic Reviews 2002, issue 2*, Art. No. CD003288.

Mitchell, C.G.B. (2000) 'Some implications of road safety for an ageing population', in *Transport trends 2000*, London: DETR, pp 26-34.

Mountain, G. and Buri, H. (2005) *Report of the evaluation of pilot local housing options advice services for older people*, Sheffield: Sheffield Hallam University for Care & Repair England.

Munro, J., Nicholl, J., Brazier, J., Davey, R. and Cochrane, T. (2004) 'Cost effectiveness of a community based exercise programme in over 65 year olds: cluster randomised trial', *Journal of Epidemiology and Community Health*, vol 58, pp 1004-10.

NAO (National Audit Office) (2002) *Tackling pensioner poverty: Encouraging take-up of entitlements: Report by the Comptroller and Auditor General*, London: The Stationery Office.

NAO (2003) *Developing effective services for older people: Report by the Comptroller and Auditor General*, London: The Stationery Office.

NICE (National Institute for Clinical Excellence) (2004) *Falls: The assessment and prevention of falls in older people*, Clinical Guideline 21, London: NICE.

Noble, B. (2000) 'Travel characteristics of older people', *Transport trends 2000*, London: DETR, pp 9-25.

Nocon, A. and Baldwin, S. (1998) *Trends in rehabilitation policy: A review of the literature*, London: King's Fund and Audit Commission.

Notter, J., Spijker, T. and Stomp, K. (2004) 'Taking the community into the home', *Health and Social Care in the Community*, vol 12, no 5, pp 448-53.

Observer, The (2005) 'Free enterprise', 23 January.

ODPM (Office of the Deputy Prime Minister) (2003) *Preparing older people's strategies: Linking housing to health, social care and other local strategies*, London: ODPM.

Oliver, D. and Masud, T. (2004) 'Preventing falls and injuries in care homes', *Age and Ageing*, vol 33, no 6, pp 532-5.

Pain, R. (2000) 'Place, social relations and the fear of crime: a review', *Progress in Human Geography*, vol 24, pp 365-87.

Parker, G., Bhatka, P., Katbamna, S., Lovett, C., Paisley, S., Parker, S., Phelps, K., Baker, R., Jagger, C., Lindesay, J., Shepperdson, B. and Wilson, A. (2000) 'Best place of care for older people after acute and during sub-acute illness: a systematic review', *Journal of Health Services Research*, vol 5, no 3, pp 176-89.

Parkinson, P. and Pierpoint, D. (2000) *Preventive approaches in housing: An exploration of good practice*, Kidlington: Anchor Trust.

Patel, N. (1999) 'Black and minority ethnic elderly: perspectives on long-term care', in Royal Commission on Long-Term Care (ed) *With respect to old age: Long term care – Rights and responsibilities. The context of long-term care policy. Research volume 1*, London: The Stationery Office, pp 257-304.

Phillipson, C. and Scharf, T. (2004) *The impact of government policy on social exclusion among older people: A review of the literature for the Social Exclusion Unit in the breaking the cycle series*, London: ODPM.

Philp, I. (2004) *Better health in old age*, London: DH.

Pollack, C. and von dem Knesebeck, O. (2004) 'Social capital and health among the aged: comparisons between the United States and Germany', *Health and Place*, vol 10, no 4, pp 383-91.

Powell, J., Wilkins, D., Leiper, J. and Gillam, C. (2000) 'Stay on your feet safety walks group', *Accident Analysis and Prevention*, vol 32, no 3, pp 389-90.

Ram, F., Wedzicha, J., Wright, J. and Greenstone, M. (2004) 'Hospital at home for patients with acute exacerbations of chronic obstructive pulmonary disease: systematic review of evidence', *British Medical Journal*, vol 329, no 7461, pp 315-18.

Rankin, J. (2004) *Mental health in the mainstream: Developments and trends in mental health policy*, London: IPPR.

Raw, M., McNeil, A., Watt, J. and Raw, D. (2001) 'National smoking cessation services at risk', *British Medical Journal*, vol 323, no 7322, pp 1140-1.

RCLTC (Royal Commission on Long-Term Care) (1999a) *With respect to old age: Long term care – Rights and responsibilities. Alternative models of care. Research volume 2*, London: The Stationery Office.

RCLTC (1999b) *With respect to old age: Long term care – Rights and responsibilities*, London: The Stationery Office.

Reijneveld, S., Westhoff, M. and Hopman-Rock, M. (2003) 'Promotion of health and physical activity improves the mental health of elderly immigrants: results of a group randomised controlled trial among Turkish immigrants in the Netherlands aged 45 and over', *Journal of Epidemiology and Community Health*, vol 57, no 6, pp 405-11.

Richards, S. and Coast, J. (2003) 'Interventions to improve access to health and social care after discharge from hospital: a systematic review', *Journal of Health Services Research and Policy*, vol 8, no 3, pp 171-9.

Riseborough, M. and Jenkins, C. (2004) *Now you see me … now you don't: How are older citizens being included in regeneration?*, London: Age Concern England.

Roberts, E. (2002) 'Age discrimination in health', in Help the Aged (ed) *Age discrimination in public policy: A review of evidence*, London: Help the Aged, pp 48-70.

Robertson, M.C., Gardner, M.M., Devlin, N., McGee, R. and Campbell, A.J. (2001) 'Effectiveness and economic evaluation of a nurse delivered home exercise programme to prevent falls. 2: Controlled trial in multiple centres', *British Medical Journal*, vol 322, no 7288, pp 701-4.

Roderick, P., Low, J., Day, R., Peasgood, T., Mullee, M., Turnbull, J., Villar, T. and Raftery, J. (2001) 'Stroke rehabilitation after hospital discharge: a randomized trial comparing domiciliary and day-hospital care', *Age and Ageing*, vol 30, no 4, pp 303-10.

Roe, B., Daly, S., Shenton, G. and Lochhead, Y. (2003) 'Development and evaluation of Intermediate Care', *Journal of Clinical Nursing*, vol 12, no 3, pp 341-50.

Rowland, D. and Pollock, A. (2004) 'Choice and responsiveness for older people in the "patient-centred" NHS', *British Medical Journal*, vol 328, no 7430, pp 4-5.

Satre, D., Mertens, J., Areán, P. and Weisner, C. (2004) 'Five-year alcohol and drug treatment outcomes of older adults versus middle-aged and younger adults in a managed care program', *Addiction*, vol 99, pp 1286-97.

Sauer, J., Tabet, N. and Howard, R. (2004) 'Alpha lipoic acid for dementia', *The Cochrane Database of Systematic Reviews 2004, issue 1*, Art. No. CD004244.

Scharf, T., Phillipson, C., Smith, A. and Kingston, P. (2002) *Growing older in socially deprived areas: Summary report*, London: Help the Aged.

Secretary of State for Health (1998) *Modernising social services: Promoting independence, improving protection, raising* standards, Cm 4169, London: The Stationery Office.

SEU (Social Exclusion Unit) (2004a) *Breaking the cycle: Taking stock of progress and priorities for the future*, London: ODPM.

SEU (2004b) *Mental health and social exclusion*, London: ODPM.

SEU (2005) *Excluded older people: Social Exclusion Unit interim report*, London: ODPM.

Seymour, P. (1997) *Evaluation of very sheltered housing: Lewisham social services: Strategy for services for elderly people. 1996-2001*, Lewisham: Lewisham Social Services.

Shaw, F., Bond, J., Richardson, D., Dawson, P., Steen, I., McKeith, I. and Kenny, R. (2003) 'Multifactorial intervention after a fall in older people with cognitive impairment and dementia presenting to the accident and emergency department: randomised controlled trial', *British Medical Journal*, vol 326, no 7380, p 73.

Shepperd, S. and Iliffe, S. (2001) 'Hospital at home versus in-patient hospital care (Cochrane Review)', *The Cochrane Library, issue 4, 2004*, Chichester: John Wiley & Sons Ltd.

Shepperd, S., Harwood, D., Gray, A., Vessey, M. and Morgan, P. (1998) 'Randomised controlled trial comparing hospital at home care with inpatient hospital care. Ii: Cost minimisation analysis', *British Medical Journal*, vol 316, no 7147, pp 1791-6.

Sink, K., Holden, K. and Yaffe, K. (2005) 'Pharmacological treatment of neuropsychiatric symptoms of dementia: a review of the evidence', *Journal of the American Medical Association*, vol 293, no 5, pp 596-608.

Sippings, M. (2000) *Benefits Agency Better Government for Older People evaluation report*, London: Benefits Agency.

Slaets, J., Kauffmann, R., Cuivenvoorden, H., Pelemans, W. and Shudel, W. (1997) 'A randomised trial of geriatric liaison intervention in elderly medical inpatients', *Psychosomatic Medicine*, vol 59, pp 585-91.

Smith, B., Appleton, S., Adams, R., Southcott, A. and Ruffin, R. (2001) 'Home care by outreach nursing for chronic obstructive pulmonary disease', *The Cochrane Database of Systematic Reviews 2001, issue 3*, Art. No. CD000994.

Speer, D. and Schneider, M. (2003) 'Mental health needs of older adults and primary care: opportunity for interdisciplinary geriatric team practice', *Clinical Psychology: Science and Practice*, vol 10, no 1, pp 85-101.

Steiner, A. (2001) 'Intermediate Care – a good thing?', *Age and Ageing*, vol 30, suppl 3, pp 33-9.

Steiner, A., Walsh, B., Pickering, R., Wiles, W., Ward, J. and Brooking, J. (2001) 'Therapeutic nursing or unblocked beds? A randomised control trial of a post-acute intermediate care unit', *British Medical Journal*, vol 322, no 7284, pp 453-60.

Steultjens, E.M.J., Dekker, J., Bouter, L.M., Jellema, S., Bakker, E.B. and van den Ende, C.H.M. (2004) 'Occupational therapy for community dwelling elderly people: a systematic review', *Age and Ageing*, vol 33, no 5, pp 453-60.

Stiggelbout, M., Popkema, D., Hopman-Rock, M., de Greef, M. and van Mechelen, W. (2004) 'Once a week is not enough: effects of a widely implemented group based exercise programme for older adults: a randomised controlled trial', *Journal of Epidemiology and Community Health*, vol 58, no 2, pp 83-8.

Stroke Unit Trialists' Collaboration (1997) 'Collaborative systematic review of the randomised trials of organised inpatient (stroke unit) care after stroke', *British Medical Journal*, vol 314, no 7088, p 1151.

Stuck, A.E., Siu, A.L., Wieland, G.D., Adams, J. and Rubenstein, L.Z. (1993) 'Comprehensive geriatric assessment: a meta-analysis of controlled trials', *The Lancet*, vol 342, no 8878, pp 1032-6.

Stuck, A.E., Walthert, J., Nikolaus, T., Bula, C., Hohmann, C. and Beck, J. (1999) 'Risk factors for functional status decline in community living elderly people: a systematic review', *Social Science and Medicine*, vol 48, no 4, pp 445-69.

Thomson, H., Petticrew, M. and Morrison, D. (2001) 'Health effects of housing improvement: systematic review of intervention studies', *British Medical Journal*, vol 323, no 7306, pp 187-90.

Tinker, A. (1999) 'Helping older people to stay at home: the role of supported accommodation', in Royal Commission on Long-Term Care (ed) *With respect to old age: Long term care – Rights and responsibilities. Alternative models of care for older people. Research volume 2*, London: The Stationery Office, pp 265-98.

Tinker, A., Wright, F., McCreadie, C., Askham, J., Hancock, R. and Holmans, A. (1999) *With respect to old age: Long term care – Rights and responsibilities. Alternative models of care for older people. Research volume 2*, London: The Stationery Office.

Trickey, H., Turton, P., Harvey, I., Wilcock, G. and Sharp, D. (2000) 'Dementia and the over-75 check: the role of the primary care nurse', *Health and Social Care in the Community*, vol 8, no 1, pp 9-16.

van Haastregt, J.C.M., Diederiks, J.P.M., van Rossum, E., de Witte, L.P., Voorhoeve, P.M. and Crebolder, H. (2000) 'Effects of a programme of multifactorial home visits on falls and mobility impairments in elderly people at risk: randomised controlled trial', *British Medical Journal*, vol 321, no 7267, pp 994-8.

Vaughan, B. and Lathlean, J. (1999) *Intermediate Care: Models in practice*, London: King's Fund.

Welsh Assembly Government (2003) *The strategy for older people in Wales*, Cardiff: Welsh Office.

Wild, R., Pettit, T. and Burns, A. (2003) 'Cholinesterase inhibitors for dementia with Lewy bodies', *The Cochrane Database of Systematic Reviews 2003, issue 3*, Art. No. CD003672.

Wilkinson, P., Landon, M., Armstrong, B., Stevenson, S., Pattenden, S., Fletcher, T. and McKee, M. (2001) *Cold comfort: The social and environmental determinants of excess winter deaths in England, 1986-1996*, Bristol: The Policy Press.

Wilson, A., Parker, H., Wynn, A. and Spiers, N. (2003) 'Performance of hospital-at-home after a randomised controlled trial', *Journal of Health Services Research*, vol 8, no 3, pp 160-4.

Wistow, G., Waddington, E. and Chiu, L. (2002) *Intermediate Care: Balancing the system: Final report*, Leeds: Nuffield Institute for Health, University of Leeds.

Wistow, G., Waddington, E. and Godfrey, M. (2003) *Living well in later life: From prevention to promotion*, Leeds: Nuffield Institute for Health.

Part 3:
Tackling health inequalities: developing an evidence base for public health

It is important that policies designed to address health inequalities are based on reliable evidence. Throughout the course of this book we have examined evidence on the effectiveness of intervention activities targeting a wide range of pathways and processes that give rise to health inequalities across different stages of the lifecourse. To this end, we have drawn on a variety of evidence, supplementing review-level findings with other published literature and grey literature. According to the formal evidence base, remarkably little actually 'works'. By contrast, the 'view from the ground' suggests that local interventions can make a difference to health inequalities. This produces quite a dilemma for local policy makers and practitioners who are encouraged to draw on the highest-quality evidence in formulating local policies and projects. Experience and local knowledge may tell them one thing, but the formal evidence base another. There is growing concern among public health researchers and policy makers that this says more about the methods used in the field of evidence-based public health than the potential effectiveness of public health interventions themselves.

Chapter Fourteen begins by exploring the growing critique of the narrow, hierarchical approach to evidence in public health which continues to be dominated by the systematic review. It finds a number of limitations of this approach, including the questionable relevance of results yielded in controlled, scientific and well-resourced conditions to routine service delivery; the lack of evidence that has been forthcoming about the cost-effectiveness of public health and preventative policies; the lack of information about process, affecting ability to distinguish between evaluation failure and programme failure and between the contributions of different programme elements; and the lack of evaluation focusing on what works for particular socio-economic or vulnerable groups. There has, moreover, been a bias towards interventions with a medical rather than a social focus, and those that target individuals rather than communities or populations; an overwhelming focus on publication in English, mitigating against international comparison; and a failure to control adequately for context, undermining the extent to which the current evidence base offers lessons that are either practically applicable or transferable.

Such concerns have given rise to a search for alternative strategies. These emphasise the need for methodological pluralism, including more descriptive and/or qualitative information, an explicit acknowledgement of the importance of context, and a move away from linear thinking about cause and effect to non-linear models that seek to understand the association and interaction between different factors. Most leading health inequalities researchers also emphasise a need to shift from the current focus on downstream policies or discrete interventions to upstream policies that target the wider determinants of health such as income distribution, employment, education, access to key services and laws and regulations pertaining to health-damaging exposures. The current approach to gathering evidence is ill equipped to assess the effects of different policy and organisational arrangements in these broad domains.

Insofar as they provide scope for the analysis of different legislative, social, political and economic structures, we suggest that natural policy experiments that draw on evidence from other countries offer a potentially promising approach to the gathering of evidence on upstream policies. However, the focus of international work to date has tended towards country-specific descriptive case studies or de-contextualised systematic reviews, neither of which yield firm conclusions about key factors that might influence observed differences in policy approaches or outcomes. To improve the utility of natural policy experiments, we propose that research on international public health policies and interventions should at the very least involve a systematic assessment of the structures and institutional arrangements that both give rise to health variations and shape the formation, implementation and effectiveness of policies and interventions designed to reduce health inequalities. It is against this background that Chapter Fourteen sets out a new research agenda for evidence-based public health, one that, drawing on methods developed within comparative social policy, involves the analysis of *public health regimes*. For single country studies, this approach lends itself to comprehensive analysis of interventions at *all* levels of the policy framework. More ambitiously, international comparative analysis of public health regimes lends itself to the identification of policies and interventions that are effective in different contexts and therefore potentially generalisable and those that are conditionally successful, depending on contingent contextual factors.

Examining significant dimensions of the public health regime in the UK (with a particular focus on England) and comparing these to key domains and indicators relating to the reduction of nutritional inequalities in Finland, we question whether the UK government's strategy for reducing health inequalities is as far-reaching as policy rhetoric would have us believe. The 2004 Public Health White Paper *Choosing health* (HM Government and DH, 2004) suggests that the core elements of the government's health inequalities strategy remain highly behavioural and individualistic in orientation, raising important questions as to whether this government's approach to the lifestyle factors that contribute to health inequalities departs from that of its Conservative predecessor. Care should also be taken in distinguishing the rhetoric surrounding the government's wider social policies (which suggests that it has a good understanding of the underlying factors that give rise to health inequalities) and its record in this respect (a failure to fundamentally change such factors). Analysis using a public health regime framework, with its explicit attention to indicators of structural reform, suggests that the UK has a long way to go before developing the social, political, cultural and economic structures that, on the basis of Scandinavian evidence, are key to promoting health equity.

Reference

HM Government and DH (Department of Health) (2004) *Choosing health: Making health choices easier,* White Paper, London: HM Government and DH.

Towards a new framework for evidence-based public health

The evidence base in public health

During the course of this book we have examined a vast array of evidence pertaining to the effectiveness of interventions targeting key public health issues. This includes several hundred non-experimental studies which do not meet the strict criteria for inclusion in systematic reviews but which, nevertheless, throw important light on the complexities of implementing interventions and on the factors that may contribute to successful outcomes. Such studies, however, are not generally considered to be robust enough to provide the basis for definitive policy guidance. Thus, we have also drawn on a formal evidence base. This includes over 125 systematic reviews (36 of which were Cochrane Reviews consulted individually as opposed to information accessed via reviews of reviews) and 29 reviews of reviews. A conservative estimate suggests these are underpinned by a minimum of 1,800 experimental and quasi-experimental trials. As we discuss below, these different sources of evidence offer very different conclusions with respect to 'what works'.

What works in addressing health inequalities? A summary of the formal evidence base

A table summarising the findings of systematic reviews has been presented in each of the policy/practice chapters. These suggest that the current evidence base is stronger for interventions implemented during adulthood than during earlier periods of the lifecourse. However, this is overwhelmingly accounted for by interventions targeting lifestyle factors at the individual level (diet, physical activity and smoking). By contrast, the evidence base for interventions that address the wider determinants of health (for example, housing, crime and employment) is very weak. There is a similar focus on interventions targeting lifestyle factors in earlier ages. Smoking and alcohol in childhood and adolescence, smoking cessation and nutrition in pregnancy and early life and, to a lesser degree, parenting education and support are the only other areas where the evidence base seems extensive (with consideration given to at least 50 trials). Thus, broadly similar areas of concern dominate across the lifecourse.

Even within the body of evidence focusing on lifestyle factors, disaggregation by topic area reveals how small the specific evidence base often is. With reference to breastfeeding, for example, most training courses for health professionals have not been formally evaluated, with research identifying only one randomised controlled trial (RCT) alongside two UK 'before and after' studies (NHS CRD, 2000). In other areas the evidence base per se is far more limited. In large part this impression reinforces the (non-age-specific) recommendations made by the Health Development Agency (HDA) as to areas where the evidence for public health interventions is strong and the likelihood of success is high. Here, recommendations relating to tobacco, obesity and nutrition and physical activity were most frequently described (alongside interventions to prevent accidents) while housing showed the least promise.

Finally, and of particular significance to this book, the existing evidence base tells us very little about the effectiveness of interventions in addressing health inequalities. Throughout, there is a lack of evaluation focusing on what works for particular socio-economic, ethnic or vulnerable groups and those subject to multiple risks. One consequence is that there is a lack of understanding of features that might make an intervention appropriate for such groups – what would increase smoking cessation among heavy smokers and women of lower socio-economic class, for example? Another is that the evidence base looks as if it has relatively few answers to offer when what it is frequently saying is that for the population as a whole, this intervention is not going to be effective. Chapter Five, for example, highlights the fact that, while review-level evidence militates against the *routine* use of iron supplementation as part of a population-based policy, this does not mean that it is ineffective in addressing the relationship between maternal anaemia during early pregnancy and preterm birth. In virtually every area for which we have drawn up a summary table, reviewers have recommended that more attention should be paid to taking into account the needs of those groups most at risk and key dimensions such as ethnicity and socio-economic status. The same applies to cost-effectiveness.

Limitations of systematic reviews

For some commentators, the difficulty of distilling guidance about the scope for addressing health inequalities says more about the methods used in the field of evidence-based public health than the potential effectiveness of public health interventions themselves. As we discussed in Chapter Three, these have tended to reflect the approach taken in evidence-based medicine, which places particular value on systematic reviews that synthesise the findings of experimental/quasi-experimental and observational studies that fulfil robust statistical criteria. We have already introduced a critique of the systematic review, focusing on the hierarchy and logic of the review process, where the tendency to underplay the role of theory and to select studies on the basis of the quality of research rather than the quality of the intervention have been identified as problems (see Chapter Three). Here, we draw on our experience of assessing the public health evidence base to extend this critique, focusing in particular on problems relating to the quality of implementation.

One reason for the gaps in evidence identified earlier is that methodologically sound studies for systematic review have been found to be 'disappointingly scarce' (Harden et al, 1999, cited in Boaz et al, 2002). Included studies are frequently criticised for failing to report on the content, duration and intensity of the intervention, or to discriminate between the contributions of different programme elements. For example, parenting programmes are indicated by review-level evidence (see Chapter Five) as capable of making a significant contribution to the short-term psychosocial health of mothers, but it is still not possible to assess *which* factors contribute to the successful outcomes (Barlow and Coren, 2003). Similarly, none of the reviews undertaken of home visiting programmes have been able to establish which components were effective in reducing childhood injury in the home (Lucas, 2003). Yet, as the HDA emphasised:

> Home visiting is not a single or uniform intervention – it is a mechanism for the delivery of a variety of interventions directed at different outcomes. Home-visiting programmes are diverse in their goals, target recipients, mode and timing of their delivery and their theory and content. They may provide parent training/education, psycho-social support to parents, infant stimulation, and infant and maternal health surveillance. The programmes may be provided by nurses, midwives or lay people within different professional bases. Home visiting may vary in when it begins, how long it lasts and how many times within this period it occurs. A programme may be provided to all families with a new baby, to families in disadvantaged circumstances, to parents or children with particular problems, or parents of children defined as 'at risk'. (Bull et al, 2004, p 1)

Neglect of key confounding variables such as gender, ethnicity, family composition, age, socio-economic status or education is an additional problem. This is compounded by poor or inconsistent definition of terms. Control groups, for example, are normally described as receiving 'usual care', without the provision of any details. Yet, this will vary from country to country and may be different at the time of the trial from that now prevailing. In the UK, for example, usual postnatal care includes a visit from a midwife for the first 10 days after birth and a routine visit from a health visitor at 10 days, an intensive level of intervention for a control compared to many other countries. Similar reservations apply to many other areas. The term 'breastfeeding', for example, is used without commonly accepted definitions for initiation or continuation and without distinction between partial or exclusive feeding. Similarly smoking is often treated as a dichotomous variable, without acknowledging the very different experiences of heavy and light smokers (Amir and Donath, 2002). There are also problems relating to measurement. Systematic reviews refer frequently to the unreliability of self-report in healthcare settings. For example, self-reported measures of diet and physical activity are often weak estimates of actual behaviour and prone to distortion when subject to long periods of recall. In areas such as smoking cessation doubts have thus been cast on the potential contribution of studies which do not validate smoking status (Lumley et al, 2001).

Critically, systematic reviews have very little to say about inequalities or inequities (Petticrew et al, 2004), and there is a lack of understanding as to the ways in which different segments of the population respond to similar interventions. In part this is because the most rigorous evidence is often gathered from "simple interventions and from groups that are easy to reach in a population" (Rychetnik et al, 2002, p 125) rather than interventions targeted at disadvantaged groups. Further, very few studies focus on wider determinants of health inequalities. As noted in Chapter Three, much of the evidence available is located far down the causal chain, focusing on 'downstream' proposals to address health behaviours and clinical issues rather than the broader social determinants of health.

Such methodological limitations and neglect of key issues are compounded by technical problems such as randomisation and allocation concealment (impossible, for example, in interventions relating to housing and regeneration), low participation, high rates of attrition and an uneven proportion lost to follow-up between control and intervention groups. In one study of day care included in a systematic review, attrition rates were 81% (Zoritch et al, 2000). Attrition and recruitment display a socio-economic bias. Review-level evidence of smoking cessation programmes, for instance, shows it to be highest among those on a low income and among the most mobile (Lumley et al, 2001). Similar attributes, including poverty, high levels of stress, high levels of child conduct disorder and minority ethnic status, apply to attrition from parenting programmes. Patients who do not adhere to interventions also tend to differ in respects that are related to prognosis (Juni et al, 2001). It is unclear whether studies always take full account of such challenges when analysing results (Barlow and Parsons, 2003).

There is also a range of ethical problems relating to the ability to give informed consent or to unexpected side-effects that effectively prevent randomisation and blinding in many public health-related interventions. The ethical problems associated with randomising mothers' feeding choices mean, for example, that case-control and cohort study experimental designs tend to be the only practical methodological option (Nicoll and Williams, 2002). Practical problems in turn relate to the fact that many RCTs are based in hospitals or clinics. Question marks thus remain as to how to translate the results of controlled, scientific and well-resourced conditions to routine service delivery (Kelly, 2004). Evidence suggests, for example, that smoking cessation interventions in pregnancy are often less favourable in real-life settings than those conducted in clinical trials (Bull et al, 2003).

Further questions have been raised as to the effectiveness of the quality assurance mechanisms applied to the primary raw material of systematic review, that is, papers published in peer-reviewed journals. This is a process that is traditionally seen as a guarantee of research quality (Grayson, 2002). However, journal conventions are now recognised as capable of distorting the review process by excluding accounts of programme failure, minimising contextual information and providing information on selective positive outcomes. Their focus too is overwhelmingly on publication in English, militating against international comparisons (Egger et al, 2001). In particular, debate has been engendered as to the relevance of North American findings for UK policy.

There is a tendency, too, to ignore empirical evidence from non-evaluation sources. The problem is compounded with the move to health and social policy because a smaller proportion of potentially relevant studies appears in peer-reviewed sources than in medical research (Grayson, 2002). There is also a more diverse literature, a greater variety and variability of secondary bibliographical tools, an increasing availability of material on the Internet and a less precise terminology (Grayson and Gomersall, 2003). Researchers have begun to develop new tools to appraise qualitative research identified for inclusion in reviews (Popay et al, 1998). For example, Harden et al (1999, cited in Boaz et al, 2002) developed separate tools for the qualitative and quantitative studies identified for inclusion in their systematic reviews. However, more is required than the ability to synthesise qualitative and quantitative research. A methodology capable of assessing the impact of clusters of interventions and admitting the complex context of governance, delivery and policy problems that extend beyond a single department is also needed.

A corollary of the lack of theoretical underpinning is a lack of information about process. "Important features of the intervention design may not be known ... thereby reducing the ability of practitioners to adopt the methods" (Speller, 1998, cited in Kelly et al, 2004). Reviewers and policy makers alike also need to be able to distinguish between evaluation failure and programme failure (and whether the latter was caused by inadequacy in the intervention itself [that is, theory]) or poor implementation. It has been suggested that greater emphasis is, however, now being placed on causal factors rather than the typical 'black box' use of epidemiology "that placed more weight on research methods and outcomes than on intervention theory" (Rychetnik et al, 2002, p 122).

What works in addressing health inequalities? A view from the ground

Recognising the limitations of relying on review-level findings alone, our investigation into 'what works' has also drawn on other published research and the grey literature. The advantage of this methodological pluralism, particularly its admittance of descriptive, qualitative work, is that it brings us closer to the normative basis of policy making (see Chapter Three). It admits power, politics, and above all the views of people as to what works, that is, not just the views of clinicians or strategic decision makers but of front-line staff, users and carers. It reports from a world where a variety of goals exist in tandem and where the organisational and operational environment are complex and subject to rapid flux. In its focus on the local, it often provides information about both process and context. It can provide a social focus to counter the medical and an insight into the divide between what may be clinically appropriate and what may be practically applicable. It also gives access to information on a range of vulnerable groups.

While systematic reviews tend to focus on the lifestyle issues of diet, physical activity, smoking and alcohol, the evidence relating, for example, to housing, crime and employment is sparse and equivocal. A wider view of what works, drawing heavily on the perceptions of the people involved, suggests this is not the end of the story and that local interventions can make a difference to health inequalities. Care and Repair schemes, welfare benefits advice and Sure Start are examples from quite different contexts and institutional structures (respectively passive, permissive and enabling), where the view from the ground suggests interventions at the local scale can work.

The HDA, as noted earlier, suggested housing interventions show least promise in terms of reducing health inequalities and, as Table 13.1 stressed, it is an area where review-level evidence remains silent. Yet home, particularly for older people, can be either a critical source of independence/quality of life or potentially disabling. Low-intensity services such as housing adaptations and home repair schemes are designed to enable older people to maintain independence in their own homes (see Chapter Thirteen). Research suggests they can be a cost–effective substitute for and supplement to formal care, and particularly valuable to those rendered vulnerable by lack of resources, including family support. Packages such as Care and Repair, hospital discharge schemes and housing option schemes, while essentially simple in construct, are multidimensional. They are about identifying real needs, getting the physical environment (such as kitchens and bathrooms) right, providing low levels of preventative help and personal care and developing and maintaining links to the local community and informal support networks. They coincide exactly with the rhetoric of the National Service Framework (NSF) for Older People (DH, 2001), providing a timely response to need, person-centred care, interventions that are supportive of health and quality of life, and interventions that revolve around partnership. Yet they remain located in the voluntary sector, insecurely funded, tenuously connected to mainstream services and inadequately evaluated.

Government policy is more proactive when it comes to the enhancement of income for those below the poverty threshold (see Chapter Three). The need to increase benefit uptake among entitled groups was one of the recommendations of the Acheson Report (1998), and efforts have been made nationally to overcome the problems; witness, for example, the introduction of Pension Credit and of the benefit entitlement checks introduced as part of the Warm Front Scheme (see Chapter Thirteen). At the local level the provision of welfare advice in non-traditional settings, most particularly within primary healthcare (again, as advocated by the Acheson Report), is another example of an intervention with a clear health inequalities dimension that seems to work on the ground. It frequently targets either older people or chronically disabled people, groups known to have low levels of benefit take-up and high levels of poverty. In common with the housing interventions discussed above, it has also been introduced, in various permutations, across the country, enabling researchers to potentially isolate what works in the UK, rather than what works in the US.

While few projects (see Chapter Eleven) have yet been subject to an experimental design, research suggests several positive outcomes. Awareness and uptake of benefits (and hence income) increases: a function variously of raised awareness among patients and staff, access to advice workers (including home visits), and a reduction in perceived stigma because of legitimisation within the health service. Evaluation of welfare support services in primary care settings in Wales suggests, for example, that almost £3.5 million of additional income was raised for low-income clients in one year of operation (CAB, 2005). The availability of such advice may also lead to an improvement in the health and quality of life of patients and reduced use of National Health Service (NHS) resources, with services reducing the mental stress and frustration of dealing with the benefits system. Research suggests that the potential exists to integrate such advice into a variety of different settings, depending on the target group, and the potential to deliver such advice as part of an holistic intervention ranging from health promotion through to structural issues such as education, employment and housing.

Anecdotal reports point to very high levels of user satisfaction. However, like low-intensity housing services it is an area where delivery is primarily voluntary (through Citizens' Advice Bureaux [CABx]) and where mainstream support, in England at least, remains limited. *Choosing health* (HM Government and DH, 2004) 'encourages' primary care trusts (PCTs) to work with local partners to provide access to welfare advice and support in health and outreach services. CAB alone now provides such access in nearly 1,000 health-related locations, chiefly general practitioner (GP) surgeries and health centres. However, such developments remain piecemeal and ad hoc, with some PCTs still offering no such access. In contrast, the 'Better Health, Better Wales' programme provides for a CAB service in primary care settings in each of the nation's 22 local authorities, backed by mainstream funding (CAB, 2005).

Finally, Chapter Five found a variety of review-level evidence favouring parenting education and support. There remains, however, a lack of review-level evidence as to the role of such programmes in primary prevention as opposed to treatment, the efficacy of relational interventions and the effectiveness of individual components. Sure Start (see Chapter Three) has the potential to answer many of these questions. Unlike the two interventions discussed above, it has a significant dedicated budget and staff resource; it is the subject of a national evaluation (with each local programme also producing research outputs); and includes a built-in intention to mainstream. It is also located within a supportive political environment that focuses attention on the early years. It has encountered many problems in implementation, not least the involvement of the most disadvantaged, and a suggestion that interventions work better in the least deprived communities. Nevertheless, early research does also suggest that targeted, community-based preventative interventions for the early years can be effective in providing parenting and family support if well-resourced and sustained, with targets often failing to capture the real difference that such programmes make to individual lives.

It is therefore ironic that the act of mainstreaming has seen Sure Start captured by the employability agenda (see Chapter Five). An increased emphasis on childcare has replaced the earlier child-centred focus and concern for community development principles. Sure Start settings, as noted in Chapter Three, are expected to become Sure Start Children's Centres over the next few years and a feature of every community by 2010. In the process the focus on those most in need will be dissipated, the level of funding that was central to the programmes reduced and health services reverted to the mainstream (Glass, 2005).

The need for alternative approaches to evidence-based public health

Given the growing critique that has been levelled at the use of systematic reviews, it is hardly surprising that much of the more formal evidence reviewed in this book gives little indication of what policy makers can do to address health inequalities. Impossibly stringent criteria for success (for example, programmes providing positive changes in favour of the experimental group, in all trials, in all contexts), make inevitable the finding that nothing works (Pawson and Tilly, 1997, p 9). This is a dangerous conclusion as it legitimises political inertia. It is also misleading. As we have noted above, a view from the ground suggests that local interventions can make a difference. One problem about distilling such local evidence for use in formal guidance, however, is that as some interventions will work for certain groups, under certain conditions, and in certain contexts, they may not work in others. That is, they are conditionally 'successful' (Pawson and Tilly, 1997). This is not easily captured by the narrow, hierarchical approach to evidence in public health.

Against this background, there has been a search for alternative strategies. These tend to admit the case for methodological pluralism and the 'softer' qualitative methods used within social sciences (Grayson, 2002). Context is also accorded importance, particularly where policies relate to services and governance. For example, Rychetnik et al (2004) advocate the need to move from the current emphasis on *type 1* evidence that identifies risk–disease relations and *type 2* evidence that identifies the relative effectiveness of specific interventions (Brownson et al, 1999) to *type 3* evidence. This includes more descriptive and/or qualitative information about the design and implementation of an intervention; the contextual circumstances in which the intervention was implemented; and information on how the intervention was received.

Such thinking informed the decision by the national evaluation team of the Health Action Zone (HAZ) initiative to apply a Theories of Change approach to assess the complex, local partnerships that were set up to tackle inequalities in health (Sullivan et al, 2003). In contrast to systematic reviews and experimental evaluation with their focus on outcomes, theory-based evaluation aims to 'surface' the implicit theory that links intervention activities with desired outcomes in the short, medium and long term (Connell and Kubisch, 1998; Barnes et al, 2003). One of the advantages of this approach is that it allows one to unpack the black box and focus on the *process* by which an initiative works or fails rather than the outcomes themselves (which may not be measurable in the life-span of an initiative or its evaluation).

In application, however, the HAZ evaluation recognised the theoretical limitations associated with a bottom–up approach that prioritises the theories of those participants involved in the design and delivery of the programme (rather than drawing from wider bodies of theories that could help link specific actions and outcomes), and the impossibility of catching the complexity of such programmes within one overarching theory (Barnes et al, 2003). They therefore made increasing reference to a number of other approaches, including realistic evaluation and complexity theory, in an attempt to bring effective theory to the evaluation process. The HDA was also receptive to this approach, running national evaluations that required more sophisticated, 'realistic' approaches to understanding what works, where and for whom (Bowers et al, 2003, cited in Kelly et al, 2004).

Realistic evaluation

Realistic evaluation assumes that the transmission of lessons occurs through a process of theory building rather than assembling empirical generalisations. The 'conceptual backbone' to realistic evaluation is defined by the formula 'context + mechanism = outcome' (Pawson and Tilley, 1997). The causal power of an initiative thus lies in its underlying mechanism, essentially the basic theory about how programme resources will influence the subject's actions or what it is about the programme that actually makes it work. Whether this mechanism is actually triggered then depends on context, the characteristics of both the subjects and the programme locality.

According to this perspective it is not 'programmes' that work; rather, it is the underlying reasons or resources that they offer subjects that generate change

(Pawson, 2001). The result, it is suggested, is not a master theory or a catalogue of inconsistent results or even a 'best buy' (approach 'x' or case 'y' seems to be the most successful), but "a typology of broadly based configurations" (Pawson and Tilley, 1997, p 126), based on constant project refinement that suggests "what works for whom, when and how?; or what kind of evidence works for what kind of problem/policy in what context and for whom?" (Parsons, 2002, p 57).

Pawson uses the example of nicotine replacement therapy (NRT), introduced in Chapter Five, to illustrate his argument. Here the focus was on incentives, with an initial free supply of patches expected to substitute for cigarettes and the money saved made available to support further patch purchases in ensuing weeks. The intended programme mechanism is one of an initial rational calculation building itself into long-term behaviour. The outcomes of such programmes are ambiguous, however. Pawson suggests one decisive contextual condition seems to be the budget balance. The programme theory assumes that household finances will be tight, but not that they will be debt-ridden and potentially chaotic (Pawson, 2001). On such occasions, he suggests, policy makers and practitioners tend to retreat to the drawing board to debate the utility of 'two weeks free' as opposed to 'free NHS prescriptions'. Realist synthesists may focus instead on having achieved a little learning and developed an incipient theory about the contextual constraint of the chaotic. Significantly, the approach also admits errors with the pursuit of successful policy recognised as depending as much on avoiding previous errors, as on imitating successes.

Complexity theory

Complexity theory has some similarities to realistic evaluation in that it moves away from linear thinking about cause and effect to non-linear models that seek to understand the association and interaction between factors, arguing that intervention in similar circumstances will result in different outcomes because of a difference in detail. However, there the similarities end, with complexity theory focusing on the role of chaos and difference (emergent properties that cannot be understood by reference to the component parts) rather than the ability to determine transferable programme theories.

It is based on the notion that complex dynamic social systems act in an unpredictable manner that defies any attempt at defining cause and effect in a linear manner and is incapable of control from the centre (Sanderson, 2002). Policy makers need, therefore, to help develop individuals, organisations and communities that are capable of self-organisation, continuous adaptation, the use of local knowledge and learning experiences (Parsons, 2002). The emphasis, in such a model, it has been suggested, is not on using better evidence to improve control but on improving communications and reducing distortions, with periphery-periphery learning likely to offer better opportunities than the official policies of the centre.

This requires the active participation and reflective learning of those who design and implement specific programmes in specific contexts. It accords a vital role to phronesis or practical wisdom (Sanderson, 2002). It also focuses attention on key institutional structures and governance regimes, requiring them to be open, porous and decentralised, able to thrive on diversity and to adapt to radical innovation (Bentley, 2002, cited in Parsons, 2002).

Stacey, for example, draws on complexity theory to develop an agreement certainty matrix to suggest appropriate management mechanisms. Where levels of both agreement and certainty are high, the field is ready for the development of planning and control mechanisms such as guidance, application of standards of practice, and performance management. In complex systems where either dimension is low, changes in practice will follow from other approaches such as experimentation and local innovation (Stacey, 1999, cited in Kelly et al, 2004). In such a context it can be seen that the attempt to impose central controls on supposedly innovatory initiatives such as HAZs through the imposition of targets and performance management frameworks has "a destabilizing effect on them, moving them closer to the 'rigid' end of the continuum" and "undermining their capacity to adapt" (Barnes et al, 2003, p 278).

Evaluation and policy

While evaluation per se has become an increasingly common component of the evidence base, it can be seen that, like the extension of the RCT and systematic review, it too is confounded by practical, political and theoretical problems. Often the theoretical base remains undeveloped and the result is a series of ad hoc initiative-specific reports rather than the accumulation of knowledge relating to a particular type of policy intervention. However, the refinement and utilisation of theory relating to complex community initiatives also remains in its infancy, particularly in terms of its ability to generate lessons for policy makers.

A more pragmatic challenge, but one constantly evidenced in this book, is the way in which policies move ahead of evidence, with the length of parliaments and ministerial tenures (often two years) conspiring against long experiments. The New Deal policies examined in Chapters Nine and Eleven, for example, proceeded with full or extended implementation long before the end of piloting, so key policy decisions were typically informed by fairly elementary monitoring and early results from process evaluations (Walker, 2001).

A similar challenge relates to policy characteristics. These typically include multiple, imprecisely defined objectives, frequently contested between different departments, and a mode of implementation that is often not determined in advance. In experimental evaluation each variant would reduce the effective sample size or require a larger and hence more expensive pilot. The process of revising a policy in the light of early experience is also common. In such circumstances pilots have been dismissed as inherently exceptional, tending to be better resourced than normal policies and likely to attract risk takers and opinion leaders among staff and programme participants (Walker, 2001). In contrast, proponents of theory-based realistic evaluation would argue that they enable the examination of yet another context–mechanism–outcome configuration that has the potential to add to the knowledge base.

Towards a new framework for evidence-based public health

Given the reservations that surround each source of evidence individually, it is not surprising that policy makers appear to be drawing on a mixed economy of evidence, combining elements from the range of approaches described above. The HDA, for example, developed a series of effective action briefings in an attempt to involve practitioners such as health visitors, school nurses, teachers, medical practitioners, managers and civil servants in producing guidance in "a more integrated, systematic and empirical way" (Kelly et al, 2004, p 5). This, they suggested, favoured a 'theories of change' approach, with an emphasis on developing the theoretical understanding of how work will lead to change and the theory-driven selection of outcome indicators to demonstrate this. They also utilised Stacey's agreement certainty matrix (see above) to guide judgements about the general types of activities likely to be effective under particular circumstances, helping them to understand when to use evidence, when to concentrate on policy changes, and when to use practice development approaches (Kelly et al, 2004).

The need to develop a 'mixed economy' of evidence, in which policy relevance is given greater priority than an obsession with methodological rigour, was also highlighted in a recent study of senior policy makers' perceptions of current research (Petticrew et al, 2004), and in a companion study of the views of current research leaders in the health inequalities field (Whitehead et al, 2004). In the latter, the case was made for a diversity of sources. Thus, in addition to formal observational studies and controlled evaluations of interventions, the value of qualitative evidence (particularly when paired with quantitative data), historical evidence and natural policy experiments that draw on evidence from other countries or regions was acknowledged. By creatively assembling an evidence 'jigsaw' from such diverse sources, far more valuable policy-relevant information tends to be yielded than from a single piece of evidence (Whitehead et al, 2004).

Use of such methods could therefore address one of the key failings of current evidence-based assessments: their focus on individualised interventions. Most leading health inequalities researchers emphasise the need to develop *upstream* policies that target the wider determinants of health inequalities such as education, employment, housing and income distribution (Acheson, 1998; Davey Smith et al, 1999, 2001; Hertzman, 1999; Townsend, 1999; Mackenbach and Stronks, 2003). Public health interventions should include "policies of governments and non-governmental organisations; laws and regulations; organisational development;

community development; education of individuals and communities; engineering and technical developments; service development and delivery; and communication" (Rychetnik et al, 2004, p 540). The current approach to gathering evidence is ill equipped to assess the effects of different policy and organisational arrangements within these broad domains.

International studies of public health interventions

Insofar as they provide scope for the analysis of different legislative, social, political and economic structures (national fiscal policies, labour market policies, legislation regarding harmful substances, food subsidies, and so on), international studies offer a promising approach to the gathering of evidence on upstream policies (and indeed to improving our understanding of the role that wider context plays in shaping the effectiveness of down- and midstream interventions). As observed earlier, however, the evidence that does exist on public health interventions is not only narrow in its tendency to focus on 'downstream' initiatives. There is also a strong bias in the literature towards studies published in the English language, particularly those that emanate from the US. Against this background, the aims of the European Network on Interventions and Policies to Reduce Inequalities in Health are significant. Members of this interdisciplinary group prepared structured descriptions of policies that explicitly addressed socio-economic inequalities in health in their own country between 1990 and 2001, and searched for empirical evidence of the effectiveness of specific policies and interventions to reduce health inequalities (Mackenbach and Bakker, 2003).

Rather than yielding comparative data across a range of indicators or leading to conclusions about key factors that might have influenced observed differences in policy approaches or outcomes, this approach mainly resulted in the description of a range of country-specific case studies. As the Network's coordinators observed, however, differences in policy content and context made direct comparison difficult. For example, different countries were in widely different phases of awareness of, and willingness to take action on, inequalities in health. Variations also existed in the extent to which country-specific initiatives were replicable on grounds of practical and political feasibility (Mackenbach and Bakker, 2003).

These are legitimate problems to raise. However, the difficulty of making cross-national comparisons also reflected research design. The Network did not set out to analyse policies within an explicitly comparative framework. The use of formal databases in the search strategy for literature on effective interventions also led to the exclusion of grey reports and studies published in national journals, and to an overwhelming reference to the types of research (RCTs and controlled experiments, for example) that have been criticised for their individualised focus and failure to acknowledge the importance of context. Thus, when the Network did attempt to carry out cross-national work on specific domains, this mainly resulted in systematic policy reviews that were largely de-contextualised (for example, Hogstedt and Lundberg, 2002; Mielck et al, 2002; Paterson and Judge, 2002; Platt et al, 2002; and, with the exception of their case studies of food and nutrition policies in Finland and the Netherlands, Prättälä et al, 2002). One exception was a descriptive review of income maintenance policies, which, drawing on the seminal work of Esping-Andersen (1990), highlighted important differences between policies associated with different welfare regimes (Diderichsen, 2002). However, although this study highlighted important contextual features, it did not yield clear conclusions about the implications of different welfare systems for the prevention of health inequalities.

If the Network was limited in the extent to which it could carry out comparative analysis, its descriptions of national experiences did allow its coordinators to identify examples of innovative approaches to reducing health inequalities that were supported by some empirical evidence of effectiveness. In the Netherlands, for example, the use of national targets relating to intermediate outcomes in the areas of poverty, labour participation of chronically ill people, smoking and heavy physical labour was considered to have been effective. Compared to England, strong employment protection and active labour market policies for chronically ill citizens in Sweden were identified as effective ways of protecting vulnerable groups from labour market exclusion, while mandatory occupational health services in France provide an effective setting for the delivery of preventive activities, including smoking cessation. With respect to health-related behaviours such as food consumption, developments in Finland were highlighted, including the provision of free or subsidised meals at school and in the workplace. Universal access to effective healthcare was considered to be an important strategy for addressing social disadvantage. Finally, the use of territorial approaches or area-based initiatives (ABIs) (such as the English HAZs) was identified as an innovative and possibly effective approach (Mackenbach and Bakker, 2003).

Some care should be taken in accepting this as an 'evidence-based' list of effective upstream initiatives. The Network itself acknowledged that its evidence of effectiveness might not always fulfil the highest scientific standards. Moreover, interpreting the experiences of other countries in terms of the country with which we are most familiar is a recognised pitfall of international research on social policy (Cochrane et al, 2001). Many English commentators would take issue with the claim that HAZs have made a significant difference to the health of disadvantaged populations and, while the UK government's strategy for reducing health inequalities acknowledges the role of a comprehensive range of social policies, the way in which that strategy has been implemented does not necessarily support the Network's conclusions (Mackenbach and Bakker, 2002, p 341) that Britain is at a more advanced stage with regard to coordinating health inequalities policies than its European counterparts.

Towards a new framework for evidence-based public health: the public health regime

The Network's experience suggests that the utility of natural policy experiments can be improved in a number of ways. First, single-country case studies would be strengthened through the systematic assessment of a common set of structures and institutional arrangements, the identification of which is theory based. It is generally accepted that, although a wide range of health-damaging exposures and behaviours can be identified at the individual level, these are embedded within the wider socio-economic context. Policy responses to health inequalities should therefore also target wider determinants of health inequalities (that is, through the development of *upstream* policies). What is less often acknowledged is that structural factors (relating to society, economy, culture and policy) also shape the formation, implementation and effectiveness of *mid-* and *downstream* interventions. Thus, in order to understand the potential of public health strategies at a national level, context should be a central focus of interest.

Given the progress that has been made in understanding the pathways that give rise to health inequalities throughout different stages of the lifecourse, well-designed single-country studies should lend themselves to an assessment of the potential policy effectiveness by using a theory-based approach – for example, by 'surfacing' the implicit theory that links intervention activities with desired outcomes in the short, medium and long terms (Connell and Kubisch, 1998). However, in order to identify examples of policies that work regardless of context, or to clarify the conditions necessary for the transfer of effective policies from one context to another, contextualisation *and* comparison is required.

From welfare regimes to public health regimes

In order to develop a framework for international comparative public health research, useful lessons can be drawn from comparative welfare state research, in particular the work of Esping-Andersen (1990). Acknowledging the link between the political ideology of a state and its welfare-related policies and institutional arrangements, this work not only provided a theoretical typology of state responses to the provision of welfare. In its use of large-scale aggregate data, it allowed for an examination of the relationship between different welfare arrangements and key outcomes such as the degree to which social policies enable individuals to enjoy an acceptable standard of living without paid employment (Esping-Andersen, 1990, p 37).

Esping-Andersen's work is not without its critics, however. It is narrow in its geographical focus, and its conclusions regarding the linkages between ideal type regimes and welfare outcomes have been questioned. For example, subsequent analysis suggests that although they are both classified as liberal welfare states (that is, offering low levels of state benefit), Britain and Canada provide welfare benefits of middling generosity. Indeed, Canada scores more closely to 'conservative' France and 'socio-democratic' Finland than it does to 'liberal' Australia or the US (Scruggs and Allen, 2004). Although several studies have uncritically treated Esping-Andersen's typology as a more or less permanent characterisation of welfare state variation, welfare regimes and the core political values that underpin them have also been subject to significant change since the 1980s. In today's globalised world, the US-influenced liberal model has become highly influential, and pressures to reform and restructure welfare are international. Thus, even in Scandinavia, where the social democratic model remains intact, emphasis has been placed on the need to contain costs and place restrictions on the extent of public social expenditure. Greater European integration has also impacted on welfare systems. Such factors suggest that, rather than continuing to be characterised by diversity, different welfare regimes are subject to increasing convergence.

In fact, pressures of globalisation provide an additional contextual feature that should be factored into any analysis of the potential of public health strategies to reduce inequalities. However, the impact of globalisation on Western welfare capitalism should not be exaggerated. A significant proportion of the national wealth of all Western European countries is still invested in welfare. Moreover, important differences remain between countries in levels of expenditure and in the way in which welfare arrangements are configured. We therefore propose that welfare regimes still provide a useful starting point for the systematic analysis of different welfare arrangements. They allow for explicit examination of the wider economic, social and political frameworks in which social policies are embedded. They lend themselves to comparative analysis, for example, of the inputs, instruments and outcomes of different welfare systems. The notion of the welfare regime can also be applied to a far wider range of welfare policies than Esping-Andersen's own focus on income maintenance. Indeed, we suggest that the concept of a welfare typology can be usefully applied to the field of public health.

Public health regimes: an analytical framework

The proposed framework (Figure 14.1) has been influenced by a range of sources, including realist evaluation with its attention to the relation between context, mechanisms and outcomes (Pawson and Tilley, 1997); complexity theory, with its interest in associations and interactions between factors (Sanderson, 2002); and our own research presented in this book on the pathways that give rise to health inequalities and the way in which interventions designed to address such pathways are socially embedded. We suggest that a range of wider contextual factors will affect inputs, processes and outcomes relating to the reduction of socio-economic inequalities in health. These, which we call the broad *domains* of public health regimes, include political, legal, social, cultural, economic and organisational structures. With the exception of the cultural, each of these domains can be linked to a core set of beliefs and values along a spectrum ranging from a belief in individual self-determination and the role of the market, a tolerance of inequality and an antipathy to government intervention to a belief in equality, social justice and solidarity and a strong role for the state.

A second feature of the framework is its use of *indicators* to construct a summary of each domain in a country's public health regime. Providing that they lend themselves to comparative analysis, indicators may be qualitative or quantitative. Choice of indicator should be theory based (that is, indicators are linked to either causal factors that give rise to health inequalities or contextual factors that shape the effectiveness of interventions). In practice, this demand for deriving theory-based indicators suggests that the approach will be easier to apply to interventions targeting specific risk factors (for example, smoking and nutrition), or preventable diseases and conditions, than to a general examination of health inequalities. Thus, a third feature of the framework is the extent to which it can be *tailored* for different uses, a characteristic reflected in Figure 14.1, which illustrates the framework with respect to the analysis of policies and interventions targeting nutritional inequalities.

Although indicators are used to depict relative position on the spectrum of core political principles, we do not assume that there is an automatic correlation between ideological orientation and public health outcomes. Domains and composite indicators are merely used to provide a contextual framework for either single-country studies of key structures, institutions and outcomes relating to public health, or for international comparative analysis. For single-country studies, the proposed framework allows comprehensive analysis of interventions at *all* levels of the policy framework (that is, the up-, mid- and downstream), which can be assessed on a theoretical basis using existing knowledge of the pathways that give rise to health inequalities. More ambitiously, international analysis provides a vehicle with which to identify regularities and differences in the outcomes of public health interventions and ask questions about the role and impact of different structural factors in reducing health inequalities. For example, what are the key differences and similarities in national structural, policy and organisational arrangements pertaining to public health? Are some regime types and domains more conducive to the promotion of health equity than others? Is it possible to distinguish between interventions that are effective across different public health regimes (and therefore generalisable) and those where success occurs under certain – identifiable and potentially replicable – conditions and contexts? What scope is there for local action to address health inequalities in the absence of enabling structures at national level? The framework can thus be used to generate series of *hypotheses* about contexts, mechanisms and outcomes regarding the reduction of health inequalities, a fourth important feature.

Fifth, through the generation of hypotheses that are subjected to empirical evaluation, we propose that analysis of public health regimes would enhance our

Figure 14.1: An analytical framework of public health regimes

Indicative framework for policies and interventions targeting nutritional inequalities

Domain	Sample indicators	Political ideology		
		Political right		Political left
Political				
Welfare regime	Qualitative description	Liberal	Corporatist	Social Democratic
	Gross public social expenditure relative to GDP	<20%		>40%
Role of state in welfare funding and provision	Net public social expenditure relative to GDP (that is, adjusting for tax and benefit systems)	<20%		>30%
	Decommodification score	<15		>35
Access to welfare services	Access to free school meals, employment-based catering	Safety net	Subsidised	Universal provision
Core political values	Qualitative descriptions of core political values	Markets, individualism, choice		Equality, social justice, solidarity
Legal				
Strength of legislation	Nature of controls on food advertising, food standards etc	Minimum	Voluntary	Compulsory
Social				
Social structure	Income distribution	High inequality		Low inequality
	Relative poverty rates	High		Low
	Educational performance and inequalities	High disadvantage		Low disadvantage
	Qualitative description of key social divides			

(continued)

Figure 14.1: An analytical framework of public health regimes (continued)

Domain	Sample indicators	Political ideology	
		Political right	**Political left**
Economic			
Level of marketisation/ consumer orientation	Food price, subsidy and tax policy measures	Weak	Strong
	Degree of trade liberalisation	Tendency towards liberalisation	Tendency towards protectionism
Relative power of statutory and commercial interests	Ratio of statutory:commercial spend on food promotion	Low	High
Organisational			
Degree of policy development and coordination	Mechanisms for food policy coordination (for example, national/local food policy councils)	Weak	Strong
	Focus of key task forces (including biological/environmental, ethical etc)	Narrow	Holistic
	Range of stakeholders involved in policy coordination and implementation	Narrow	Wide
Cultural			
Socio-cultural meanings of food	Qualitative analysis		
Traditional and contemporary food patterns	Data from surveys and surveillance systems		
Extent of globalisation regarding food preferences	Analysis of food imports etc		

understanding of the relative role of different domains in determining the effectiveness of policies and interventions to tackle health inequalities. Taking the example of policies designed to target nutritional inequalities, obvious questions arise about the relative power of statutory and commercial interests in shaping food preferences. A simple comparison of the advertising spend on food by industry with the food campaign spend by government in the UK suggests that consumerism is entrenched in this country. In 2003, commercial advertising of food, soft drink and chain restaurants was in the range of £743 million. By contrast, the government's spend in 2004 was only £7 million (HM Government and DH, 2004, p 32). In addition, the School Fruit and Vegetable Scheme and Five-a-day community initiatives have respectively received £42 million and £10 million of New Opportunities Funding. Thus, even when the two main components of the government's flagship initiative promoting healthy eating are taken into account, public sector expenditure on food promotion is dwarfed by that of industry. The relative power of commercial farming and public health interests in the UK also appears to be strongly balanced in favour of the former. In Scandinavia, by contrast, public health and environmental interests have been successfully fused with food and agricultural policy, although again there are concerns that closer European integration and globalisation are undermining existing policies and legislation (Lang, 2002).

At this stage, it would be premature to assume that trade liberalisation and consumerism necessarily conflicts with public health interests. For example, recent increases in fruit and vegetable consumption have been positively influenced by importation of foods. However, the current lack of knowledge about the relative role of key domains and their interactions is worrying as it undermines understanding of the conditions that are necessary for policies to operate effectively. We propose that analysis of policies and interventions using the public health regime framework could not only address this gap in knowledge. It may, in the longer term, provide a basis on which to apply *weightings* to different indicators and domains (expressed, for example, by different line widths when marking position along the spectrum or core values). Such an approach could usefully highlight the complex and often ambiguous status of different countries' welfare and public health regimes. As we discuss below, the UK is a case in point.

Single-country analysis: the UK as a public health regime

As noted above, the public health regime approach can be applied to either single-country studies or international comparative analysis. In both cases, one of the potential benefits of the approach is its ability to capture the complexity of modern political systems, the mixed nature of welfare regimes, and the fact that any one country can comprise both enabling and constraining structures with respect to the promotion of health equity. There is, for example, considerable debate about the current UK government's philosophy and the effects of its policies on the nature of the welfare state. Confusion about the ideological orientation of New Labour may in part reflect the ongoing power struggle between re-distributive and neo-liberal factions. However, as we concluded in Chapter Three, ideological ambiguity has also been a defining characteristic of New Labour's 'Third Way'. In the shift in emphasis away from a concern with equality to a focus on opportunity, with which comes *responsibility*, there are elements of the individualising and privatising stance that marked the Thatcher years. The welfare state must offer a hand-up, not a hand-out. New Labour also appears to agree with the Conservatives' belief that large-scale government bureaucracies are not the most efficient way of delivering services. Thus, partnerships with the private sector have been actively sought. Against this, the government believes in promoting equality of opportunity and ensuring that lower-income or disadvantaged groups are protected from poverty and social exclusion. This acceptance of the need to tackle inequality is more characteristic of thinking on the political left (Baldock et al, 2003).

Upstream initiatives

Similar ambiguity is evident in the UK government's approach to promoting public health. With its emphasis on the need to target the underlying causes of health inequalities and to achieve this through cross-sectoral action, New Labour would appear to be at the more advanced ('comprehensive coordinated policy') stage on the action spectrum pertaining to health inequalities (Mackenbach and Bakker, 2002, p 341). In its Programme for Action for tackling health inequalities, the government identifies a number of policies that it has developed to address the more structural determinants of health (see Chapter Three). This suggests that its approach to public health is underpinned by an explicit recognition of the link between socio-economic and health inequalities and a commitment to social justice, beliefs that are traditionally linked with a collectivist ideology that values equality. The introduction of targets to monitor progress relating to key dimensions of inequality also suggests that the government is taking health inequalities seriously. Yet, although New Labour's use of targets and publicly available 'evidence' suggests a willingness to be politically transparent and to be held to account, the dysfunctional effects of targets (including the use of deliberately low benchmarks to demonstrate success) have been well documented (Smith, 1995). Questions have also been raised about the extent to which the policy-making process and the evaluation of New Labour's policies have been subject to genuinely independent research (Walker, 2001). When a government sets the terms for the evidence that it uses to justify its policies and to evaluate its achievements, real questions should be asked about its policy record. Thus, to properly evaluate the extent to which current policies will succeed in creating a more equal society, it is necessary to look beyond the 'spin'.

Closer examination suggests that, with respect to key domains of the public health regime, New Labour has made considerably less progress towards equality and social justice than its policy rhetoric and headline indicators imply. In Chapter Three, for example, we found that neo-liberalism is evident in the government's support for wider economic forces that favour socio-economic inequality. Thus, while incomes and earnings at the very top have increased the fastest since 1997, and median income is up 17%, the poorest are only 10% better off (*New Statesman*, 2005). In reality, a reduction in overall income inequality is *not* an aim of the current government, although if the government had left the tax and benefit system as it was when it took power, the inequality gap between rich and poor would be far greater than today (Joseph Rowntree Foundation, 2005). Instead, it has tolerated growing economic rewards for the richest sections of the population and focused on the relative poverty of selected groups (families with children and pensioners) in a way reminiscent of the Victorian distinction between the 'deserving' and 'undeserving' poor. Since 1997, relative poverty rates for those of working age without children have increased – to a record level in 2002-03. Moreover, as relative child poverty levels are still greater than the average for the (pre-enlargement) European Union, even the most prominent anti-poverty strategy suggests room for improvement (Joseph Rowntree Foundation, 2005).

In other areas, too, the impact of government policies on key dimensions of inequality falls somewhat behind rhetoric. Although the official unemployment rate is now the lowest in recorded history, there has been a sharp rise in claimants of Incapacity Benefit who, in the North East and North West of England, account for more than 10% of the working population. Particularly high rates of claimants are found in areas of industrial decline, rates among men aged 16-64 in 2001 exceeding 25% in the former coalfield areas of Easington, County Durham and Merthyr, South Wales (Select Committee on Work and Pensions, 2003). Against this background, interpreting the possible significance of recent trends in unemployment rates to health inequalities is very difficult.

Similarly, improvements to housing are claimed through reductions in the numbers of substandard homes. Yet, the gulf between the rich and poor in terms of property wealth is now wider than at any time since the Victorian era (Thomas and Dorling, 2004). Growing segregation in the housing market in part reflects the government's reluctance for the state to interfere in the operation of the property market. Policy regarding the social housing sector which, since its decline in the 1980s, serves a safety net function to a far greater degree than in other European countries, also has a role to play (Stephens et al, 2002). New Labour has done little to change this function. Indeed, there have been proposals to extend Thatcher's 'Right to Buy' policy to housing association properties (*The Observer*, 2005a), a move that would be expected to exacerbate the residual function of the rented social housing sector.

Education also continues to be characterised by large social class differences. With respect to access to university places (which is increasingly important for success in the workplace), the gap appears to have widened. Between the early

1980s and late 1990s, the proportion of children from the richest quarter of families who had completed a degree by the age of 23 increased from 20% to almost a half. Over the same period, the number of graduates among the poorest quarter of families increased from 6% to just 9% (*The Observer*, 2005b). At the other end of the educational spectrum, the government has made the early years a priority focus for policy. Its *Ten-year strategy for childcare* (HM Treasury et al, 2004) provides a very sound analysis of some of the tensions surrounding parents' needs to balance work and family life, as well as good evidence about the benefits of supporting development in the early years. It acknowledges that the UK lags well behind some other countries in the support that is offered to parents and the qualification levels of the childcare workforce, and presents strategies that, in the context of current provision, appear quite radical (for example, the deployment of graduate qualified early years' professionals in full day care settings).

Yet, although evidence suggests that the relatively few well-resourced state nurseries offer higher-quality education and care than private and voluntary providers, the government's childcare strategy continues to base expansion of early years' childcare on a system of regulation and inspection rather than direct state provision. With the exception of early education for three- and four-year-olds, which is universally funded but only on a part-time basis, the new strategy does not focus strongly on the supply side. Instead, the emphasis is on using additional investment to develop mechanisms to ensure that providers improve training and quality and on the use of demand-side subsidies. Working Tax Credits (WTCs) will continue to be the main focus of investment here. These are awarded on a sliding scale (referred to as 'progressive universalism') to help parents meet the costs of childcare. In practice, however, the support provided requires parents to make far greater contributions to childcare expenses than in countries such as Sweden, where childcare places continue to be very heavily subsidised. The policy is also targeted at working parents, which means that many disadvantaged children who could benefit from high-quality day care have no effective access.

There is, of course, more than one way to improve early years provision. The government remains convinced that its use of private and voluntary sector involvement within a regulatory framework offers the best means of achieving 'choice and flexibility, availability, quality and affordability' (the strategy's key themes). International evidence that high-quality, accessible services tend to be associated with a high level of state involvement suggests that this assumption should be more robustly tested.

Midstream initiatives

Moving from the upstream to the government's midstream initiatives to tackle health inequalities, the results of several high-profile programmes have been very mixed, giving rise to changes in both policy and continuation funding. Thus HAZs, highlighted by the European Network on Interventions and Policies to

Reduce Inequalities in Health as a potentially innovative and effective approach to addressing health inequalities, have been allowed to quietly wither. Despite its popularity, the government's Sure Start scheme also faces uncertainty about long-term funding for existing projects, although the initiative will be sustained through the development of Children's Centres that provide parenting and health support, information and advice (although not necessarily direct childcare).

HAZs and Sure Start are but two of a number of high-profile projects (including Education and Employment Action Zones) that have been targeted at deprived areas and subsequently axed or merged into mainstream provision, giving rise to charges of 'initiativitis'. The plethora of ABIs that has been launched by the government has stretched the capacity of local organisations, which have been drawn into different funding and performance mechanisms, targets and timescales. Short-termism and a lack of central coordination between schemes have also proved to be extremely demoralising (McGregor et al, 2003).

Downstream initiatives

Against an uneven record with respect to the impact of up- and midstream initiatives on tackling health inequalities, the recent publication of the Public Health White Paper *Choosing health: Making healthier choices easier*, demonstrates a strong interest on the part of government in focused interventions that address lifestyle factors at an individual level. Proposals within the White Paper include the development of a service to provide information on health choices by telephone, online, and digital television information services; the use of NHS trainers to provide advice to individuals on how to improve their lifestyle; and the development of personalised health guides. Using the results of a public consultation, the underlying assumption of the government's public health strategy is that "Health is a very personal issue. People do not want to be told how to live their lives or for government to make decisions for them" (HM Government and DH, 2004, p 12). The major thrust of the White Paper is thus on the need to support individuals – as consumers – to make healthier choices. It suggests that, in a market economy, the role of government should take a similar form to that of commerce in promoting its own business – that is, it becomes a matter of 'marketing health' or increasing awareness of the benefits and supply of healthy options.

This largely individualistic and behavioural approach is embedded within a wider framework, albeit one wedded to the operation of the market as opposed to a strong state. For example, the government proposes to work with industry to promote 'corporate social responsibility' (for example, around the development, labelling, promotion and pricing of healthy foods). Voluntary restrictions on the advertisement of junk foods to children are encouraged. Similarly, the government intends to work with industry to develop a voluntary social responsibility scheme for alcohol producers and retailers to encourage more responsible drinking by young people. While proposed restrictions on the advertising of tobacco are tighter, only a partial ban on smoking on pubs and restaurants is proposed (although this is one area where, in response to objections from the health sector, a further tightening of restrictions has since been announced).

With respect to direct state benefits, the White Paper proposes the use of means testing and targeting (as opposed to universalism), strategies normally associated with liberal welfare regimes. For example, eligible pregnant women, breastfeeding mothers and young children in low-income families are to be issued with vouchers that can be exchanged for fresh fruit and vegetables, milk and infant formula. While this strategy addresses concerns about the importance of diet for optimum development in the early years, like other means-tested policies, it may be affected by low take-up due to stigmatisation. The provision of school meals is another key area in which evidence suggests that benefits could accrue from direct investment in universal services. At present, government guidelines exist for the type of food that should be served in schools, as well as targets to reduce the amount of unhealthy food eaten. However, these do not deliver healthy meals. According to the Soil Association's Food for Life Programme, the 'Best Value' approach to the management of school catering contracts results in gross under-investment in children's school lunches. As has been highlighted by a high-profile campaign run by the celebrity chef, Jamie Oliver, in 2004, the daily amount spent was as low as 37 pence, which is simply insufficient for a balanced, healthy meal. Responding to this campaign, the government has promised to increase funding per meal to 50 pence. However, its strategy still focuses on the provision of guidance, training and support in order to improve public–private partnerships between food procurers and caterers in schools and local food providers. The current crisis in school dinner provision has been attributed to the end of the universal system set up by the 1944 Education Act and replaced by a system of local pricing and competitive tendering. There is therefore some doubt as to whether the government's confusing mix of a universalist and consumerist philosophy can deliver the healthy meals that children deserve (Wilson, 2005).

The discussion above suggests that the new Public Health White Paper provides another example of ambiguity in the current UK government's policies concerning welfare in general and public health in particular. Like so many policy documents, it is strong on analysis. Yet the way in which the government outlines policy problems does not always automatically map onto the solutions it desires. Its belief that modernisation through public–private partnership and the promotion of individual responsibility holds the key to meeting the health challenges of the 21st century appears to be more strongly based on ideology than objective evidence. On balance, then, core political values underpinning policy development at upstream, midstream and downstream levels appear to be more strongly influenced by the political right than the political left.

This assessment provides an important contextual backdrop against which to

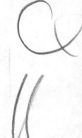

assess policies and interventions targeting health inequalities on a theoretical basis. We know, for example, that financial insecurity (often associated with poor educational qualifications and employment prospects) is associated with a range of risk factors, from smoking and maternal stress during pregnancy to exposure to poor parenting, psychologically stressful family environments, low educational expectations, and so on, during childhood and youth. This raises the question of whether parenting programmes, for example, would be more effective if embedded within the broader framework of income (and ultimately educational) equality. Similarly, evidence suggests that unhealthy lifestyles cannot be simply attributed to a lack of knowledge or a lack of money, but may reflect a more complex response to the way in which people manage their experience of poverty (Wardle and Steptoe, 2003). Against this background, inequalities in health behaviours may be less effectively addressed by the information campaigns or interventions targeting access to and affordability of healthy choices than by policies that explicitly address the way in which individual behaviours relate to interactions between the psychosocial environment and material deprivation.

Linking what we know about the pathways that give rise to health inequalities with a structured assessment of the role of structures and institutions in shaping these pathways, and interventions designed to target them, can throw light on the potential effectiveness of the UK's health inequalities strategies on a theoretical level. However, until the public health outcomes of its 'Third Way' regime are held up to genuine comparison with other regimes, the extent to which the government's professed goal of promoting greater health equity is likely to be achieved remains open to question. It is beyond the scope of this book to undertake detailed comparison of the UK's health inequalities policies with those of other countries. However, reference to just a few of the domains and indicators included in the analytical framework suggests that the approach does lend itself to the identification of key contextual features that turn potential into successful outcomes.

From single-country studies to international comparative analysis

Taking food and nutrition policies in Finland as an example, although gross public social expenditure in this 'social democratic' regime is significantly higher than in the UK, net expenditure – at 25.6% and 24.6% of gross domestic product (GDP) respectively (Adema, 2001) – hardly differs. Yet a tradition of direct welfare provision, together with a strong state role in steering cooperative action, has meant that significant progress has been made in ensuring that efforts to promote better nutritional health are 'joined-up'.

Within the political domain, for example, universalism, which has been a guiding welfare principle in Finland, has provided good opportunities to embed nutritional interventions into key social institutions. A good example has been the Finnish approach to developing catering services (Prättälä et al, 2002). Free school meals are available at all levels of primary and secondary education; meals for university students are subsidised; and a significant proportion of working-age adults (22% in 1997) benefit from meals provided by workplace canteens, many of which are state-subsidised. In contrast to other parts of the world where eating outside the home tends to contribute to unhealthy diets, special dietary guidelines are used to ensure that lunches served at outlets such as staff canteens in Finland are healthy. For example, fish dishes are served regularly, and the hot meal is always accompanied by a free selection of salads and vegetables. Staff using workplace canteens have been found to consume higher amounts of fish and vegetables. However, uptake of these facilities tends to be higher within the capital and by workers of a higher socio-economic status (Roos et al, 2004).

Universalism may also shape the relative effectiveness of more focused 'downstream' initiatives. A wide range of public sector agencies is involved in nutritional education. School and student healthcare services, occupational health services, maternity and child health clinics, health centres, hospitals and home care nursing facilities have all been charged with providing nutritional education as part of their everyday activities. Within schools, nutrition education is incorporated into home economics studies, biology and environmental studies and health education studies. All girls and boys in the 7th grade (around age 13) receive three hours per week of home economics for one year, and older pupils can take this subject as an elective. Nutrition education is also given in vocational courses relating to the food industry, hotel, restaurant and catering services, home economics and cleaning services, and social and healthcare services (Lahti-Koski, 2001).

Within the legal domain, Finland's regulations in food legislation were among the strictest in the world. It is important to note, however, that, with closer integration with the European Union and a national political and economic shift towards fiscal efficiency, decentralisation and a more competitive, consumer-oriented market, there has been a loosening of previously strict regulations in food legislation. For example, although the salt content of food is still labelled, it is no longer treated as an additive and is today only limited in baby foods. Efforts continue to be made, however, in developing pricing and quality requirements favourable to a healthy diet. For example, a national agricultural strategy has been developed with input from a range of stakeholders that aims to ensure that while food production is customer-orientated, the safety of foodstuffs, as well as ethical and ecological quality, remain high.

Key dimensions of Finland's social structure may be responsible for the reduction of nutritional inequalities. Educational standards in the country are very high, recent research placing Finland in third place in the international education league table, behind only Japan and Korea. In terms of relative educational disadvantage (the extent of difference between children at the bottom and middle of the achievement range), Finland is ranked first. It is also one of only four countries (with Norway, Sweden and Denmark) to have driven illiteracy among

16- to 25-year-olds to below 5% (UNICEF, 2002). As higher levels of education tend to be associated with healthier diets, the impact of education policy in Finland is likely to have been both absolute (in terms of improving general consumption) and relative (in terms of reducing nutritional inequalities according to socio-economic status).

Economically, the Finnish government has a strong history of actively involving the private sector in government policy. As far back as the 1970s, the food industry had responded to officially endorsed nutritional recommendations, increasing the availability of low-fat dairy products, high-fibre breads, vegetable oils and special dietary items, and reducing the amount of salt in its products. Since this period, the typical Finnish diet changed quite dramatically towards the higher consumption of fresh vegetables, cheese, poultry and non-alcoholic beverages. This has been linked to significant improvements in key health indicators. For example, between 1972 and 1992, Finnish male mortality from coronary heart disease (CHD) declined by 55% (Pietinen, 1996). It is important to note, however, that, with a national political and economic shift towards fiscal efficiency, decentralisation and a more competitive, consumer-oriented market, the approach to upstream policy making and implementation has become less strongly centralist (Milio, 1998). Deregulation of the market (with greater emphasis on consumer choice and the influx of foreign products) has been linked with reversal of previous improvements in key nutritional indicators such as dietary fat context, sugar consumption, dental health and obesity among children and adolescents (Lahti-Koski and Mervi, 2004).

Conclusion

As continuing changes in Finnish food preferences suggest, health inequalities interventions – however well designed – operate within complex social systems. It is evident that all of the potential variables that affect the implementation and impact of an intervention cannot be realistically controlled. Acknowledging that the effectiveness of similar interventions can vary according to context, the key challenge is to distinguish instead between potentially generalisable and conditionally successful interventions and, for the latter, to tease out the key contextual features that turn potential into successful outcomes. Much of the qualitative evidence presented in this book is useful to this end and should be read in conjunction with the results of more narrow systematic reviews.

We also propose that international comparison of policies and interventions adopted by different public health regimes provides a useful analytical framework. The next challenge is to analyse policies and interventions more systematically within this framework. We strongly recommend that search strategies for information on public health interventions are 'opened up' to include qualitative as well as quantitative material; grey reports and studies published in national journals as well as research published in international peer-reviewed journals;

and work that explicitly considers process as well as inputs and outcomes. There is also a growing body of international comparative data (descriptive and statistical) that could be better exploited and that would lend itself well to an analysis of the relationship between different public health arrangements and key public health outcomes. The potential exists to develop and implement an exciting research agenda within the field of evidence-based public health. A key question is whether the researchers and policy makers in public health are ready to accept the limitations of the current hierarchical approach to informing policy and practice, and to accord analysis using the concept of public health regimes the status of 'evidence'.

References

Acheson, D. (1998) *Independent Inquiry into Inequalities in Health*, London: The Stationery Office.

Adema, W. (2001) *Net social expenditure* (2nd edn), Labour Market and Social Policy Occasional Papers No 52, Paris: OECD.

Amir, L. and Donath, S. (2002) 'Does maternal smoking have a physiological effect on breastfeeding? The epidemiological evidence', *Birth*, vol 29, no 2, pp 112-23.

Baldock, J., Manning, N. and Vickerstaff, S. (2003) 'Social policy, social welfare and the welfare state', in J. Baldock, N. Manning and S. Vickerstaff (eds) *Social policy*, Oxford: Oxford University Press, pp 3-28.

Barlow, J. and Coren, E. (2003) 'Parent-training programmes for improving maternal psychosocial health (Cochrane Methodology Review)', *The Cochrane Library*, Chichester: John Wiley & Sons Ltd.

Barlow, J. and Parsons, J. (2003) 'Group-based parent-training programmes for improving emotional and behavioural adjustment in 0-3 year old children (Cochrane Review)', *The Cochrane Database of Systematic Reviews 2003*, Chichester: John Wiley & Sons Ltd.

Barnes, M., Matka, E. and Sullivan, H. (2003) 'Evidence, understanding and complexity: evaluation in non-linear systems', *Evaluation*, vol 9, no 3, pp 265-84.

Bentley, T. (2002) 'Letting go: complexity, individualism and the left', *Renewal*, vol 10, no 1, pp 9-26.

Boaz, A., Ashby, D. and Young, K. (2002) *Systematic reviews: What have they got to offer evidence based policy and practice?*, Working Paper 2, London: ESRC UK Centre for Evidence-based Policy and Practice.

Bowers, H., Secker, J., Llanes, M. and Webb, D. (2003) *The gap years: Rediscovering mid-life as the route to healthy, active ageing*, London: Health Development Agency.

Brownson, R., Burney, J. and Land, G. (1999) 'Evidence-based decision making in public health', *Journal of Public Health Management Practice*, vol 5, no 5, pp 86-97.

Bull, J., Mulvihull, C. and Quigley, R. (2003) *Prevention of low birth weight: Assessing the effectiveness of smoking cessation and nutritional interventions*, London: Health Development Agency.

Bull, J., McCormick, G., Swann, C. and Mulvihill, C. (2004) *Ante- and post-natal home-visiting programmes: A review of reviews*, London: Health Development Agency.

CAB (Citizens' Advice Bureau) (2005) 'Citizens advice bureau can help deliver health improvements' (www.citizensadvice.org.uk/press50311).

Cochrane, A., Clarke, C. and Gewirtz, S. (2001) 'Comparing welfare states', in A. Cochrane, C. Clarke and S. Gewirtz (eds) *Comparing welfare states*, London: Sage Publications in association with Open University Press, pp 1-28.

Connell, J. and Kubisch, A. (1998) 'Applying a theory of change approach to the evaluation of comprehensive community initiatives: progress, prospects and problems', in K. Fulbright-Anderson, A. Kubisch and J. Connell (eds) *Theory, measurement and analysis: New approaches to evaluating community initiatives 2*, Washington, DC: The Aspen Institute, pp 15-44.

Davey Smith, G., Ebrahim, S. and Frankel, S. (2001) 'How policy informs the evidence', *British Medical Journal*, vol 322, no 7280, pp 184-5.

Davey Smith, G., Dorling, D., Gordon, D. and Shaw, M. (1999) 'The widening health gap: what are the solutions?', *Critical Public Health*, vol 9, pp 151-70.

DH (Department of Health) (2001) *National Service Framework for Older People*, London: DH.

Diderichsen, F. (2002) 'Income maintenance policies: determining their potential impact on socio-economic inequalities in health', in J. Mackenbach and M. Bakker (eds) *Reducing inequalities in health: A European perspective*, London: Routledge, pp 53-66.

Egger, M., Dickersin, K. and Davey Smith, G. (2001) 'Problems and limitations in conducting systematic reviews', in M. Egger, K. Dickersin and G. Davey Smith (eds) *Systematic reviews in health care: Meta-analysis in context*, London: BMJ Publishing Group, pp 43-68.

Esping-Andersen, G. (1990) *The three worlds of welfare capitalism*, Cambridge: Polity Press.

Glass, N. (2005) 'Surely some mistake?', *The Guardian*, 5 January.

Grayson, L. (2002) *Evidence based policy and the quality of evidence: Rethinking peer review*, Working Paper 7, London: ESRC UK Centre for Evidence-based Policy and Practice.

Grayson, L. and Gomersall, A. (2003) *A difficult business: Finding the evidence for social science reviews*, Working Paper 19, London: ESRC UK Centre for Evidence-based Policy and Practice.

Harden, A., Weston, R. and Oakley, A. (1999) *A review of the effectiveness and appropriateness of peer delivered health promotion interventions for young people*, London: EPPI-Centre.

Hertzman, C. (1999) 'Population health and human development', in D. Keating and C. Hertzman (eds) *Developmental health and the wealth of nations*, New York, NY and London: The Guilford Press, pp 21-40.

HM Government and DH (Department of Health) (2004) *Choosing health: Making healthy choices easier*, White Paper, London: HM Government and DH.

HM Treasury, DfES (Department for Education and Skills), DWP (Department for Work and Pensions) and DTI (Department of Trade and Industry) (2004) *Choice for parents, the best start for children: A ten-year strategy for childcare*, London: The Stationery Office.

Hogstedt, C. and Lundberg, I. (2002) 'Work-related policies and interventions', in J. Mackenbach and M. Bakker (eds) *Reducing inequalities in health*, London: Routledge, pp 85-103.

Joseph Rowntree Foundation (2005) *Findings: Policies towards poverty, inequality and exclusion since 1997*, London: Joseph Rowntree Foundation.

Juni, P., Altman, D. and Egger, M. (2001) 'Assessing the quality of randomised controlled trials', in M. Egger, K. Dickersin and G. Davey Smith (eds) *Systematic reviews in health care: Meta-analysis in context*, London: BMJ Publishing Group, pp 87-108.

Kelly, M. (2004) *The evidence of effectiveness of public health interventions – and the implications*, London: Health Development Agency.

Kelly, M., Speller, V. and Meyrick, J. (2004) *Getting evidence into practice in public health*, London: Health Development Agency.

Lahti-Koski, M. (ed) (2001) *Nutrition report 2000*, Helsinki: National Public Health Institute.

Lahti-Koski, M. and Mervi, S. (2004) *Nutrition report 2003*, Helsinki: National Public Health Institute.

Lang, T. (2002) 'Should the UK have a food policy council? A briefing for the agri-food network', Unpublished paper, London: Institute of Health Sciences, City University.

Lucas, P. (2003) 'Home visiting can substantially reduce childhood injury' (www.whatworksforchildren.org.uk), What Works for Children Group, Evidence Nugget, April.

Lumley, J., Oliver, S. and Waters, E. (2001) 'Interventions for promoting smoking cessation during pregnancy (Cochrane Review)', *The Cochrane Library*, Oxford: Update Software.

McGregor, A., Glass, A., Higgins, K., MacDougall, L. and Sutherland, V. (2003) *Developing people – Regenerating place: Achieving greater integration for local area regeneration*, Bristol: The Policy Press.

Mackenbach, J. and Bakker, M. (eds) (2002) *Reducing inequalities in health: A European perspective*, London: Routledge.

Mackenbach, J. and Bakker, M. (2003) 'Tackling socio-economic inequalities in health: analysis of European experiences', *The Lancet*, vol 362, pp 1409-14.

Mackenbach, J. and Stronks, K. (2003) 'A strategy for reducing health inequalities in the Netherlands', *British Medical Journal*, vol 325, pp 1029-32.

Mielck, A., Graham, H. and Bremburg, S. (2002) 'Children, an important target group for the reduction of socioeconomic inequalities in health', in J. Mackenbach and M. Bakker (eds) *Reducing inequalities in health: A European perspective*, London: Routledge, pp 144-68.

Milio, N. (1998) 'European food and nutrition policies in action: Finland's food and nutrition policy: progress, problems and recommendations', *WHO Reg Publ Eur Ser*, vol 73, pp 63-75.

New Statesman (2005) 'Why we need a strong state more than ever', vol 17, January, pp 6-7.

NHS CRD (National Health Service Centre for Reviews and Dissemination) (2000) 'Promoting the initiation of breastfeeding', *Effective Health Care*, vol 6, no 2, pp 1-12.

Nicoll, A. and Williams, A. (2002) 'Breastfeeding', *Archives of Disease in Childhood*, vol 87, no 2, pp 91-2.

Observer, The (2005a) 'Milburn fuels "Right to Buy" row', 16 January.

Observer, The (2005b) 'Class divisions bar students from university', 16 January.

Parsons, W. (2002) 'From muddling through to muddling up – evidence based policy making and the modernisation of British government', *Public Policy and Administration*, vol 17, no 3, pp 43-60.

Paterson, I. and Judge, K. (2002) 'Equality of access to health care', in J. Mackenbach and M. Bakker (eds) *Reducing inequalities in health: A European perspective*, London: Routledge, pp 169-87.

Pawson, R. (2001) *Evidence based policy: Ii. The promise of 'realist synthesis'?*, Working Paper 4, London: ESRC UK Centre for Evidence-based Policy and Practice.

Pawson, R. and Tilley, N. (1997) *Realistic evaluation*, London: Sage Publications.

Petticrew, M., Whitehead, M., Macintyre, S., Graham, H. and Egan, M. (2004) 'Evidence for public health policy on inequalities: 1: The reality according to policymakers', *Journal of Epidemiology and Community Health*, vol 58, no 10, pp 811-16.

Pietinen, P. (1996) 'Trends in nutrition and its consequences in Europe: the Finnish experience', in P. Pietinen, C. Nishida and N. Khaltaev (eds) *Nutrition and quality of life: Health issues for the 21st century*, Geneva: WHO, pp 67-71.

Platt, S., Amos, A., Gnich, W. and Parry, O. (2002) 'Smoking policies', in J. Mackenbach and M. Bakker (eds) *Reducing inequalities in health: A European perspective*, London: Routledge, pp 125-43.

Popay, J., Rogers, A. and Williams, G. (1998) 'Rationale and standards for the systematic review of qualitative literature in health services research', *Qualitative Health Research*, vol 8, pp 341-51.

Prättälä, R., Roos, G., Hulshof, K. and Sihto, M. (2002) 'Food and nutrition policies and interventions', in J. Mackenbach and M. Bakker (eds) *Reducing inequalities in health: A European perspective*, London: Routledge, pp 104-24.

Roos, E., Sarlio-Lähteenkorva, S. and Lallukka, T. (2004) 'Having lunch at a staff canteen is associated with recommended food habits', *Public Health Nutrition*, vol 7, pp 53-61.

Rychetnik, L., Frommer, M., Hawe, P. and Shiell, A. (2002) 'Criteria for evaluating evidence on public health intervention', *Journal of Epidemiology and Community Health*, vol 56, no 2, pp 119-27.

Rychetnik, L., Hawe, P., Waters, E., Barratt, A. and Frommer, M. (2004) 'A glossary for evidence based public health', *Journal of Epidemiology and Community Health*, vol 58, no 7, pp 538-45.

Sanderson, I. (2002) 'Making sense of "what works": evidence based policy making as instrumental rationality?', *Public Policy and Administration*, vol 17, no 3, pp 61-75.

Scruggs, L. and Allen, J. (2004) 'Welfare state decommodification in eighteen OECD countries: a replication and revision', Unpublished paper (downloaded from http://userpages.wittenberg.edu/jallan/jesp1.1.pdf).

Select Committee on Work and Pensions (2003) *Hidden unemployment*, London: UK Parliament.

Smith, P. (1995) 'On the unintended consequences of publishing performance data in the public sector', *International Journal of Public Administration*, vol 18, pp 277-310.

Speller, V. (1998) 'Quality assurance programmes: their development and contribution to improving effectiveness in health promotion', in D. Scott and R. Weston (eds) *Evaluating health promotion*, Cheltenham: Stanley Thornes, pp 75-91.

Stacey, R.D. (1999) *Strategic management and organisational dynamics: The challenge of complexity*, New York, NY: Financial Times/Prentice Hall.

Stephens, M., Burns, N. and MacKay, L. (2002) *Social market or safety net? British social rented housing in a European context*, Bristol/York: The Policy Press/Joseph Rowntree Foundation.

Sullivan, H., Barnes, M. and Matka, E. (2002) 'Building collaborative capacity through "theories of change"', *Evaluation*, vol 8, no 2, pp 205-26.

Thomas, B. and Dorling, D. (2004) *Know your place: Housing wealth and inequality in Great Britain 1980-2003 and beyond*, London: Shelter.

Townsend, P. (1999) 'A structural plan needed to reduce inequalities of health', in D. Gordon, M. Shaw, D. Dorling and G. Davey Smith (eds) *Inequalities in health: The evidence presented to the Independent Inquiry into Inequalities in Health, chaired by Sir Donald Acheson*, Bristol: The Policy Press, pp xiv-xxi.

UNICEF (United Nations Children's Fund) (2002) *A league table of educational disadvantage in rich nations*, Florence, Italy: UNICEF Innocenti Research Centre.

Walker, R. (2001) 'Great expectations: can social science evaluate New Labour's policies?', *Evaluation*, vol 7, no 3, pp 305-30.

Wardle, J. and Steptoe, A. (2003) 'Socioeconomic differences in attitudes and beliefs about healthy lifestyles', *Journal of Epidemiology and Community Health*, vol 57, pp 440-3.

Whitehead, M., Petticrew, M., Graham, H., Macintyre, S., Bambra, C. and Egan, M. (2004) 'Evidence for public health policy on inequalities: 2: Assembling the evidence jigsaw', *Journal of Epidemiology and Community Health*, vol 58, no 10, pp 817-21.

Wilson, B. (2005) 'Please sir, can I have some more?', *The New Statesman*, 18 July, supplement, pp x-xi.

Zoritch, B., Roberts, I. and Oakley, A. (2000) 'Day care for preschool children', *The Cochrane Library*, Chichester: John Wiley & Sons Ltd.

Index

Note: Page numbers followed by *tab* indicate information is to be found only in a table.

A

abortion and teenage pregnancies 300
abuse *see* child abuse; domestic violence
access to health services 395–8, 456
  older age 490–4, 495
    age discrimination 476, 493–4, 534
    policy and practice 531, 534–44, 546*tab*,
      547–8
accidental injury
  childhood and youth 220, 221–3, 236, 294
    policy and practice 250–8, 273*tab*
  early life 120, 130
  falls in older age 484, 487, 542
    policy interventions 511, 512–17, 532
accidental injury review 62
accumulation models 44–5, 374, 386, 389
Acheson Report (1998) 1, 32–3, 57, 153, 333,
  507
  recommendations and responses 66, 70–92,
    113, 167–8, 450, 458, 570–1
Action Heart programme 341, 427
Action on Smoking and Health (ASH) 157–8,
  293, 428
Action Teams for Jobs 449
admission rates 396, 397
adulthood and health inequalities 373–401
  early life influences 374–7, 398–9
  material deprivation 389–98, 399–401
  policy and practice 398–401, 417–63
  psychosocial factors 384–9, 399–400, 431–43
  socio-economic status and risk 374–7, 378–
    98
advertising and smoking behaviour 292–3, 430
advocacy for homeless people 457
Age Concern 529
age discrimination 476, 493–4, 534
agreement certainty matrix 575, 576
air pollution 118–19, 393–4
alcohol consumption
  adulthood 382, 429, 430–1, 462*tab*
  childhood and youth 293–6, 337–8
    mortality in young people 223, 294, 338
    policy interventions 339, 343–4, 348–9,
      362–3*tab*
    and socio-economic status 295–6, 311
  early life risk factor 114, 115, 123
Alcohol Harm Reduction Strategy for England
  348, 349, 431
alcoholism 295–6, 338
Anchor Trust 518, 521, 523
antenatal depression 125, 126, 127, 137, 178–9
antioxidant supplements 481, 482, 543
antisocial behaviour

and material deprivation 388, 440
  and mental health 225–6, 249, 259–60, 268
Anti-Social Behaviour Act (2003) 270
Anti-Social Behaviour Unit 271
anxiety disorders 224–5, 228–9, 231, 262
  see also depression; mental health
APPLES study 329
area effects 93, 123, 387–9
  see also neighbourhood effects
area-based initiatives (ABIs) 20, 92–8, 272, 361,
  417, 588
  education 83
  employment 88–9
  health 66, 67
  neighbourhood renewal 437–40
artefact explanation 24–5
Asian cookery club in Luton 420
Attention Deficit/Hyperactivity Disorder
  (ADHD) 224, 231–2, 264
attrition rates in research 568
Audit Commission 266–7, 270, 519, 527, 529,
  543
Avon Longitudinal Study of Parents and
  Children (ALSPAC) 5, 23, 114, 115, 116–
  17, 119, 128

B

Baby Friendly Hospital Initiative (BFHI) 163
Barker, D.J.P. 40, 41, 42, 43, 112, 113, 114, 115,
  118, 135
Barker Report (2004) 91, 92
Beacon Programme 420
behavioural explanations 26–8
behavioural problems
  childhood and youth
    behaviour therapies 260, 261–2, 264, 266,
      270, 274*tab*
    conduct disorders 224, 225–8, 249, 260–1,
      299
    delinquency reduction policies 249, 259–64,
      265, 268–71, 274*tab*
    costs to society 172
    early detection 171–2, 226
    parent education programmes 172–83, 260–1,
      270
behavioural therapy 260, 261–2, 264, 266, 270,
  274*tab*
  and smoking cessation 427, 462*tab*
Bell Farm Estate 455
benefits
  Acheson recommendations 71, 73, 570–1
  disabled claimants 89, 534
  for older people 78, 529, 533, 570–1